REALITIES OF CANADIAN NURSING

Professional, Practice, and Power Issues

3rd Edition

REALITIES OF CANADIAN NURSING

Professional, Practice, and Power Issues

Marjorie McIntyre, RN, PhD
Associate Professor
University of Victoria
Victoria, BC

Carol McDonald, RN, PhD
Associate Professor
University of Victoria
Victoria, BC

 Wolters Kluwer | Lippincott Williams & Wilkins
Health

Philadelphia · Baltimore · New York · London
Buenos Aires · Hong Kong · Sydney · Tokyo

Acquisitions Editor: Hilarie Surrena
Managing Editor: Helen Kogut
Director of Nursing Production:
  Helen Ewan
Senior Managing Editor /
  Production: Erika Kors
Production Editor: Mary Kinsella
Art Director, Design: Holly Reid
  McLaughlin
Art Director, Illustration: Brett
  McNaughton
Manufacturing Coordinator: Karin
  Duffield
Production Services / Compositor:
  Cadmus, a CENVEO Company

3rd Edition

9 8 7 6 5 4 3 2

Printed in China

Library of Congress Cataloging-in-Publication Data

Realities of Canadian nursing : professional, practice, and power issues / [edited by] Marjorie McIntyre, Carol McDonald. — 3rd ed.
    p. ; cm.
  Includes bibliographical references and index.
  ISBN 978-0-7817-8981-3
  1. Nursing—Canada. 2. Nurses—Canada. I. McIntyre, Marjorie, RN, PhD. II. McDonald, Carol.
  [DNLM: 1. Nursing—Canada. 2. Nurses—Canada. WY 16 R288 2009]
  RT6.A1R435 2009
  610.730971—dc22

                                                                    2008040427

Care has been taken to confirm the accuracy of the information presented and to describe generally accepted practices. However, the authors, editors, and publisher are not responsible for errors or omissions or for any consequences from application of the information in this book and make no warranty, expressed or implied, with respect to the currency, completeness, or accuracy of the contents of the publication. Application of this information in a particular situation remains the professional responsibility of the practitioner; the clinical treatments described and recommended may not be considered absolute and universal recommendations.

The authors, editors, and publisher have exerted every effort to ensure that drug selection and dosage set forth in this text are in accordance with the current recommendations and practice at the time of publication. However, in view of ongoing research, changes in government regulations, and the constant flow of information relating to drug therapy and drug reactions, the reader is urged to check the package insert for each drug for any change in indications and dosage and for added warnings and precautions. This is particularly important when the recommended agent is a new or infrequently employed drug.

Some drugs and medical devices presented in this publication have Food and Drug Administration (FDA) clearance for limited use in restricted research settings. It is the responsibility of the health care provider to ascertain the FDA status of each drug or device planned for use in his or her clinical practice.

FOR MARY (HUFFMAN) McDONALD, 1926–2005.

Calgary General Hospital School of Nursing, Class of 1948.

An inspiration in our work, a continued presence in our lives.

About the Authors

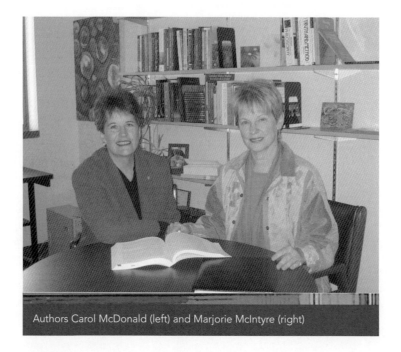

Authors Carol McDonald (left) and Marjorie McIntyre (right)

Marjorie McIntyre, RN, PhD, attended the Royal Alexander School of Nursing in Edmonton and practised in both acute care and community settings. She earned a BN at the University of Victoria, an MN at the University of British Columbia, and a PhD at the University of Colorado in Denver. As an associate professor, she currently teaches at the University of Victoria, where her interests include issues in health and health care, leadership in nursing education and curriculum design.

Carol McDonald, RN, PhD, is currently an associate professor at the University of Victoria School of Nursing. Following a 20-year practice career in mental health nursing Carol earned a PhD in nursing from the University of Calgary. Among her current interests are nursing education, philosophical hermeneutics and issues for non-heterosexual people in the health care system.

Contributors

Pat Armstrong, PhD
Professor
Department of Sociology
York University
Toronto, Ontario
Chapter 17

Anne Bruce, RN, PhD
Assistant Professor
School of Nursing
University of Victoria
Victoria, BC
Chapter 25

Laurel Brunke, RN, MSN
Executive Director
College of Registered Nurses of
British Columbia
Vancouver, BC
Chapter 8

W. Dean Care, BN, MEd, EdD
Associate Professor
Faculty of Nursing
University of Manitoba
Winnipeg, MB
Chapter 13

Christine Ceci, RN, PhD
Assistant Professor
Faculty of Nursing
University of Alberta
Edmonton, Alberta
Chapter 20

Wanda M. Chernomas, RN, PhD
Associate Professor
Faculty of Nursing
University of Manitoba
Winnipeg, MB
Chapter 13

Heather F. Clarke, RN, PhD
Principal
Health and Nursing Policy
Research and Evaluation Consulting
Vancouver, BC
Chapter 5

Noreen Frisch, RN, PhD
Professor and Director
School of Nursing
University of Victoria
Victoria, BC
Chapter 12

David Michael Gregory, RN, PhD
Professor
School of Health Sciences
University of Lethbridge
Lethbridge, Alberta
Chapter 13

Laurie Hardingham, RN, MA
Clinical Ethicist
St. Joseph's Health Care London
London, ON
Chapter 18

Fjola Hart-Wasekeesikaw, RN, MN
Past-President
Aboriginal Nurses Association of
Canada
Winnipeg, Manitoba
Chapter 24

Karen MacKinnon, RN, PhD
Assistant Professor
School of Nursing
University of Victoria
Victoria, BC
Chapter 2

Kathryn McPherson, PhD
Professor History and Women's
Studies
York University
Toronto, Ontario
Chapter 10

Dorothy Pringle, RN, PhD
Professor
Faculty of Nursing
University of Toronto
Toronto, ON
Chapter 14

Margaret Scaia, RN, MN
School of Nursing
University of Victoria
Victoria, BC
Chapter 10

Judith Shamian, RN, PhD
President and Chief Executive
Officer
Victorian Order of Nurses Canada
Ottawa, ON
Chapter 6

Linda Silas, RN, BScN
President
Canadian Federation of Nurses
Unions
Chapter 17

Judith Skelton-Green, RN, PhD
President
TRANSITIONS: HOD Consultants,
Inc.
Penetanguishene, ON
Chapter 6

Janet L. Storch, RN, PhD
Professor Emeritus
School of Nursing
University of Victoria
Victoria, BC
Chapter 3

Sally Thorne, RN, PhD
Professor and Director
School of Nursing
University of British Columbia
Vancouver, BC
Chapter 11

Colleen Varcoe,RN, PhD
Associate Professor
School of Nursing
University of British Columbia
Vancouver, BC
Chapter 23

Michael J. Villeneuve, RN, MSc
Senior Nurse Consultant
Canadian Nurses Association
Ottawa, ON
Chapter 6, 7, 26

Reviewers

Nancy Archibald, RN, BScN, MN
Nursing Instructor
Red Deer College
Red Deer, AB

Yolanda Babenko-Mould, RN, BScN, MScN, PhD(c)
PhD candidate and School of
  Nursing faculty member
The University of Western Ontario
London, ON

Sandra Bassendowski, EdD, RN
Associate Professor
College of Nursing, University of
  Saskatchewan
Regina, SK

Susan Beiderwieden, RN, BSN, Med
Long term sessional instructor,
  School of Nursing
University of Victoria
Victoria, BC

Stephanie Buckingham, CD, RN, BSN, MA
University-College Professor
Malaspina University-College
Nanaimo, BC

Eleanor Calder, BSN, MS
Sessional Instructor
University of Victoria
Victoria, BC

Greta Cummings, RN, PhD
Assistant Professor, Faculty of
  Nursing
University of Alberta
Edmonton, AB

Isolde Daiski, RN, BScN, MEd, EdD
Associate Professor
York University
Toronto, ON

Anne Dewar, RN, BA, BScN, MHP, PhD
Associate Professor School of
  Nursing
University of British Columbia
Vancouver, BC

Suzanne Dupuis-Blanchard, BScN, MN, PhD
Assistant Professor
School of Nursing – Université de
  Moncton
Moncton, NB

Lenore Duquette, RN, BScN, MEd, EdD
Nursing Professor
Humber ITAL
Toronto, ON

Denise M. English, RN, BN, MN
Nurse Educator
Centre for Nursing Studies
St. John's, NL

Wendy Fostey, RN, BHScN, MHScN
Professor of Nursing, BScN
  collaborative program
Sault College
Sault Ste. Marie, ON

Mary Haase, RPN, RN, BScN, PhD
Instructor
Grant MacEwan College
Edmonton, AB

Margaret Hadley, RN, MN
Instructor
Grant MacEwan College
Edmonton, AB

Carole-Lynne Le Navenec, RN, PhD
Associate Professor
Faculty of Nursing, University of
  Calgary
Calgary, AB

Sister Rosemary MacDonald, BScN, MDiv, STB, DMin
Assistant Professor
UPEI School of Nursing
Charlottetown, PEI

Pertice Moffitt, RN, BSN, MN, PhD
Senior Instructor, Nursing
Aurora College
Yellowknife, NT

Dan Nagel, RN, BScN, MSN
BSN Faculty
Douglas College
Coquitlam, BC

Aroha Page, RN, BA, BScN, MPhil, PhD, FCNA
Professor/Nursing
Nipissing University
North Bay, ON

Dawn Prentice, RN PhD
Assistant Professor
Brock University
St. Catharine's, Ontario

Louise Racine, RN, BScN, MScN, PhD
Assistant Professor
University of Saskatchewan, College
  of Nursing
Saskatoon, SK

Julianne Sanguins, RN BScN MS(N) PhD
Research Associate & Sessional
  Instructor
University of Manitoba & Athabasca
  University
Winnipeg, MB

Susan Wynne, RN, CNCC(C), ENC(C)
Clinical Instructor
Trent University
Peterborough, ON

Preface

In 2000, when we were approached by Margaret Zuccarini, who, at the time, was a senior acquisitions editor for Lippincott Williams & Wilkins, we could never have imagined the enthusiastic response that the text would receive from students, teaching faculty, and practicing nurses. Nor could we have foreseen that in 2006 we would release the second edition of the text. Needless to say, we are thrilled at the success of the first two editions and the apparent resonance of the text with nurses across the country. As we put the final touches on the third edition, complete with both new and revised chapters, we find ourselves once again curious about how our latest creative endeavor will be received in the nursing community.

One of the biggest challenges in writing an issues textbook is the nature of issues as emerging and evolving. While many of the issues that we address in health care have been with us over time, others can be seen as uniquely located in the realities of our current situation. At the outset of this third edition, we imagined some revisions to the text arising from changes in political and practice realities as well as from feedback received from reviewers. Specifically, we responded to the reviewers request for the inclusion of a chapter on the nursing shortage. New topics have emerged from our own teaching and research experiences, among these issues related to holistic health, health care for those in rural settings and for people of non-heterosexual orientations. We are delighted to open space in this edition for the contribution of new scholars, Karen MacKinnon and Margaret Scaia, as well as welcoming the valued work of respected scholars. Among these accomplished contributors are Kathryn McPherson, Pat Armstrong, Colleen Varcoe, and Noreen Frisch. From a national perspective, the work of Canadian Nurses Association (CNA) writer in residence Michael Villeneuve and the Canadian Federation of Nurses Union (CFNU) president Linda Silas add significantly to the impact of this third edition.

Books are written for many reasons, and the first edition of *Realities of Canadian Nursing: Professional, Practice, and Power Issues* was no exception. At first glance, it might seem that the decision to edit a book on nursing issues was simple. On one level, we convinced ourselves that a new and different book for teaching nursing issues was needed. On another level, we were looking for a book that would do more than provide the material needed to understand issues; we wanted to prepare and inspire students to participate in political action alongside the generations of nurses who have already taken the lead. We imagined a book that would engage readers in such a way that they would be prepared to work with others in addressing the long-standing barriers to many of the issues that confront nurses and the people who seek nurses' services. We further speculated that, in addressing these issues, nurses who understood the barriers to resolving these issues were in the best position to make significant contributions to their resolutions. We wanted to dispel the many myths that question the need for nurses to be political and the notion that others will act on our behalf.

We hope that the third edition of *Realities of Canadian Nursing: Professional, Practice, and Power Issues* will not only influence students to engage with nursing issues in new ways but that its chapters will stimulate new writing among Canadian scholars on nursing issues. An additional goal of this book is to disrupt the notion that changes to nursing and health care will happen without informed political action on the part of nurses: We hope to instill in more nurses the obligation to use their regulatory power, collectively and individually, to influence decision making in professional associations, collective bargaining units, government, and workplaces.

The intention of *Realities of Canadian Nursing: Professional, Practice, and Power Issues* has been, from its inception, to provide readers with a critical analysis of the tensions and contradictions that exist between nurses' legislated authority to self-regulate and the changing nature and realities of nurses' work. The changing conditions of nurses' workplaces, the changing settings and contexts of nurses' work, and the realities of contemporary society that challenge, on a daily basis, nurses' practice are all covered, as is the centrality of nurses' work and its contribution to the health of Canadians. Additionally, reference to earlier publications on professional regulation, health care systems, leadership, education, research, ethics, and legal issues is also included. Drawing on feminist and other forms of critical analysis, our contributors offer strategic points of resistance to dominant discourses by attributing significance to that too often considered insignificant—the underlying experiences and unheard concerns of nurses. Thoughtful exploration of these issues calls us all, nurses and non-nurses, to reflect on the ways in which we disrupt and maintain complicity in dominant discourses and on how we can deliberately use our knowledge to break through barriers and act strategically to resolve issues.

On a closing note, we would like to acknowledge the change in contributors for the third edition. While we are very pleased with the new contributors to this edition, we recognize too the work of previous contributors. In particular we deeply appreciate Betty Thomlinson's participation in the conceptualization and authorship of the first edition of this text.

Contents

 PART 1 • NURSES, NURSING, and the HEALTHCARE SYSTEM 1

CHAPTER 1 Nursing Issues: A Call to Political Action 3

Marjorie McIntyre and Carol McDonald

Significance for Nurses 5 • Significance for the Profession 5 • Nursing Practice as Political Action 6 • Framing the Topic 7 • Analyzing the Issue 8 • Barriers to Resolution 10 • Devising Strategies for Resolution 10 • Summary 14

CHAPTER 2 Rural Nursing in Canada 17

Karen MacKinnon

• Situating the Topic: Framing the Issue 18 • Understanding the Issues 19 • Resolution: Constraints and Possibilities 26 • Summary 28

CHAPTER 3 Canadian Healthcare System 34

Janet L. Storch

• The Importance of Understanding Canada's Healthcare System 35 • The Canada Health Act 35 • So What does this Mean? 47 • What Lies Ahead? 49 • Nurses Leading to Influence Change 50 • Summary 51

CHAPTER 4 Issues in Contemporary Nursing Leadership 56

Marjorie McInytre and Carol McDonald

• Situating the Topic: The Nature of the Issue 57 • Historical Analysis 60 • Social Analysis 60 • Economic Analysis 61 • Ethical Analysis 61 • Political Analysis 61 • Barriers to Resolving the Issue 62 • Strategies to Resolving the Issue 62 • Summary 66

CHAPTER 5 Health and Nursing Policy: A Matter of Politics, Power, and Professionalism 68

Heather F. Clarke

• Policy, Politics, Power, and Professionalism 69 • History and Background: Perspectives on Policy 72 • Conceptualizing the Policy Design Process 81 • Impact on Nursing: The Relevance of a Nursing Perspective 84 • Future Implications: Challenges and Strategies 85 • Summary 87

CHAPTER 6 Policy: The Essential Link in Successful Transformations 91

Michael J. Villeneuve, Judith Shamian, and Judith Skelton-Green

• The Challenge: Avoiding Critical Situations 93 • High-Quality Evidence 95 • Effective Research–Policy Linkages 96 • Planned Change: Why does it Happen ... Or Not? 97 • Policy Cycle 99 • Political Acumen: The Drive Behind Policymaking 104 • Overcoming Barriers: Lessons from those Who have Walked Before 106 • Overcoming Barriers and Initiating Action 108 • Summary 109

 PART 2 • REGULATORY POWER 115

CHAPTER 7 The Canadian Nurses Association and the International Council of Nurses 117

Michael J. Villeneuve

• The Canadian Nurses Association: The National Voice of Nurses in Canada since 1908 118 • CNA's Strategic Responses to Priorities and Challenges Confronting Canadian Nursing in the 21st Century 123 • The International Council of Nurses: A Historical Perspective 135 • The ICN in the 21st Century 142 • Summary 143

CHAPTER 8 Canadian Provincial and Territorial Professional Associations
and Colleges 147

Laurel Brunke

• Regulation 148 • Regulation of Nursing 149 • Issues in Regulation 152 • Summary 163

CHAPTER 9 The NP Movement: Recurring Issues 166

Carol McDonald and Marjorie McIntyre

• Situating the Topic: The Nature of the Issue 167 • Articulating the Topic as an Issue 167
• Analyzing the Issue: Ways of Understanding 167 • Barriers to Resolution 173 • Strategies 175
• Summary 176 • Glossary of Terms 177

PART 3 • NURSING KNOWLEDGE: How We Come to Know What We Know 181

CHAPTER 10 Challenges and Change in Undergraduate Nursing Education 183

Margaret Scaia and Kathryn McPherson

• Roots and Wings: Issues in Undergraduate Nursing Education 185 • Prepared to Care? 187
• Constructing Bodies: Who Becomes a Nurse? 187 • Active Education: Connecting the Global and
the Local 190 • Advocating for Nursing: Change is Political 191 • Workplace Blues 192
• Looking Forward; Looking Back 194 • Historical Issues in Undergraduate Nursing Education 195
• The Future: New Old Issues? 198 • Summary 199

CHAPTER 11 Graduate Education 203

Sally Thorne

• History of Graduate Nursing Education in Canada 204 • Practice Realities and Challenges for
Graduate-Prepared Nurses 208 • Issues and Controversies in Graduate Education 210 • Challenges
for Graduate-Prepared Nurses 214 • Strategies for Advancing Graduate Education 215 • Summary 218

Chapter 12 The Challenges of Holistic Nursing Practice 223

Noreen Frisch

• What is Holistic Nursing? 224 • Holism in Nursing: 20th Century Developments 225 • Modern
Holistic Nursing: A Three Country Comparison 229 • Practicing Holistic Nursing Today: Issues and
Challenges 232 • Summary 234

CHAPTER 13 Nursing, Technology and Informatics: Understanding the Past and
Embracing the Future 238

W. Dean Care, David Michael Gregory, and Wanda M. Chernomas

• Relationship between Nursing and Technology 240 • Nursing Informatics 241 • Applications of
Nursing Informatics and Technology in Practice 242 • Issues in the Application of Biomedical
Technology and Nursing Practice 246 • Issues in the Allocation of Technology in Education 247
• Issues in Adopting Technology in Nursing Education 250 • Future of Technology in Education and
Practice 252 • Summary 254

CHAPTER 14 The Realities of Canadian Nursing Research 259

Dorothy Pringle

• The Evolution of Nursing Research in Canada 260 • Influence of Research on Nursing Practice and
Education 268 • Contribution of Nursing Research to the Health and Healthcare of Canadians 273
• Issues Facing Nursing Research 274 • The Future of Nursing Research 276 • Summary 277

PART 4 ● WORKPLACE REALITIES 281

CHAPTER 15 Issues Arising From the Nature of Nurses' Work and Workplaces 283

Carol McDonald and Marjorie McIntyre

● The Nature of Nurses' Work 284 ● The Nature of Nurses' Workplaces 284 ● The Significance of Nurses' Work Issues 285 ● Issues Arising in Nurses' Work and Workplaces 286 ● Barriers to Resolving Work and Workplace Issues 296 ● Strategies for Resolving Work and Workplace Issues 297 ● Summary 300

CHAPTER 16 The Nursing Shortage: Assumptions and Realities 303

Marjorie McIntyre and Carol McDonald

● Nature of the Nursing Shortage 304 ● Framing and Analyzing the Issue 304 ● Historical Analysis of the Nursing Shortage 305 ● Social and Cultural Analysis of the Nursing Shortage 307 ● Economic Analysis of the Nursing Shortage 309 ● Political Analysis of the Nursing Shortage 310 ● Critical Feminist Analysis of the Nursing Shortage 311 ● Status of Nursing Knowledge 311 ● Status of Nurses' Work 312 ● Identifying Barriers to Resolution of the Nursing Shortage 312 ● Devising Strategies to Resolve Selected Issues 313 ● Summary 314

Chapter 17 Taking Power: Making Change and Nurses' Unions in Canada 316

Pat Armstrong and Linda Silas

● Historical Influences 317 ● Organizing Practices of Professional Nurses 319 ● Emergence of Union Practices 320 ● Transformations in Healthcare 320 ● Transformations in Unions 321 ● CNA Influences on the Move to Unionization 322 ● Changes in Nurses' Thinking about Collective Bargaining 324 ● The Gendered Nature of Issues Surrounding Collective Bargaining 324 ● Nurses' Workplaces 326 ● Collective Bargaining 329 ● Moving Ahead 330 ● Unions Today and Tomorrow 331 ● Summary 333

CHAPTER 18 Ethical and Legal Issues in Nursing 337

Laurie Hardingham

● Story: The Winnipeg Nurses 338 ● What is Ethics? What is Bioethics? 339 ● Recognizing Ethical Issues 339 ● Identifying and Articulating Ethical Issues 340 ● Ethical or Legal Issue? Alike but Different 343 ● Issues of Moral Integrity 345 ● Barriers to Resolving Ethical and Legal Issues 349 ● Strategies for Resolution of Ethical and Legal Issues 351 ● Summary 352

CHAPTER 19 Issues of Gender and Power: The Significance Attributed to Nurses' Work 355

Carol McDonald

● Gender and Power: Articulating the Issue for Nursing 356 ● The Effects of Gender in Nurses' Lives 361 ● Barriers to and Strategies for Issue Resolution 365 ● Summary 366

CHAPTER 20 When Difference Matters: The Politics of Privilege and Marginality 369

Christine Ceci

● A Philosophical Approach to Understanding Difference 370 ● The Challenge of Difference 373 ● Theorizing Difference 374 ● Difference as Deviance: A Case of Biologic Determinism in Practice 376 ● Difference as Relationship 379 ● The Distinct Realities of Others 382 ● Summary 384

CHAPTER 21 Orientating to Difference: Beyond Heteronormative Sexualities 387

Carol McDonald

● Beyond Heteronormative Sexualities: Articulating the Topic for Nursing 388 ● Articulating the Topic as an Issue 390 ● Analyzing the Issue: Ways of Understanding 391 ● Barriers to Resolution 395 ● Strategies for Resolution 396 ● Summary 396

CHAPTER 22 Environmental Health and Nursing   400

Carol McDonald and Marjorie McIntyre

• Historical Links between Environment and Health 402 • Environmental Health Hazards 403
• Barriers and Strategies 409 • Summary 410

CHAPTER 23 Interpersonal Violence and Abuse: Ending the Silence   414

Colleen Varcoe

• The Many Forms of Interpersonal Violence 416 • Historical Perspectives on Violence and Abuse 418
• Statistics in the Canadian Context 419 • Understanding Violence: Theoretical Perspectives 424
• Impact on Health and the Healthcare System 425 • Issues for Nurses and the Nursing Profession 426
• Barriers to Resolution 427 • Strategies for Resolution 428 • Summary 429

CHAPTER 24 Challenges for the New Millennium: Nursing in First Nations   435

Fjola Hart Wasekeesikaw

• Diversity of the First Peoples 436 • European Relationship with First Nations 437 • Cultural
Resurgence of First Nations and Community Development 439 • Miyupimaatissiium: Being Alive
Well 440 • Healthcare in Northern and Isolated Communities 442 • Climate for Change: Nursing
in First Nations Communities 444 • Summary 451

CHAPTER 25 Opening Conversations: Dilemmas and Possibilities of Spirituality and Spiritual Care   455

Anne Bruce

• Introduction to the Topic: Opening the Conversation about Spirituality 456 • Situating the Topic:
Personal and Professional Assumptions 457 • Situating the Topic: Understanding Spiritual Practices
Historically 457 • Significance of the Topic for Nursing: Embracing the Tensions 458
• Articulating the Topic as an Issue: Practice Dilemmas 459 • Identifying Barriers: Furthering Our
Understanding 467 • Generating Strategies: Future Possibilities 467 • Summary 467

Chapter 26 Looking Back, Moving Forward: Taking Nursing toward 2020   470

Michael J. Villeneuve

• Studying the Future 471 • Summary 479

Index   483

NURSES, NURSING, and the HEALTHCARE SYSTEM

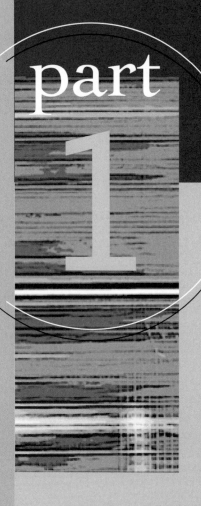

part

1

Undergraduate student nurses from the University of Victoria participate in the Western Region Canadian Association of Schools of Nursing. (Photography by Chris Marshall. Used with permission from University of Victoria.)

Nursing Issues: A Call to Political Action

Marjorie McIntyre
Carol McDonald

Critical Questions

As a way of engaging with the ideas in this chapter, consider the following:

1. What comes to mind when you think of political action?

2. Do you think of yourself as a social activist?

3. Would you consider nursing practice a political act?

Chapter Objectives

After completing this chapter, you will be able to:

1. Distinguish between problem solving and the process of issue articulation and resolution.

2. Use a framework for the articulation and analysis of an issue.

3. Describe strategies for addressing barriers and moving issues toward resolution.

Nurses across Canada are grappling with what seems at times to be irresolvable issues embedded in healthcare delivery, nursing practice, and education. Nurses struggle to solve recurring problems within a context of inadequate resources and insufficient support. In this text, we raise the questions of how we might understand these problems differently. How might we move beyond a short-term problem-solving approach, in which problems are viewed in isolation, to facilitate an understanding of issues as complex and interrelated, with a breadth and scope not accounted for in a problem-solving approach? How might we benefit from a new approach to issue articulation and issue resolution? The premise of this chapter and, in fact, of this entire book is that reconceptualizing short-term, seemingly irresolvable problems as issues situated in political, material, and social contexts opens us to the realities and possibilities previously obscured. It is important for nurses to question the ways in which issues are conceptualized because how a nursing situation is understood by nurses and other decision makers will have implications for how it is likely to be addressed. The many issues affecting nurses, the profession, and the healthcare system can be understood and articulated as political issues in that they ultimately involve influencing others for the purpose of quality patient care.

Thoughtful exploration of these political questions calls us all, nurses and non-nurses, to reflect on that which constrains—and enables—the ways we can communicate and think about nursing. When nurses find themselves unable to nurse as they had envisioned, as they believe they can or should, or when their interpretations of what is occurring in healthcare are excluded from policy discussions, a sense of being incorrect, in some essential sense, in their understanding of themselves and their work, comes into play. A profound dissonance emerges between what one believes one is called on to be and do and what the world, and one's relationship to it, allows. This distress deepens when it remains unheard, when what is of concern to nurses remains stubbornly invisible to others (Ceci & McIntyre, 2001). The ability to articulate and act on issues is one of the means of preparing nurses for political action. Box 1.1 presents a healthcare issue identified by nurses.

BOX 1.1 Healthcare Issue: Political Action Results in Screening Program

Four community nurses working with homeless people suspected there was an increase in tuberculosis (TB) based on several cases of active TB and an increase in positive skin tests among their patients. However, when they approached the public health department, they were informed that the statistics did not indicate an increase. Although the nurses asked that TB screening be conducted in homeless shelters and drop-in centers, the health department refused.

The nurses believed that TB was increasing and, therefore, decided to press the health department to initiate a screening program. They proceeded with the following steps:

- Calling a meeting with other healthcare workers, shelter and drop-in staff, and homeless people
- Forming an action group
- Educating group members about TB
- Researching the experiences of other cities
- Making representations to health departments
- Offering to assist with screenings

These efforts resulted in a major screening program that demonstrated the increased numbers of people with TB. The group then expanded its focus to include other issues.

From Canadian Nurses Association. (2000) *CNA Today, 10(2)*, 11. Used with permission.

This chapter introduces nursing issues and provides an overview of issue articulation and its significance to nursing. Specifically, it provides a framework to explore, articulate, analyze, and generate possibilities for increased understanding and, when feasible, for resolution of nursing issues. Examples of barriers to issue resolution and specific strategies to generate possibilities for resolution are also discussed.

SIGNIFICANCE FOR NURSES

What is the significance of understanding problems in healthcare as complex and multilayered issues? Issues are best served by an approach that questions and interrogates the taken-for-granted view of the particular subject. Rather than a move to solve problems, an in-depth analysis of issues includes an exploration of barriers that makes visible the complexity of the issue. This exploration moves us past the notion that any one strategy could move an issue to resolution. To articulate an issue fully means to consider the political, historical, social, and economic realities on and through which issues are constructed.

The nursing shortage is an excellent example of how we might distinguish between issue analysis and resolution and problem solving. If we think of the shortage as a problem of not enough nurses—a problem of numbers—the shortage could be solved by producing more nurses. If we think of the shortage as reflecting nurses' dissatisfaction with their work, we might move to improve nurses' salaries and other contractual issues. However, regardless of what might be accomplished by addressing these individual problems in the short term, studies have shown that it is not one but many problems, and the relationships between them, that contribute to the shortage (Baumann et al., 2001). The recurrence of the nursing shortage over time suggests that it would be more beneficially analyzed and addressed as a complex issue including many overlapping and interconnected problems.

Analyzing the nursing shortage as a political issue raises many questions. How might we account for the cycle of surplus and shortages historically? What constitutes a shortage of nurses? Who is the authority on what counts as a shortage? How do the prevailing attitudes in society about what it means to be a nurse contribute to the shortage? What of the status of nurses' work and nursing knowledge in the recruitment and retention of nurses? Is it possible that nursing shortages are created? Who might benefit from such a shortage? Who suffers? What are the economic implications of a shortage for nurses, for the healthcare system, and for the health of Canadians? Moving the shortage past the idea of individual problems to be solved to the depth and scope of a political issue illuminates the potential barriers for resolution. Barriers to resolving the nursing shortage include the incongruity between the complex nature of nursing practice and the lesser status attributed to nurses' work and nursing knowledge, the reality that many decisions made about nurses' work are not made by nurses, and the use of nurses as temporary workers prepared to fill a gap in services. Strategies that emerge from such an analysis would necessarily include the multiple stakeholders involved and consideration of these barriers so that solutions are long term.

SIGNIFICANCE FOR THE PROFESSION

The significance of clear articulation of issues for the profession goes beyond the individual nurse to include the organization of nurses and their ideas into a larger collective. To be effective in supporting political action within the profession, nurses need to speak in unison on issues and organize themselves to act provincially and territorially, nationally, and internationally. In 1977, Mussallem (1977, p. 156) claimed what is still true today: In the context of state-provided healthcare, the link between healthcare and political action is inseparable. The *raison d'etre* of nursing is healthcare. The quality of healthcare depends to a large extent on the nature of the nursing component determined by four elements:

- standards of education and preparation for those entering the profession
- quality of care provided by the practitioner—a quality closely associated with education and preparation
- number of nurses available—a determination considered in modern times largely by the social and economic status the profession offers its members
- milieu in which care is offered.

If nurses are concerned about healthcare, they must accept responsibility for safeguarding these four dynamic elements of nursing practice. This safeguarding can be achieved only by the participation of nurses in political action.

NURSING PRACTICE AS POLITICAL ACTION

The need for problem-solving and decision-making abilities has been ingrained in the discipline of nursing since its inception. Although many problems are amenable to deductive thinking and problem solving, nurses face increasingly complex issues in a continually expanding array of practice settings. And so, although nursing practice and education have historically privileged a deductive approach to decision making, the changing world in which practice occurs and the advancing education level of nurses underscore the need for more inductive, interpretive approaches. In recent years, there has been an increased focus on nurses' advocacy. Legislative changes in the scope of practice and in the code of ethics have contributed to the politicization of nursing practice. While once many nurses were identified as nonpolitical, today, political awareness, political action, and social justice are increasingly—and necessarily—embedded in nursing education and nursing practice. The advancement of nursing education underpins the movement of nurses into leadership positions in the healthcare system and in education. Concurrent with their increasing social consciousness, nurse leaders experience an awareness of the limitations of approaching complex social-political issues with short-term approaches to change. The recently released Canadian Nurses Association (CNA) "Code of Ethics for Registered Nurses (2008 Centennial Edition)," explicitly states that "there are broad aspects of social justice that are associated with health and well-being and that ethical nursing practice addresses. Nurses should endeavor as much as possible, individually and collectively, to advocate for and work toward eliminating social inequities" (p.20).

In the face of a healthcare system in which there are seemingly continual therapeutic and technological advances, it is easy to think of healthcare and indeed of nursing practice as progressively advancing. However, the reality for many Canadians is diminished access to nursing and healthcare services. Perhaps more than ever before, nurses are in a position to bring attention to the healthcare needs of underserved populations. Increasing numbers of nurses are employed in the community, in home-care work, and in agencies and institutions providing care to elderly individuals (Canadian Nurses Association, 2004). In these work environments, nurses face issues of health and healthcare that are mediated by the social and material realities of the lives of the people to whom they provide care. Community and home-care nursing magnifies our awareness of the realities of poverty, lack of education, inadequate housing, and isolation and their influence on the health of Canadians. Although we can expect that many people would have intellectual awareness of these impoverished circumstances within our society, nurses, through their privileged access to underserved populations in the provision of care, live alongside this knowledge in practice. Nurses are, then, caught in the tension of knowing what is needed, yet also knowing that these resources are not forthcoming. This disparity is what incites the political will to challenge existing structures and processes that limit access to health and healthcare for underserved Canadians.

 ## FRAMING THE TOPIC

To begin examining and acting on an issue, one identifies the topic of interest and from this selects a particular issue and articulates, or expresses, it clearly. An issue can be expressed as a dilemma, conundrum, question or series of questions, or simple statement. Box 1.2 summarizes the steps used in articulating and analyzing an issue.

Situating the Topic

One situates the topic by making explicit the assumptions that are held about the topic. An assumption is an idea that is held to be true without any support or substantiation; all of us operate from day to day under assumptions. Part of situating the topic is looking to the literature to find out what is known about the topic within the discipline and in some cases in literature outside the discipline. The literature review is intended to help establish the particular issue that will be addressed within the topic. For example, within the topic of the nursing shortage, one might articulate the issue for analysis as the particular way in which the nursing shortage has been conceptualized or presented to the public.

The following are some questions to ask when situating the topic:

- What is already known about this topic?
- Who has generated this knowledge?
- What assumptions are held about this topic?
- What issue within this topic would you like to explore?

Articulating the Issue

Once the issue to address has been identified, ask the following questions:

- What makes this issue a nursing issue?
- In what ways are nurses involved in the issue?
- Who are the other participants and what is their involvement in the issue?
- Who first became concerned with the subject?
- Who began to raise the subject as an issue and why?

 ## BOX 1.2 Articulation and Analysis of an Issue

1. Identify the topic of interest.
2. Select a particular issue and articulate it clearly. Define your own beliefs and assumptions about the issue.
3. Proceed with the analysis by addressing appropriate frameworks.
4. Identify barriers to resolution.
5. Explore strategies for resolution.

ANALYZING THE ISSUE

Once the issue is articulated clearly, the analysis may proceed as outlined in the following section. Some issues call for a particular approach to analysis, but most issues benefit from more than one approach. However, it is unlikely that all approaches to analysis would be undertaken with every issue. The categories of analysis are intended to generate rather than limit possibilities for discussion. The purpose of asking these questions is to increase understanding of all aspects of the issue and to move the discussion toward resolution.

Historical Analysis of the Issue

An historical analysis of issues brings us the opportunity to reopen our nursing and healthcare history. This reopening is more than a return to the history that has been dominantly recorded; rather, it can be seen as an opportunity to excavate the historical understandings that have been silenced, diminished, or erased. This approach to history reminds us that each telling of history is necessarily situated in the standpoint or the assumptions of the one who recounts the story. Each telling of our past is, in some sense, a partial and incomplete interpretation. In this way, history is understood as multiple histories; each account presents a reality, although only a limited depiction of our recorded past. McPherson (1996), a nurse historian, points out that events from nursing history are understood quite differently depending on who has been responsible for the documentation or analysis of the event. For example, in her discussion of the subordination of nurses, McPherson highlights the difference in viewing historical events through a lens of class analysis, gender analysis, or academic and professional analysis. The view of a particular issue through different lenses for analysis reveals different historical realities, each of which contributes to a full understanding of the issue. The questions below are intended to guide a historical analysis:

- When did the issue originate?
- What are the conditions that led to the development of the issue?
- How have these conditions changed over time?
- What is the source of the historical accounts of the issue?
- What might have influenced this perspective of the history?
- What has contributed to the stance taken by participants in the issue?
- What have been the barriers to resolution?
- What strategies for resolution have already been tried?

Ethical and Legal Analysis of the Issue

The CNA's "Code of Ethics for Registered Nurses (2008 Centennial Edition)" outlines the responsibilities and obligations for the provision of professional practice of safe, compassionate, competent, and ethical care. In addition to the values and responsibilities in the "Code of Ethics," it addresses broad aspects of social justice that are associated with health and well-being. For this reason, the code itself provides a framework for an ethical analysis of issues for nurses' professional relationships with individuals, families, groups, students, colleagues, and other healthcare professionals.

In addition to consulting the "Code of Ethics," you may ask the following questions:

- What are the laws that influence this issue?
- What professional codes or legislative acts mandate participants' responses to this issue?
- What professional, organizational, and governmental (municipal, provincial and territorial, and national) documents inform, constrain, or influence the issue? In addition to the CNA's "Code of

Ethics," possibilities include the provincial and territorial standards of practice, the British North America Act, the Health Professions Act, and the Canada Health Act.

Social and Cultural Analysis of the Issue

Every issue develops in a societal context that shapes the issue and influences the possibilities for resolution. An analysis of the social and cultural context explores the prevailing attitudes, the values and priorities, and the privileging of the dominant culture. The questions below provide guidance in analysis:

- What social and cultural contexts shape this particular issue?
- What are the prevailing attitudes or assumptions in society about this issue?
- What values and priorities of the dominant culture influence this issue? In what ways, if any, do these values and priorities privilege the dominant culture over other members of society?

Political Analysis of the Issue

A political analysis asks questions that explore the location of power and influence within particular issues. In other words, whose knowledge, whose voice is able to influence either the barriers to or the strategies for resolution of an issue? Specifically, what is the relationship between knowledge and power in this situation? Questions to guide the political analysis include:

- Who benefits from the issue staying the same?
- Who is resisting change and satisfied to maintain the status quo?
- Who is advocating for change regarding this issue?
- Who benefits from the issue being resolved?
- Whose interests are being served?
- Are there hidden agendas or less visible influences affecting this issue?
- How do ageist, sexist, racist, and ableist ideologies influence our understanding of this issue?

Critical Feminist Analysis of the Issue

A critical feminist approach asks questions that challenge the taken-for-granted assumptions of gender that are prevalent in society. The intention is not to privilege the position of one gender over the other but to question the way in which notions of gender have been attached to issues influencing nurses, patients and clients, and relationships with others in the healthcare system. More often than not, a critical feminist analysis does not relate to the gender of a particular person, but rather to the ways that traditional structures based on gender divisions of power have influenced or shaped issues or events. The following questions could be included in a critical feminist analysis:

- Are there errors or myths about women's or men's abilities or realities contained in this issue?
- Is this issue influenced by the power inequities or the hierarchical or patriarchal structures of institutions over nurses or patients and clients?
- In this situation, is expert power given authority over personal power and the right to be the subject of one's own life?

Economic Analysis of the Issue

In today's healthcare systems, questions of economics are prevalent in relation to nearly every identified issue. The discourses that we hear and repeat are replete with the language of economic constraint, efficiency and cost effectiveness, and scarcity of resources. An economic analysis asks difficult questions that challenge the source of these pervasive discourses and asks how things could be otherwise. Questions for the economic analysis might include:

- Who is the author of the economic discourses we hear?
- What knowledge, besides economic goals, might influence the issue?
- Who benefits from the dominance of economic discourses over other knowledge affecting this issue?
- In what ways are the forces of supply and demand at work in this issue?

 ## BARRIERS TO RESOLUTION

One of the most important strategies for moving an issue toward resolution is identifying barriers that may impede the resolution process. Once the barriers are identified, there may be an increased opportunity for resolution through mediation, collaboration, or negotiation. The following are some potential barriers to resolution of nursing issues:

- Limited accessibility to resources, such as human and financial resources, knowledge, or expertise, may obstruct resolution.
- Issues are not clearly understood or are understood in a limited way. For example, a barrier to resolving the nursing shortage is conceptualizing the issue as only a problem of the numbers of nurses entering the profession.
- Irresolvable differences or competing interests between participants may block the resolution of issues.
- Circumstances in which some participants benefit from the issue remaining unresolved limit the opportunity for resolution.
- Power inequities between parties invested in the issue can contribute to resistance to resolution.
- Participants in the issue may experience unconscious resistance to change.
- Key stakeholders in the issue may lack tolerance for multiple viewpoints.
- Stakeholders may ascribe to differing underlying assumptions or beliefs that influence the way the issue is understood and the way resolution is undertaken.
- Alienation from coworkers, hostility from bureaucratic and administrative officials, and fear of job loss may isolate nurses from the supports needed for resolution.
- Lack of time, energy, role models, and mentors seriously undermines possibilities for effective resolution.

 ## DEVISING STRATEGIES FOR RESOLUTION

After an issue relevant to the profession of nursing or healthcare is articulated and analyzed, multiple strategies can be implemented to address and resolve the issue. Essential to the success of any effort is the communication of a well-developed plan of action. Strategies for resolution include, but are not limited to, the following:

- formation of lobby groups
- preparation of resolutions for presentation to agencies, associations, and organizations
- establishment of a letter-writing campaign
- involvement of the news media through letters to the editor and articles that solicit public support.

The use of any of these strategies depends on the following:

- people affected by the issue
- interest that is generated
- time available
- human and financial resources available.

To generate the maximum amount of support, it is important to enlist the assistance of as many people as possible who are affected by the issue. A greater response and resolution can be anticipated if the affected parties are unified in their efforts to address the specific issue. The following sections include specific, detailed examples of strategies that have been employed by individuals from multiple segments of the population in their efforts to create change and to address issues of relevance to them.

Lobbying Strategies

Although lobby groups are usually associated with persuading elected officials to vote a certain way on an issue or to carry an issue forward for debate, change within an organization can be promoted by lobbying key individuals. Regardless of whether the issue is of national or international importance, or whether the issue affects nurses and healthcare on a particular unit or in a particular agency, the same techniques are available and applicable.

Lobbying may occur through direct contact with people who are in positions to address the issue and through indirect methods by which others influence the officials (Hood, 1998). Table 1.1 provides a comparison of direct and indirect strategies.

Nurses must keep several key points in mind when initiating a lobby and planning meetings with key officials, including the following:

- Become informed about the issue by reading newspapers, documents, scholarly articles and reports; searching the Internet; and knowing the professional associations' positions.
- Use simple statistics and avoid percentages. The clearer the statistics, the more attention they will generate. Then apply the numbers in human terms, and illustrate the statistics with personal stories.
- Be sure to articulate clearly why the issue is an issue and identify its importance.
- Know what other people are saying about the issue.
- Keep in mind that the more people supporting the issue, the more effective the lobby.

Table 1.1	Comparing Direct and Indirect Lobbying Strategies
DIRECT STRATEGIES	**INDIRECT STRATEGIES**
Engaging in letter, phone call, and e-mail campaigns to elected officials or others in power	Writing reports, articles, and books
Meeting with key people professionally	Enlisting the support of key people
Taking opportunities to meet key people socially	Using the media through news announcements on the radio and on television, in newspaper and magazine columns, and in advertisements
Submitting resolutions to professional organizations and unions	

- If you are lobbying government officials or bodies, remember to include members of the opposition parties.
- Follow meetings with written submissions that are accurate and succinct.

LETTERS TO OFFICIALS

One popular and well-used lobbying strategy is writing letters. Prepare the letter so it outlines a selected issue and the possibilities for resolution. Send the letter to a public official such as the dean of your school or faculty, the unit manager in your facility or organization, a city councilor, members of the legislative assembly of your provincial government, or members of parliament of the government of Canada. Consider sending a copy of the letter to other stakeholders and interested parties, and keep a copy of letters for your own files. See Box 1.3 for an example of a lobbying letter, and see the Appendix for additional samples of written documents.

BOX 1.3 Lobbying and Letter Writing: An Example

Whether you are writing to your MP or to the minister of health or finance, adapt these letters to fit your own situation. Personalized letters have more impact. The sample letter presented here is to the minister of health.

The Honorable _____, P.C., M.P. Minister of Health

House of Commons Ottawa, Ontario K1A OA6

Dear Minister,

At the CNA Biennial Convention in Ottawa in June, you noted that "since Jeanne Mance set foot in this land, nurses have been caring for this country, and now, more than ever, it is time for Canada to show how much it cares for nurses." I thank you for these words and am writing you today to encourage you to demonstrate your willingness to invest in the nursing profession.

Canadians are worried about the state of the healthcare system and associate the declining quality of care with the decreasing availability of nurses. (Note: Add a personal example from your own area as appropriate.) As you are aware, Canada faces a severe shortage of nurses with the knowledge and skills to meet the future health needs of Canadians. Care is becoming increasingly complex and technologically advanced. As you work to create an integrated continuum of care, Canadians will require highly qualified nurses to plan and deliver that care.

As the federal government examines its fiscal priorities and resources for the coming year, the nurses of Canada urge you to take a leadership role in making sustainable investments in the healthcare system, including:

- Increasing federal transfer payments
- Expanding the continuum of care to include accessible home and community care
- Making a modest investment of $200 million over 5 years to support nursing recruitment, retention, research, and the dissemination and uptake of evidence to provide the best patient care

The nurses of Canada are looking to the federal government to demonstrate the strength of your commitment to ensure that all Canadians continue to enjoy ready access to the best healthcare system in the world.

Sincerely,

[Your name & address]

From Canadian Nurses Association. (1998). *The quiet crisis in healthcare*. Lobby Kit. Ottawa: Author. Used with permission.

LETTERS TO THE EDITOR

To be published, letters to the editor should comment on a public issue, and they usually are a response to a particular article or editorial published in the newspapers. An example may be a letter that responds to an editorial discussing the next federal budget, which is expected to be a "health budget." Keeping the letter short and punchy will enhance its chances of being published. Remember to sign the letter and add a daytime telephone number in case the editor wants verification or more information from you. Information on where to send letters is usually found in the letters section of the newspaper.

NEWS RELEASES

A news release is much like a letter but does not have a salutation. Information should include relevant facts—the who, what, when, where, why, and how of the issue that you want to highlight. The release should also include the name and telephone number of a person whom the media can contact for further comments or to arrange for an interview. The following example of a news release may be adapted to fit various needs:

> *In* (name of region), *registered nurses will be meeting with politicians and holding events, such as news conferences, to build support for the nursing investment. A meeting with* (name of politician) *will be held* (insert date) *at* (insert place). *A photo opportunity and brief statement by the nursing group will follow at* (time and place). *The event is scheduled in response to a public meeting held* (insert when and where), *when nurses joined their voices with the growing number of Canadian nurses calling for a federal investment in healthcare. Canadian nurses are warning the government that Canadians will soon be deprived of care if action is not taken to avert a massive nursing shortage.*
>
> *"Nurses make up 75% of health professionals. Without registered nurses at the bedside, who will care for Canadians?" asked* (insert name). *"You can't open beds in hospitals or deliver quality home care if there are no nurses."*
>
> *Earlier, in Ottawa, in meetings with members of parliament and government officials, the Canadian Nurses Association (CNA) called on the federal government to support recruitment and retention of registered nurses, nursing research, and the dissemination and uptake of evidence. The CNA estimates the federal government investment should be $40 million a year over the next 5 years. "Our support of this is essential. We know firsthand the impact of the nursing shortage on patient care," said* (insert name).

RESOLUTIONS

Prepare a written resolution for presentation at a professional organization's annual general meeting, such as one for a provincial association, a college of nursing, or the CNA. To be most effective, resolutions should be submitted in writing before the meeting date, so be sure to check deadlines, as resolutions received after the deadline may not be able to be considered by the resolutions committee. Although resolutions can usually be presented from the floor of the meeting, this means that time for consideration and discussion may be limited. You will be most effective if you allow participants time to formulate their own responses and opinions on the topic.

A resolution is an original main motion written with great formality. A resolution generally has two parts: a preamble (optional) and the resolution.

The preamble states the reasons for making the resolution and is the equivalent to debating the question before it is on the floor. Each paragraph begins with the word "*Whereas*"—underscored or in italics and followed by a comma—and each paragraph closes with a semicolon. Additionally, the word after "*Whereas*" begins with a capital letter (i.e., "*Whereas*, The"). There is no limit to the number of times you use "*Whereas*."

BOX 1.4 What to Ask About Resolutions

1. Does each *Whereas* support the resolution?
2. Does the resolution conflict with the act under which the association is legislated?
3. Have you indicated who will carry out the action (e.g., a taskforce of members, a staff person)?
4. Have you projected the cost of the resolution (e.g., will the resolution for a lobby be limited to one letter from the association to a minister, or will the campaign be expanded to a major letter-writing campaign involving all members [10,000 × 0.48 = 4,800], for mail plus paper, envelopes, staff time, and phone for a total of 6,000)?
5. Have you included supporting documentation for the resolution, if appropriate?
6. Have you indicated a deadline for completion?
7. If the action requires reporting back, have you identified to whom and when?
8. Have you considered the intended effect of your resolution, political implications, and so forth?

A resolution is introduced with the word "*Resolved*," and, as with "*Whereas*," the word is underscored or put in italics and followed by a comma. Additionally, the word after "*Resolved*" begins with a capital letter (i.e., "*Resolved*, That"). You may have more than one "resolved" sentence.

All proposed resolutions must include supporting documentation, including the financial implications relevant to the proposal. Also, it is helpful if the proposed resolution includes an implementation date. An example follows:

Whereas, *The biennial meeting will be held in Ottawa; and*

Whereas, *There will be business, education sessions, and special awards; therefore*

Resolved, That all the members of the Canadian Nurses Association be encouraged to attend the 2008 Biennial meeting from June 16 to 18, 2008.

Each resolution must be moved and seconded.

Questions regarding the preparation of a resolution can usually be answered by contacting the association office to which you will be submitting the resolution. Box 1.4 summarizes the resolution process. See the Appendix for an example of a complete resolution.

Additional Resources and Political Action

Nurses can obtain information to assist with political action from their national and provincial nursing associations. The use of electronic media has made resources available to nurses across the country; most associations can be accessed through the Internet.

Other sources of information include nursing unions. The Web sites and e-mail addresses for several nursing unions can be found in Chapter 17.

SUMMARY

This chapter addresses the significance of nurses understanding the inherently political nature of nursing and being able to articulate clearly the relevant issues in nursing, in healthcare, and in advocating for the health of Canadians. Articulation of an issue involves selecting the particular issue from a topic of interest. The nature of the issue is articulated by asking such questions as: Who are the participants in the issue? What makes this a nursing issue? Who first raised this as an issue and why?

Beliefs and assumptions inform an understanding of the issue, and the importance of articulating these assumptions is the first step of issue analysis. A framework for the analysis of issues includes raising questions of historical, ethical-legal, social-cultural, political, critical feminist, and economic natures. The purpose of asking these questions is to increase understanding of all aspects of the issue and to move the discussion toward resolution. The categories of analysis are, however, not intended to be exclusive; pertinent questions may arise during the analysis process.

Identifying barriers to the resolution of an issue is an important step in moving the issue toward resolution. Potential barriers to resolution include inaccessibility of resources, irresolvable differences or competing interests between participants, and differing underlying assumptions on the part of key stakeholders.

Essential to the success of any effort in issue resolution is the communication of a well-developed plan of action. Strategies for resolution include, but are not limited to, formation of lobby groups; establishment of letter-writing campaigns; submission of letters to the editor; distribution of news releases to print and Internet sources; and preparation of resolutions for presentation to agencies, associations, and organizations.

Add to your knowledge of this issue:		Online
Canadian Journal of Nursing Research	**www.cjnr.nursing.mcgill.ca/ archive/30/30_4_Baumgart.html**	
Canadian Nursing Association	**aiic.ca/cna/documents/pdf/publications/ Nursing_Political_Act_May_2000_e.pdf**	
Canadian Student Nurses' Association	**www.cnsa.ca**	

REFLECTIONS on the Chapter...

1 From your practice experience, identify examples of nursing as political action.

2 There is evidence to suggest that nurses take a variety of stances in relation to using their knowledge and influence to address relevant issues in their practice. How might you account for these differences?

3 Identify at least one issue in your practice experience. Using the questions highlighted in the chapter, begin to explore the nature of this issue and possibilities for why it has remained an issue. Identify your own assumptions and beliefs that influence your interpretation of this issue.

4 What are the barriers to this issue being resolved?

5 Review the strategies for issue resolution offered at the end of the chapter, and discuss the advantages and limitations of each for the issue you have selected.

References

Banks, P. (1988). Lobbying: A legitimate, critical nursing intervention. *RNABC News, 12*(5), 31–32.

Baumann, A., O'Brien-Pallas, L., & Armstrong-Strassen, B., et al. (2001). *Commitment and care: The benefit of healthy work places for nurses, their patients and the system. A policy synthesis.* Canadian Health Research Foundation. Ottawa: Government of Canada.

Canadian Nurses Association. (1997). *Code of ethics.* Ottawa: Author.

_____. (1998). *The quiet crisis in healthcare. Lobby kit.* Ottawa: Author.

_____. (2000). CNA Today. *Canadian Nurse, 10*(2), 11.

_____. (2004). *Highlights of the 2003 nursing statistics.* Ottawa: Author.

_____. (2008). *Code of ethics for registered nurses (2008 centennial edition).* Ottawa: Author.

Ceci, C. & McIntyre, M. (2001). A "quiet" crisis in healthcare: Developing our capacity to hear. *Nursing Philosophy, 2*(2), 122–130.

Hood, L. (1998). The professional nurse's role in public policy. In S. Leddy (Ed.), *Conceptual bases of professional nursing* (4th ed., pp. 275–298). Philadelphia: Lippincott Williams & Wilkins.

Manitoba Association of Registered Nurses. (1997). *Directions for a pharmaceutical policy in Canada.* Report prepared for the National Forum on Health. Winnipeg: Author.

McPherson, K. (1996). *Bedside matters: The transformation of Canadian nursing 1900–1990.* Don Mills: Oxford University Press Canada.

Mussallem, H. (1977). Nurses and political action. In B. LaSor & R. Elliott (Eds.), *Issues in Canadian nursing.* Ontario: Prentice Hall.

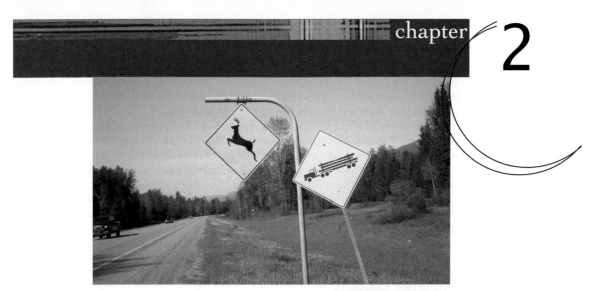

chapter 2

Realities of working in rural settings. (Used with permission of photographer Karen MacKinnon.)

Rural Nursing in Canada

Karen MacKinnon

You know that you are rural if there is no Starbucks or Second Cup . . . You know you are remote if there is no Tim Horton's.

J. Roger Pitblado, 2005

Critical Questions

As a way of engaging with the ideas in this chapter, consider the following:

1 What do you already know about rural nursing work? What knowledge and skills are required?

2 What do you think it would be like to work as a nurse in a rural, remote, or northern community?

3 How does the rural setting of practice influence nursing work? What are the similarities and differences between rural, remote, northern, and Aboriginal health services?

4 What social and institutional factors affect rural nursing work?

Chapter Objectives

After completing this chapter, you will be able to:

1 Identify relevant issues in relation to rural nursing work.

2 Articulate selected ways of understanding these issues, including historical, political, economic, social and cultural, critical feminist, ethical, and legal.

3 Appreciate how different understandings of rural issues (including urban-centric perspectives) affect rural nursing work and health service provisions.

4 Identify past and current barriers that influence rural nursing work.

5 Identify possibilities for providing nursing care in rural communities that enhance community capacity and ensure the provision of safe, accessible, and affordable healthcare services as close to home as possible.

Rural Canadians have been identified as a vulnerable group because they lack access to health services and have overall poorer health outcomes (Ministerial Advisory Council on Rural Health, 2002). Rural geography is varied across Canada but weather, mountain ranges, coastal hazards, and large distances pose significant barriers to health service access and delivery. In addition, more than half of Canada's Aboriginal people (including First Nations, Métis, and Inuit people) live in rural, remote and northern Canada. Aboriginal people face unique health challenges (Smith, Varcoe, & Edwards, 2005) that are explored later in this volume. (See Chapter 24.)

Historically, nurses living and working in rural communities have taken on additional responsibilities to ensure that the health needs of rural Canadians have been addressed. The complexity, variability, and lack of resources supporting nursing practice in rural and remote locations have also been documented (MacLeod et al., 2004; Ulrich, 2001). This chapter will explore the nature of rural nursing work, the knowledge and skills required, the experiences of rural nurses, and the influence of the rural setting for nursing practice. In addition, historical, political, economic, social, legal, and ethical factors that affect nursing work will also be considered. Finally, barriers that influence rural nursing work will be identified along with strategies for working towards a more sustainable future for health service delivery to rural Canadians.

 ## SITUATING THE TOPIC: FRAMING THE ISSUE

No universally agreed on definitions of "rural" exist in the literature but population counts indicate that the percentage of Canadians living in rural communities ranges from 21% to 30% (Hanvey, 2005). How rural is defined for statistical purposes is important because it affects health service decision making and the allocation of resources. Small, geographically isolated towns that may not meet the common definition of rural (less than 10,000 people) are also experiencing acute stress in providing appropriate health services (MacKinnon, 2007). MacLeod, Browne, and Leipert (1998, p. 72) have proposed a more encompassing practice definition of rural that focuses on the "skills and expertise needed by practitioners who work in areas where distance, weather, limited resources and little backup shape the character of their lives and professional practice." The shortage of available healthcare providers who are able and willing to work in rural, northern, and remote communities across Canada continues to worsen (Iglesias et al., 1998; Stewart et al., 2005). In 2001, less than 18% of Canada's nurses were providing nursing services in rural communities (Canadian Institute for Health Information, 2002). The intensifying nursing shortage and increasing regionalization of healthcare services require new and creative approaches to providing nursing and health services for rural Canadians (MacLeod et al., 2004; McBride & Gregory, 2005).

So what do we mean by rural nursing? Rural nurses work in a variety of settings across Canada and their nursing work reflects this diversity. Examples of rural nursing practice include working as a public health nurse, a home-care nurse, or a hospital nurse in rural communities and geographically isolated small towns. Nurses also work in more remote and/or northern communities, sometimes alone as the only healthcare provider in an "outpost" setting. Outpost nurses provided essential health services to isolated and northern communities who have little or no access to medical care. Examples of remote or outpost nursing include working in the northern territories and for the First Nations and Inuit Health Branch.

Anne, a band-employed nurse in southern Ontario, has worked with community members to develop residential workshops on learning to live with diabetes. June, a home care-nurse and the only healthcare practitioner in a small southern prairie community, helped a drop-in client to her weekly footcare clinic to gain a timely referral to an urban specialty clinic. The clinic confirmed June's assessment of advanced congestive heart failure. Barbara, a nurse in a small hospital in a coastal community, tells about travelling by snowmobile to the site of a violent crime and having to attend to both victim and perpetrator—neighbors of hers— in a snowstorm. Claire, a nurse in northern Canada, tells about how she and her colleague, the only nurses in a small community, handled a cardiac arrest by drawing on the only resources available, including the patient's adult children, to perform CPR and the "attending" physician, 600 km away on the speakerphone (MacLeod et al., 2004, p. 27).

Stories like these help us to understand the nature of nursing practice in rural and remote Canada. It is important to be aware that rural settings can be very different across the country and that the context for nursing work becomes increasingly significant as the size of the community decreases (MacLeod et al., 2004). The nature of nursing work in settings where the nurse is the sole healthcare provider differs considerably from nursing work in small towns where peer support and mentoring are more available (Andrews et al., 2005). Although rural and remote nursing can be very different, there are also important commonalities across rural settings of practice. Historically, nurses living and working in rural communities have taken on additional responsibilities to ensure that the health needs of rural Canadians have been addressed. Rural nurses have been described as "expert generalists" who demonstrate an increased sense of responsibility for and commitment to addressing the health needs of people living in their community (MacLeod et al., 2004; MacKinnon, 2007; Ulrich, 2001). Rural nurses have also demonstrated considerable creativity mobilizing community resources and developing/delivering local programs and health services (Bushy, 2002; MacKinnon, 2008). Currently, much debate is ongoing about whether rural nursing is a specialty (Canadian Association for Rural and Remote Nurses [CARRN], 2008) and about whether remote nursing requires advanced practice or Nurse Practitioner (NP) competencies for the provision of primary healthcare services (Bushy, 2002). Another commonality that has been identified by rural nurses is a sense of marginalization or a lack of understanding about rural nursing issues from nurses and educators working in urban and suburban settings (Jackman, 2008; Medves & Davies, 2005).

UNDERSTANDING THE ISSUES

What is it like to be a rural nurse? In the last few years, the nature and experience of rural nursing has been studied by nurse researchers (MacKinnon et al., 2007; MacLeod et al., 2004; Scharff, 2006). "Nursing practice in rural and remote Canada is characterized by its variability, complexity, and the need for a wide range of knowledge and skills in situations of minimal support and few resources" (MacLeod et al., 2004, p. 2). Rural nurses are also expected to do the work of both nonprofessionals, such as housekeepers and dietary aids, and other professionals, such as physiotherapists and pharmacists, particularly on night shifts and weekends when these workers are not available (CARRN, 2007; MacKinnon et al., 2007; Rosenthal, 2005).Based on her research, Jane Ellis Scharff (2006) has eloquently described the meaning of being a rural nurse:

> *Being rural means being a long way from anywhere and pretty close to nowhere. Being rural means being independent or perhaps just being alone. Being a rural nurse means that when a nurse saves a life, everyone in town recognizes that she or he was there, and that when a nurse loses a life, everyone in town recognizes that she or he was there. Being rural means turning inward for answers, because there may be nobody to turn to outward. Being rural means that when a nurse walks into the emergency room, it may be her or his spouse or child who needs a nurse, and at that moment, being a nurse takes priority over being anyone else. Being rural means being able to deal with what she or he has got, where she or he is, and being able to live with the consequences (p. 181).*

Rural nurses' work as "expert generalists" in both hospital and community settings has also been described (MacLeod et al., 2004; Winters et al., 2006):

> *On most days, I guess, I love the generalist model. I always have. I love the variety of the day. And that's really challenging and it keeps me fresh and I don't get bored very easily. The down side of*

that some days I just want to be a specialist. I just want to be responsible for one area and really sink my teeth into that one area and really feel completely confident and competent in that area. Because when you're responsible for everything, that's challenging too (Focus group, PHNs; MacKinnon et al., 2007).

The characteristics of the local community, including local demographics; available resources, amenities, and people; and community needs directly influence nursing work in these settings. Rural nurses have described needing to know who lives in their community, what their skills are, and whether they are available to address local health needs and respond in emergency situations (MacKinnon, 2008; MacLeod et al., 2004). Although privacy concerns were acknowledged by rural nurses, rural nurses consistently described knowing the people in the community as a way to enhance local health services. Studies of the experiences of rural nurses reveal that rural nursing is rewarding work. Rural nurses are proud of the work they do and demonstrate passion, commitment, and creativity in their everyday work. This commitment can lead to an increased sense of responsibility for ensuring that people living in their communities have access to the health resources they need. One nurse described this sense of responsibility as follows:

We are very responsive in our community because we see those people in our churches and in our grocery stores. And so, you know, we try to be all things to all people—maybe that is kind of bad. But in the end we are the ones who see these people outside of our work life too (MacLeod et al., 2004, p. 13).

Rural nurses' sense of responsibility and commitment to their local communities is evident in how they practice nursing in their communities. For example, in one relatively isolated small town the two remaining operating room nurses in the community worked out between themselves an informal on-call system so that one or the other would always be available should a local woman require an emergency Caesarean delivery (MacKinnon, 2008). Sometimes this commitment was visible in the willingness of rural nurses to learn new things, such as learning how to work with women suffering from postpartum depression, to better meet the needs of people living in their community. Rural nurses have consistently identified mobilizing community strengths by knowing about and living alongside the people in their communities. Some rural nurses have developed creative programs by practicing intersectoral collaboration such as the creative "Girls Night Out" program developed by public health nurses (PHNs) for high school students in one rural community (Masters, 2005). Rural nurses have also described the centrality of building, promoting, and maintaining relationships in the work they do. Feminist researchers (DeVault, 1991; 1999) have described "relationship work" as a form of important, yet invisible, work done by women in our society. This kind of nursing work is grounded in knowing their rural community. The centrality of relationships in rural nursing work and the importance of knowing their community also makes visible the difficulties of practice models where nurses "from away" are flown into isolated rural and remote communities for relatively brief periods of time (Binmore et al., 2005; Minore & Boone, 2002). Vudic and Keddy (2002) have also described invisible aspects of rural nursing work such as "integrating into an indigenous setting." One PHN, who resides in a rural community, talked about how her work there intersects with her life as a parent. As this nurse told us this story about her work she did a wonderful pantomime of changing hats:

When you're in the small community, especially something like Public Health, where we're talking about healthy lifestyles and we're talking about good decisions and all this sort of stuff, you sort of have to be more of a "walk the walk" sort of person (Focus group, PHNs; MacKinnon et al., 2007).

Nurses working in small rural communities also need to be skilled in maintaining professional boundaries between their home and their work responsibilities. Rural nurses have consistently told researchers that the complexity of their work is vastly underestimated (MacLeod et al., 2004). In a recent study of rural nurses providing maternity care, rural hospital nurses were able to clearly identify situations in which their work required advanced assessment and decision-making skills, such as delivering the baby, when they were the most skilled healthcare providers available and resuscitating and stabilizing the ill neonate for long periods of time before the neonatal transport team arrived (MacKinnon et al., 2007). Having to perform complex tasks, even if only rarely—such as inserting an umbilical artery catheter—requires accessible skill rehearsal continuing education programs, preferably in an interprofessional format. Areas identified as particularly challenging for rural nurses working in hospital settings included providing emergency and maternity care and dealing with complex mental health challenges (MacKinnon, 2008). Working alone can also mean being the designated maternity nurse in a small rural hospital. Being alone can be a scary experience, particularly for new and less experienced registered nurses (RNs):

> If you have someone else that's working (somewhere in the rural hospital) who's done OB then I always feel better. Especially as a new nurse, I think I would always like to have someone else there in case something happens, right (RN18, MacKinnon 2008)?

Many of the more experienced maternity nurses expressed concerns about not having the time they needed to mentor new nurses (MacKinnon et al., 2007). Understanding the knowledge and skills required by rural nurses makes the experiences of new nurses understandable and provides support for the need for nursing internships models (MacKinnon, 2007). The influence of the rural setting of practice on nurses' work is most readily apparent in the many settings where rural nurses work alone. In 2000, Canadian Institute for Health Information (CIHI) data revealed that there were 399 communities across Canada in which the nurse was the only healthcare provider (CIHI, 2002, p. 39). Tarlier, Johnson, and Whyte (2003) described outpost nursing as a form of community health nursing that is grounded in the competencies needed for primary healthcare. Building skills in settings without direct mentoring opportunities requires considerable creativity. Nurses could benefit from "telehealth" links to facilitate peer or interprofessional consultations (Andrews et al., 2005). Some PHNs working in rural communities also described reaching out to their colleagues who were working alone with more remote First Nations' communities (MacKinnon et al., 2007). Many of the policies and practice guidelines that influence rural nursing work are developed for urban and suburban practice settings (MacLeod et al., 2004). For example, the number of required continuing education programs and certifications for nurses in generalist practice can be overwhelming. Educational programs that utilize "train-the-trainer" models may also be difficult to implement in settings where the nursing resources are stretched to capacity (MacKinnon, 2007). The following section explores some of the factors influencing rural nursing work in more detail.

Understanding the Issues Historically

The Victoria Order of Nursing (VON) was founded in 1897 by the National Council of Women of Canada. These women were convinced that the lack of medical and nursing services for pioneer women contributed to high maternal and infant mortality rates. VON began by providing prenatal and postnatal care in small cottage hospitals across Ontario and visiting nurse services in country districts. Although the rural program was not continued because of the lack of secure funding, this early work convinced health and medical officials that nurses were able to provide care for women in the home and therefore improve the health of rural families. VON also established "training homes" in Ottawa, Montreal, Toronto, and Halifax, which provided nurses with the opportunity to take a formal course in public health and visiting nursing in Canada. Because employment in this nursing specialty required skills beyond those obtained in hospital training programs, PHNs were later counted among the profession's elite (McKay, 2005). The first PHNs in rural and northern Canada often worked alone, were assigned to large geographic districts where travel was difficult, and were more likely to be expected to provide emergency medical care. Nurses' stories about early rural public health nursing speak to the difficulties nurses experienced travelling in rural and remote communities. "Nurses travelled on foot, by car, on horseback, by dogsleds, on airplanes and trains, and on snow-shoes. They braved dangerous road and weather conditions to travel to families in need of care" (McKay, 2005, p. 109).

Unlike their counterparts in urban settings, the first rural PHNs were often generalists. They delivered programs in health education, dental health, communicable disease control, prenatal and postnatal care, prevention of chronic illness, and medical/surgical nursing. In addition, they delivered babies and provided emergency medical, dental, and even veterinary assistance on the frequent occasions when these professionals were not available. Although the work was arduous and seemingly never-ending, the sense of satisfaction in both a career and a way of life was sufficient reward for many nurses (McKay, 2005, p. 119). After World War I (WWI), interest grew in the role nurses could play improving the health of Canadians. Concerns were once again raised about Canadians living in rural and remote areas of the country where public health programs were not available. Although there was also a need for primary care services in rural communities, local governments did not have the resources to fund child welfare nurses. Nurses who had struggled to establish themselves in rural communities knew that when they left the rural community nobody was going to take their places. Their exit meant the end of both public health programs and essential primary healthcare services (McKay, 2005). Prior to the introduction of the Hospitals Act and medical care funding, which positioned doctors as the "gatekeepers" to the Canadian healthcare system, most "graduate" nursing work was community-based practice (McPherson, 2003). Outpost nursing began as early as the 1890s and was well established in Canada by the 1920s (Dodd et al., 2005). Outpost nurses provided essential health services to isolated and northern communities who had little or no access to medical care. Following WWI, the Canadian Red Cross Society set up a chain of outpost nursing stations and hospitals in remote areas with 43 outposts eventually being established in Ontario alone. Similar services, modelled after the pioneering work of VON, were established in Newfoundland, Labrador, Alberta, and Quebec. These pioneering programs also demonstrated that public funding was needed to ensure access to essential health services in remote and, typically, poor communities which could not afford or were unable to attract a physician. Because of need, outpost nurses frequently undertook tasks that were beyond the sanctioned scope of nursing practice and gained gratitude and respect from their local communities. In Alberta, the Public Health Nurses Act of 1919 granted nurses the authority to practice midwifery in remote areas where no doctors were available. The work of outpost nurses included managing deliveries, suturing victims of farm accidents, battling epidemics of influenza and diphtheria, and holding makeshift "clinics" at local dances to provide opportunities for rural people to consult the nurse about their health concerns. These nurses were on call 24 hours a day to provide advice and treatment, sometimes consulting with distant physicians. Outpost nurses also organized travelling dental, eye, and tonsil clinics, bringing needed health services to their remote communities (Dodd et al., 2005). Beginning in 1904, the Canadian government, because of its responsibilities for Aboriginal healthcare, placed a few outpost nurses in arctic and sub-arctic regions of Canada. This placement was deemed necessary "for humanitarian reasons. . .and to prevent the spread of disease to the white population" (Dodd et al., 2005, p. 144). Maternity care was one of the primary motivators for establishing outposts but posed problems because midwifery was illegal in most provinces. The federal government preferred to hire nurses with midwifery experience (usually from Britain) to provide care in northern communities partly because they were less expensive than PHNs. Few outpost nurses received obstetrical training and many simply learned on the job or from "lay" midwives in the community.

Because the needs of the community commonly shaped the roles and responsibilities of the community-based nurse, the boundaries between district, outpost, and public health nursing have always been blurred. PHNs, however, focused their efforts primarily on the prevention of illness and the promotion of health rather than on the provision of direct nursing care (McKay, 2005, p. 107). Because much rural nursing work was directed at reducing maternal and infant mortality rates, the history of midwifery in Canada should not be forgotten. Aboriginal midwifery predates colonization; young Aboriginal girls were chosen to work as apprentices, learning the skills of the sacred nature of childbearing (Benoit & Carroll, 2005). Some settlers to Canada also brought with them midwifery experiences and skills. However, physicians wielded considerable power in colonial times and introduced laws restricting the practice of midwifery to physicians. This move was problematic in rural and remote communities where physicians were not available. The gap was filled by nurse-midwives in many communities and for most of the twentieth century nurse-midwives were the only legally sanctioned midwives allowed to practice in Canada. Although nurse-midwives provided an essential service in rural, remote, and northern Canada, this exclusionary policy has also contributed to political tensions between nursing and midwifery in Canada today.

Understanding the Political Nature of the Issue

Midwifery is being reintroduced into the Canadian healthcare system. Although the numbers of Registered Midwives (RMs) across Canada are increasing, relatively few are currently working in rural and remote locations. However, when they are living and working in small towns and rural communities, good working relationships with nurses are developing (MacKinnon, 2007; Zimmer, 2006). One of the tensions currently being explored is how to better integrate midwives into small communities where the numbers of births are relatively low. Many of these communities are currently being served by more generalist rural or outpost nurses. NPs are also being educated to provide primary healthcare services so that interprofessional teams might be able to work collaboratively in rural and remote communities. Although rural nursing is practiced locally, it is affected by political decisions usually made in larger urban centres. Drury, Francis, and Dulhunty (2005) reported a perceived devaluing of the work of rural nurses by nurses working in urban centres. One Canadian example of an urban-centric practice was the decision recently made in British Columbia to remove the "management of normal labor" from the scope of practice for RNs (College of Registered Nurses of British Columbia [CRNBC], 2006). This decision meant that a special certification program had to be developed and all nurses regardless of their previous experience would be expected to certify. Nurses, working in rural settings where they had done this work for decades, rallied to protest this decision. As the list of required certifications and mandatory education programs grows for RNs, we need to be aware of the implications for generalist rural nurses working in resource-limited facilities and communities.

Economic Understandings

In the late 1990s reductions in federal spending on healthcare resulted in regionalized healthcare services and, consequently, health services were centralized for fiscal reasons (Klein, Christilaw, & Johnston, 2002; Pauly, 2004). Although it may make economic sense to centralize some acute and/or highly specialized services, we must remember the costs that are borne by Canadians living in rural and remote communities. These costs include travel to and from regional referral centres—and the dangers associated with travel, particularly in winter months—and the emotional, social, and family costs of leaving their home communities (Kornelsen & Grzybowski, 2005a; Moffitt & Vollman, 2006).

For example, since 2000, maternity services were closed in 17 communities across British Columbia, echoing a trend that has also occurred in Ontario, Nova Scotia, and abroad (Kornelsen & Grzybowski, 2006). Although maternity care can be thought about as a "specialized" health service, the need to provide care for healthy women and families and the unpredictability of childbirth also makes maternity care an essential component of primary healthcare services (Multidisciplinary Collaborative Primary Maternity Care Project [MCP²] Final Report June 2006; Ontario Maternity Care Expert Panel, 2006). Although some of these closures may help contribute to sustainable maternity care in slightly larger communities (i.e., small towns), such decisions need to be made with a more complex understanding of the effects of decision making on rural communities and awareness of the contribution of maternity care to the sustainability of small communities (Klein et al., 2002). Primary healthcare services, including primary maternity care, need to be available as close to home as possible (Kornelsen & Grzybowski, 2005b; Ontario Maternity Care Expert Panel, 2006). Leipert et al. (2007) studied the challenges of providing essential home-care services in rural settings. Issues of weather, travel, and geography resulted in significantly higher travel costs and the need for seasonal adjustments in timing of home-care visits. When supervisors and dispatchers were located centrally in urban centres, the result was inappropriate scheduling of nurses and other healthcare providers.

Social and Cultural Understandings

RNs make an important contribution to Aboriginal health services in many rural and remote First Nations and Inuit communities (Kulig, MacLeod, & Lavoie, 2007, p. 14). "Since 1994 the First Nations and Inuit Health Branch (FNIHB) of Health Canada has been committed to handing over responsibility for direct service delivery to First Nations and Inuit people." Although there are some required components, such as public health, this decentralization has resulted in more local flexibility to deliver health services that are tailored to Aboriginal health needs. For rural nurses this means that more RNs will be employed by First Nations' communities and fewer by FNIHB. Because not all nurses working with Aboriginal communities are First Nations or Inuit people, rural nurses need to be culturally competent and aware of the need to practice cultural safety (Browne, 2005). They also need to be prepared for working in a "politically charged organizational environment" (Kulig, MacLeod, & Lavoie, 2007). Increasing the proportion of Aboriginal nurses working with First Nations' communities has also been suggested as an important strategy for providing culturally relevant health services in these communities (Kulig et al., 2006).

Nursing, too, has a culture. Much of the leadership for the profession originates in educational institutions and professional organizations, which tend to be organized around urban and suburban centres. Areas of practice have been contested within nursing but the trend has been for increasing education and specialization. For example, the Canadian Nurses Association (2008) currently recognizes and provides certification for 17 nursing specialties. (Box 2.1). Some researchers have described nurses working in rural hospitals as having "multi-specialist" roles (Rosenthal, 2000; Lindsey, 2007).

Nursing education also has been affected by economic downsizing and a looming worldwide shortage of nurses. Although more nursing students are entering education programs, this influx has resulted in increasing pressures to find appropriate practice opportunities for pre-registration nursing students. Preparing generalist nurses within an increasingly specialized healthcare environment is a growing challenge. Nowhere is this more apparent than in maternity care, which is both a nursing speciality and an essential component of primary healthcare services (MacKinnon, 2007).

Critical Feminist Understandings

Women living in rural and remote areas of Canada have reduced access to healthcare resources during pregnancy and childbirth compared to their urban counterparts (Klein et al., 2002). Recent research suggests that rural childbearing women want local access to primary maternity services and that the health and social costs of the lack of access are significant (Kornelsen & Grzybowski, 2005a, 2005b). Researchers have identified that rural residence precipitates a unique set of risks and responses

BOX 2.1   Nursing Specialties Currently Recognized by the Canadian Nurses' Association

Cardiovascular Nursing	Community Health Nursing	Critical Care Nursing
Critical Care Pediatrics	Emergency Nursing	Gastroenterology Nursing
Gerontology Nursing	Hospice/Palliative Care	Nephrology Nursing
Neuroscience Nursing	Occupational Health	Oncology Nursing
Orthopaedic Nursing	Perinatal Nursing	Perioperative Nursing
Psychiatric/Mental Health	Rehabilitation Nursing	Rural Nursing

and have identified women living in rural and remote areas of Canada as a vulnerable population (Kornelsen & Grzybowski, 2005c). West (2006) has described how childbearing women living in rural settings strategize for safety. Women's and family health services are also lacking in many rural and remote communities. Paluck et al. (2006), studied the health promotion needs of women living in rural Saskatchewan. These researchers found that dealing with stress and emotional problems, exercise, and smoking cessation were among the top concerns of rural women. They also identified that women living in rural areas have very limited access to programs and facilities that promote physical and mental health and that services for older women were also lacking. Across the U.S. border in Montana, Bales (2006) interviewed women living in communities with 850 people or less. These women described navigating distance as both a way of life and as a disadvantage in an emergency. These women also described putting the health of their children first coupled with a desire for preventive, holistic health services and "reasonable access" to medical care. Leipert (2006) has documented how rural women develop resiliency to manage this vulnerability. The gendered nature of family caregiving has been well described in the feminist literature (DeVault, 1991; 1999). Many healthcare services are constructed around assumptions made about families (Smith, 1999) in which women are expected to provide care for family members throughout their lives. Rural women have verbalized their concerns about how the shift from institutional care to the community and the home has increased their work yet provided little recognition for the stresses placed on women caregivers (Petrucka & Smith, 2005). Recognizing women's family caregiving contributions as work (MacKinnon, 2006) makes access to respite care and home support services important considerations for health service planners.

Ethical and Legal Understandings

The fact that both successes and failures in nursing practice are more visible in small rural and remote communities has been documented. Stories of moral distress experienced by nurses who lost a community member in the emergency or a baby in the delivery room have surfaced in studies of nurses' experiences with working and living in rural and remote communities (MacKinnon, 2008; Scharff, 2006). Although most rural nurses report good relationships with physicians and other healthcare providers, tensions can arise when others do not respond to the nurses' calls for assistance or do not respect the nurses' knowledge and skills. NPs have also been shown to experience ethical dilemmas in rural and remote practice settings (Turner, 1996). Previous research has also documented that healthcare providers and rural and remote community members may have different understandings of risk—including legal risks. Within medicine and nursing, taking risks during childbearing or with the lives of neonates and children is understood as an unacceptable practice (MacKinnon, 2005). In many remote and northern communities across Canada, childbearing women are routinely evacuated in the last month of pregnancy so that they can give birth in larger, regional hospitals (Moffitt & Vollman, 2006). Because nurse-midwives are less available to provide care in small outpost settings today, some nurses also feel less confident about supporting normal childbirth. Tensions arise when First Nations' women, who understand birth as a "community, social and spiritual act" (Daviss, 1997, p. 441), want to reclaim birth in their communities. Nurses can experience ethical distress when they are caught between wanting to advocate for community needs and their own beliefs about "acceptable" risks. Currently, the predominant discourses of legal risk are very loud (MacKinnon & McCoy, 2006), discouraging nurses from taking professional risks by stepping outside the sanctioned scope of nursing practice. Outpost nurses also face overwhelming workloads and isolation when working as the sole health service providers in Inuit and First Nations communities (Andrews et al., 2005; Daviss, 1997). Lack of adequate staff, backup, and resources increase rural nurses' concerns about their legal and ethical risks. In Montana, Bales, Winters, & Lee (2006, p. 63) interviewed people living in rural communities and identified a theme they described as "informed risk." "Informed risk means that individuals are aware of the risks or consequences of their decisions, but desire for quality of life outweighs the risks presented." The problems with understanding risk simply as informed choice, particularly when selecting from predetermined options, is that it creates women as consumers and as personally respon-sible for the outcomes of the choices they make (Lippman, 1999; MacKinnon & McIntyre, 2006). Quality-of-life discourses may also mask the multiple circumstances that surround decisions about living and working in rural and remote communities. However, strong social support networks in rural communities have been identified as one powerful mediating factor. Rural women have been shown to strategize for safety (West, 2006).

RESOLUTION: CONSTRAINTS AND POSSIBILITIES

This final section focuses on identifying barriers that influence rural nursing work and creative possi-bilities or solutions that may address some of these concerns. A global crisis in health and human resources has once again brought attention to the lack of nurses and other healthcare providers who are willing and able to work in rural and remote settings across Canada (Canadian Women's Health Network, 2008). Internal migration patterns of Canadian-educated rural RNs have recently been stud-ied (Pitblado, Medves, & Stewart, 2005). Using information from the Registered Nurses Database and a national survey, researchers learned that British Columbia has the highest proportion (40.3%) of rural and remote nurses who received their initial education and training in another province or ter-ritory of Canada. Saskatchewan was identified as the province least able to retain RNs who were edu-cated in the province. These researchers also learned that most RNs who leave their rural community for work or for school do not return home. They concluded that "mobility may be even more impor-tant than retirement with respect to the loss of nursing-care providers. There [in small and vulnera-ble rural communities], the losses consist of not only healthcare providers but also community members who directly contribute to the social and economic well-being and therefore the sustainabil-ity of those communities" (Pitblado, Medves, & Stewart, 2005, p. 119).

Proposed recruitment and retention strategies then, involve investing in local communities and investing in local healthcare providers (Table 2.1). Nurses educated in rural communities or small towns are more likely to stay in their communities (Bushy & Leipert, 2005; Courtney et al., 2002). Another strategy that has been proposed to recruit more rural nurses is providing opportunities to live, learn, and work in a rural community as part of pre-registration professional education programs (Neill & Taylor, 2002; Van Hofwegan, Kirkham, & Harwood, 2005). Several creative interprofessional opportunities for nursing, midwifery, and education have also been developed (Interprofessional Network of B.C., 2008; Queen's University Patient-Centred Education Direction [QUIPPED], 2008). Communities have rallied around these projects, sometimes providing accommodation and support for students (Fraser Annett, 2008). Because local resources are limited, providing support for rural RNs as preceptors of nursing students has also been identified as essential to ensuring success for rural placements (Yonge, 2007). Creating a consortium that allows nursing students and new graduates to rotate between different rural and remote health services to gain experience has also been recom-mended (Hegney et al., 2002a).

Rural nurses place high value on building and maintaining competency in clinical skills, partic-ularly in being able to perform even rarely used emergency skills (Hegney et al., 2002b). Continuing education opportunities, then, become an important retention strategy for rural and remote nurses. Barriers to continuing education that have been identified include staffing shortages and the result-ant inability to replace rural nurses so that they can attend education sessions (MacKinnon et al., 2007). Other barriers include the lack of employer or administrative support, workplace budget constraints, family responsibilities and limited access to childcare, and time and financial con-straints for tuition and travel (Penz et al., 2007). Kosteniuk et al. (2006) proposed that employers can facilitate access to information and knowledge exchange by providing education, travel support, opportunities for knowledge-sharing, and promoting physical access to peripheral information sources (such as the Internet and journals) during work time. Scholarships and bursaries for both

Table 2.1	Articulating the Challenges and Recognizing the Possibilities for Supporting Rural Nursing Work

CHALLENGES	POSSIBILITIES
Lack of recognition for the variability and complexity of the work	Listening to the voices of rural nurses who know their work and their communities
Lack of resources including nursing staff & opportunities for continuing education	Creative recruitment incentives and flexible distance/blended learning opportunities
Urban-centric policies, guidelines, and educational programs	Developing policies and programs that reflect the realities of rural nursing practice
Being visible in the community and feeling responsible for needed health services	Developing creative programs based on knowing their community, knowing how to mobilize resources, and knowing how to promote intersectoral collaboration
Difficulty working together when conflict is experienced in interprofessional relationships	Relationship building opportunities, nursing leaders who support "new" nurses, and opportunities for interprofessional education
Generalist/specialist tensions, particularly in hospitals	Building areas of "expertise" within generalist practice over time

nursing students and rural and remote nurses have been recommended (MacLeod et al., 2004). Supporting nurses through providing opportunities for continuing professional education in their local communities has been identified as an important retention strategy for rural nurses. Lindsey (2007) conducted interviews and focus groups with rural nurses from across British Columbia to develop an education program that was tailored to the needs and concerns of rural nurses. The rural nursing certificate program was then developed collaboratively with participation from nurse leaders, nurse educators, and front-line nurses working in rural and remote communities. This module-based, distance education program uses blended learning technologies to deliver educational opportunities as close to home as possible. (See the University of Northern British Columbia's Web site for further details.) Kulig (2005) noted that a number of nursing education programs with a rural focus are being developed across Canada. Recruitment and retention of rural nurses has become an important priority for employers, and a variety of recruitment incentives are being proposed and used. Specific challenges include physical isolation, heavy workloads, fewer social amenities or opportunities for spousal employment, smaller professional networks, fewer treatment services, and increased costs of living in rural and remote communities (Kosteniuk et al., 2006). These incentives include student loan repayment incentives, housing and northern cost of living allowances, and systems that facilitate relocation of spouses and partners. The local provision of maternity care has been identified as one incentive for the relocation of young nurses to rural communities (MacKinnon, 2008). Marketing a rural lifestyle and the advantages of community support might also be an effective recruitment strategy (Hegney et al., 2002). Nurses working as the only healthcare provider warrant special consideration. A recent study of 412 RNs working alone in rural and remote Canada described these nurses and the communities they work in and identified predictors of work satisfaction (Andrews et al., 2005). Barriers to continuing education and emotional stressors associated with high workloads were identified as negatively related to job satisfaction. Face-to-face contact with other healthcare providers (not necessarily RNs) and "decision latitude," or the discretion needed to make decisions, organize their work, and use their skills, were positively related to work satisfaction. Given the importance of continuity of care and relationships in remote communities, this study has important implications for employers who recruit and attempt to retain nurses who work alone. MacLeod et al. (2004, p.3) also identified the need to pay special attention to supporting nurses working with Aboriginal communities "as well as to the ways in which continuity of care and culturally appropriate care can be provided." Creative models with respite from isolated remote communities may also be required (Aboriginal Nurses Association of Canada, 2000; Minore, Boone, & Hill, 2004). Henderson-Betkus and MacLeod (2003) have also identified strategies for retaining PHNs in rural British Columbia. Nursing regulations and scope of practice documents also influence nursing practice in rural and remote communities. Negotiations around scope of practice and "who can do what" are also political acts that tend to ignore the impact of these decisions on rural and remote communities. PHNs working in northern British Columbia identified a number of barriers (including economic, scope of practice limitations, and power relations) as barriers to their ability to offer health promotion and early risk identification for women living in their communities (Leipert, 1999). These rural PHNs believed that their ability to listen, to respect, and to provide care in a nonjudgmental way meant that they could provide more comprehensive and holistic women's health services, including sexual health services and PAP screening. Flexible boundaries and overlapping scopes of practice may be more appropriate for healthcare providers working in rural and remote communities. Interprofessional willingness to embrace new and creative models for collaborative practice may come from carefully listening to the experiences and concerns of all rural healthcare providers. Union and management structures and practices can also be a barrier in rural settings. The disappearance of front-line nursing leaders (a.k.a. head nurses) within hospital administrative structures has made visible the need for front-line leadership for nurses working in rural communities. For example, negotiating a delay in a "routine" induction when skilled nursing staff is not available may be difficult for inexperienced rural nurses who do not have the support of a more experienced nurse available to them (MacKinnon & Yearley, 2007). However, closer relationships between managers, nurses, and other healthcare providers in local rural and remote communities also increase the possibilities for collaborative resistance against centrally imposed cutbacks in personnel or health services (MacKinnon, 2008). Within nursing education there are also competing priorities between community health and acute care nursing and between specialty practice as needed for urban and suburban settings and primary healthcare that may be more appropriate for nursing in rural and remote communities. Nursing education programs that focus on rural and remote health services are being developed in several locations across the country, which may allow more sustained attention to the knowledge needed for rural and remote nursing practice. Along with embracing the full scope of nursing practice, creative programs that provide educational opportunities for advanced practice nurses with specialized skills to address rural health needs, such as Clinical Nurse Specialists (CNSs), and with additional skills in primary healthcare, such as NPs, are also being developed to address health needs in rural and remote communities (Smith Higuchi et al., 2006; Tilleczek, Pong, & Caty, 2005).

SUMMARY

Rural communities are extremely different from one another (MacLeod et al., 2004a), so it is likely that "one-size-fits-all" solutions will not work for all rural and remote communities across Canada. Learning to listen well to rural nurses, other healthcare providers, and community members and sustaining attention through rural health research should help to ensure that policies and practices that influence health and health services in rural communities are identified. Working collaboratively with health planners and decision makers in partnership with rural communities to provide essential and needed health services as close to home as possible can help ensure that

Canadians living in rural and remote communities across Canada are also recipients of our global attention to "Health for All" (World Health Organization, 2008).

Add to your knowledge of this issue:	
Aboriginal Nurses Association of Canada	http://www.anac.on.ca/
Canadian Association for Rural and Remote Nurses (CARRN)	http://www.carrn.com/
Canadian Journal of Rural Medicine	http://www.cma.ca/cjrm/index.htm
Canadian Rural Health Research Society	http://crhrs-scrsr.usask.ca/
Nursing Practice in Rural and Remote Canada	http://ruralnursing.unbc.ca/
Online Journal of Rural Nursing and Healthcare	http://www.rno.org/journal/index.php/online-journal
Rural and Remote Health: The International Electronic Journal of Rural and Remote Health Research, Education, Practice and Policy.	http://www.rrh.org.au/home/defaultnew.asp

Online

REFLECTIONS on the Chapter...

1 Is rural nursing a specialty? If so, what kinds of education and experience do rural nurses need?

2 What does it mean to practice the "full scope" of nursing in rural and remote communities?

3 How can we make continuing education programs for rural nurses affordable and accessible?

4 What role do/could advanced practice nurses, such as NPs or CNSs, play to address health needs in rural and remote communities?

5 How are advanced practice nursing roles being integrated into the healthcare system in rural and northern communities?

6 How can nurses provide "culturally safe" care when working with First Nations' communities?

7 How could interprofessional teams of healthcare providers work together to ensure that rural health services are available as close to home as possible for Canadians living in rural and remote communities?

8 What assumptions are currently being made about women's family caregiving work in rural and remote communities? How could women and families be better supported?

9 What assumptions are currently being made about rural nursing work and what can we learn from nurses working in rural and remote communities?

References

Aboriginal Nurses Association of Canada. (2000). *Survey of nurses in isolated First Nations communities: Recruitment and retention issues.* Ottawa, ON: ANAC.

Andrews, M., Stewart, N., Pitblado, R., et al. (2005). Registered nurses working alone in rural and remote Canada. *Canadian Journal of Nursing Research, 37*(1), 14–33.

Bales, R. (2006). Health perceptions, needs, and behaviors of remote rural women of childbearing and childrearing age. In H. Lee & C. Winters (Eds.), *Rural nursing* (2nd ed, pp. 66–78). New York: Springer Publishing.

Bales, R., Winters, C., & Lee, H. (2006). Health needs and perceptions of rural persons. In H. Lee & C. Winters (Eds.), *Rural nursing* (2nd ed., pp. 53–65). New York: Springer Publishing.

Benoit, C. & Carroll, D. (2005). Canadian midwifery: Blending traditional and modern practices. In C. Bates, D. Dodd & N. Rousseau (Eds.), *On all frontiers: Four centuries of Canadian nursing* (pp. 27–41). Ottawa, ON: University of Ottawa Press.

Binmore, B., Boone, M., Katt, M., et al. (2005). The effects of nursing turnover on continuity of care in isolated First Nations communities. *Canadian Journal of Nursing Research, 37*(1), 86–99.

Browne, A. (2005). Discourses influencing nurses' perceptions of First Nations patients. *Canadian Journal of Nursing Research, 37*(4), 62–87.

Bushy, A. (2002). International perspectives on rural nursing: Australia, Canada, USA. *Australian Journal of Rural Health, 10,* 104–111.

Bushy, A. & Leipert, B. (2005). Factors that influence students in choosing rural nursing practice: A pilot study. *Rural and Remote Health (online)*, 387. Retrieved March 31, 2007 from http://www.rrh.org.au.

Canadian Association for Rural and Remote Nurses. (2008, January). *Rural and remote nursing practice parameters: Discussion document.* Retrieved February 28, 2008 from http://www.carrn.com/files/NursingPracticePararmeters.pdf.

Canadian Institute for Health Information. (2002). *Supply and distribution of Registered Nurses in rural and small town Canada.* Ottawa, ON: CIHI.

Canadian Nurses Association. (2008). *Certification for nursing specialities.* Retrieved February 28, 2008 from www.cna-aiic.ca/CNA/nursing/certification/specialities/html.

Canadian Women's Health Network. (2008). *Thinking women series.* Retrieved February 28, 2008 from http://www.cwhn.ca/indexeng.html.

Cartwright, E. & Thomas, J. (1996). Constructing risk: Maternity care, law and malpractice. In R. Devries, C. Benoit, E. Van Teijlingen, et al. (Eds.), *Birth by design: Pregnancy, maternity care, and midwifery in North American and Europe.* New York: Routledge.

College of Registered Nurses of British Columbia. (2006). *Scope of practice for Registered Nurses: Standards, limits, conditions.* Retrieved July, 2006 from www.crnbc.ca.

Courtney, M., Edwards, H., Smith, S., et al. (2002). The impact of rural clinical placement on student nurses' employment intentions. *Collegian, 9,* 12–18.

Daviss, B. (1997). Heeding warnings from the canary, the whale and the Inuit. In R. Davis-Floyd & C. Sargent (Eds.), *Childbirth and authoritative knowledge* (pp. 441–473). Berkeley, CA: University of California Press.

DeVault, M. (1991). *Feeding the family: The social organization of caring as gendered work.* Chicago: University of Chicago Press.

DeVault, M. (1999). Comfort and struggle: Emotion work in family life. *The Annals of the American Academy of Political and Social Science, 561,* 52–63.

Dodd, D., Elliott, J., & Rousseau, N. (2005). Outpost nursing in Canada. In C. Bates, D. Dodd, & N. Rousseau (Eds.), *On all frontiers: Four centuries of Canadian nursing* (pp. 139–152). Ottawa: University of Ottawa Press.

Douglas, M. (1992). *Risk and blame: Essays in cultural theory.* New York: Routledge.

Drury, V., Francis, K., & Dulhunty, G. (2005). The lived experience of rural mental health nurses. *Online Journal of Rural Nursing and Healthcare, 5*(1), 19–27.

Fraser Annett, J. (2008, February). *In the land of the Hamastza.* Western Region Canadian Association of Schools of Nursing Conference, Victoria, BC.

Hanvey, L. (2005, September). *Rural nursing practice in Canada: A discussion paper.* Ottawa, ON: The Canadian Nurses Association.

Hegney, D., McCarthy, A., & Rogers-Clark, C., et al. (2002a). Why nurses are attracted to rural and remote practice. *Australian Journal of Rural Health, 10*(3), 178–186.

Hegney, D., McCarthy, A., & Rogers-Clark, C., et al. (2002b). Retaining rural and remote area nurses. *Journal of Nursing Administration, 32*(3), 128–135.

Henderson-Betkus, M., & MacLeod, M. (2003). Retaining public health nurses in rural British Columbia: The influence of job and community satisfaction. *Canadian Journal of Public Health, 95*(1), 54–58.

Iglesias, S., Grzybowski, S., & Klein, M., et al. (1998). Rural obstetrics: Joint position paper on rural maternity care. *Canadian Family Physician, 44*, 831–837.

Interprofessional Network of BC. (2008). *Vancouver Island interprofessional education project.* Retrieved February 28, 2008 from http://www.in-bc.ca/.

Jackman, D. (2008, February). *The effects of marginalization on the role of nursing within rural populations.* Western Region Canadian Association of Schools of Nursing Conference, Victoria, BC.

Klein, M.C., Christilaw, J., & Johnston, S. (2002). Loss of maternity care: The cascade of unforeseen dangers. *Canadian Journal of Rural Medicine, 7*(2), 120–121.

Klein, M.C., Johnston, S., & Christilaw, J., et al. (2002). Mothers, babies, and communities. Centralizing maternity care exposes mothers and babies to complications and endangers community sustainability. *Canadian Family Physician, 48*, 1177–1179.

Kornelsen, J. & Grzybowski, S. (2005a). The costs of separation: The birth experiences of women in isolated and remote communities in British Columbia. *Canadian Woman Studies, 24*(1), 75–80.

_____. (2005b). Is local maternity care an optional service in rural communities? *Journal of Obstetrics and Gynaecology of Canada, 27*(4), 327–329.

_____. (2005c). Safety and Community: The maternity care needs of rural parturient women. *Journal of Obstetrics and Gynaecology of Canada, 27*(6), 247–254.

_____. (2006). The reality of resistance: The experiences of rural parturient women. *Journal of Midwifery & Women's Health, 51*(4), 260–265.

Kosteniuik, J., D'Arcy, C., Stewart, N., et al. (2006). Central and peripheral information use among rural and remote Registered Nurses. *Journal of Advanced Nursing, 55*(1), 100–114.

Kulig, J. (2005). What educational preparation do nurses need for rural and remote Canada? *The Nature of Rural & Remote Nursing 2.* Retrieved from http://www.ruralnursing. unbc.ca/factsheets/factsheet2.pdf.

Kulig, J., MacLeod, M., & Lavoie, J. (2007). Nurses and First Nations and Inuit community-managed primary health services. *The Nature of Rural & Remote Nursing 5.* Retrieved from http://www.ruralnursing.unbc.ca/factsheets/factsheet5.pdf.

Kulig, J., Stewart, N., Morgan, D., et al. (2006). Aboriginal nurses: Insights from a national study. *The Canadian Nurse, 102*(4), 16–20.

Leipert, B. (1999). Women's health and the practice of Public Health Nurses in northern British Columbia, *Public Health Nursing, 16*(4), 280–289.

_____. (2006) Rural and remote women developing resilience to manage vulnerability. In H. Lee & C. Winters (Eds.), *Rural Nursing* (2nd ed., pp. 79–95). New York: Springer Publishing.

Leipert, B., Kloseck, M., & McWilliam, C., et al. (2007). Fitting a round peg into a square hole: Exploring issues, challenges, and strategies for solutions in rural home care settings. *Online Journal of Rural Nursing and Healthcare, 7*(2), 5–20.

Lindsey, E. (2007). *Rural focused nursing education: Post-basic nursing education in northern and rural British Columbia* (Phase 2 Report). Prepared for the B.C. Nursing Directorate.

Lippman, A. (1999). Choice as a risk to women's health. *Health, Risk & Society, 1*(3), 281–291.

MacKinnon, K. (2005). *The social organization of women's preterm labour experiences.* Doctoral dissertation, University of Calgary, Calgary, AB.

_____. (2006). Living with the threat of preterm labor: Women's work of keeping the baby in. *Journal of Obstetrical Gynecologic & Neonatal Nursing, 35*(6), 700–708.

_____. (2007, November). *Learning maternity nursing work: The "scary" experiences of new RNs working in rural hospitals in B.C.* Canadian Association of Schools of Nursing, Nurse Educator's Conference, Kingston, ON.

_____. (2008, February). *Celebrating and supporting rural nursing work.* Western Region Canadian Association of Schools of Nursing Conference, Victoria BC.

MacKinnon, K. & McCoy, L. (2006). The very loud discourses of risk in pregnancy! In P. Godin (Ed.), *Risk and nursing practice* (pp. 98–120). Basingstoke, UK: Palgrave Publishers.

MacKinnon, K. & McIntyre, M. (2006). From Braxton Hicks to preterm labour: The constitution of risk in pregnancy. *Canadian Journal of Nursing Research, 38*(2), 52–72.

MacKinnon, K. & Yearley, J. (2007, October). *Labouring to nurse: The work of rural nurses who provide maternity care in B.C.* Association of Women's Health, Obstetrics and Neonatal Nurses Canada 18th National Conference. Halifax, NS.

MacKinnon, K., Yearley, J., & Ondrik, C., et al. (2007). *Pilot study for rural nurses' experiences with the provision of maternity care.* Report prepared for the B.C. Medical Services Foundation, the Canadian Nurses' Foundation and the Nursing Care Partnership Program.

MacLeod, M., Browne, A., & Leipert, B. (1998). Issues for nurses in rural and remote Canada. *Australian Journal of Rural Health, 6,* 72–78.

MacLeod, M., Kulig, J., & Stewart, N., et al. (2004). *The nature of nursing practice in rural and remote Canada.* Retrieved September 21, 2006 from www.chrsf.ca.

_____. (2004). The nature of nursing practice in rural and remote Canada. *Canadian Nurse, 100*(6) 27.

Masters, A. (2005). Girls' night out. *Nursing B.C. (June),* 8–11.

McBride, W. & Gregory, D. (2005). Aboriginal health human resource initiatives: Towards the development of a strategic framework. *Canadian Journal of Nursing Research, 37*(4), 89–94.

McKay, M. (2005). Public health nursing. In C. Bates, D. Dodd, & N. Rousseau (Eds.), *On all frontiers: Four centuries of Canadian nursing* (pp. 107–123). Ottawa: University of Ottawa Press.

McPherson, K. (2003). *Bedside matters: The transformation of Canadian Nursing. 1990–1990.* Toronto: University of Toronto Press.

Medves, J., & Davies, B. (2005). Sustaining rural maternity care: Don't forget the RNs. *Canadian Journal of Rural Medicine, 10*(1), 29–35.

Ministerial Advisory Council on Rural Health. (2002). *Rural health in rural hands: Strategic directions for rural, remote, northern, and Aboriginal communities.* Ottawa, ON: Health Canada.

Minore, B. & Boone, M. (2002). Realizing potential: Improving interdisciplinary professional/paraprofessional healthcare teams in Canada's northern Aboriginal communities through education. *Journal of Interprofessional Care, 16*(2), 139–147.

Minore, B., Boone, M., & Hill, M. (2004). Finding temporary relief: Strategy for nursing recruitment in northern Aboriginal communities. *Canadian Journal of Nursing Research, 36*(2), 148–163.

Moffitt, P. & Vollman, A. R. (2006). At what cost to health? Tlicho women's medical travel for childbirth. *Contemporary Nurse, 22*(2), 228–239.

Multidisciplinary Collaborative Primary Maternity Care Project. (2006). *Final Report.* Retrieved February 28, 2008 from http://www.mcp2.ca/english/documents/FinalReport-HealthCanada.pdf.

Neill, J. & Taylor, K. (2002). Undergraduate nursing students' clinical experiences in rural and remote areas: Recruitment implications. *Australian Journal of Rural Health, 10,* 239–243.

Ontario Maternity Care Expert Panel (2006). *Maternity care in Ontario 2006: Emerging crisis, emerging solutions.* Toronto: Ontario Women's Health Council.

Paluck, E., Allerdings, M., & Kealy, K., et al. (2006). Health promotion needs of women living in rural areas: An exploratory study. *Canadian Journal of Rural Medicine, 11*(2), 111–116.

Pauly, B. (2004). Shifting the balance in the funding and delivery of healthcare in Canada. In J. Storch, P. Rodney, & R. Starzomski (Eds.), *Toward a moral horizon: Nursing ethics for leadership and practice* (pp. 191–208). Toronto: Pearson/Prentice Hall.

Penz, K., D'Arcy, C., & Stewart, N., et al. (2007). Barriers to participation in continuing education activities among rural and remote nurses. *The Journal of Continuing Education in Nursing, 38*(2), 58–66.

Petrucka, P. & Smith, D. (2005). Select Saskatchewan rural women's perceptions of health reform: A preliminary consideration. *Online Journal of Rural Nursing and Healthcare, 5*(1), 59–73.

Pitblado, J. R. (2005). So, what do we mean by "rural," "remote," and "northern"? *Canadian Journal of Nursing Research, 37*(1), 163–168.

Pitblado, J., Medves, J., & Stewart, N. (2005). For work and for school: Internal migration of Canada's rural nurses. *Canadian Journal of Nursing Research, 37*(1), 102–121.

Queen's University Patient-Centred Education Direction. (2008). *Interdisciplinary education in Canada.* Retrieved March 2, 2008 from http://meds.queensu.ca/quipped/literature.

Rosenthal, K. (2000). Rural nursing. *American Journal of Nursing, 100*(4), 24A–24B.

_____. (2005). What rural stories are you living? *Online Journal of Rural Nursing and Healthcare, 5*(1), 37–47.

Scharff, J. (2006). The distinctive nature and scope of rural nursing practice: Philosophical basis. In H. Lee & C. Winters (Eds.), *Rural nursing* (2nd ed., pp. 177–196). New York: Springer Publishing.

Smith, D. (1999). The standard North American family: SNAF as an ideological code. In D. Smith (Ed.), *Writing the social: Critique, theory, and investigations.* Toronto: University of Toronto Press.

Smith, D., Varcoe, C., & Edwards, N. (2005). Turning around the intergenerational impact of residential schools on Aboriginal people: Implications for health policy and practice. *Canadian Journal of Nursing Research, 37*(4), 38–60.

Smith Higuchi, K., Hagen, B., & Brown, S., et al. (2006). A new role for advanced practice nurses in Canada: Bridging the gap in health services for rural older adults. *Journal of Gerontological Nursing, 32*(7), 49–55.

Stewart, N., D'Arcy, C., & Pitblado, J., et al. (2005). A profile of registered nurses in rural and remote Canada. *Canadian Journal of Nursing Research, 37*(1), 163–168.

Tarlier, D., Johnson, L., & Whyte, B. (2003). Voices from the wilderness: Interpretive study describing the role and practice of outpost nurses. *Canadian Public Health Association Journal, 94*(3), 180–184.

Tilleczek, K., Pong, R., & Caty, S. (2005). Innovations and issues in the delivery of continuing education to Nurse Practitioners in rural and northern communities. *Canadian Journal of Nursing Research, 37*(1), 146–162.

Turner, L. (1996). Rural nurse practitioners: Perceptions of ethical dilemmas. *Journal of the American Academy of Nurse Practitioners, 8*(6), 269–274.

Ulrich, C. (2001). *The nature of public health nursing practice: Finding coherence in complexity.* Unpublished Master's Thesis, University of Northern British Columbia, Prince George, BC.

Van Hofwegan, L., Kirkham, S., & Harwood, C. (2005). The strength of rural nursing: Implications for undergraduate nursing education. *International Journal of Nursing Education Scholarship, 2*(1), 1–13.

Vukic, A., & Keddy, B. (2002). Northern nursing practice in a primary healthcare setting. *Journal of Advanced Nursing, 40*(5), 542–548.

West, K. (2006). Strategizing safety: Perinatal experiences of rural women. In H. Lee & C. Winters (Eds.), *Rural nursing* (2nd ed., pp. 96–109). New York: Springer Publishing.

Winters, C., Thomlinson, E., & O'Lynn, C., et al. (2006). Exploring rural nursing theory across borders. In H. Lee & C. Winters (Eds.), *Rural nursing* (2nd ed., pp. 27–39). New York: Springer Publishing.

World Health Organization. (2007). *The World Health Report: Conclusions and recommendations.* Retrieved February 29, 2008 from http://www.who.int/whr/2007/ conclusion/en/index.html.

Yonge, O. (2007). Preceptorship rural boundaries: Student perspectives. *Online Journal of Rural Nursing and Healthcare, 7*(1), 5–12.

Zimmer, L. (2006). *Seeking common ground: Experiences of nurses and midwives.* Doctoral dissertation, University of Alberta, Edmonton, AB.

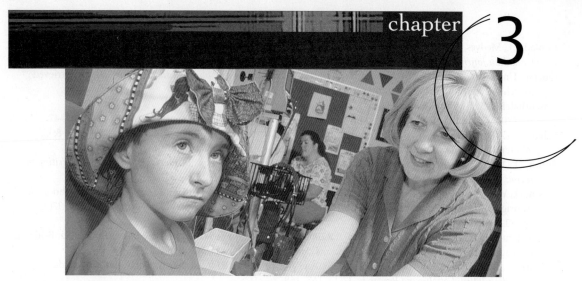

chapter 3

Nurses find more meaning and reward in their work when they can care for their patients as professionals and when the conditions of work support the scope of practice gained through education and experience. (Used with permission, Faculty of Nursing, University of Calgary.)

Canadian Healthcare System

Janet L. Storch

Critical Questions

As a way of engaging with the ideas in this chapter, consider the following:

1 What views do you hold of the Canadian healthcare system and how have you come to hold those views?

2 In what ways does the healthcare system support the health of Canadians?

3 What are your thoughts about how the healthcare system structures nursing practice?

4 In your view, what is the major challenge facing those who manage the healthcare system?

Chapter Objectives

After completing this chapter, you will be able to:

1 Recognize the history in our current challenges in healthcare.

2 Appreciate the underlying tensions of issues in healthcare.

3 Understand the system's impact on Canadian nursing.

4 Recognize the need for nursing leadership in maintaining all that is good about healthcare and making changes to correct deficiencies.

5 Identify future possibilities for nurses in the healthcare system.

Nurses' practice is influenced by social, cultural, and historical realities worldwide, and Canadian nursing practice is no exception to this fact. These influences underlie the context within nurses' practice, a context that affects their everyday lives as nurses.

THE IMPORTANCE OF UNDERSTANDING CANADA'S HEALTHCARE SYSTEM

In 2007, the Premier of British Columbia implemented a plan for public consultations focused on healthcare with the stated goal of making improvements to British Columbia's healthcare programs as informed by the residents of the province. At one of the many sessions held throughout the province, issues related to sustainability of the current healthcare system were raised by the facilitators, who were young men best acquainted with the forest industry. These facilitators questioned the value of Canada's approach to healthcare, that is, using tax dollars to fund medical care and hospital services for all individuals who are residents of Canada. They supported the idea of opening these same services to a market-based system, in which individuals and families could choose from a range of services, including private, public, and quasi-governmental services.

In response to their comments, one participant in the conference said that he recalled his parents (prior to the implementation of Medicare and hospital insurance programs in Canada) raised funds for a neighbor who required surgery. The young facilitators responded with disbelief, wondering why his parents would have been involved in such fundraising. Even when the reasons were explained to them, i.e., that the family could not afford to pay for the surgery and the hospital stay, the facilitators were puzzled, seemingly unable to imagine such a situation.

The reality is that for anyone under the age of 60, living in Canada without full coverage of medical and hospital care has not been part of their experience. Canada's national Medicare program came into being between the late 1960s and the mid-1970s and was reaffirmed in the Canada Health Act (CHA) of 1984. That means that national health insurance programs in Canada are about 45 years old. It is no wonder, then, that the majority of younger adults have limited or no understanding of what life without national healthcare insurance programs would look like. In 1987 Malcolm Taylor, a rigorous historian writing about Canada's healthcare programs, stated:

> It is impossible for anyone under the age of forty today, protected as we now are with a full panoply of social insurance programs, to appreciate, or perhaps even to comprehend, the threats to individual and family independence and integrity that characterized the thirties and extended, to a declining degree, into the forties and fifties. But to millions the threats had been real and, for hundreds of thousands, had come to pass (Taylor, 1973, p. 2).

This chapter aims to provide nurses with an understanding of the healthcare system in which they work. To do so, reference will be made to the CHA. This act replaced two key federal acts in effect previously, i.e., the Hospital Insurance and Diagnostic Services Act first introduced by the Canadian government in 1957 and the Medical Care Act introduced in 1967. It was designed to affirm the four principles of the Medicare program and to add a fifth principle, "access to care" or accessibility. The CHA also placed a ban on physicians charging their patients extra monies for medical services provided, i.e., charging patients funds over and above what the provincial government paid per patient visit. Such "extra billing" of patients is forbidden (Rice & Prince, 2000).

THE CANADA HEALTH ACT

As a way of examining the strengths and limitations of Canada's approach to healthcare, the principles of the CHA will be used to frame this analysis. Each of these five principles will be examined, beginning with *comprehensiveness,* followed by *universality* and *portability, accessibility, and public administration.* It is hoped that by using the principles as a framework for discussion, readers will be attuned to the strengths of our healthcare system, the challenges involved in preserving the best of the system, and be better informed and equipped to work to make changes and improvements to address its limitations. Readers will be reminded about nursing's involvement in healthcare reform (past and present) and the nursing leadership needed to make a difference in this complex federal-provincial healthcare system.

As each principle is highlighted, its definition in the CHA will be provided. This definition will be followed by an analysis and discussion focusing on assessing the adequacy of Canadian healthcare in conforming to the principles as well as those areas of healthcare not covered by the act (based upon its definitions).

We begin with the principle of comprehensiveness. Is the Canadian healthcare system comprehensive? Does it meet the needs of Canadians? If not, what services are privileged, and what services are missing?

Comprehensiveness

> . . . the health insurance plan of the province must ensure all insured health insured services provided by hospitals, medical practitioners or dentists, and where the law of the province so permits, similar or additional services rendered by other health care practitioners.
>
> Canada Health Act, 1984, c.6, s.9

The wording of what constitutes comprehensive in the CHA, with its focus on "medically necessary" services, spells out some of the limitations of this principle and explains some of the fragmentation of the current health system. Excluded from the specified services in the definition, for example, are nursing services, public health services, communicable disease control, home care, pharmacare, chronic care and any number of other health services as well as a focus on primary healthcare.

The original *draft* of a comprehensive health and social insurance plan for Canada was much broader in concept and design. As long ago as the mid-1940s, while the country's efforts were focused on World War II (WWII), a broad plan was developed to include unemployment insurance, health insurance, and a full range of services for prevention, diagnosis, treatment, and care. This plan was in response to evidence that by the time Canada had entered WWII, healthcare needs continued to exceed the supply of any type of comprehensive healthcare. Infant and maternal mortality rates were high, and morbidity and mortality from communicable diseases were of grave concern (Taylor, 1973, p. 5). One third of the men who were examined for military service were unfit for service, with one third of that group rejected because of "psychiatric disorders" (Cassidy, 1947, p. 51). There was also a growing sentiment that Canada owed a comprehensive package of social programs to its returning troops (Rice and Prince, 2000), and that some type of publicly funded health insurance was inevitable. After all, Canadian soldiers returning from abroad had come to know that other countries were developing these types of programs.

The draft plan or *blueprint* for Canadian health and social programs reflected a postwar idealism fostered by international influences such as the freedoms outlined in the Atlantic Charter (Marsh, 1975; Taylor, 1973). This plan recognized that all are deserving of adequate social supports for living (Marsh, 1975). However, due to economic realities and political dissension, this comprehensive plan was not approved by Parliament, and what followed was a piecemeal implementation of programs and services over a 20-year period using the draft plan (blueprint) as a general guide. The effect of this piecemeal, politically expedient approach led to a poorly integrated health system that can scarcely be called a 'system'. Thus, in the 21st century, *poor integration of services* remain highly problematic (Leatt, Pink & Guerriere, 2000).

NATIONAL HEALTH GRANTS AND THE PUBLIC'S HEALTH

Some of the first programs the Canadian government took from the blueprint were designed to bolster health and healthcare in the provinces. Thus, the federal government began to offer targeted cost-sharing grants to the provinces to enable them to enhance their health services. To accept the federal government's offer each province would have to agree to pay roughly 50% of the costs. Needs in these post-war years (1945 and onwards) are quite clear, based upon the named grants offered. These annual grants included general public health, venereal disease control, mental health, tuberculosis control, cancer control, crippled children funds, professional training, public health research, and grants for hospital construction (Taylor, 1973, p. 163). Organizational charts in provincial ministries of health reflected these grant categories, showing a Deputy Minister in charge of a string of programs aligned with the grants and with seemingly limited attempts to integrate program services (Defries, 1962).

The hospital construction grants that constituted part of the 50–50 offer set in motion an agenda of building hospitals, and, by default, minimizing attention to primary healthcare in Canada. Some have speculated that if the original comprehensive plan developed in the 1940s had been implemented, Canada would have set in motion a different course of action, one with an emphasis on basic health services that would have included primary healthcare.

PRIMARY HEALTHCARE

There was a strong background for *primary healthcare* in Canada. Between World War I (WWI) and WWII, public health activities, carried out mainly through the work of competent nurses, increased significantly in an attempt to address deficiencies in health services (Hastings & Mosley, 1980, pp. 149–150). But this growth threatened many physicians and was opposed by them because ". . . these nurses worked semi-independently in the community" (Coburn, 1988, p. 443). The continuation of this structured medical profession dominance led to significant delays in full implementation of expanded roles for nurses, such as the role of nurse practitioner (NP). For example, Angus and Bourgeault (1999) described the rise and fall of NPs in between the late 1960s and mid-1980s. Their rise occurred largely due to a perceived physician shortage; however, once that supply was replenished, organized medicine stood in opposition toward urban-based NPs in particular (p. 63). Over the past decade progress has been made in the preparation and utilization of NPs, yet there continue to be barriers to NP extended practice (MacDonald et al., 2006).

In implementing interdisciplinary primary healthcare, similar barriers exist today. The concept of a primary healthcare center was widely discussed and debated in the 1970s, when a community health center project was underway in Canada. John Hastings (1972) described a model of primary healthcare and provided examples of its application. In essence he and his colleagues were promoting interdisciplinary healthcare as a point of first contact as well as continuing care. His concept of healthcare involved different members of the healthcare team taking leadership, contingent upon the needs of the person seeking assistance. The opposition by organized medicine to this team-care model was widespread, and for a period of time this community health-centered approach to primary healthcare waned. In the late 1990s, the federal government again attempted to stimulate development of primary healthcare, using ideas similar to those proposed in the community health center report. Unfortunately, in some provinces monies intended for pilot projects involving interdisciplinary team members were utilized instead to augment primary care services provided by physicians, and this development again faltered.

Organized nursing, largely through the Canadian Nurses Association (CNA), has been a steady, informed advocate of primary healthcare. In 1979, for example, in response to a federal commission called the Health Services Review, CNA developed a submission entitled "Putting Health Back into Health Care" (CNA, 1980), recommending that:

- the existing legislation underlying the hospital and medical insurance programs be revised to allow the emergence of a health insurance program that would stimulate the development of primary health services, permit the introduction of new entry points, and promote the appropriate utilization of qualified health personnel
- provincial legislation be revised to enable qualified nurses and other prepared health personnel to undertake activities currently defined as medical acts

- remuneration of all health personnel be salaried
- the Health Services Review '79 strongly support the initiation of better preventive, diagnostic, and ambulatory care programs through various community-based points of entry
- the federal government be requested to reinstitute a national health survey that would provide the necessary information on which to build and evaluate a healthcare system to meet the needs of the people of Canada
- all governments and health profession organizations be urged by this Health Services Review to adopt, as a priority, better and broader health education programs to sensitize consumers to the cost of acute-care services.

The CNA's input was well received by the Commissioner and constituted a major part of his report. However, this more comprehensive approach to healthcare and healthcare insurance has continued a slow development. In the late 1990s, CNA focused renewed attention on primary healthcare in publications, position statements, and "backgrounders" about primary healthcare. *Primary care* was described as "provider-driven; based in clinical diagnosis and treatment; institutionally oriented; individually focused; and emphazing service provision" (CNA Backgrounder, October 2005). In contrast, *primary healthcare* was described as offering a continuing and organized supply of essential health services available to all people without unreasonable geographic or financial barriers (or, "accessible"); involving public participation; focusing on health promotion to enable people to increase control over and to improve their health; utilizing appropriate technology; and involving intersectoral cooperation, i.e., commitment from all sectors (p. 1).

CARE OF THE CHRONICALLY ILL

Another sector of healthcare not covered adequately through the CHA definition of comprehensive is the care of the chronically ill, both institutional care and home care. In 2007, an entire issue of *Healthcare Papers* was devoted to the topic of the inadequacy of the healthcare system to address the multiple chronic diseases that those who are living longer endure. With the majority of attention in healthcare focused on acute, episodic care, those citizens needing continuing and comprehensive care to manage their chronic disease commonly "fall through the cracks" or are "lost in transition" (Morgan, Zamora, & Hindmarsh, 2007, p. 8). As Morgan, Zamora, and Hindmarsh note, "Canadians with chronic illness deserve a transformed healthcare system that provides coordinated, comprehensive care—a system that results in fewer visits to the emergency departments, fewer complications and a better and longer quality of life (p. 21)."

One important approach to optimizing health and reducing hospital admissions for chronically ill patients is self-management education. Recognizing the contribution that patients and clients with chronic conditions can make to their own healthcare is a significant step forward in addressing chronic illness. This approach is neither simply "passing the buck" to the patient nor is it simply providing patients with information. It is about providing both information and support in an intensive and interactive manner by training patients to monitor themselves and by using written care plans that are tailored to individual lifestyles and needs. But, as researchers caution, "self-management education programs should be seen as part of a larger strategy for improving care for people with chronic disease" that includes a team of coordinated health professionals. Only in this way can patients be given the tools and treatments they need to lead better and healthier lives (Canadian Health Services Research Foundation [CHSRF], June 2007, p. 2). Visit www.chsrf.ca/research_themes/ safety_ephp for more information.

"SUPERBUGS" AND PATIENT SAFETY

Communicable disease control and patient safety has rapidly become another critical issue for Canadian healthcare. Topping the headlines in many current daily newspapers is the emergence of "superbugs" (Harnett, 2008; Priest, 2008). For example, the incidence of hospital-acquired *Clostridium difficile,* methicillin-resistant *Staphylococcus aureus,* and other such infectious microorganisms is alarming. It has been noted that many adverse events might be prevented by appropriate staffing with well-educated nurses—versus reducing nursing staff to a minimum due to cutbacks in healthcare (Storch, 2005). In a similar manner, there is reason to believe that cutbacks and contracting out poorly supervised cleaning services in hospitals can lead to an increase in these organisms flourishing in hospitals and nursing homes. Handwashing alone in a filthy environment will not likely effect the decrease in these microorganisms needed to ensure that patients who are chronically ill, as well as those in acute care, are protected from the invasions of these superbugs.

Influenced by a major report from the Institutes of Medicine in the United States (1999), attention has focused on all manner of hospital-acquired injury or infection. Many Western countries have established organizations to focus on this new threat to the health status of their citizens. In Canada, the Canadian Patient Safety Institute (CPSI) was announced by the federal government in December 2003 and became operational in 2005, with its headquarters in Edmonton, Alberta. The purpose of CPSI is "to provide national leadership in building and advancing a safer Canadian health system" (Canadian Patient Safety Institute, 2007, p. 1). Within a short time, CPSI engaged in a campaign to decrease adverse events in healthcare through involvement of teams of health professionals across Canada. Although initiatives started in acute care, CPSI has widened its gaze to include patient safety and home care as well as supporting research that probes numerous specific concerns in patient safety and seeks to influence policy.

THE RESURGENCE OF COMMUNICABLE DISEASE AND PUBLIC HEALTH SERVICES

Despite the influx of federal monies to the provinces through the cost-shared programs instituted in the late 1940s, attention to public health services has lagged behind acute care in its continuing development. The rise of communicable disease and the threat of outbreaks, epidemics, and pandemics highlights the vulnerability of Canadians. This awareness has given rise to federal and provincial actions to enhance public health services. The outbreak of sudden acute respiratory syndrome in Toronto in the spring of 2003 served as a "wake-up call" to restore public health services. One might correctly guess that the lack of specific mention of public heath services in the statement of comprehensiveness in CHA, and the fact that most Canadians take public health services for granted until some major public health problem develops, had allowed opportunities to reduce budgets in public health. If ever there was a call for a universal approach to health, threats of diseases that cross all borders and the threat of pandemics surely have emphasized that need.

In 2004, the Public Health Agency of Canada (PHAC) was created as a national presence to address some of these pressing issues. Their mission is "to promote and protect the health of Canadians through leadership, partnership, innovation and action in public health" (www.phac-aspc.gc.ca). PHAC has been effective in uniting Canadian efforts in pandemic planning, as well as in addressing other national issues, and serves as a prime contact for the World Health Organization (WHO) for such international work. "The creation of the Public Health Agency of Canada marks the beginning of a new approach to federal leadership and collaboration with provinces and territories on efforts to renew the public health system in Canada and support a sustainable health care system (www.phac-aspc.gc.ca)." However, even with PHAC in place, the ability of this federal body to take action can still be impeded by Canada's constitutional provisions for federal and provincial responsibilities in healthcare. Thus, we move on to discuss the CHA's principles of universality and portability.

Universality and Portability

> . . . *in order to satisfy the criterion respecting universality, the health care insurance plan of a province must entitle one hundred per cent of the insured persons of the province to the insured health services provided for by the plan on uniform terms and conditions.*
>
> Canada Health Act, 1984, c.6, s.10

... in order to satisfy the criterion respecting portability, the health care insurance plan of a province must not impose any minimum period of residence in the province, or waiting period, in excess of three months before the residents of the province are eligible to insured health services ...

... must provide for the payment of amount for the cost of insured health services provided to insured persons while temporarily absent from the province...

Canada Health Act, 1984, c.6, s.11

One of the challenges in maintaining and sustaining Canadian healthcare is the difficulty the federal government encounters in influencing national policy and national standards. This difficulty tends to be a puzzling matter for many who study Canadian healthcare but only until they recall or realize that Canada's constitution dictates that health is the major responsibility of the provinces. That means that the principles of the CHA, including universality and portability, cannot easily be enforced by the federal government.

BARRIERS IMPOSED BY THE BRITISH NORTH AMERICA ACT

The Fathers of Confederation, who were the developers of Canada's constitution, are notable mainly for what they did not know—and what they could not have known—about future healthcare needs. When these leaders set out the terms of the British North America (BNA) Act of 1867, which continues to form a part of Canada's current Constitution Act, they had no idea how trends in industrialization and urbanization would affect healthcare needs (Cassidy, 1947; Hastings & Mosley, 1980; Wallace, 1950). Thus, they wrote of what they knew and outlined very basic responsibilities of the federal government, leaving wide room for the provinces to be the key players in the provision of healthcare and believing that individuals could and should be self-reliant.

The federal and provincial responsibilities influencing healthcare (and universality in health programs) were stated in Section 91 (federal responsibilities) and Section 92 (provincial responsibilities), and included the following (Van Loon & Whittington, 1976):

Sec. 91—taking of the census, ... collecting statistics (birth, marriage, death), establishing quarantine regulations and hospitals for those in quarantine, and taking responsibility for Canada's native peoples.

Sec. 92 (7)—The Establishment, Maintenance and Management of Hospitals, Asylums, Charities, and Eleemosynary Institutions in and for the Province, other than Marine Hospitals.

This division of federal and provincial responsibilities has created permanent tension between the federal government, who collect most of the taxes, and the provincial governments, who have seen their mandate for the provision of health services growing each year (Lindenfield, 1959). Much of what might be titled 'federal-provincial wrangling' over healthcare funding is based upon this distribution of powers.

The result of Sections 91 & 92 in relation to healthcare is that the federal government has limited ways to introduce national health and social service programs. Only three ways are open to them. They can change the constitution for a specific program they wish to introduce, they can offer cost-sharing programs that allow them to establish initiatives (as they did with the 50–50 cost-sharing health grants in 1947–1948), and they can set national standards with penalties for lack of adherence to such standards (as in the case of the CHA). Inevitably, this limitation requires some compromise on the part of the federal government as well. For example, the federal government compromised some of the blueprint for federal programs by developing a single-payer system (the public) utilizing the tax base to pay for health services (health insurance) that would be supplied by autonomous or semiautonomous "private" providers such as physicians and hospitals (Fuller, 1998).

Because each province still has a *choice* about joining a cost-shared program or forfeiting penalties to maintain its autonomy, it typically took several years before all provinces bought into various national programs, including hospital insurance, medical care insurance, and any number of other social programs. The consequence was, for example, that citizens of Quebec were late beneficiaries of many of the national programs. In Quebec, the longstanding tradition of Catholic charity (Cassidy, 1947), ties to the "Old World," a commitment to maintaining an identity, and a lag in industrial development (Lindenfield, 1959) were some of the barriers that precluded easy adoption of federal programs.

With such potential and real diversity in provincial uptake of health and social programs (or not), issues such as universality and portability remain contingent upon a province "buying in" to national initiatives. The Health Council of Canada, a national body formed in 2003 to monitor and report on healthcare towards improving the health status of Canadians, continues to highlight the disparities across provinces in terms of national initiatives. Their 2005 annual report contains information tables that summarize by jurisdiction the status of home care, of primary healthcare reforms, of drug programs, of human resource initiatives, and other topics of comparison. These tables exemplify the disparities across provinces.

FRAMEWORKS FOR HEALTH PROMOTION

Despite the limitations of the BNA Act, Canada has made unique contributions to public health worldwide. Just before WWI, the president of the Vancouver Medical Society, J. W. McIntosh (1914), delivered a paper at the Royal Sanitary Conference in Vancouver on the topic of the interrelationship of physician, citizen, and state to public health. He provided a conceptual framework to describe the disabilities affecting many Canadians, classifying them as hereditary, personal or self-imposed, or environmental—"the gift of our neighbors and surroundings" (McIntosh, 1914, p. 454). Years later, his framework would resonate with the writing of a federal civil servant named Laframboise (1973). Laframboise's article was the basis of a prominent Canadian report known as the Lalonde Report (1974), named after the Minister of Health, Marc Lalonde, during whose tenure this report was released.

The Lalonde Report, titled "A New Perspective on the Health of Canadians," marked Canada as a leader in formulating a four-point policy framework that considered heredity, environment, lifestyle, and health services as critical to health. This report was considered an attempt to break away from the medical approach to health and move toward a more holistic approach (LaBonte, 1994, p. 74). Almost 10 years later, the new concept of public health began to focus on healthy policies and healthy cities and communities. The concept of healthy cities and communities was designed to incorporate citizen participation and to press local governments to cooperate in bringing about healthy outcomes.

In 1986, a compelling framework for health promotion was developed under the leadership of Jake Epp (1986) in a document titled, "Achieving health for all: A framework for health promotion." With the goal of achieving health for all Canadians, three key areas were identified: health challenges, health promotion mechanisms, and implementation strategies (Rootman & O'Neill, 1994, p. 141). Health challenges called for a reduction in inequities, increasing prevention, and enhancing coping. Health promotion mechanisms included self-care, mutual aide, and healthly environments. Implementation strategies involved fostering public participation, strengthening community health services, and coordinating health pubic policy (p. 141).

With the cutbacks to healthcare in Canada in the late 1980s and early 1990s, implementation of these ideals of public health was seriously impacted. By the mid-1990s, cutbacks to the public health system had created a high degree of vulnerability for all Canadians. For example, the quality of the water supplies in many cities and towns in several provinces was found to be faulty (Pike-MacDonald, 2007). As the years have progressed, many municipalities have had to put their citizens on an unsafe water supply alert for a temporary period. The advent of mad cow disease (bovine spongiform encephalopathy), West Nile virus, and many other threats to public health found the system wanting.

As some of the earliest advances in maintaining health and preventing disease in early Canadian history had to do with improving water supply, sanitation, and conducting meat inspections, it is somewhat alarming to think that we may have returned to situations somewhat akin to preconfederation days. When basic pillars for health promotion and preservation are removed from the health system, there are bound to be serious threats to health. Public health measures such as these have been taken for granted by most Canadians, and the warnings are clear: A public health system cut to the bone is not able to safeguard the health of Canadians.

GOVERNMENT STUDIES AND AGREEMENTS

In 1994, the federal government established a National Forum on Healthcare (1997) to make recommendations about the "crisis in healthcare." This eight-member committee studied various aspects of healthcare and came out in strong support of the merits of current Canadian health programs, adding to them the need to enhance home-care services as well as to improve coverage of pharmaceutical costs. Most of the forum's recommendations have yet to be implemented as other political agendas shift the emphasis in healthcare reform.

In 1999, the federal and provincial governments signed the Social Union Agreement, the purpose of which was to define the principles "for the design and development of social policies and programs" (CNA, 2000a). The principles include citizen engagement and accountability, and the agreement reconfirmed the conditions (principles) of the CHA of 1984.

Yet regional variations in the availability and caliber of services remain problematic within each province. Further, data released by the Canadian Institutes for Health Information indicate mounting evidence of wide gaps in healthcare benefits across the provinces. In May 2001, for example, the press reported on a survey suggesting that the likelihood of surviving a heart attack varied from 9% mortality during a hospital stay in Alberta to 18% in Newfoundland. Further evidence of regional variation is seen in the erosion of the principle of portability of the CHA.

As noted earlier, pharmacare or reimbursement for outpatient prescription drugs is not mandated by the CHA or any other federal legislation. In a recent Canadian study, researchers compared provincial prescription drug plans and their impact upon patients' annual drug expenditures. Wide variations were found across the provinces, including drug plans with different criteria for reimbursement, deductibles, copayments, premiums, and maximum annual beneficiary contributions (Demers et al., 2008, p. 405-406). Researchers concluded, "Given the differences in reimbursement according to age, income level, marital status and province of residence, prescription drug reimbursement in Canada is manifestly un-equal. Although current provincial drug plans provide good protection for isolated groups, most Canadians still have unequal coverage for outpatient prescription drugs (p. 409)."

In this case, adherence to both the principles of universality and portability are unenforceable in this highly costly, but typically medically necessary, healthcare need.

Accessibility

> ... the health care insurance plan must provide for insured health services on uniform terms and conditions and on a basis that does not impede or preclude, either directly or indirectly whether by changes made to insured persons or otherwise, reasonable access to those services by insured persons ...
>
> Canada Health Act, 1984, c.6, s.12

From the outset, concerns about rising costs, about socialized medicine interfering with doctor–patient relationships, and any number of other reasons were put forward to promote the private operation of health services. In Alberta in particular, physicians moved to bill patients extra for the care they received based on the premise that limited Medicare funds restricted their right to adequate compensation for services. This practice, known as *extra billing* or *balance billing*, set the stage for a national drama as the federal health minister, Monique Begin, took a highly public stance against the Alberta government on this issue. With a change in the funding formula from the federal to the provincial governments (i.e., the transfer of tax points to the provinces), the federal government had lost some leverage in its insistence that the provinces adhere to the national standards for Medicare.

The outcome was the passage of a new federal act meant *to enforce the principles* of Medicare, namely, the CHA.

In early April 2001, Roy Romanow, a former premier of Saskatchewan, was commissioned by an Order in Council of the federal government to inquire into and undertake policies and measures respectful of the jurisdictions and powers in Canada required to ensure, over the long term, the sustainability of a universally accessible, publicly funded health system that offers quality services to Canadians and strikes a balance between these investments in prevention and health maintenance and those directed to care and treatment (Commission on the Future of Healthcare in Canada, 2002, p. iii).

The report was tabled in November 2002 after one of the most extensive public consultations in Canadian history. Through these consultations Romanow was able confirm that

- Canadians remain attached to the values at the heart of the system
- Medicare has served Canadians extremely well
- the system is as sustainable as Canadians want it to be
- Canadians want and need a truly national healthcare system
- Canadians want and need a more comprehensive healthcare system
- Canadians want and need a more accountable healthcare system
- the Canadian system is based on values (Commission on the Future of Health Care in Canada, 2002, p. xvi-xix).

Romanow offered numerous recommendations in his 356-page report, almost all supported by strong research evidence secured through commission staff and commissioned papers. His key recommendations centered on the need for an infusion of funds into healthcare with calls for a dedicated health transfer payment to the provinces; a Canada healthcare covenant; modernizing the CHA; a home-care transfer for post-acute, palliative, and mental healthcare; a catastrophic drug transfer; and a rural and remote access fund. He also recommended the formation of a Health Council for Canada (mentioned earlier), reminiscent of the Dominion-Provincial Health Council formed in the 1940s, and he advised *against* for-profit delivery of health services.

Meanwhile, the Senate of Canada was also busily engaged in parallel activity by authorizing a committee led by Senator Michael Kirby to examine the fundamental principles on which Canada's publicly funded system is based, its historical development, the pressures and constraints on the system, and the role of the federal government in Canada's healthcare system. Kirby recommended no change to the CHA and to set funding priorities on service-based funding for hospitals. He also urged that greater responsibility be given to regional health authorities for delivering or contracting out publicly insured health services. As priorities, he recommended primary healthcare reform, a healthcare guarantee, coverage of catastrophic prescription costs, and home care. Kirby did not address Canadian values, and he left the door open to more private sector involvement. As Roberge (2003) observed:

> One of the ironies of the current crisis and the nature of the debate is that it was the desire to ensure access that led to the creation of public health insurance in Canada in the first place. Now it appears that a desire to ensure access is being used as an argument to move away from a public system. Public health insurance was designed to shift the burden from the individual to the collective through government funding. Now the financial burden of healthcare on governments has led to reduced access and there is pressure to shift the burden, at least in part, back to the individual (p. 14).

Whereas Romanow's findings were based on public consultation with over 40,000 Canadians, Kirby could only boast 400 voices.

Some argue that portraying Kirby as the proponent of privatization and Romanow as the champion of a public system creates a false polarity (Chodos & MacLeod, 2004), but both Kenny (2004), an ethicist, and Deber (2004), an economist, disagree. Kenny suggests that the difference lies in Kirby's suggestion to let the market decide for itself, while Romanow sees healthcare as a moral enterprise, not a business venture. Deber concludes that very limited benefits are likely to arise from an increase in the delivery of for-profit clinical services. She suggests that, "This does not mean that they should be outlawed, or that one should be comfortable with the status quo. But neither does it present any reason why they should be encouraged. . . . Improving care delivery, particularly more careful attention to best practices, communication and coordination, appears essential (pp. 59–60)."

In part as a consequence of these two reports, in February 2003, a Healthcare Renewal Accord was passed by the First Ministers' conference to reaffirm their commitment to the five principles of health insurance in Canada (the principles of the CHA). In this accord, they called for a standard of care that would include:

- access to a healthcare provider 24 hours a day, 7 days a week
- access to diagnostic procedures and treatments
- reduction in duplication of patient histories and testing for every provider they visit
- access to quality home and community care services
- access to quality care no matter where they live
- a healthcare system that is efficient, responsive, and adapting to changing needs (Healthcare Renewal Accord, 2003).

To reach these goals, the federal government agreed to establish a long-term Canada Health Transfer to include a portion of the current cash and tax points corresponding to provincial expenditures and with predictable annual increases.

Preceding and subsequent to this accord, surgical waiting lists became the pressing problem of healthcare professionals and government officials as well as private entrepreneurs. The latter offered their services of surgical day care settings, as a solution to the problems of accessibility. Once again, the provincial and federal governments challenged physicians who were seen to be extra-billing patients through these surgical for-profit centres.

In late spring 2004, the case of *Jacques Chaoulli et al. v. Attorney General of Quebec* raised the issue of "whether there is an infringement of Charter rights that occurs when the public system is unable to provide timely access to needed services while simultaneously prohibiting individuals from purchasing these services using their own resources" (Chodos & MacLeod, 2004, pp. 24–25). Two years later, "the Supreme Court of Canada decided in a 4–3 judgment to invalidate Quebec's prohibition against the sale of private insurance for core medical services provided through Medicare on the grounds that it violated the guarantee of rights to life and to personal inviolability in Quebec's Charter of Human Rights and Freedoms" (Crawford, 2006, p. 92). This, if adopted by other provinces, would in effect negate the accessibility clause in the CHA that protects consumers from paying extra (either through private insurance or out-of-pocket expenditure) for publicly funded services. Since this Quebec decision, many have expressed concern about other legislated acts that might be impacted by this decision. They question, for example, its impact upon free trade agreements. Since the Canadian government did not negotiate the exclusion of private health insurance from the terms of the North American Free Trade Agreement (NAFTA), market access might become open to other insurers beyond public health insurance (Crawford, 2006, pp. 93–95).

As scholars, health professionals, bureaucrats, and media took up the issue of wait times, it was noted that, "Waiting for elective surgery is the hottest political issue facing Canadian healthcare today. In fact, it's no exaggeration to say that how wait lists are managed—or not—could seal the fate of Medicare" (Priest, Rachlis, & Cohen, 2007)."

Considerable attention has been focused on wait times and wait lists, often with limited outcomes. In 2006, *HealthcarePapers* 7(1) was devoted to wait-time strategy, with reports of some success in reducing wait times in select areas of surgical treatment and related diagnostics. Those commenting on these successes reminded readers that excluded from these wait-time considerations are wait times for home care (Shamian, Shainblum, & Stevens, 2006) and many other less dramatic services. In British Columbia, Priest, Rachlis, & Cohen (2007), writing for the Canadian Center for Policy

Alternatives, analyzed the issue of wait lists. They highlighted the main reasons for wait lists and recommended attention to these barriers to time-appropriate surgeries. These recommendations include having a single common waiting list, improving current organizational processes, focusing on team-based care, offering presurgical programs, and using electronic information systems. In that many of these recommendations involve changes in ways of practice by many people (from surgeons to operating room nurses, to administrators and the public), implementation of solutions to the problem of wait lists may take some time to be realized. Delays in the introduction of electronic patient records and other patient information systems to allow healthcare providers ready access to information for care provision and planning is considered to be a major need for best practices in the Canadian healthcare system. But many provinces have been seriously delayed in adopting these innovative approaches.

Other issues of substance in late 2007 were those related to errors in pathology and histology laboratories. The main impetus for this news was the inaccurate results of lab tests in Newfoundland and Labrador, but the concerns about potential error rates in laboratories soon spread across Canada (Porter, 2008; Peritz, 2008). Accessibility to accurate test results, as well as the human cost of inaccurate lab results, became alarming concerns for most Canadians. Questions about national standards and supervision to ensure adherence to these standards were paramount in these discussions.

Equally alarming findings of a study focused on adherence to standards and subsequent outcomes of intensive care unit care and cardiac care on evenings and weekends, compared to adherence to standards and subsequent outcomes on the five weekdays, were newsworthy (Peberdy et al., 2008). Researchers found that ". . . survival to discharge following in-hospital cardiac arrest was lower during nights and weekends compared with day and evening times on weekdays, even after accounting for many potential confounding patient, arrest events, and hospital factors" (p. 788).

These are only a few examples of the many issues arising in healthcare in Canada. Some of these issues can be linked to previous and current cost-cutting measures and inattention to quality assurance, all leading to undesirable patient outcomes. Many of these issues are being used to question the sustainability of the Canadian healthcare system, particularly the financing of our publicly insured programs. Despite evidence to the contrary, many believe that the problem with the Canadian healthcare system is due to *public funding* and *public administration*, which they see as the problem rather than the solution (CHSRF, 2007b, p. 1).

Public Administration

> . . . the health care insurance plan of a province must be administered and operated on a non-profit basis by a public health authority appointed or designated by the government of the province . . .
>
> Canada Health Act, 1984, c.6, s.8

Canada does, in fact, have a mix of public and private for-profit care, with the private for-profit element normally linked to certain sectors of care. Roughly 70% of total health expenditures in Canada are paid by public sector funding, with 30% financed privately through supplementary insurance, employer-sponsored benefits, or direct out-of-pocket expenditures (Health Canada, 2002). For example, dental and orthodontic care falls outside the publicly funded health services in most provinces. There are also numerous private for-profit nursing homes because these are outside the acute care and medically oriented emphasis of Canada's health programs, and complementary medicine is not normally covered. Many of the fastest rising expenditures in healthcare fall outside of Medicare. Drug expenditures are paid for by combinations of private insurance plans and public funds, often with added out-of-pocket expenditures. These costs have often tripled their share of the gross domestic product over the last twenty years (CHSRF, 2007b).

Calling Canada a "learning disabled nation," Lewis (2007) comments on our obsession with sustainability when the facts based upon 2007 data from the Organization for Economic Cooperation and Development are so clear. He states that when comparing Canadian financial figures in healthcare to 19 other nations, that ". . . our cumulative rate of spending increases has been unexceptional; our fiscal houses are in order; and our economy is humming. It's hard to imagine a less daunting sustainability situation" (p. 21). Lewis maintains that preoccupation with sustainability arises from "three sources of inspiration" (p.22). One is the growing proportion of provincial dollars consumed by healthcare, the second is that the aging population will bankrupt the healthcare system, and the third is the ideology of those who want to privatize the system.

Many Canadian families have a strong historical bias toward privatization. After the two World Wars ended, and Canada began to prosper in the 1950s, many private medical insurance plans were developed by the provinces. With the popularity of these private medical insurance plans (particularly in the eyes of physicians and business leaders), and with hospitals available for use, the federal government was reluctant to rush to introduce the long-promised Medicare program that was the final part of the blueprint. At that point another study (a Royal Commission) was conducted on the feasibility of introducing a Medicare program. Contrary to governmental expectations, when the commissioners considered the total package of healthcare services needed by a Canadian family, they recommended that it was cost effective to subsidize the 10 health insurance programs in Canada (Taylor, 1973).

The final plank of Canada's healthcare system, a national Medicare program, was then put in place in the mid-1960s. It would seem natural that the battle for Medicare fought in Saskatchewan would pave the way for a relatively easy introduction of a similar program in Canada. However, such was not the case because many provinces had already established systems of private medical insurance they believed were superior to any national plan, and at least three provinces paid all or part of the costs of health insurance for those considered poor risks while leaving the majority of the population who could afford voluntary insurance to the private sector (Taylor, 1987).

Following implementation of the major programs featured in the Canadian blueprint, governments began to study the effects of the Canadian Health Insurance programs. The economic downturn in the late 1980s (noted earlier with respect to public health services) began to seriously threaten Canada's federal–provincial healthcare programs. The political climate of the Western world was strongly influenced by the dominant neo-conservative ideology of political leaders in England, the United States, and Canada. The development of large corporations, a concentration of wealth, and free trade were outcomes of this ideology, which included adopting a business model for healthcare delivery, identifying people as deserving and undeserving, and the growing attempts of governments to withdraw from involvement in comprehensive public programs and to promote private sector providers. Several provinces, Alberta and Quebec in particular, took the lead in downsizing healthcare through sudden and severe budgetary cutbacks.

Thus began massive layoffs of hospital workers—particularly nurses. Included in these cutbacks was the removal of one or two levels of nurse managers from the system, an action that ensured no one was there to advocate for professional nursing care. The effects of these actions are most evident today in serious nursing shortages and the absence of clinical nurse leaders to mentor and support nurses entering practice and those changing practice settings (Broughton, 2001; Canadian Nursing Advisory Committee, 2002; Shamian & LeClair, 2000).

Part of the downsizing strategy included a push toward healthcare reform that promoted healthcare as just another "business" and promoted greater regionalization of health services. In regionalization, the downsizing of the provincial health departments was one consequence because centralized policies and services were considered to be no longer required. The loss of intellectual ability, experience, and wisdom in public-sector management and in healthcare policy development was immeasurable.

Many health regions also implemented program management, an approach adopted from the business world that is built on product-line management strategies. The goal in program management is the integration of care through "seamless systems" that would be devoted to one similar focus of care, such as heart health, to include the spectrum from prevention to tertiary care (Leatt, Lemieux-Charles, & Aird, 1994). However, adopting this business way of thinking overlooks the unique aspects of healthcare, including the fact that patients, for example, do not fit into neat categories like product lines such as shoes or cars. This view might be described as the "false simplification of human life"

(Saul, 1995). Although there is a cry for evidence-based practice, the evidence to support dismantling many good systems that were put in place to promote high-quality care is lacking.

The Canadian Health Services Research Foundation (2004, 2007) has regularly pointed out that drawing money from another source additional to government funding does not make the system more affordable, because Canadians still have to pay for it. Further, sustainability is not only about money. Included in measures to sustain the system are changes that must be made in the system and are typically changes that have been resisted, such as a greater focus on primary healthcare, better home-care services, more focused preventive services, more interdisciplinary teamwork, and salaried physicians. As Kenny (2002, p. 29) points out, if these and similar recommendations to sustain the system are "eminently sensible and obviously necessary for maximum efficiency, why have they not been implemented? Who benefits from the status quo?" Another very serious question in this decade is who benefits from the push toward greater private health insurance? As has been noted, "When governments cut taxes, any public program, including health services, can be unsustainable. Fiscal sustainability, therefore, is a matter of governments choice, but more fundamentally the public's choice. . . . Medicare is as sustainable as Canadians want it to be" (CHSRF, 2007b).

SO WHAT DOES THIS MEAN?

Despite all its flaws, Canada's system of healthcare is well worth saving. While respecting its limitations, one can make a few general statements about the system's virtues. People in Canada do not have to be as fearful about their access to care and about the devastating costs of an illness or surgery as do many in the United States. And Canadian patients have considerably more choice in the selection of their doctors—and even their hospitals—than many of their neighbors to the south. Many managed care plans in the United States, for example, offer extremely limited choices to consumers, reserving considerable choice for the managers of the plans whose goal is to purchase the most cost-efficient services for their patient groups.

Physicians in Canada have freedom to choose their practice locations without restriction and they can set their work pace and manage their scheduling. Canadian national programs have also allowed for an enviable collection of data about hospital stays, patients' conditions, and physician services. And the programs still have the support of the majority of the public. Some observations still seem beyond challenge. Access to healthcare based solely on need is the core value that gave rise to and sustains Medicare, and the advent, through Medicare, of universal, publicly funded physician and hospital services substantially reduced disparities in access to, and outcomes of, healthcare based on socioeconomic status. But despite those gains, disparities remain—factors other than need continue to influence access to and use of services (Hutchison, 2007).

The serious pressures on the system in the 21st century need to be carefully considered both in relation to our historical legacy and to the wider context of international capital in which our healthcare system and other countries' healthcare systems are embedded (Coburn & Rappolt, 1999). Problems arising from this legacy are our failure to develop a comprehensive system of care and our failure to recreate, re-energize, and renew our systems based on known evidence. These problems also represent our failure to change traditional practices, to move to primary healthcare, and to utilize all health professionals well. All of these problems might well be included in what Coburn and Rappolt (1999) describe as the "logic of Medicare."

So what has our history, our heritage, told us about our current situation in healthcare and the need and potential for change?

1. We continue to operate under the terms of the BNA Act provisions (now incorporated into the Constitution Act) for determining federal and provincial responsibilities in healthcare, meaning that we still operate with the same division of federal and provincial responsibilities

in healthcare as seemed appropriate in 1867. Such a division of responsibility leaves room for provinces to assert their authority when it suits their particular situations, and it forces the federal government to work through three main alternate approaches to influence healthcare. More importantly, it leaves room for each level of government to blame the other for failure to take action (e.g., in areas such as pollution or home care) and to leave the public waiting—and often lobbying—for the impasse to be overcome.

2. We continue to talk about social determinants of health but have yet to deal with those determinants in a comprehensive and committed way. Governments and the public both are responsible for the lack of attention to these matters, yet conditions like full employment, a guaranteed annual income, stamping out poverty, and other such fundamental health-promoting conditions could have a significant effect on improving the health status of all and decreasing expenditures in tertiary healthcare.

3. Medicare continues to enjoy a high level of public support, although that level is slipping as corporate claims of better, more efficient care by for-profit medicine woo the public to their way of thinking. This persuasion is often accomplished by scare tactics, which distort the facts about current and projected public healthcare spending (CHSRF, 2007b).

4. As our history shows, in implementing federal and provincial programs, we have continued to compromise on what should be included and how the systems should operate. In the mid-1940s, we did not adopt a comprehensive approach to health and social security as had been suggested by Marsh and Heagerty. Instead, we chose to implement publicly appealing programs selectively (Armstrong et al., 2000). This approach had the effect of setting us up for rising costs because many of these programs were oriented toward high-technology medicine (e.g., the hospital insurance and diagnostic services program) and took the focus away from holistic patient care. Further, these programs excluded funding for many services, such as nursing homes, home care, and pharmaceutical coverage, and thereby disadvantaged elderly and poor people. Later, during the introduction of Medicare, Saskatchewan and then the federal government abandoned the concept of all-on-a-salary and gave in to doctors' demands for fee-for-service payments instead. This capitulation also paved the way for cost increases for healthcare and closed the door to a more level playing field in power relationships among physicians, nurses, and other health professionals, which has had a serious effect on women and on nursing.

5. The majority of nurses work in hospitals or other institutions where their autonomy is more limited than that of their counterparts working in the community. Relationships between physicians and nurses are not ideal, and this does not create the best environment for high-quality care.

6. The promise of health reform has yet to be realized; in fact, reforms such as regionalization may have added to the shortfall in comprehensive care as different regions make different decisions about what services they are prepared to offer.

7. Canada has failed to manage the growth of medical technology in a rational way. We have been unable to set limits on professional desires and public expectations.

8. We have yet to develop primary healthcare services, to make better legislative provisions for new entry points to the system, or to promote better use of qualified health personnel. Health promotion and disease prevention are key recommendations critical to current population needs.

9. We need to question whose interests are being served in keeping the system relatively unchanged since the 1960s. We need to ask what effect free trade and increased moves to globalization have had on maintaining a system characterized by medical dominance, an emphasis on technology without limits, unequal access to care, and marginalization of many health professionals and patient groups.

10. It is also necessary to ask what effect ideologies of individualism and egalitarianism have had on our inability to see the socioeconomic barriers that prevent patients from taking personal responsibility for their health (Anderson & Reimer-Kirkham, 1998).

11. There is no question about the need to work toward greater coordination and efficiencies in healthcare, as in any line of work. But, at the end of the day, the questions remain: Where else is the money going? What other corporate demands are driving healthcare? Who is profiting by maintaining the status quo in healthcare?

WHAT LIES AHEAD?

Several analysts (Armstrong et al., 2000; Coburn & Rappolt, 1999) provide insights for understanding the context of healthcare today and prospects for tomorrow. They suggest that the gradual rise in medical dominance over the past decades in Canada and the implementation of Medicare by the governments in Canada were the last keys in the welfare state. In their analysis, Coburn and Rappolt (1999) see this as representing the triumph for labor and for the state (the government). However, they suggest that the gradual decline of medical dominance in healthcare and a decline in government involvement in healthcare has occurred as the result of a " . . . major transformation of national and international political economies towards the internationalization of capital" (p. 142). This transformation has led to an increase in business power and a decrease in the relative autonomy of the state.

Coburn and Rappolt (1999) suggest that the " . . . welfare state, and particularly anything to do with labour market policy, is brought under fierce attack from a newly united right and its international and national agents in the business community, in neoliberal international institutions such as the International Monetary Fund, in national neoconservative policy institutions and think tanks, as well as the conservatively skewed media" (p. 152). Labeling this relatively recent phenomena as the "internationalization of capital" or "global capitalism," Coburn and Rappolt note how the International Monetary Fund, the World Bank, and the new ideologic unity between large and small business have had substantial influence on domestic business interests. This influence has enhanced the power of business with Canadian governments (both federal and provincial) and has particularly strengthened the hand of American influences on governments. Thus, free trade agreements are viewed as the inevitable costs of keeping Canada competitive, even though they have the potential to undermine Canadian social programs.

The potential scenario here is that governments' gradual undermining of social programs causes the public to see these programs as inadequate or outdated for 21st century needs. One has only to cut costs to particular services for so long before the public comes to believe that there must be no more money and, therefore, there is "no choice" except to welcome private, for-profit healthcare services. The effect has been one of transformation with new " . . . structures of class, state, welfare state, health care, health profession interaction [taking] one form under the particular dynamics of monopoly capitalism and [assuming] a new form under the somewhat different structure of global capitalism" (Coburn & Rappolt, 1999, p. 160). The overall impact has been designed " . . . to produce powerlessness . . . making citizens powerless within their own countries" (p. 160).

Yet when Coburn and Rappolt (1999) examine how "global" globalization really is, they point out that within the three major trading blocs in the world, the greatest influence on Canada is from the United States; the effect on healthcare is that we are harmonizing downward toward this partner (p. 161). (This strong United States influence has become even more apparent since the September 11, 2001 terrorist attacks on the World Trade Center in New York, as many cherished Canadian policies in areas outside of healthcare, such as border guards carrying firearms in Canada, changed because of United States demands.) By altering the balance of power in Canada, the Free Trade Agreement (the agreement between the United States and Canada for free trade) and NAFTA (the free trade agreement that includes Mexico) have far-ranging consequences for Canada's social fabric and its social policies (p. 161). But even Coburn argues that there are " . . . degrees of freedom and openings for resistance to neoliberal doctrines" (p. 160). To suggest that there is no choice left and that we cannot expect our social programs to continue is to adopt a fatalistic view that flies in the face of the power of individual and collective action to make a difference. A documentary called *The Corporation*, which was shown in theaters across the country in 2004, makes this point most clearly.

During the 2008 U.S election primaries and presidential campaign, Canadians were once again reminded that 47 million Americans have no, or inadequate, insurance coverage for healthcare. These citizens of the United States choose to either go without care, rely on charitable donation for their care, or go into serious debt to pay for necessary healthcare. Other Americans realize that their healthcare spending is high compared to that of other countries (Kuttner, 2008), yet it does not lead to better health overall. In one critique of the U.S. system, which is balanced toward privatization of healthcare based upon the premise of a market economy model with consumer choice, one author argued for *justice* to be included in a framework for the election candidates' healthcare debates. Given different concepts of justice, she noted that ". . . we do not have to agree on a theory of justice to be revolted by injustice" (Crowley, 2008).

The history and current status of Canadian healthcare make it clear that many of the important ideas and services in healthcare came about through struggle and persistence. A commitment to change is a commitment to engage in a political struggle that accompanies the change (Anderson & Reimer-Kirkham, 1998). One Canadian reality worth remembering is that the Canadian Constitution establishes that the federal government is responsible for making " . . . Laws for the Peace, Order and good Government of Canada" (Van Loon & Whittington, 1976, p. 480). This concept is in contrast to that of the U.S. Constitution, which centers on individual liberties and freedoms. This difference set the stage for enacting Canadian legislation that emphasized the common (collective) good evident in values that promote Canada's social programs.

NURSES LEADING TO INFLUENCE CHANGE

If nurses are to be effective leaders in influencing change both individually and through collective action, some homework is needed. Nurses need to understand the history and structures of the healthcare system in Canada, to educate themselves to the needs of their patients, and to set goals and work together to achieve those goals.

What Nurses Need to Know

Individually, there is a need for nurses to know about the history of Canadian healthcare, or at least to be aware of basic programs and structures that have been put in place over time. This awareness includes some understanding of the historical ideologic debates and how those same debates continue to play out in healthcare today. This knowledge and understanding should not only give nurses confidence in stating their case but also ensure that they are not susceptible to being silenced by others' rhetoric. Additionally, nurses must be clear about some of the international and national pressures on the healthcare system and be ready to push against the perceived inevitability of a greater uptake of the business orientation that might diminish the effectiveness of healthcare delivery.

Second, nurses need good—and updated—information, including keeping up to date with public debates in the media and elsewhere and also digging deeper to uncover reliable facts and other viewpoints. Professional nursing associations, educational institutions, public libraries, and the Internet can be helpful resources for nurses. CNA's development of NursingOne can be a useful internet access for all nurses. (Visit www.nursingone.ca for more information.)

Other information needed by nurses includes keeping abreast of the influence of trade agreements on healthcare and professional practice as well as on basic needs for the public's health, such as an adequate supply of clean water, clean air, security, and other essentials of life. Knowledge of ethics in nursing practice is critical to reflection on these issues (Storch, Rodney, & Starzomki, 2004). Nurses also need to know about their professional associations, including the freedom and responsibilities of self-regulation and the importance of collective action.

What Nurses Need to Be

Above all, nurses need to be well educated, good listeners, and sensitive caregivers. Nurses need to see and respond to the many people who are marginalized in society—Aboriginal peoples, immigrants, different ethnic groupings, women—particularly single mothers and their children—those living in poverty, elderly people, and so forth.

We also need to see and critically think about the dominant players in healthcare and seek to understand their views as well as direct our attention toward ways to broaden and influence their thinking (e.g., Pauly, 2004; Varcoe, 2004). Despite the difficulties nursing faces today with regard to being valued, we need to keep on caring without regard for race, color, creed, religious persuasion, or political alignments. In short, we need to continue to be role models of caring practices. It is not surprising that the CNA chose "be the change" as the slogan for their Centennial Year.

What Nurses Need to Do

Collectively, nurses need to be willing to work together to reach good outcomes for their patients and for themselves. Canada has fine examples of nurses involved in collective action to make a difference through both provincial nursing organizations and through the CNA, including specific foci during provincial and federal elections.

Nurses also need to use the knowledge gained through nursing education and nurse–patient relationships to focus attention on the determinants of health. Frank and Mustard (1994), and many before them, demonstrated the relationships between illness and socioeconomic factors. In addition to noting how the job hierarchy influences health, these authors suggested that " . . . an individual's sense of achievement, self-esteem, and control over his or her work and life appears to affect health and well-being" (p. 9). As nurses come to know their patients, they see the effects of these variables on patient well-being and on their own health. That is important knowledge to be utilized in dialogue with politicians or bureaucrats.

Working collectively toward the goal of primary healthcare for all is also critical work for nurses today. Nurses in advanced nursing practice make a difference in patient care and can improve the health system overall. The persistence of nurses in moving toward patient-centered goals continues to make a difference within specific areas and has a spillover effect over time (Pauly et al., 2004).

Individually, nurses can also be ready to speak, to question, and to spread hope (Broughton, 2001). As nurses, we may not have all the answers but we do know most of the questions. With regard to information about the political economy discussed earlier in this text, an individual nurse may not have complete knowledge but can question politicians and government bureaucrats, as well as other civil servants, neighbors, friends, and colleagues to make them think and potentially to influence their actions however large or small they may be. This is to move against a place of powerlessness.

SUMMARY

Nurses need to understand what drives today's healthcare system, particularly in regard to the underpinnings of Medicare, the international economic manipulation of resources available for healthcare, and the related disempowerment of healthcare professionals.

The same value conflicts that we see today were inherent in the development of Canadian policies and programs since their inception: a focus on individual responsibility and self-reliance versus collective responsibility; a free market system versus more socially oriented collective policies and programs in healthcare (the privatization debate); an emphasis on scientific discovery and techno-logic imperatives versus humanism and care for the disadvantaged; and those who believe that all have equal opportunities to healthcare versus the reality that gender, race, and class differences affect the way in which healthcare is delivered.

These are some of the influences that keep Canada's healthcare system focused on primary care as opposed to primary healthcare: "*Primary care* is a medical concept referring to a situation wherein the physician provides diagnosis, treatment, and follow-up for a specific disease or problem" (CNA, 2000b). *Primary healthcare*, as adopted by WHO in 1978 as the basis for the delivery of health services, most effectively involves both "a philosophy and an approach" to the way health services are delivered. It includes health promotion, disease prevention, curative services, rehabilitative care, and supportive or palliative care (CNA, 2000b). Primary healthcare involves a shift from traditional practices and power dynamics in healthcare to a system in which all health professionals are utilized to their maximum potential to effect good patient outcomes in care. NPs, advanced practice nurses, and staff nurses alike are able to practise to their full scope of practice in this model.

This is the model of care Canadian nurses have sought for almost three decades, and it continues to be a model worth pursuing. In fact, it is one of the CNA's two key goals in this millennium; the other goal is achieving improved quality of work environments for nurses.

Nurses can influence change by attending to the history, current status, and future projections for healthcare; by being listening and caring caregivers; and by taking action individually and collectively to promote greater attention to social determinants of health and better healthcare provision for their patients.

As nurses, we need to be clear about our own values and opinions and be able to stand by them so our voices can help shape better approaches to healthcare. If we are not prepared to do so, nursing and nurses will have little to say in the healthcare system of tomorrow.

Add to your knowledge of this issue:		Online
Canadian Nurses Association	**www.cna-nurses.ca**	
Health Canada	**www.hc-sc.gc.ca**	
Canadian Health Services Research Foundation	**www.chsrf.ca**	

REFLECTIONS on the Chapter...

1 In what ways do you think the Canadian healthcare system would have been different and less subject to political influence if the Fathers of Confederation had chosen to assign principal responsibility for healthcare and education to the federal government rather than to the provinces?

2 If medical care insurance had been introduced before the introduction of hospital insurance, what differences might we have seen in the formation of health facilities? What contributions do you think this might have made in controlling the costs of technology? Would primary healthcare likely have become the norm?

3 Do you believe that healthcare costs are out of control? Why or why not?

4 In reflecting on what you know about nurses' individual or collective actions to influence better healthcare, what types of knowledge have they utilized to influence change?

5 To what degree have you felt powerless or powerful against business interests in healthcare? Why have you felt that way?

References

Achbar, M. (Producer/Director), Abbot, J. (Director/Editor), & Simpson, B. (Producer). (2003). *The Corporation.* [Motion Picture]. Canada: Big Picture Media Corporation.

Anderson, J. & Reimer-Kirkham, S. (1998). Constructing nation: The gendering and racializing of the Canadian health care system. In V. Strong-Boag, S. Grace, A. Eisenberg, et al. (Eds.), *Painting the maple: Essays on race, gender, and the construction of Canada* (pp. 242–261). Vancouver: UBC Press.

Angus, J. & Bourgeault, I.L. (1999). Medical dominance, gender and the state: The nurse practitioner initiative in Ontario. In D. Coburn, S. Rappolt, I. Bourgeault, & J. Angus (Eds.), *Medicine, nursing and the state* (p. 55). Aurora, ON: Garamond Press Ltd.

Armstrong, P., Armstrong, H., Bourgeault, I., et al. (2000). *"Heal thyself": Managing health care reform.* Aurora, Ontario: Garamond Press.

Badgely, R.F. & Wolfe, S. (1967). *Doctors' strike: Medical care and conflict in Saskatchewan.* Toronto: Macmillan of Canada.

Bliss, M. (1975). A preface. In L. Marsh (Ed.) *Report on social security for Canada.* Toronto: University of Toronto Press.

Broughton, H. (2001). *Nursing leadership: Unleashing the power.* Ottawa: Canadian Nurses Association.

Canadian Health Services Research Foundation. (2004). *Myth: For profit, ownership of facilities would lead to a more efficient health care system.* Ottawa: Author.

Canadian Health Services Research Foundation (CHSRF). (2007a). Self-management education to optimize health and reduce hospital admissions for chronically ill patients. *Evidence Boost for Quality.* Ottawa: Author.

_____. (2007b). Myth busters. *Canada's system of healthcare financing is unsustainable.* Ottawa: Author.

Canadian Nurses Association. (1980). *Putting "health" back into health care.* Submission to the Health Services Review '79. Ottawa: Author.

_____. (2000a). *The Canada Health Act.* Ottawa: Author.

_____. (2000b). *The primary health care approach.* Fact sheet. Ottawa: Author.

_____. (2005). *CNA backgrounder: Primary health care: A summary of issues.* Ottawa: Author.

Canadian Nursing Advisory Committee. (2002). *Our health, our future: Creating quality workplaces for nurses.* Final report. Ottawa: Health Canada.

Canadian Patient Safety Institute (CPSI). (2007). Patient safety: New heights, higher standards. Edmonton: Author.

Cassidy, H.M. (1947). The Canadian social services. *The Annals of the Academy of Political and Social Sciences, 253*(September), 190–201.

Chodos, H. & MacLeod, J.J. (2004). Romanow and Kirby on the public/private divide in healthcare: Demystifying the debate. *HealthcarePapers, 4*(4), 10–25.

Coburn, D. (1988). The development of Canadian nursing: Professionalization and proletarianization. *International Journal of Health Services, 18*(3), 437–456.

Coburn, D. & Rappolt, S. (1999). The "logic of medicare": Variants of capitalism and medical dominance. Contextualizing profession-state relationships. In D. Coburn, S. Rappolt, I. Bourgeault, et al. (Eds.), *Medicine, nursing and the state* (pp. 139–167). Aurora, Ontario: Garamond Press.

Commission on the Future of Healthcare in Canada. (2002). Commissioner R.J. Romanow. Ottawa: Health Canada.

Crawford, M. (2006). Interactions: Trade policy and healthcare reform after Chaoulli v. Quebec. *Healthcare Policy, 1*(2), 90–102.

Crowley, M. (2008). Justice as a frame for health reform. *Hastings Center Report, 38*(1), 3.

Deber, R.B. (2004). Cats and categories: Public and private in Canadian healthcare. *HealthcarePapers, 4*(4), 51–60.

Defries, R.D. (1962). *The federal and provincial health services in Canada* (2nd ed.). Toronto: Canadian Public Health Association.

Demers, V., Melo, M., Jackevicius, C., Cox, J., Kalavrouziotis, D., Rinfret, S., Humphries, K.H., Johansen, H., Tu, J.V., & Pilote, L. (2008). Comparison of provincial prescription drug plans and the impact on patients' annual drug expenditures. *Canadian Medical Association Journal, 178*(4), 405–409.

Evans, R. (1984). *Strained mercy: The economics of Canadian health care.* Toronto: Butterworths.

Frank, J.W. & Mustard, J.F. (1994). The determinants of health from a historical perspective. *Daedalus,* Fall, 1–19.

Fuller, C. (1998). *Caring for profit: How corporations are taking over Canada's health care system.* Vancouver: New Star Books.

Hall, E.M. (1980). *Canada's national–provincial health program for the 1980s: A commitment for renewal.* Justice E.M. Hall, Special Commissioner. Ottawa: Department of National Health and Welfare.

Harnett, C.E. (2008). Superbug spreading in hospitals, communities. *Times Colonist,* March 3, A1, A4.

Hastings, J.E.F. (1972). *Report of the community health centre project to the health ministers.* Toronto: Canadian Public Health Association.

Hastings, J.E.F. & Mosley, W. (1980). Introduction: The evolution of organized community health services in Canada. In C.A. Meilicke & J.L. Storch (Eds.), *Perspectives on Canadian health and social services policy: History and emerging trends* (pp. 145–155). Ann Arbor, Michigan: Health Administration Press.

HealthcarePapers. (2006). *New models for the new healthcare. 7*(1). Entire issue.

Health Canada. (2002). Canada's health care system. Retrieved on October 21, 2008 from http://www.hc-sc.gc.ca/.

Health Care Renewal Accord. (2003). First ministers accord on healthcare renewal. Available from http://www.hc-sc.gc.ca/english//hca2003/accord.html.

Health Council of Canada (2005). *Health care renewal in Canada.* Ottawa: Author.

Hutchison, B. (2007). Editorial: Disparities in healthcare access and use: Yackety-yack Yackety-yack. *Healthcare Policy. 3*(2), 10–13.

Institute of Medicine. (1999). *To err is human: Building a safer health care system.* Washington, DC: National Academics Press.

Kenny, N. (2002). *What good is health care?* Ottawa: CHA Press.

_____. (2004). Value(s) for money? Assessing Romanow and Kirby. *HealthcarePapers, 4*(4), 28–34.

Kuttner, R. (2008). Market-based failure—A second opinion on U.S. health care costs. *New England Journal of Medicine, 356*(6), 549–551.

LaBonte, R. (1994). Death of program, birth of metaphor: The development of public health in Canada. In A. Pederson, M. O'Neill, & I. Rootman (Eds.), *Health Promotion in Canada: Provincial, National and International Perspectives* (pp. 72–90). Toronto: W.B. Saunders Canada.

Lalonde, M. (1974). *A new perspective on the health of Canadians.* Ottawa: Information Canada.

Laframboise, H.L. (1973). Health policy: Breaking the problem down into more manageable segments. *Canadian Medical Association Journal, 108*(February), 388–393.

Lalonde, M. (1974). *A new perspective on the health of Canadians.* Ottawa: Information Canada.

Leatt, P., Lemieux-Charles, L., & Aird, C. (1994). *Program management and beyond: Management innovations in Ontario hospitals.* Ottawa: Canadian College of Health Service Executives.

Leatt, P., Pink, G.H., & Guerriere, M. (2000). Towards a Canadian model of integrated healthcare. *HealthcarePapers, 1*(2), 13–35.

Lewis, S. (2007). Can a learning-disabled nation learn healthcare lessons from abroad? *Healthcare Policy, 3*(2), 19–28.

Lindenfield, R. (1959). Hospital insurance in Canada: An example in federal–provincial relations. *Social Services Review, 33,* 148–160.

MacAdam, M. (2000). Home care: It's time for a Canadian model. *HealthcarePapers, 1*(4), 9–36.

MacDonald, M., Regan, S., Davidson, H., Schreiber, R., Crickmore, J., Moss, L., Pinelli, J., & Pauly, B. (2006). Knowledge transfer to advance the nurse practitioner role in British Columbia. *Healthcare Policy, 1*(2), 80–89.

Marsh, L. (1975). *Report on social security for Canada 1943.* Toronto: University of Toronto Press.

McIntosh, J.W. (1914). Inter-relation of physician, citizen and state to public health. *The Public Health Journal, 5*(July 14), 451–455.

Morgan, M.W., Zamora, N.E., & Hindmarsh, M.F. (2007). An inconvenient truth: A sustainable healthcare system requires a chronic disease prevention and management transformation. *HealthcarePapers, 7*(4), 6–23.

National Forum on Health Care. (1997). *Canada health action: Building the legacy.* Ottawa: Health Canada.

Pauly, B. (2004). Shifting the balance in funding and delivery of health care in Canada. In J. Storch, P. Rodney, & R. Starzomski (Eds.), *Towards a moral horizon: Nursing ethics for leadership and practice* (pp. 181–208). Toronto: Pearson Education Canada.

Pauly, B., Schreiber, R., MacDonald, M., et al. (2004). Dancing to our own tune: Understandings of advanced nursing practice in British Columbia. *Journal of Nursing Leadership, 17*(2), 47–57.

Peberdy, M.A., Ornato, J.P., Larkin, G.L., Braithwaite, R.S., Kashner, T.M., Carey, S.M., Meaney, P.A., Gen, L., Nadkarni, V.M., Praestgaard, A.H., & Berg, R.A. (2008). Survival from in-hospital cardiac arrest during nights and weekends. *JAMA, 299*(7), 785–792.

Peritz, I. (2008). Technician faces trial over false blood-test results. *The Globe and Mail,* February 6, A7.

Pike-MacDonald, S., Best, B.G., Twomey, C., Bennett, L., & Blakeley, J. (2007). Promoting safe drinking water. *Canadian Nurse, 103*(1), 15–19.

Porter, S. (2008). St. John's lab plagued by staffing problems, report finds. *The Globe and Mail,* February 21, A7.

Priest, L. (2008). Ottawa targets hospital superbugs. *The Globe and Mail,* February 4, A1, A6.

Priest, A., Rachlis, M., & Cohen, M. (2007). *Why wait? Public solutions to cure surgical waitlists.* Vancouver: Canadian Centre for Policy Alternatives BC.

Registered Nurses Association of Ontario (RNAO). (1999). *Putting nurses back into health care: Who will respond?* Toronto: Author.

Rice, J.J. & Prince, M.J. (2000). *Changing politics of Canadian social policy.* Toronto: University of Toronto Press.

Roberge, G. (2003). A four part paper on health policy and management implications of the Romanow and Kirby reports. Unpublished paper. Faculty of Human and Social Development, University of Victoria, Victoria, British Columbia.

Rootman, I. & O'Neill, M. (1994). Developing knowledge for health promotion. In A. Pederson, M. O'Neill, & I. Rootman (Eds.), *Health Promotion in Canada: Provincial, National and International Perspectives* (pp. 139–151). Toronto: W.B. Saunders Canada.

Royal Commission on Health Service (Vols. I, II). (1964, 1965). Justice E. Hall, Commission Chair. Ottawa: Queen's Printer.

Saul, J.R. (1995). *The unconscious civilization.* Concord, Ontario: Anansis.

Shamian, J. & LeClair, S.J. (2000). Integrated delivery systems now or . . . ? *HealthcarePapers, 1*(2), 66–75.

Shamian, J., Shainblum, E., & Stevens, J. (2006). Accountability agenda must include home care and community based care. *HealthcarePapers, 7*(1), 58–64.

Storch, J.L. (2005). Patient safety: Is it just another bandwagon? *Nursing Leadership 18*(2), 39–55.

Storch, J.L., Rodney, P., & Starzomski, R. (2004). *Towards a moral horizon: Nursing ethics for leadership and practice.* Toronto: Pearson Education Canada.

Strategies for population health: Investing in the health of Canadians. (1994). Prepared by the Federal, Provincial and Territorial Advisory Committee on Population Health for the Meeting of the Ministers of Health, September 14–15.

Taylor, M.G. (1973). The Canadian health insurance program. *Public Administration Review, 33*(January-February), 31–39.

_____. (1987). *Health insurance and Canadian public policy* (2nd ed.). Montreal: McGill Queens University Press.

Van Loon, R.J. & Whittington, M.S. (1976). *The Canadian political system: Environment, structure and process* (2nd ed.). Toronto: McGraw-Hill Ryerson.

Varcoe, C. (2004). Widening the scope of ethical theory, practice, and policy: Violence against women as an illustration. In J. Storch, P. Rodney, & R. Starzomski (Eds.), *Towards a moral horizon: Nursing ethics for leadership and practice* (pp. 414–432). Toronto: Pearson Education Canada.

Wallace, E. (1950). The origins of the social welfare state in Canada, 1867–1900. *Canadian Journal of Economics and Political Science, 16*, 383–393.

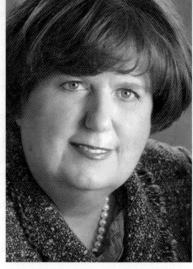

chapter 4

Dr. Judith Shamian's leadership has been instrumental in influencing and developing professional policy to move forward the agenda of nursing and patient care, influencing healthcare all levels. (Used with permission.)

Issues in Contemporary Nursing Leadership

Marjorie McInytre and
Carol McDonald

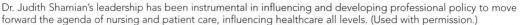

The authors acknowledge the work of previous contributors, Deborah Tamlyn and Sandra Reilly.

Critical Questions

As a way of engaging with the ideas in this chapter, consider the following:

1 Drawing on your student experience in nursing practice, how do you understand leadership in nursing and its impact on the healthcare system?

2 In what ways do you think about yourself as a leader?

3 How would you assess the potential for leadership in others?

Chapter Objectives

After completing this chapter, you will be able to:

1 Identify relevant issues in relation to nursing leadership.

2 Describe the relationship between leadership and management.

3 Describe the attributes of contemporary nurse leaders.

The premise of this chapter is that nursing leadership is challenged by the competing goals that currently influence professional nursing practice. Nurse leaders are increasingly called to account for the economic goals of the business model crowding out the professional goals of nursing practice. As a discipline, goals for professional practice arise from an ethic of care; these goals, however, are not necessarily aligned with the goals of the institutions and organizations in which professional nursing practice takes place.

Typically the tensions that are generated through this misalignment of goals become the responsibility of people in administrative positions in organizations: the designated managers and leaders. As the complexity and intensity of this tension increases, it becomes even more important that all professional nurses explore how they can participate in the leadership needed to mediate this dissonance.

In reading this chapter you will have the opportunity to reflect on your own potential for leadership as well as your capacity to participate with and support others who are in leadership positions. Nursing, like every discipline, has its outstanding leaders; in this chapter we recognize some of the leaders who have made significant contributions to professional nursing practice. That said, in the enactment of ethical practice each of us faces daily decisions in which we have the opportunity to exercise leadership. As you begin reading this chapter, take a moment to reflect on your own life; who has exemplified leadership qualities that you value? What is it about those qualities that you hold as important? Are you able to see those qualities in yourself, or can you imagine that those are qualities that you would like to develop?

SITUATING THE TOPIC: THE NATURE OF THE ISSUE

Although there are many ways to talk about or understand leadership, one distinction that seems important to point out is the difference between the idea that leadership is something that happens to us, rather than something that each of us participates in. We would suggest that not only is it possible for us to participate in nursing leadership, but that professional nursing leadership is a shared project in which we are obligated to participate.

One way to participate in the leadership endeavor is to follow or accept the authority of the designated leader and to take the "lead from the leader." This approach is similar to what has traditionally been thought of as a mentorship model. In this case the mentor typically possesses—or at least is thought to possess—the knowledge and skills the person being mentored hopes to acquire. A second way of being in a leadership relationship is to participate reciprocally. Here the strengths of each person are drawn on and responsibilities are negotiated. Typically, nursing teams and interdisciplinary teams operate in this way. A third way of being in a relationship with leaders is to take a position to be willing to critique the leaders or even challenge decisions and practices when, in your view, existing practices might benefit from new knowledge and approaches. This approach creates space for people outside of the traditional hierarchy of leadership, such as students, new graduates, or new persons on the team, to make important contributions to nursing leadership. The ability of others to create space for the leadership contribution of this group of people (students and new graduates) is in itself a sign of leadership excellence.

Leadership and Management

In their book, *The New Leadership Challenge: Creating the Future for Nursing*, Grossman and Valiga (2005) critique the literature that conflates leadership with management. Their criticism of textbook titles that include "leadership and management" is that "a great deal of attention is given to management and very little to leadership" (p. 4). Instead, they make the point that "leadership is not necessarily tied to a position of authority and each of us as a professional nurse has the potential and perhaps the responsibility to provide leadership" (p. 4). (Table 4.1).

Table 4.1	Differences between Leadership and Management	
	LEADERSHIP	MANAGEMENT
Position	Position is one selected or allowed by a group.	Position is one appointed by someone higher in the organization.
Power	Power comes from knowledge, credibility, and ability to motivate others.	Power arises from the position of authority.
Goals/visions	Goals and visions arise from personal interests and passion and may not be synonymous with the goals of the organization.	Goals and visions are those espoused or prescribed by the organization.
Risk level	High-risk level, high-risk creativity, and innovation are involved.	Low risk, balance, and maintaining the status quo are involved.
Degree of order	Relative disorder seems to be generated.	Rationality and control prevail.
Nature of activities	Activities are those related to vision and judgment.	Activities are those related to efficiency and cost effectiveness.
Focus	Focus is on people.	Focus is on systems and structure.
Perspective	Long-range perspective, with an eye on the horizon is critical.	Short-range perspective, with an eye on the bottom line often dominates.

While these distinctions may appear dualistic, they are for the purpose of illustration. In many situations, managers also serve as leaders and many leaders enact managerial abilities. (Source: Modified from Grossman, S., & Valiga, T. (2005). *The new leadership challenge: Creating the future of nursing.* Philadelphia: Davis.)

Although the distinctions between leadership and management illustrated in Table 4.1 are important, Hibberd & Smith, (2006) caution against creating a dichotomous distinction between leadership and management. They remind us that "leaders who lack management skills, are as much of a liability to modern organizations and the communities they serve as are managers who lack the vision of leadership" (2006, ix).

Attributes of Contemporary Nursing Leaders

According to Rodger (2006) herself a notable Canadian nurse-leader, leadership requires four primary attributes. In her chapter on leadership in the third edition of the Hibberd and Smith text, Rodger suggests successful leaders display an ability to translate a *vision* into reality; they possess the *knowledge* and the *confidence* to deal with uncertainty; and, at the same time, they demonstrate a commitment to maintain their *visibility* as nurses. Goldman (1997) refers to these attributes as characteristics of emotionally intelligent individuals.

TRANSLATING VISION INTO ACTION
Successful nursing leaders demonstrate vision when their ideas successfully bond the mission of the organization with the larger purposes of society and the ideals of the profession. That is, nurses expect a high order of satisfaction from their work. Successful nursing leaders take their insights and create a vision that compels the participation of others. In so doing, nursing leaders actually stimulate innovation because of their ability to envision what will happen in the long run.

KNOWLEDGE

For the transformation of the healthcare sector to occur with minimal disruption, successful nursing leaders also have to possess comprehensive knowledge about the larger society as well as about different areas of the healthcare system. In combining knowledge of the healthcare needs of society, knowledge of the healthcare system, and knowledge of professional nursing practice, nurse leaders are able to envision needed changes and, importantly, to assist others in embracing this vision. In order to do so, nurse leaders must have the skills to influence others without polarizing team members along professional, departmental, or specialty lines.

CONFIDENCE

Confidence represents the most personal and least tangible of the attributes associated with successful leadership. According to Rodger (2006, p. 504), "nursing needs confident leaders who have self-esteem and are able to live with insecurity." Not only do they "think outside the box" but they also possess the fortitude to express ideas that run counter to the prevailing wisdom. For example, although public participation represents a fundamental tenet of the "new public health," consultation between communities and providers largely represents a yet-to-be-realized goal. A successful nursing leader challenges those practices that do not align with professional practice goals of the discipline.

VISIBILITY

An equally important attribute of successful nursing leadership is visibility. Here we have one of those paradoxes so typical in this period of transformation. At the same time that healthcare reforms have downgraded the role of professionals (Storch & Stinson, 1988), the complexity of healthcare tells us that professionals consistently play an essential role and that they require the support of healthcare organizations. It is ironic, then, as Rodger (2006, p. 504) reminds us, that healthcare organizations continue to eliminate "nursing positions at the policy and senior-management levels of healthcare agencies." Although nurses still hold management portfolios, now they more often function as healthcare leaders, not necessarily as nursing professionals. This omission of their professional credentials from the administrative work of nurses has serious consequences. For certain, nursing runs the risk of becoming "invisible and disposable." And this diminished profile of nursing can lead to lower standards of care.

Whether one agrees or disagrees that such changes devalue professionals, it seems obvious that professional assessments—at least for individual patients—count for less. This conundrum raises another important question for nursing leaders: How does the system deliver services efficiently without compromising the effectiveness of these services? When people in positions of authority, regardless of their discipline, make decisions about clinical practice based on something other than the goals of professional practice there is the potential to reduce the individual needs of the client or patient to a system of classification.

ARTICULATING THE ISSUE

The issue for nurse leaders and leadership—everyone participating in the leadership enterprise—is that the goals of professional nursing practice are frequently misaligned with the goals of the institutions where professional practice takes place and the government organizations that fund that practice. In addition, it is often the institutions and governments who exert influence on the decision making for leaders and leadership in nursing practice. These competing goals for professional nursing practice are further complicated by the internal tensions within practice among nurses with differently informed goals. That is to say that nurses themselves align with different loyalties in their professional practice.

HISTORICAL ANALYSIS

A historical analysis asks the questions: Under what conditions did the current situation originate and what has contributed to the evolution of the issue over time? In an historical analysis it is also useful to ask: What has influenced the position that people have taken on this issue?

Like their colleagues in medicine, psychology, pharmacy, and social work to name a few, nurses at the turn of this century find themselves without their traditional sense of purpose and autonomy (Storch & Stinson, 1988). Efficiency too often replaces effectiveness as a standard of practice. For example, many nurses now come under the direct authority of business managers with financial agendas. In these circumstances, nurses find themselves measured against outcomes that bear little resemblance to the profession's ideological values. The accompanying loss of purpose and autonomy has untoward consequences on the quality of care and delivery of services.

We are not the first to recognize that the current situation in nursing calls for attention (Nunn, 2001). Nevertheless, unless these problems are addressed, patient care suffers as nurses become demoralized by a pervasive sense of mistrust in the system. This mistrust likely accounts "for decreased commitment and job performance" (Corey-Lisle, Tarzian, & Cohen et al., 1999, p. 36). Regrettably but understandably, the consequence is that fewer nurses seem willing to assume leadership roles. In other words, at the same time nursing faces significant challenges, it lacks a cadre of leaders ready to provide direction to the largest group of well-educated professionals in the entire healthcare system.

SOCIAL ANALYSIS

Changes to the Canadian healthcare system became commonplace in the 1990s. Many practicing nurses still remember how, as students, they received their training in a hospital system with express religious and paramilitary overtones. Supported by the scientific management principles of Frederick Taylor (1947), training emphasized the command-control practice model, which employed a strict hierarchical approach and invested all authority in physicians. By the 1990s, memories of these practices became increasingly distant. And it seems the paradigm shift from such linear, top-down, deterministic thinking has only just begun.

Sometime after World War II, North America began changing from an industrial to a service economy. This change, with its emphasis on meeting human needs, began a transformation that questioned the century-old conviction in measuring human success solely by scientific, industrial, and material progress. Instead of extolling reason and order, society began, certainly by the 1960s, to place increasing importance on the rights and needs of individuals.

Social commentator Alvin Toffler (1980) believes that the self-help and wellness movements represent tangible evidence of how these changes have affected the practice of healthcare. Instead of behaving strictly as passive consumers of healthcare, individuals now behave as active "prosumers," which Toffler describes as a combination of producer and consumer. According to his logic, as patients assume more responsibility for their own care, we can expect a decrease in paternalistic, authoritative, physician-centered thinking (Bulger, 1999).

Certainly, as patients gain a greater role in decisions about their care, they often turn to alternative providers. The emergence of nurse practitioners testifies to a public willingness for nurses to expand their scope of practice. Because patients often perceive nurses as social and economic equals, nurses enjoy special access in helping patients become informed consumers and managers of their health. Of course, this access extends to entire communities where public health nurses have a long history of working with diverse population groups.

Nurses can reasonably expect that the transformation of society and the healthcare sector will present increased opportunities and challenges to provide more comprehensive care for patients. In such an environment, nurses can expect their traditional job titles, with their well-defined scopes of responsibilities, to disappear as healthcare systems devise new, multiskilled teams (Spitzer, 1998).

The changes facing nursing reflect those occurring in the wider society, which appears ready to change the essence of healthcare delivery. Albeit challenging, the question is simple enough: How can the Canadian healthcare system operate efficiently and effectively, especially when an aging population, with heightened expectations of healthcare, makes greater demands of a system with limited resources?

 ## ECONOMIC ANALYSIS

Economic challenges are not new to nurse leaders. "Since the post-war years, at least nurses in Western industrial countries have had to negotiate among the sometimes-conflicting demands and obligations of their employers, healthcare organizations and those for whom they care" (Ceci, 2006, p.56). However, as economic constraints intensify, nurses in professional practice find themselves with limited resources to respond to client situations and with a "limited capacity to exercise control over their practice" (p.56). In her analysis of the effects of economic discourses in home-care practice, Ceci reveals the difficulties that home-care nurses have in sustaining views of themselves as professionals when they experience such limited opportunity to direct their practice. It seems that even in the face of the assessed needs of their clients these nurses felt "obliged to implement organizational priorities that seemed increasingly distant from the best interest of the clients" (p. 56). Nurse leaders, in turn, are caught in the tension between professional practice needs and the economic demands of the institution or organization.

 ## ETHICAL ANALYSIS

Nursing ethics is concerned with the delivery of professional nursing practice and the influence of broad societal issues on the health and well-being of Canadians (Canadian Nurses Association [CNA], 2008). The Canadian Nurses Association recently released the "Code of Ethics for Registered Nurses (2008 Centennial Edition)." The code is intended to serve as "an ethical basis from which nurses can advocate for quality work environments that support the delivery of safe, compassionate, competent and ethical care" (p. 2). The responsibilities outlined in the code obligate nurses to act within the values outlined in the code. However, the dominance of political and economic discourses commonly overrides the opportunity for professional practice questions to be addressed through an ethical framework. Too often it seems that the taken-for-granted assumptions driving decisions are those based on so-called "economic realities" or the privileging of dominant groups in society. Despite the constraints of limited resources and the dissonance of professional practice with organizational goals, the "Code of Ethics" directs nurse leaders and managers "to advocate for and work toward eliminating social inequities" (p. 20).

POLITICAL ANALYSIS

In a political analysis, questions are posed about the connection between knowledge and power, asking how, for example, racist, ageist, and ableist ideologies influence our understandings of particular issues. In this analysis we are interested in how understandings of these ideologies influence nurse leaders and managers. Although there are many examples we could draw on, we will return to Ceci's (2006) research on a current situation in home care in western Canada. In her work, Ceci notes that despite the fact that the largest portion of home-care nurses' clients was made up of older people and people with disabilities, nurses reported being directed to steer "scarce" resources to another significantly smaller cohort: those having the most acute medical needs. In other words, despite the expert knowledge of the nurses and their direct access to observing this client group, their knowledge is dismissed; decisions to direct care are informed by powerful ideologies that value acute care and undervalue people with disabilities and older adults. Ceci suggests and supports through her research the idea that rather than accepting these decisions as inevitable, that we "do, in fact, have choices about how we will conduct ourselves and . . . that our present system is no more, but no less, than a humanly constructed set of possibilities" (p. 67). Given the evidence this research offers, nurse leaders and managers run the risk of being caught between two realities: the professional practice knowledge of nurses and the privileged knowledge reflecting organizational goals.

BARRIERS TO RESOLVING THE ISSUE

If a sense of undervaluation and underutilization lies at the center of nurses' dissatisfaction, it also represents the major challenge facing nursing leaders. As one nursing leader questioned, how can the system reinvent itself so as to re-establish trust with nurses so that they become meaningful partners in the Canadian healthcare system (Shamian, 2000)?

1. Barriers to excellence in nursing leadership arise when there is dissonance between goals and visions of the organization and those of professional nursing practice, for example, when a goal of efficiency and cost effectiveness overrides a vision of safe, compassionate, competent, and ethical care.
2. Leaders and managers face complex decisions of where and with whom to align themselves. Although leaders may theoretically wish to support the goals of professional nursing practice, they may feel obligated to support conflicting goals of the organization, if that is the source of the leader's power and authority.
3. Over-focus on short-term problem solving, rational decision making, and the need to keep things under control can inhibit the leadership strengths of creativity, vision, and the ability to reside in uncertainty.

STRATEGIES TO RESOLVING THE ISSUE

In many ways, the situation for nurses is emblematic of the system-wide problems in healthcare. Better educated and increasingly expected to increase their effectiveness and efficiency, nurses face restrictions that hinder their efforts. Without innovative models for alternative kinds of practice, nurses likely face the ongoing dilemma of how to actualize the self-care and wellness movements. For example, consider the challenge that nurses face in educating policymakers and the public that a comprehensive healthcare system includes not only health protection but also health promotion. Heavily invested in a hospital system, organized around body parts and diseases, governments appear reluctant to challenge the traditional medical approach. In short, nursing leaders have to divest policymakers of the belief that healthcare means sickness care.

Healthcare is extraordinarily complex and requires that providers simultaneously pay attention to the person, the environment, and the system. Regrettably, the system remains highly compartmentalized and too often unresponsive. Yet unless the professions address this failure, they face uncertain futures. According to Spitzer (1998, p. 168), any profession that fails to redefine itself during this transformation "can be consumed, reduced, transformed or expelled out of the system as it reorganizes and adapts."

A recognized nursing leader and past president of the CNA, Ginette Lemire Rodger looks at this crisis as vindication for all the reforms asked for by nurses over the past 20 years. These reforms include:

● concentrating on "health, not just healthcare"
● arranging for more "health services in the community, not just in hospital"

- developing "multidisciplinary networks of practitioners, educators, researchers, and managers, not just solo players" with something to offer patients
- welcoming "public participation in shaping the system, not just public consultation"
- focusing on "inter-sectoral health, not just healthcare"
- using "appropriate technology, not just 'high tech'"
- directing attention to "ecology, not just environment" (Hibberd & Rodger, 1999, p. 261).

Nursing history also serves to teach us that challenges, albeit daunting, are not insurmountable. About 40 years ago, nursing leaders, who long ago recognized the dangers of routinizing nursing practice, envisioned nursing practice as more collaborative. They advocated abandoning the 100-year-old hospital-based training system, with its adherence to the militaristic principle of obedience to authority. In its place, they proposed that a baccalaureate education become the entry point for nursing. These leaders faced serious opposition, and the struggle continues. Nursing requires visionaries who understand the importance of advanced education in preparing nurses for expanded responsibilities in reshaping the healthcare system.

As we celebrate the significant contributions of current and past nursing leaders in Canada, one of the most important strategies we can consider is the cultivation of new leadership. A recent example is the Canadian Nurses Student Association Leadership Boot Camp, held at their National Conference in Winnipeg in January 2008. Co-facilitators of this important leadership development opportunity were Dr. Judith Shaman (President and CEO, Victoria Order of Nursing) and Krista Kamstra RN, BScN (National Career and Leadership Development Officer, 2007–2008). Discussions focused on the views expressed by the Conference keynote speakers in addition to the student's own ideas about leadership (Canadian Nurses Student Association, 2008).

Celebrating Our Leaders

Fortunately, for nearly 38 years the government of Canada, through the office of the governor general, has recognized the outstanding achievements and lifetime contributions of those Canadians, including many nurses, who have made significant contributions to our society. Created in 1967, the Order of Canada lies at the center of Canada's system of honors. Divided into three levels, the Order of Canada includes, in ascending order: members, officers, and companions. Of the nurses who received the order, 36 are members, 13 are officers, and 1 is a companion (Table 4.2).

The only recipient of the highest level of the Order of Canada is Dr. Helen K. Mussallem. Her accomplishments make her emblematic of the innovative contributions of all the nurses who have received the order. Highlighting only some of those instances in which Dr. Mussallem had the distinction of being first or truly innovative makes the point that nurses have made sizeable and innovative contributions to healthcare.

Dr. Mussallem stands as the first Canadian nurse to earn a doctoral degree in nursing. Her published dissertation, from Teachers College, Columbia University, provided the impetus for subsequent significant innovations in Canadian nursing education. In addition, she holds the distinction of being the first nurse to address the Annual Assembly of the Canadian Medical Association. She also conducted a survey for the Royal Commission on Health Services (Hall Commission) and a national survey of Canadian schools of nursing. She served as chair (and the only Canadian) on both the World Health Organization Scientific Group on Research in Nursing and on the Economic Council of Canada. She worked on the formation of the Commonwealth Nurses Foundation and received a Commonwealth Lectureship. She also completed international assignments in 37 developing countries under the auspices of the World Health Organization, the Pan American Health Association, the Commonwealth Foundation, and the Canadian International Development Agency (CNA, July 23, 2001).

Other leaders have received national recognition. They include recipients of the Ethel Johns Award (Table 4.3), given by the Canadian Association of Schools of Nursing, and the prestigious Jeanne-Mance Award (Table 4.4), given by the CNA.

Table 4.2	Nurse Leaders Who Are Recipients of the Order of Canada (1969–2003)		
NAME	DATE APPOINTED	NAME	DATE APPOINTED
Moyra Allen, O.C.	1986	Louise Y. Maheu, C.M.	1992
Myra M. Bennett, C.M.	1973	Edith E. Manuel, C.M.	1990
Barbara Bromley, C.M.	2000	Helen McArthur, O.C.	1971
Susan Calne, C.M.	2001	Maura McGuire, O.C.	1967
Rae Chittick, C.M.	1975	Marvelle McPherson, C.M.	1994
Christina Cole, C.M.	1991	Cécile J.G. Montpetit, C.M.	1990
M. Dorothy Corrigan, C.M.	1978	Helen K. Mussallem, C.C.	1992
Lyle Creelman, O.C.	1971	Margaret Ruth Page, C.M.	1997
Jeanne d'Arch Bouchard, C.M.	2008	Evelyn Agnes Pepper, C.M.	1996
Beverly Witter Du Gas, C.M.	2001	Margot Phaneuf, C.M.	2003
Josephine Gibbons, C.M.	1992	Edith B. Pinet, C.M.,	1979
Alice Girard, O.C.	1968	Edith May Radley, C.M.	1978
Helen Preston Glass, O.C.	1988	Helena F. Reimer, C.M.,	1974
Jean Goodwill, O.C.	1991	Vera Roberts, C.M.	1986
Patricia T. Guyda, C.M.	1992	Ginette Lemire Rodger, O.C.	2007
Margaret Hillson, C.M.	2003	Margaret Sinn, C.M.	1976
E. Prudence Hockin, C.M.	1980	Harriet (Halle) Sloane, C.M.	2003
Margaret M. Hunter, C.M.	1984	Verna Huffman Splane, O.C.	1995
Jane L. Hutchings, C.M.	1972	Juliette A. St.-Pierre, C.M.	1976
Audrey Jakeman, O.C.	1968	Shirley Stinson, O.C.	2002
Jean Cecilian Leask, O.C.	1973	Margaret M. Street, C.M.	1976
Denise Lefebvre, O.C.	1983	Constance Alexa Swinton, C.M.	1987
Marie Lemire, O.C.	1969	F. Elva Taylor, C.M.	1991
Clara Yee Lim, C.M.,	1979	Eveline Tremblay, C.M.	2000
Millicent Loder, C.M.	1982	Sheila Weatherill, C.M.	2006
Kathleen Mary Jo Lutley, C.M.	1986	Anne Wieler, C.M.	2007
Dorothy A. Macham, C.M.	1980	D. Ethel Williams, C.M.	1984

Legend:
C.M. **Members of the Order of Canada** are recognized for distinguished service in or to a particular group, locality, or field of endeavor.
O.C. **Officers of the Order of Canada** are recognized for national achievement and merit of a high degree.
C.C. **Companions of the Order of Canada** are recognized for outstanding achievement and merit of the highest degree, especially service to Canada or humanity at large.

Table 4.3	Nurse Leaders Who Received the Ethel Johns Award (1988–2004)		
DATE	**NAME**	**DATE**	**NAME**
1988	Dr. Dorothy Kergin	1998	Dr. Susan E. French
1990	Professor Joan Gilchrist	1999	Dr. Helen Glass
			Dr. Marilyn Wood
1992	Sister Jeanne Forest	2000	Dr. Shirley Stinson
1993	Professor Marie France Thibaudeau	2001	Dr. Carol Jillings
1994	Dr. Moyra Allen	2002	Edith Côté
			Louise Chartier
1996	Dr. Alice Baumgart	2003	Dr. Margaret Hart
		2003	Dr. Peggy Anne Field
1997	Dr. Denise Alcock	2004	Dr. Janet Storch
		2005	Dr. Carole Orchard
		2006	Diana Davidson Dick
		2007	Dr. Anita Molzahn

Table 4.4	Nurse Leaders Who Received the Canadian Nurses Association Jeanne-Mance Award (1971–2004)		
DATE	**NAME**	**DATE**	**NAME**
1971	Dr. Helen McArthur	1986	Dr. Dorothy Kergin
1974	Dr. Lyle Creelman	1988	Dr. Maria Rovers (posthumous)
	Dr. Alice Girard	1990	Dr. Shirley Stinson
	E.A. Electa MacLennan	1992	Dr. Helen Glass
1977	Dr. Rae Chittick	1994	E. Louise Milner
1979	Moyra Allen	1996	Margaret Neylan
	Dr. Huguette Labelle	1998	Peggy Anne Field
1980	Dr. Helen K. Mussallem	2000	Dr. Dorothy Pringle
1982	Dr. Verna Huffman Splane	2002	Dr. Janet Rush
1984	Dr. Florence Emory	2004	Dr. Ginette Lemire Rodger
	Sister Denise Lefebvre	2006	Dr. Linda O'Brien- Pallas
		2008	Judith Oulton

SUMMARY

This chapter explores one of the central issues that arise for nurse leaders and managers, that is, the decisions to be made when there is dissonance between the goals of professional practice and the goals of the organization or institution through which the leader obtains her or his power and authority. In addition to a historical, political, social, and ethical analysis of this issue, we look at the relationship between leadership and management, the attributes of contemporary nurse leaders, and the need for the development of leadership in future generations of professional nurses. Regarding the latter, we suggest that leadership should be cultivated within each one of us with the intention of fuller participation of all professional nurses in the leadership endeavor.

Add to your knowledge of this issue:	
Canadian Nurses Association	**www.cna-nurses.ca**
Canadian Association of Schools of Nursing	**www.casn.ca**
Health Canada	**www.hc-sc.gc.ca**
Order of Canada	**www.gg.ca/honours/order_e.asp**
Canadian Nursing Students' Association	**www.cnsa.ca**
Nursing Strategy for Canada	**www.hc-sc.gc.ca/english/pdf/nursing.pdf**
The National Office on Nursing Policy	**www.hc-gc.ca/onp-bpsi/english/ about_us/index_e.html**

Online

REFLECTIONS on the Chapter...

❶ What issues, other than the one focused on in this chapter, can you identify for nurse leaders?

❷ In your practice experience this far, what attributes can you identify in nurse leaders?

❸ In your experience, what barriers can you identify to effective leadership?

❹ Provide an example of goals of efficiency and cost effectiveness overriding the provision of ethical, competent care. Any thoughts on how this situation might be addressed?

❺ Of the four analytic approaches used in this chapter, which seems the most relevant to the issues of leadership?

References

Bulger, R. J. (1999). What will healthcare look like in the future? In E. J. Sullivan (Ed.), *Creating nursing's future issues, opportunities and challenges* (pp. 14–31). St. Louis: Mosby.

Canadian Nurses Association. (2001). Communication Services, July 23. Ottawa: Author.

———.(2008). *Code of ethics for registered nurses* (2008 centennial edition). Ottawa: Author.

Canadian Nursing Students' Association. (2008). Leadership Boot Camp. Retrieved July 24, 2008 from www.cnsa.ca.

Ceci, C. (2006). Impoverishment of practice: Analysis of effects of economic discourses in home care case management. *Canadian Journal of Nursing Leadership* 19(1), 56-58.

Corey-Lisle, P., Tarzian, A.J., & Cohen, M.Z., et al. (1999). Healthcare reform: Its effects on nurses. *Journal of Nursing Administration, 29*(3), 30–37.

Goldman, D. (1997). *Emotional intelligence.* NY: Bantam Books.

Grossman, S., & Valiga, T. (2005). *The new leadership challenge: Creating the future for nursing.* Philadelphia: Davis.

Hibberd, J.M., & Rodger, G.L. (1999). Contemporary perspectives on leadership. In J.M. Hibberd & D.L. Smith (Eds.), *Nursing management in Canada* (pp. 259–277). Toronto: W.B. Saunders.

Hibberd, J.M., & Smith, D.L. (2006). *Nursing leadership and management in Canada* (3rd ed.). Toronto: Elsevier-Mosby.

Nunn, K. (2001, February). *What about nursing leadership? A discussion paper for the nursing leadership conference.* Paper presented at the Nursing Leadership Conference, Ottawa.

Office of Nursing Policy, Health Canada. (2001). Healthy nurses, healthy workplaces. *Proceedings of the National Stakeholder Consultation Meeting.* Ottawa: Author, Health Policy & Communications Branch.

Rodger, G. (2006). Leadership challenges and directions. In JM Hibberd & DL Smith, (Eds.). *Nursing Leadership and Management in Canada* (3rd ed.). (pp. 497- 513). Toronto: Elsevier-Mosby.

Shamian, J. (2000). On the heels of Florence Nightingale: Re-energizing hospital care. *Reflections on Nursing Leadership, First Quarter,* 24–26.

Southon, G. & Braithwaite, J. (1998). The end of professionalism? *Social Science & Medicine, 46*(1), 23–28.

Spitzer, A. (1998). Nursing in the healthcare system of the postmodern world: Crossroads, paradoxes and complexity. *Journal of Advanced Nursing, 28*(1), 164–171.

Storch, J.L., & Stinson, S.M. (1988). Concepts of deprofessionalization with applications to nursing. In R. White (Ed.), *Political issues in nursing: Past, present and future* (Vol. 3, pp. 33–44). Chichester, NY: John Wiley & Sons.

Taylor, F. (1947). *Scientific management.* New York: Harper & Row.

Toffler, A. (1980). *The third wave.* New York: William Morrow.

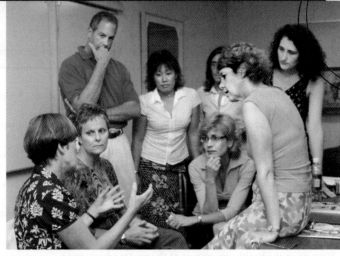

University of Victoria School of Nurse Practitioner students speak with a Ministry of Health representative.

Health and Nursing Policy: A Matter of Politics, Power, and Professionalism

Heather F. Clarke

Critical Questions

As a way of engaging with the ideas in this chapter, consider the following:

1 What comes to mind when you think about nursing policy? Consider one health or nursing policy that influences nursing practice.

2 What do you anticipate might influence or shape policy?

3 Which nurses are most effectively positioned to influence policy? What are the roles and responsibilities of those positions or the nurses in those positions?

4 What have you observed to be links between nursing and health policy and the delivery of healthcare?

Chapter Objectives

After completing this chapter, you will be able to:

1 Appreciate the real and potential contributions of nurses to health and nursing policy.

2 Understand types of policy.

3 Understand the policy process and the significance of contextual factors.

4 Identify roles, responsibilities, and opportunities for nurses in the policy process.

5 Identify challenges to nurses' involvement.

6 Determine strategies required for successful involvement.

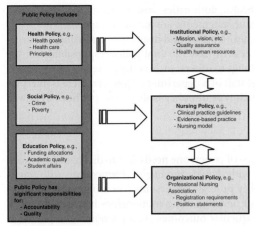

Public policy forms a basis for emerging institutional, nursing, and organizational policies.

This chapter discusses health and nursing policy and nurses' responsibilities and roles within the policy process. Policy is introduced as a process, as a product, and as an instrument. Relevant contextual and infrastructure requirements for nurses' involvement in policy are also discussed and illustrated with examples of nurses' influence in health and nursing policy.

The importance of nurses understanding policy—its development, implementation, and evaluation—cannot be overemphasized. Public policy decisions directly affect the healthcare of everyone as well as the practice of nursing. Nurses can and should become more involved with the policymaking process to ensure that decisions benefit the public at local, provincial and territorial, and national levels. Nursing leadership in the public policy arena will give nurses the best opportunities for putting forth agendas that will accomplish health goals that are in the public's interest.

POLICY, POLITICS, POWER, AND PROFESSIONALISM

Health policy, nursing policy, and institutional policy are all significant types of public policies that call for nursing involvement. A policy—a broad goal statement—has been defined as "the principles that govern action [mandates or contrains] directed towards given ends" (Titmus, 1974, p. 23).

Policy

Public policy is whatever governments choose to do or not to do (Dye, 1978). It is a conscious choice of action, inaction, decisions, and nondecisions directed toward an end—a deliberate choice between alternatives. It is based on a commonly held value, and it gives direction for action (e.g., rules, laws).

Health policy, one aspect of public policy, includes the directives and goals for promoting the health of the public. Health policy may include policy related to population health goals such as provincial health goals; healthcare system principles such as the Canada Health Act (CHA); and service priorities and accountabilities such as the British Columbia Ministy of Health 2008/09–2010/11 Service Plan. (Refer to the Online Resources section at the end of this chapter for more information.)

Nursing policy may be an aspect of, and influenced by, public policy (e.g., provincial and territorial nursing or health professions acts, and free trade agreements) as well as a component of institutional policy (e.g., clinical practice guidelines, care maps, and critical paths). Nursing policy also includes organizational policy of the nursing association (e.g., policy and position statements, nursing practice and education standards and competencies).

Organizational policies, such as those of professional nursing associations, are the rules governing and the positions taken by an organization. Some organizational policies may be determined by public policy (e.g., registered nurses [RNs] or health professions acts and scope of practice regulations), whereas others are association specific (e.g., education standards and registration and continuing competency requirements). Recent trends have been for public policy to significantly determine nursing policy that is of a regulatory nature.

Institutional policies, such as those of a hospital or healthcare agency, comprise the rules governing workplaces. Some institutional policies may be grounded in public policies (e.g., policies governing responsibility and accountability of health authorities and accreditation standards), whereas others, such as mission, vision, and core value statements, are institution specific.

The difference between public policies, such as health policy, and institutional, nursing, and organizational policies is that government does not necessarily have the total policy responsibility for the latter three types of policies. That responsibility belongs to others, such as the professional regulatory body, governance board of an agency, or managerial staff of a department. However, there is interplay and influences between these types of policies, as each type of policy is shaped by politics and power.

Distinguishing Policy From Politics

In determining how to participate in shaping any type of policy, one needs first to distinguish between political strategies and policy agendas. *Policy* deals with *shoulds* and *oughts*. *Politics* deals with *conditions* and sometimes impedes or accelerates the policy process. Politics involves using power to influence, persuade, or otherwise change—it is the art of understanding relationships between groups in society and using that understanding to achieve particular outcomes. As a phenomenon, politics is often reactive. Policy, on the other hand, is based in values, goals, or principles, even when those values may represent idiosyncratic biases (Table 5.1). Policy is more proactive, involving give and take in negotiation (Solomon & Roe, 1986).

Policy development is a value-laden process, beginning with what problems become policy issues and concluding with who decides how a policy will be evaluated. When values are in conflict, as they often are in the health and nursing policy arenas, politics necessarily comes in to play. When individuals and groups with disparate values enter into the policy process, politics, a major determinant of health policy, shapes the content and process of policy development (Mason, Talbott, & Leavitt, 1993).

People perceive politics in different ways. For some, the term evokes images of smoke-filled rooms, devious dealings, or power in the hands of a few. For others, the images have a different and more generic meaning (Ross Kerr & MacPhail, 1996). Whatever the perception, politics can be viewed as the art of influencing another person. There is no escaping politics in any arena. Many nurses recognize the importance of developing political skills, realizing that these skills are as important on the

Table 5.1	Policy and Politics: Some Comparisons	
POLICY	**POLITICS**
Deals with shoulds and oughts	Focuses on conditions
Based on values, goals, and principles	Uses power to persuade and influence
Frequently proactive—negotiable	Primarily reactive—non-negotiable
Stages of development from formation of the problem through adoption of the policy, implementation, and evaluation	Political process is the way policy is developed—requires identification of true issues and stakeholders and their goals and interests
Objective is to be evidence based (e.g., using research, epidemiology, databases in health information, surveys)	Foundation is philosophical—party oriented (e.g., liberal, conservative, socialist)
The chosen theoretical perspective with its values and principles determines details of the policy process	Shapes the content for the policy and the policy process

nursing unit as they are in other spheres of social activity where decisions must be made. For this reason, the Registered Nurses Association of Ontario held a Nursing Policy Summer Institute in 2004 and followed that up with providing online resources—*Taking Action! Political Action and Information Kit for RNs* (2006)—available to all nurses. In both the policy and political processes, individuals require the following skill and qualities:

- analytical thinking
- visionary perspective—future and goal oriented
- force of commitment
- communication of goals
- reliability and integrity.

Power

The concept of power is not generally associated with nursing. The media, the public at large, and other opinion makers refer to the power of major corporations, politicians, trade unions, medical associations, and male-dominated organizations; seldom are the nursing profession and nurses considered powerful (Ferguson, 1993). However, today's idea of empowerment replaces yesterday's notion of power (Barnum & Kerfoot, 1995), and nurses are demonstrating significant empowerment in all contexts of practice. Instead of the capacity one has to influence others to accomplish something they would not normally accomplish, empowerment is authority purposefully shared with others to increase the total amount of nurses' influence in the organization. Nurses, like anyone else, fulfill their mission better when they are empowered to work to their full capacity. The Canadian Nurses Association (CNA) facilitates this empowerment among nurses. Sources of empowerment include the following:

- expanded expertise and restructured practice aim to use each nurse's competencies and knowledge level
- nurses who are valued as scarce resources and knowledgeable workers who cannot be spared to do lower-level tasks
- new legal powers that legitimize various nurse roles, such as nurse practitioner (NP), and public acceptance of these roles integrated into the healthcare system
- new roles, such as clinical nurse specialist in informatics, that provide clinical expertise as well as contribute to system-level responsibilities, such as quality assurance, research, and evidence-based practice
- changed self-perception—accepting one's own ideas or the ideas of one's leader over those imposed by others who would create limitations (Barnum & Kerfoot, 1995).

Why should nurses pay attention to power and empowerment? Ferguson (1985) notes that:

- Nurses must be able to get things done on behalf of the people they serve—they are advocates.
- Nurse educators and nurse administrators need to make course content in schools of nursing and activities in service settings of interest and applicable to students.
- Nurses' power base is expanded as nurses encourage and support nurse candidates for political office and professional organization lobbying efforts.
- Knowledge is power. As such, it confers authority on the possessor. Knowledge, then, may be nurses' greatest source of power.

Nurses find that a number of strategies and skills increase their ability to influence policy (Grohar-Murray & DiCroce, 1997; Loveridge & Cummings, 1996; Primono, 2007). These include the following:

- Enhanced skills and knowledge—being well informed and current—are the basis for attaining credibility.

- Good working relationships with all coworkers are essential and include networking and consultation.
- The ability to convince others of the appropriateness of one's views is based on providing logical arguments and proposing positive solutions.
- Being visible and in a position to speak with groups and individuals is the basis for influencing those groups and individuals.

Professionalism

The *raison d'etre* of any profession is the contribution it makes to society. The nursing profession contributes to the delivery of care and health status of the population. The ultimate reason for enhancing nurses' political influence and empowerment, be it in the workplace, community, government, or professional organization, is to improve the healthcare received by clients—individuals, families, groups, communities, and populations who require nursing expertise (Mason & McCarthy, 1985). Nurses and their knowledge are pivotal to advocating for and ensuring that health and nursing policies promote quality client care through professional nursing practice in clinical, administrative, educational, and research domains—wherever nurses practise. Policy, politics, and power (empowerment) are essential components of professional nursing practice, just as the professional practice of nursing must inform public policy. Therefore, we need to clarify the roles and responsibilities of nurses in policy development, implementation, and evaluation.

 ## HISTORY AND BACKGROUND: PERSPECTIVES ON POLICY

Historically, nurses have influenced, and indeed initiated, public policy related to health and nursing. However, until the past decade, the study of health and nursing policy has not been part of formal nursing education. The science of policy as a domain of nursing practice has received little attention in nursing literature. There is minimal research related to nurses' involvement, the roles and responsibilities for nurses' participation, and competencies required for various contexts of policymaking. This chapter highlights anecdotal accounts of some significant nurse involvement in policy and theoretical underpinnings from a public policy perspective.

Historical Perspective

Nurse leaders, past and current, have clearly demonstrated an ability to mobilize nurses' political strength to influence health and nursing policy to change a woefully inadequate system. Florence Nightingale was a consummate politician who recognized the value of data in influencing policy (Mason et al., 1993). Her fame was widespread in the 1860s as the heroine of the Crimean War, as a foremost sanitarian and social reformer, and as an authority on the management of hospitals and training of nurses (Allemang, 2000). Dock states, "As a reformer and political activist she helped establish a new attitude toward the contributions of nurses in a military environment and the education of women" (cited in Krampitz, 1985, p. 10).

EDUCATIONAL ACHIEVEMENTS

In Canada, after the successful founding in 1874 of the first training school, based on Nightingale's work at the General and Marine Hospital in St. Catharines, Ontario, nursing schools became an essential part of the organization of large and small hospitals. Graduates became superintendents of the schools and hospitals where they influenced policy development and implementation for nursing and health (Allemang, 2000). Later in the decade, Lady Aberdeen, wife of the governor general of Canada, facilitated the development of a visiting nurse component to healthcare and repatriated Charlotte Macleod, a Canadian from New Brunswick, as the first superintendent of the Victorian Order of Nurses (VON) for Canada (Pringle & Roe, 1992). Macleod's experience as superintendent of the Waltham Training Home for District Nurses in Massachusetts was critical to the development of the Canadian VON.

SPECIALIZATION

In 1913, Mary Ard MacKenzie, national superintendent of VON and president of the Canadian National Association of Trained Nurses, brought to national attention the inadequacy of nurses' training. A national committee of nurses and two university presidents subsequently recommended that nursing schools or colleges be connected with the educational system and offer a general course and an honors course with specialization options, for example, district and public health nursing (Allemang, 2000). By 1920, nurses such as E. Kathleen Russell, director of the Department of Public Health Nursing at the University of Toronto; Margaret Moad, district supervisor with VON; and Jean I. Gunn, director of nurses at the Toronto General Hospital, successfully influenced policy to fund public health nursing certificate programs at six Canadian universities: Toronto, Western Ontario, McGill, Dalhousie, Alberta, and British Columbia (Allemang, 2000).

LEGISLATION ENACTED

In British Columbia, just before this educational policy advance, the Vancouver Graduate Nurses Association lobbied arduously for registered status so nurses would have the legal right to set standards and establish training requirements. The Nurses Registration Act became law in 1918 (Brown, 2000). Although weakened from its original form, the act formed a basis for professional legitimacy and won over opposing arguments that if nursing standards were too high, nursing service would not be affordable. Additionally, the legislation would shift control of nursing from the male-dominated medical profession, which thought it should have a greater say in decisions about the nursing profession, into the hands of graduate nurses who were, with few exceptions, women (Brown, 2000). Urged on by nurses, other provinces eventually passed similar legislation. In the last quarter of the 1900s, nurses lobbied for and got revisions to provincial and territorial nurse registration acts that gave them greater control of and accountability for standards of nursing practice, education, and continuing competency as well as protection of the use of the titles *nurse* and *RN*.

LEADERSHIP AND NATIONAL INFLUENCE

Since the early 20th century, nurses in Canada have influenced federal and provincial and territorial health and nursing policy. Some nurses have held official positions, such as "nurse advisor," "chief nurse executive," or "chief nursing officer." Others have supported their professional associations' policy advocacy efforts, and others have acted in advisory and consultative roles to government. Of particular national significance was the CNA submission, "Putting 'Health' Back Into Healthcare," to the federal government's commission for the review of the national and provincial health programs (1980). These recommendations served as the basis for the major 1984 lobbying efforts of nurses across Canada to influence amendments to the CHA (Rodger & Gallagher, 2000). For more information, see Box 5.1.

The new enabling legislation allowed nurses and health professionals other than physicians to be fully used in a reformed healthcare system inspired by primary healthcare. The primary healthcare approach is both a philosophy of healthcare and an approach to providing services (World Health Organization [WHO], 1978; WHO, 1986). Primary healthcare embraces five types of care, which are based on principles of accessibility, public participation, appropriate technology, and intersectoral cooperation. The five types of care are promotive, preventive, curative, rehabilitative, and supportive and palliative. Since then, the national, provincial, and territorial professional nursing

BOX 5.1 Nurse-Influenced Amendments to the Canada Health Act

Lobbying efforts of nurses nationwide in 1984 led to amendments to the Canada Health Act (RS. 1985 c.C-6). Amendments included the following:

1. A definition of *healthcare practitioner* that expanded the recognition of those providing health services beyond physicians and dentists:

   "Healthcare practitioner means a person lawfully entitled under the law of a province to provide health services in the place in which the services are provided by that person."

2. Inclusion of healthcare practitioners in one of the five criteria for federal funding to provinces and territories:

   "9. In order to satisfy the criterion respecting comprehensiveness, the healthcare insurance plan of a province must insure all insured health services provided by hospitals, medical practitioners, or dentists, and where the law of the province so permits, similar or additional services rendered by other healthcare practitioners."

Department of Justice Canada, Canada Health Act. Retrieved August 20, 2004. http://laws.justice.gc.ca/en/c-6/text.html

associations have been clarifying their positions on primary healthcare, a major thrust of nursing, and recommending strategies to attain health for all (Canadian Nurses Association [CNA], 2003a; Rodger & Gallagher, 2000).

Primary healthcare demonstration projects (e.g., Comox Valley Nursing Centre in British Columbia, Saskatchewan's Beechy Collaborative Practice Pilot Project, Nova Scotia's Cheticamp Primary Healthcare Project), position statements, briefs, and meetings with politicians and bureaucrats have been developed and implemented by nurses since the mid-1980s. The CNA (2000a) states that "the goal of nursing practice is to improve the health of clients. In working to that goal, nurses must apply the five principles of the primary healthcare approach. This is true for nurses involved in direct care, in education, in research, in administration, or in policy roles."

More recently, the nursing profession has been successful in obtaining legislation and educational opportunities for NPs as a strategy for increasing choice and accessibility to healthcare in Canada. While professional regulation and licensure is a provincial and territorial responsibility, a framework for national regulation and work has been recognized as an important mechanism for enabling nurses to achieve their potential in promoting the health of the public (2005b). The CNA believes that a comprehensive, proactive regulatory framework is key to maintaining the public's high level of trust in the nursing profession. Based on extensive stakeholder consultation (e.g., policymakers, governments, regulatory bodies, and unions) a national framework was developed by CNA—one that supports coordinated regulatory approaches in Canada, promotes consistent standards across the country, and eliminates barriers to the mobility of nurses across provincial and territorial borders (2007a).

Today, the policy work of nurses is more important than ever. Federal, provincial, and territorial governments are recognizing the need to have senior nurses at the policy table. In creating the Office of Nursing Policy, federal health minister Alan Rock stated, "The new position is a positive step towards finding ways to better utilize the remarkable knowledge and expertise of nurses in strengthening the health of all Canadians" (cited in Shamian, 2000). Since then, Health Canada also created in the First Nations and Inuit Health Branch an Office of Nursing Services with an executive director. Most provincial and territorial governments and the health regions and authorities have also instituted offices or positions for nursing policy and strategic planning. Such positions have also been established with First Nations Tribal Councils that have had health services transferred to their responsibilities. The proactive work of professional nursing associations and unions is increasingly recognized as an important component of public policy work.

HISTORICAL SIGNIFICANCE OF POLICY

Policies determine the context in which nurses provide and clients receive care, whether it is in an institutional or community setting, whether care is privately or publicly funded, which individuals and groups are entitled to receive care, and what resources are allocated to fund services. Policies influence nurses' roles at a number of levels: provincial and territorial; in professional associations, healthcare organizations, and units within organizations; and individual. Although nurses are generally knowledgeable about policies that guide specific nursing practices (e.g., use of restraints and incident reporting), they have less understanding of public policy (e.g., health and nursing) and its relationship to their work (i.e., practice and work environment). Yet the relationship between nursing practice and public policy is crucial when we consider that nurses' daily working lives and clients' daily lives are defined and controlled by this policy.

The CNA states that "nursing is a political act . . . a natural extension of the essence of nursing—of caring" (CNA, 2000b, p. 4). Healthcare privatization, increasing poverty, environmental pollution and destruction, and escalating violence all have clear repercussions for health and nursing. White (1995), after reviewing Carper's four patterns of knowing (1978) and Jacobs-Kramer and Chinn's critique (1998), concluded that the sociopolitical pattern of knowing was missing in the paradigm. This pattern of sociopolitical knowing causes the nurse to question the taken-for-granted assumptions about practice, the profession, and health policies and should be considered an essential nursing competency.

Regardless of the policy context—government, association, workplace, etc.—involvement of all nurses is needed to address health and nursing policy and strategic planning priorities, which include the following:

- nursing-related human resource planning and deployment
- safe, healthy, and professionally supportive work environments
- scope and models of nursing practice grounded in primary healthcare principles
- utilization and involvement of nurses in decision making and policymaking as well as in leadership roles
- nursing data requirements in clinical and administration health information systems and electronic health records
- education for lifelong learning, including undergraduate, graduate, postdoctoral, and continuing professional education.

Theoretical Perspective

Conventional wisdom holds that elected governments make health policy, that federal and provincial cabinets approve programs and policies on the advice of their minister of health, that ministers of health are advised by professional public servants working in their departments, and that Canada's parliament and provincial legislatures then formally make health policy by passing laws governing the health system (Decter, 2001). This conventional wisdom can be applied to nursing policy development at government, association, or local levels. In reality, however, the policy process is more complex and messy and is shaped and influenced by public strategies, media reports, interest groups and stakeholders, academics, and policy consultants. The policy process is not always the same or as rational and linear as logic and democratic beliefs suggest (Brooks, 1998).

Several theories, or theoretical perspectives, have been developed in an attempt to bring more logic and understanding to the policy process. A theory offers an explanation of why things happen the way they do. With respect to the policy process, theories, or theoretical perspectives, provide a map that directs our attention to particular features of the world or issue. Depending on the theoretical perspective, our attention focuses on different features of the situation we seek to understand, different stakeholders and players who will be involved, different priorities to set, and different goals to identify (Brooks, 1998). Major theoretical models include the pluralistic, public choice, and Marxist models.

PLURALISTIC MODEL

A pluralistic model of policymaking in democratic societies views the process as a competition among elites. Powerful groups influence policymakers to have their wishes applied to all (Brooks, 1998). Such groups as physicians, unions, and policy consultants have influenced health policy in the past. More recently, professional nursing associations and consumer groups have become more powerful and influential in the process, advocating for issues related to health promotion (e.g., tobacco legislation), injury and disease prevention (e.g., bicycling helmet regulations), and choice of healthcare practitioners (e.g., NPs).

PUBLIC CHOICE MODEL

The public choice model, concerned with economics and individual positions, grounds the policy process in the strategic behaviors of individuals. Individual politicians and bureaucrats act on the basis of rational self-interest, often under conditions of imperfect knowledge (Brooks, 1998). Politicians and board members seek to be elected and, once elected, to maintain themselves in power, while bureaucrats and staff seek promotion and more control of their work environments (Brooks, 1998). Policy influence is primarily at the individual-to-individual level. Thus, new government chief nurse positions are important for exerting influence on a one-to-one basis as well as within groups, bringing forward nursing issues, perspectives, and evidence-based knowledge.

MARXIST MODEL

The Marxist model is based on the belief that antagonistic relationships exist between different social and economic classes of people. This antagonism is the central factor of politics and policies (Brooks, 1998). The capitalist class, considered supreme, is the determinant of public policy decisions. The private versus public healthcare system policy debate exemplifies the Marxist model. Influencing this policy process perspective may be difficult if the issue is not framed as a social or economic class issue. For example, there is ample evidence that nurses' professional practice work environment significantly affects nurse and patient and client outcomes, yet very few policies for changing that environment have been developed and implemented. Reframing the issue as an economic or political one may be more effective for influencing policy.

Understanding the Complexity of Policy

No one theoretical perspective is consistently taken in the policy process. The perspective differs depending on a variety of factors, including the specific policy issue, timeframe for resolution, political agenda, and power relationships. What is important for nurses to understand and learn is how to become part of the process and use their knowledge and expertise to enlighten and influence specific policy processes, regardless of the theoretical perspective taken.

Policy development involves a conscious choice that leads to deliberate action or inaction. The conscious choice of selecting a particular goal requires a plan of action—or the means for achieving the goal—to be developed and put into effect. Policy goals may be actualized in such products or instruments as laws, regulations, policy or position statements, briefs, taxes, or fines.

Spheres of Nurse Involvement

"Our challenge is to exercise our power and influence and use the political process to help bring about a major change in the delivery of nursing services to society" (Rodger, 1993, p. 25). Professional nursing holds significant and plausible solutions to current crises in healthcare.

Nurse leaders are increasingly aware that all health issues, no matter how seemingly remote from nursing, will have an impact on the direction of health policy and, thus, eventually on nursing. For example, today's nursing shortage is the result of policy decisions made in the mid-1990s to reduce the number of hospital beds and at the same time reduce the number of students accepted into nursing schools. Other policy decisions, such as regionalization, reduction in funds for certain services, redefined scopes of practice, and decreased funding for equipment, have direct effects on nurses' professional practice in direct care, education, administration, and research.

WORKPLACE: THE HEALTHCARE INSTITUTION

At an institutional level, evidence-based policy is required not only to address management and financial issues (e.g., health and human resource deployment and health information systems) but also to make critical interdisciplinary clinical decisions (e.g., practice guidelines for prevention and treatment of pressure ulcers and care maps) and develop work environments supportive of quality care and professional nursing practice. Clinical practice is a political endeavor because nurses must effectively influence the allocation of scarce resources, collaborate in evidence-based clinical decision making, work in the interest of other parties (e.g., clients or clients' families), and facilitate development of health resources and supports for groups and communities. Involvement in the policy process may be related to clinical practice guidelines specific to nursing care, patient safety issues for interdisciplinary care, or system-wide quality assurance initiatives, for example. Nurses in clinical and administrative practice frequently lead interdisciplinary care teams in development, implementation, and evaluation of evidence- and outcome-based policies and guidelines as well as in advocating for practice environments supportive of quality care. The international interdisciplinary study on hospital characteristics and client and nurse outcomes has contributed to our understanding of critical relationships between the work environment and outcomes and notes areas where changes in policy are required (Clarke et al., 2001). In addition to adequate resources, nursing leadership at middle management and executive levels is crucial to improving client and nurse outcomes and contributing to related policy decision making.

A healthcare agency's or an institution's mission, vision, and core values are the foundations for operational policy and decision making as well as strategic planning. Nurses have a responsibility to contribute to the development of their institution's policy foundations and to the philosophy of nursing and client care at both institutional and unit levels. It is the role of nurse leaders and senior executive nurses to ensure that a process is in place to facilitate nurses carrying out this responsibility. Nursing practice councils are one structure that has been used to encourage and support nurses' participation in these institutional policies.

Nurses also need to be aware of their institutions' key policies: the organizational charts with their lines of communication and responsibility (i.e., power); mission statements, goals, and objectives (i.e., organizational culture); and policy and procedure manuals (i.e., expectations). Additionally, all healthcare institutions and agencies have an informal life not bound by a formal chain of command, board of directors, or committee structure. Nurses who want to influence an institution should take stock of the informal structure and processes. Those with formal titles usually have power and authority; however, others who do not have such formal titles can also wield power and influence. It is important for nurses to know where all the sources of power and influence lie.

Policies in healthcare institutions are profoundly influenced by policies and politics of government as well as by changes in the workforce and client populations and by economic and social changes within communities and professional organizations. In turn, workplace policies influence learning experiences for students, new employees, and nurses with new or different responsibilities. Important opportunities, such as mentoring, preceptoring, organizing orientations, and promoting professional development, are directly affected by clinical and institutional policies. Empowered nurses and students can influence such policies and their implementation.

GOVERNMENT

An understanding of political, demographic, epidemiologic, and other forces shaping healthcare now and in the future is necessary if nurses are to ensure that workplace policies promote the health of the public and foster a supportive environment in which healthcare is provided—healthcare that spans the continuum of care from health promotion and illness and injury prevention to rehabilitative and palliative care. One of the most pressing policy issues facing all societies today is the nurse shortage and how to plan for and maintain relevant health resources, with an appropriate mix and optimal utilization of these scarce resources.

Although nursing is a self-regulating and self-governing profession, government provides society with a legal definition of nursing and what is within or beyond its scope of practice. Nursing associations and colleges and individual nurses advocate with government to ensure that nursing legislation and subsequent rules are in the best interest of the public—that they facilitate and support the full participation of nursing practice to achieve the goal of safe and appropriate healthcare.

Government also determines who will get what kind or level of healthcare (e.g., needle exchange sites and medications). Canadian nurses have been influential, locally and globally, in advocating for healthcare policy that promotes health and prevents illness in addition to curing disease, rehabilitating, and providing palliative care. Canadian nurses have also exerted influence to ensure that quality care is accessible, universal, and equitable and is supported by qualified, professional healthcare providers who are publicly accountable. The CNA's advocacy role in federal policy and politics has been increasingly evident at the turn of the century, as has its involvement of individual members and provincial and territorial nursing regulatory and professional associations and colleges (Box 5.2).

In recent years, governments have once again recognized the need to provide infrastructure aimed at increasing nurses' input into the health and nursing policy process. At both federal and provincial levels, positions and offices are once again being created for senior nurse executives. The first federal principal nursing officer, Verna Huffman Splane, was appointed in 1968 (Splane & Splane, 1994); in 1938, Laura Holland was the first appointed nurse advisory to the British Columbia Ministry of Health (Paulson, Zilm, & Warbinek, 2000). Multiple-stakeholder federal, provincial, and territorial nursing committees and studies have also been instituted to advise government ministers and senior staff. It is absolutely critical that nurses support both these current initiatives by contributing their expertise to the policy work to be undertaken and for employers to recognize and facilitate this support as an expectation of their roles.

Through its funding priorities, government can influence which health problems will be researched and targeted for government funding and support. Without nurses' unfaltering involvement in research policy and sharing their nursing knowledge and evidence, research-funding agencies would not recognize the value of supporting nursing research. In turn, nurses would not be able to make significant contributions of knowledge to improve the health of the public. The Nursing Research Fund within the Canadian Health Services Research Foundation (CHSRF) and the Nursing Care Partnership Program are the result of lobbying by Canadian nurses and demonstrate the power of nursing knowledge (Box 5.3).

PROFESSIONAL ORGANIZATIONS AND UNIONS

Professions exist at the pleasure of society and address specific human needs (Joel, 1993). Out of respect for the complex and learned nature of its work, the public allows a high degree of internal

---

 BOX 5.2 Strengthening the Voice: The Ninth Decade of the Canadian Nurses Association

Looking back throughout each decade in its history, the Canadian Nurses Association (CNA) has made a significant impact on the advancement of the nursing profession and the promotion of quality, accessible healthcare for Canadians. The document identified below by its online address is a retrospective of the period 1990 to 1999, the ninth decade since the creation of the CNA.

Canadian Nurses Association. Retrieved March 24, 2008, from http://www.cna-aiic.ca/cna/documents/pdf/publications/ninth-decade-e.pdf

BOX 5.3 The Nursing Research Fund

The Nursing Research Fund was created as an answer to concerns raised by nursing organizations and others representing nursing interests. The CNA and other major nursing voices lobbied the federal government extensively for funding to develop nursing researchers and to support research on nursing recruitment, retention, management, and the issues emerging from health system restructuring. In 1999, the federal government responded by providing the foundation with enough funds to support research personnel, research dissemination, and research projects on nursing management, organization, and policy at a level of $2.5 million per year for 10 years. The fund supports the production of research with health system decision makers in mind, as well as training and personnel support. Nursing leadership, organization, and policy are themes of the open grants competition. In 2003, the CHSRF granted the Canadian Nurses Foundation a 5-year renewable award of $2.5 million for the administration of the Nursing Care Partnership Program (NCP) to support clinical nursing. CHSRF continues its commitment to nursing and nursing research and has demonstrated this through its 2005 report.

Canadian Health Services Research Foundation, Nursing Research Fund. Retrieved March 24, 2008, from http://www.canadiannursesfoundation.com/nursecare.htm; http://www.chsrf.ca/nursing_research_fund/index_e.php; http://www.chsrf.ca/whats_new/pdf/Nursing_week_Report_e.pdf

regulation by the profession, recognizes the complexity of professional practice, and looks to the profession as a collective to define its standards of safety and competence. Until the 1973 Supreme Court decision *Service Employees International Union v. Saskatchewan Registered Nurses Association* (SRNA), collective bargaining was a function of the professional association. The Supreme Court decision agreed with the union's contention that the SRNA could not legally represent staff nurses in Saskatchewan because of management domination. Since then, there has been a separation of professional associations and unions (Rowsell, 1982).

Today's professional organizations' decision-making bodies develop policy to meet their public mandates, move strategic plans, direct the associations' resources, guide implementation, and evaluate outcomes. It is important that their policies target issues that are critical to nurses' ability to be able to meet nursing practice standards, codes of ethic and professional guidelines and to provide clarity about the point beyond which there is no compromise. The professional associations of Canadian nurses have the potential to influence the nursing profession, health policy, and client care.

Professional nursing organizations are instrumental in shaping nursing practice. They develop standards for nursing practice, education, ethical conduct, and continuing competence. They lobby for progressive changes in the scope of nurses' practice and play a role in collective action that influences workplace policies. Whether the issue of concern is primarily nursing or healthcare, nurses have responsibilities to use their political skill and nursing expertise to contribute to their associations' leadership role in public policy development—policy that aims to improve the health of communities and to ensure the provision of high-quality nursing care.

Unions representing nursing are primarily concerned with the development of legally binding agreements that regulate staff nurses' salaries, working conditions, and other negotiable benefits. However, unions also advocate for health and nursing policy related to other issues (e.g., scope of nursing practice and primary healthcare). Nurses may be involved in union policy work—its development and implementation—as well as monitoring contractual agreements. Such involvement is essential to the promotion of work environments supportive of nurses' practice and their health.

Professional organizations and unions have some common goals, including the welfare of members and the improvement of their working conditions. They share a concern for professional ethics, although it is the professional organization that is responsible for ensuring that the standards of professional conduct reflected in the codes of ethics are practised. Although they do have common interests, professional organizations and unions are different in many ways, with different responsibilities and perspectives on public policy, including that related to health and nursing. When relevant, professional nursing organizations and unions work together to influence policy affecting the professional practice of nursing and the health of the population. Such collaboration was evident in identifying workplace issues affecting nurse retention and recruitment; enabling employment of student nurses outside their educational requirements; addressing mentor–preceptor issues; working on the Canadian Nursing Advisory Committee, which has culminated in a final report and recommendations, "Our Health, Our Future: Creating Quality Workplaces for Canadian Nurses" (Canadian Nursing Advisory Committee, 2002); and participating in the Nursing Sector Study, *Building the Future: An Integrated Strategy for Nursing Human Resources in Canada* (Nursing Sector Study Corporation, 2004). When nurses work together, their collective voice is strong.

EDUCATIONAL INSTITUTIONS

Both faculty and students have opportunities and responsibilities to be involved in public professional education policy. Such involvement may be with government-level policy (e.g., initiatives with respect to legislation, funding, scholarships and bursaries, and quality of education); within the institution level (e.g., with respect to mission, vision, curriculum, and learning opportunities); and with associations (e.g., Canadian Association of Schools of Nursing, Canadian Nursing Students' Association, and professional specialty associations) and their policies, positions, standards, and the like (Box 5.4).

COMMUNITY

As members of a community, nurses have a responsibility to promote the welfare of the community and its members. The community's resources can be invaluable assets for health promotion and healthcare delivery. Nurses' contributions through community development and participation in community initiatives provide another credible and trusted voice in the policy process. Outcomes of nurses' contributions can be witnessed in the sustainability of demonstration and pilot projects such as nursing and community health centers in a number of Canadian provinces and territories.

Nurses working with First Nations communities are especially aware of the need to work with the community to incorporate Aboriginal values, beliefs, and practices into healthcare and nursing policies. Reaching community health goals can only be achieved with true partnerships, with nurses contributing their expertise while at the same time listening to and understanding the priorities and preferences of First Nations people. The Nuu-chah-nulth Community and Human Services

---

BOX 5.4 Professional Nursing Educational Associations: CASN and CNSA

The Canadian Association of Schools of Nursing (CASN) was formed to promote desirable standards of education and research and to support the development of future university schools of nursing. Today, CASN, the official accrediting agency for university nursing programs in Canada, is a voluntary association representing all universities and colleges that offer undergraduate and graduate programs in nursing. CASN speaks for Canadian nursing education and scholarship, participates in a national network for discussion of issues in higher education, and contributers to public policy: www.casn.ca//content.php?doc=91.

The Canadian Nursing Students' Association (CNSA) is the national voice of Canadian nursing students. The aim is to increase the legal, ethical, professional, and educational aspects that are an integral part of nursing. The association is dedicated to an active and positive promotion of nurses and the nursing profession as a whole (www.cnsa.ca).

Community Health Nurses on Vancouver Island received the Advocacy for Health Award from the Registered Nurses Association of British Columbia for their advocacy in providing culturally sensitive nursing care to the people of the communities (Moore, 2001). The community health nurses have not only developed a nursing framework that defines their relationship with their clients, setting the parameters of a health partnership that recognizes Nuu-chah-nulth traditions and values, but they have also developed nursing program strategic directions, with client-focused objectives, outcomes, and measurable indicators.

CONCEPTUALIZING THE POLICY DESIGN PROCESS

Policymaking, a dynamic and cyclical process, can be conceptualized as a model of systematic and functional activities (Anderson, 1990) aimed at exploring the causal links between problems and solutions. Shamian and colleagues (2003) describe an eight-phase cycle to move from issue to policy. Although a model is useful, one must also remember that policymaking is messy, often with multiple iterations of some of the stages. There are also power differentials to take into consideration in the policy process. Some current powerful influencers of policy include characteristics of the economy and society and the recent globalization of information availability. The latter has both competition and cooperation potential because of unequal access to information technology within the country. Also, there are differential power relationships between governments (e.g., federal and provincial governments regarding federal contributions to provincial healthcare funding) as well as between governors and the governed (e.g., the professional regulatory organization and its members regarding continuing competency requirements for registration). These differences bring with them opportunities for negotiation and revisions to a proposed or existing policy.

Identifying Issues

Policy problems are identified through situations that produce needs or dissatisfaction for which relief is sought (Anderson, 1990). Policy problems must be brought to the policymakers' attention. Once there, the policy issues and theoretical perspective to policymaking are influenced by many factors (Brooks, 1998). The strengths of political and cultural influences are often determined by geographic location (e.g., rural versus urban), language (e.g., English versus French), ethnicity (e.g., majority versus minority), and values and principles (e.g., public versus private). Problem definition develops as values, beliefs, and social attitudes toward a concern are delineated and policy approaches are considered.

Setting Priorities: The Policy Agenda

Ideally, policymaking involves interested parties coming together to formulate ideas and solutions to given circumstances or problems. In reality, however, struggles for power are, and always have been, principal factors in motivating change (Hart, 1994). At provincial and federal levels, commissions have been formed to help identify policy issues, priorities, and strategies. In recent years, many provincial governments have also established healthcare commissions or *Conversations on Health* to address issues related to healthcare systems and the health profession. The 2001 Federal Commission on the Future of Healthcare in Canada, commissioned to make recommendations on sustaining a publicly funded health system that balances investments in prevention and health maintenance with those directed to care and treatment, released its final report, "Building on Values: The Future of Healthcare in Canada" (Romanow, 2002). Although such commissions provide information for decision making and priority setting, they are frequently linked to politics and the political party of the time. Thus, findings and recommendations are often not acted on because of change in government or political priorities. However, with policy advocacy from many stakeholders, including nursing organizations and individual nurses, Romanow's recommendations for a Healthcare Renewal Accord was signed by Canada's First Ministers, and a Health Council was established.

Policy issues and priorities may also arise from research. However historically, there has been a gap between research and policy—having the evidence available for policymakers when it is required, researching issues of current interest to policymakers, and having policymakers focus on evidence in decision making. More recently, attention has been given to encouraging a closer link between policymakers and researchers. Granting agencies, such as the CHSRF, promote and fund management and policy research in health services and nursing to increase the quality, relevance, and usefulness of this research for health system policymakers and managers and work with health system decision makers to support and enhance their use of research evidence when addressing health management and policy challenges (Brokering Program, 2004).

Besides gaps between researchers and policymakers and the re-examination of issues through commissions, challenges to nurses' consistent and meaningful involvement in setting policy agendas are related to the following:

- dominance of the medical profession
- culture, values, and structures of predecessor healthcare systems
- invisibility of nursing
- stability of the "iron triangle" of civil servant (bureaucrat), politician, and physician (Hart, 1994).

Uncovering the Evidence

Discovering reasons for policy involves discovering the data on which policies are based (Solomon & Roe, 1986). However, sometimes there are no data, just someone's idea of what should be. Although this situation can be found at the level of public policy as politics, it is also evident at the clinical level, where many practices have become policy for less than rational reasons.

Ideally, policy depends on data—data gathered from existing information and summarized and synthesized with a particular question in mind. Existing sources of data used in the policy process include published and unpublished reports, briefs, and research as well as public, stakeholder, or member communication. Thus, it is critical for nurses to pay attention to the development of data-gathering systems (e.g., health information systems and nursing workload and classification systems) and to learn how to make clinical knowledge and wisdom accessible and meaningful to the policy process.

During data analysis—a systematic description and explanation of causes and consequences of action and inaction—conversation among researchers and scientists and among politicians and stakeholders or advocates should be maintained (Anderson, 1990). The role of nurses in data analysis is part expert advisor and part advocate in providing their unique professional nursing perspective for policy decisions. In an open letter from the president to all members, CNA encouraged all nurses to engage decision makers about issues that affect the healthcare system and the health and well-being of all Canadians because nurses have the facts and insights relevant to the policy decisions (2007).

Choosing Instruments for Policy Formulation

The successful attainment of policy goals depends on the choice of instruments for achieving them (Brooks, 1998) and is influenced by values and the theoretical perspective taken (pluralist, public choice, or Marxist). Instruments may include passage of a law or regulation, the expenditure of money, an official speech, or some other observable act. In general, "carrots" (incentives) are less intrusive than "sticks" (commands and prohibitions) and are more likely to be preferred by those decision makers predisposed toward smaller governance structures and greater scope for individual choice.

In deciding how best to accomplish a policy goal (or set of related goals), policymakers consider a number of factors, such as the following:

- political considerations
- past experiences
- bureaucratic or staff preferences
- random factors, like personal values of key decision makers
- measures most likely to achieve the goals
- how the goals can be accomplished at the least cost.

Some of the policy instruments or products particularly relevant to nurses, but also used in other public policies, are the following:

- endorsed positions (e.g., CNA "Code of Ethics for Registered Nurses" by other nursing jurisdictions)
- briefs, position statements, and official messages (e.g., CNA response to the Health Services on Healthcare in Canada, *Putting "Health" Back Into Healthcare* [CNA, 1980])
- strategic policy (e.g., mission, vision, core values, and priorities)
- procedures (e.g., clinical practice guidelines)
- standards (e.g., practice standards and care and accreditation standards)
- rules and regulations (e.g., communicable disease control)
- legislation (e.g., nurse registration and health professions acts).

Adopting and Implementing the Policy

Adoption of the policy, or enactment of legislation, occurs before implementation of the policy. Consideration must be given to ensuring that stakeholders are aware of the policy. For example, most professional nursing organizations publish new or revised position and policy statements, practice expectations, and standards in a form that all members receive. Although it is the responsibility of the policymaker to communicate the policy, it is the responsibility of those affected, the stakeholders, to recognize and take note of any new policy and its enactment.

Implementation is about doing: accomplishing a task, achieving a goal. Policy implementation is the process of transforming the goals associated with policy into results (Brooks, 1998). However, goals established by policymakers may be extremely vague, relying on words whose meanings are ambiguous and open to interpretation. Policymakers do not always know exactly what they want; consequently, their instructions are sometimes imprecise or even conflicting (Brooks, 1998). Thus, goals must be set, well articulated, understood, and translated into programs with budget and funding appropriations. Programs are vehicles by which policies are implemented and ideally have input from those who have a stake in the issue—policymakers, interest groups, professional associations, and others (Anderson, 1990). Once a legitimate authority approves the program, it can be implemented.

Implementation involves such activities as applying the rules, interpreting regulations, enforcing laws, and delivering services. Ideally, at this time, evaluation criteria are set for determining whether a program meets policy goals and objectives. Program development and implementation are usually the responsibility of staff of an organization or government.

Communicating the Policy

Communication is tremendously important; it is a vital link between goals and implementation. Without clear and concise communication about the policy—what it means and how it is to be implemented—policy goals will never be accomplished. Furthermore, implementation and communication problems may be related to coordination within and between organizations. Virtually all programs depend on some level of joint action. As the number of separate decisions that must be made increases, the likelihood of successful implementation decreases (Brooks, 1998).

Recognizing Barriers to Implementation

Other issues confound the implementation of policy. These include the following:

- attitudes and beliefs of program administrators
- territorialism and reluctance to give up that which is considered to be one's own
- external stakeholders' interests
- political culture.

Evaluating the Outcome

A feedback or monitoring process should be included from the beginning of any policy program development. Planned evaluation should be carried out at specified intervals throughout the process to monitor the impact of the policy (outcomes evaluation) and to be certain that the policy deals with the identified needs, issues, and goals (Glass & Hicks, 2000). How do we know when a program works or whether the policy has achieved its goal? How can we be sure that the results achieved have been accomplished as efficiently as possible? Although difficult, evaluation is an important part of policy and its implementation. Successful strategies involve early partnerships among evaluators and researchers, policymakers, and program implementers as well as the identification of appropriate, measurable outcome indicators. The primary difficulties to overcome include:

- realizing that quantity does not necessarily mean quality
- accepting that policy goals may be nebulous and use language such as "promoting," "protecting," or "improving" something
- learning that some politicians have an interest in hard numbers, and others have an interest in ambiguous, or "soft," data.

Revising the Policy

Findings from the evaluation phase should identify whether a program has satisfactorily met the original concerns and should be continued. Segments of the original policy goals may remain unmet, or new issues may surface, indicating that the policy process cycle needs to start again with further clarification of the policy problem.

Given the complexity and barriers within the policy process, it is not unreasonable that nurses and others are skeptical about the actualization of policy intents or goals. However, this skepticism only emphasizes the need for nurses to be involved in *all* stages of the policy process. Whether one is a student, new graduate, seasoned expert, or leader, all nurses can play important roles in the policy process.

IMPACT ON NURSING: THE RELEVANCE OF A NURSING PERSPECTIVE

A policy perspective for nurses must be one that assumes that professional nurses pay attention to what clients need and deliver that service (Solomon & Roe, 1986; Falk-Rafael, 2005; Primono, 2007). That means health and nursing policy are part of the practice of nursing. Nurses need to shape policy in a variety of ways and in a variety of places, not the least of which are the places where they work (Mason et al., 1993). Nursing perspective and expertise are required in government and professional association policy work. Nurses who understand the institutions in which they work, the professional associations they belong to, their community organizations, and the government structures are more likely to be able to participate in the policy process effectively.

Participation in the policy process most likely involves advocacy—active pursuit of the cause. Primono (2007) found that taking a nursing course in health policy made a significant difference to students' political astuteness—awareness about health policy issues and implications for nursing, understanding of legislative and policy processes, political skills, and actual involvement in the political process. Nursing curricula that include health systems and policy may enhance nurses' ability to engage in setting political agendas and advocate successfully for healthy public policy.

Professional associations need the energy, expertise, and vision of all nurses, from students to renowned leaders. Support and influence for professional nursing organizations' policies and involvement in public policy can be expressed in many ways, including the following:

- active membership
- submission of resolutions
- membership on task forces or committees
- identification of issues
- candidacy for or membership on boards of directors
- membership or leadership in a professional specialty group
- support of lobbying efforts with letters, telephone calls, networking, and the like.

 ## FUTURE IMPLICATIONS: CHALLENGES AND STRATEGIES

What is often thought of as a challenge commonly takes on the characteristics of an opportunity requiring particular strategies. Changing one's perspective from challenge to opportunity requires a vision and a belief in one's self and the nursing profession. Thus, the challenges that follow can be thought of as nothing more than opportunities to change what existed in the past and what can exist in the future.

Challenges

Nurses often have the experience of not being listened to or not finding a suitable channel through which their voices will be heard and their contributions to policy valued. Sometimes change occurs and that change is to the detriment of nurses who have not known what the full consequences of change would be. Change also occurs when nurses feel powerless, when they believe any resistance or any attempts to effect change on a specific issue would be hopeless. This kind of change most often occurs when nurses lack the empirical evidence on which to make their cases.

Yet the clinical knowledge and expertise of nurses are their greatest assets in the policy process. Expert power is actualized in the increasing number of well-educated and degreed nurses. There is also recognition of nursing as a learned profession with the capacity for independent as well as collaborative practice and all the attendant and inherent rights, responsibilities, and accountabilities that go along with that status. Nursing curricula that include opportunities for students to learn about the policy process in a variety of contexts can help prepare nurses in the sociopolitical pattern of knowing and to gain related competencies.

Nurses need to feel empowered with the authority commensurate with this knowledge and expertise as caregivers closest to clients and proportionate to their numbers. They need power to ensure their ability to provide competent, humanistic, and affordable care to people; power to help shape health policy and alter the disproportionate leverage of physicians; and power to ensure that nursing is an attractive career option for women and men who expect to influence and improve nursing, healthcare, and health policy (Ferguson, 1993).

The fundamental source of empowerment is self-confidence—the projection of a powerful image that emanates from a sturdy self-image. The key to acquiring this lies, to a great extent, in the hands of nursing leaders and managers in decision-making roles who actualize nurses' legitimate power and have the authority to bring about change (Ferguson, 1985). The role of the governing structures in institutions and government is important in establishing and maintaining organizational and professional arrangements by which nurses control their practice and professional affairs. The workplace must be committed to ensuring that nurses have accountability for decisions affecting nursing.

Some groups are more adept at exploiting the policy process and are better placed to do so. This exploitation can pit the interest not only of one occupational group against another but also of individuals within a particular group such as nursing. An example of this can be found in the increased number of hospital nurses at a time when primary healthcare policies and directions dictate that more resources and nursing personnel be directed into community nursing. "There can be little doubt that one of the primary problems facing nurses is actually identifying what their best interests are and then arriving at strategies for advancing them" (Hart, 1994, p. 184). Not being a homogeneous group endlessly complicates the policy-influencing process, as does nurses' general position in the healthcare system pecking order. The closer nurses in all contexts of practice work together to advance policies that will improve the health of the public, and the more collaboration there is between nursing professional associations and unions, the greater will be the voice and influence of nursing in the policy process.

Strategies for Involvement

Nurses need to be sensitive to the political process. Experience shows that positive results are most often obtained by working with the system, not against it (Glass & Hicks, 2000). Working with the system requires an understanding of the political process, of the global perspective of the health system, and of issues in the local community. It is essential for nurses to be knowledgeable about current policy directions, to be aware of the expected outcomes of the programs, and to participate in the development of policy in the many sectors influencing health and nursing.

Some strategic guidelines for influencing the policy process include the following:

- Educate yourself about the issue, the decision makers, and other stakeholders.
- Vote for policymakers who support humanistic policies. Get to know your representatives personally at various levels—local, tribal and band, provincial, territorial, and federal.
- Participate in your professional nursing association's work; this participation communicates your message to the appropriate people. Hold an office. Be on a committee.
- Join a professional organization with goals and philosophies you can identify with and support in working to shape nursing and healthcare.
- Work with colleagues to transform the places in which healthcare is provided or nursing is taught.
- Involve those directly affected by an issue in planning and carrying out strategies.
- Enlist allies; mobilize a group of colleagues to address a policy issue in government.
- Participate in improving neighborhoods, schools, and communities.
- Speak from your experience as a nurse; learn how to communicate your ideas effectively using examples, analogies, and history.
- Create public support for an issue; develop the important socialization and networking skills to convey your points to the policymakers.
- Use the media (e.g., local newspapers and association newsletters); cultivate relationships with media personnel you believe will be sympathetic to your issue.

- Learn the arts of compromise and tact; sometimes, it is more advantageous to reach half your goal than lose the entire fight. See others' points of view so you understand where the opposition is coming from. Plan your strategy and reach compromise without sacrificing your beliefs.
- Volunteer to serve as a member of a local health or nursing advisory committee (CNA, 2000b, 2007b; Mason et al., 1993; Ross Kerr & MacPhail, 1996; Vance, 1993).

"Walking the corridor," meeting with departmental heads in informal ways, and contributing to policymaking and decision making through telephone calls and conversations are approaches to policy influence that need to be better developed and more readily available to nurses (Hart, 1994). Nurses are beginning to learn the benefits of collective action, mutual support, and interdependence (Beck, 1982) not just in labor issues but also in other issues that affect their ability to provide safe and effective care. Individual nurses increase the power of all nurses when they acknowledge their own expertise and that of their peers. Nurses who participate in interdisciplinary groups with consumers of healthcare services and in organizations, associations, and boards beyond nursing achieve personal growth and help others better understand nurses and nursing.

Knowledge is a strategic resource that confers authority on its possessor. Nurses who view themselves as lifelong learners will have a more potent effect on deliberations and the ultimate decision-making process than nurses who fail to devote time to their formal and informal continuing education.

In a dynamic environment, where conditions change rapidly and power and influence take on new forms, the continued acquisition of knowledge and skills is essential. Power and empowerment are gained, maintained, and expanded as nurses give sustained attention to the perfection of practice, education for practice, research to improve practice, and administrative activity to enable practice (Ferguson, 1993). As nurses compete for increased participation in management, governance, planning, and policy development in the healthcare system, they must value scholarship and continually apply it.

SUMMARY

Reconceptualizing nursing and the nursing role as a political act promotes a new understanding of the role and its relationship with policy. The growing theoretical evidence supports the notion that influencing public policy is a health promotion activity and an expression of caring (Falk-Rafael, 2005) and is particularly suited to enacting Nightingale's legacy of political action as an expression of caring. Nurses practice at the intersection of public policy and personal lives and are therefore ideally situated and, some would say, morally obligated to include political advocacy and efforts to influence health public policy in their practice. Such reconceptualizing will need to defend and expand knowledge in the fields of clinical practice, management, education, research, and policy as well as challenge the power structures that seek to devalue nurses' roles.

Nurses have gradually gained understanding of the processes and skills involved in influencing others, thereby becoming more powerful and exercising more control of the factors that influence their working lives. The nursing profession's history of political action and policy influence is something of which every nurse can be proud. Yet many more challenges in the 21st century require the policy expertise of nurses—expertise that requires political savvy and power.

Nursing and policy, with its adjuncts of politics and empowerment, are as congruent to nursing practice as are diagnosis and intervention—both require acute problem-solving and decision-making skills. Nurses are part of the policy solution to healthcare and public health problems. Nursing's history, both recent and remote, is filled with examples of nurses who have understood the inherent political and policy nature of nursing. Cathy Crowe, currently a public health nurse and street nurse in Toronto, is frequently quoted in Toronto news article stories about dehoused, homeless people. Several years ago, Cathy was instrumental in forming a coalition and having homelessness declared a national disaster (Crowe, 2000). Our individual and collective challenge is to continue such nurses' legacy of being knowledgeably engaged in the policy process.

Add to your knowledge of this issue:	
Canada Health Act	laws.justice.gc.ca/en/C-6/index.html
Health Council of Canada fosters accountability and transparency of the healthcare system.	http://www.healthcouncilcanada.ca/en/
First Ministers' Accord on Healthcare Renewal (2003)	http://www.hc-sc.gc.ca/hcs-sss/delivery-prestation/fptcollab/2003accord/index_e.html
Health Goals for British Columbia	http://www.health.gov.bc.ca/library/publications/year/1997/healthgoals.pdf
British Columbia Ministy of Health 2008/09–2010/11 Service Plan	http://www.bcbudget.gov.bc.ca/2008/sp/hlth/default.html#1
Registered Nurses Association of Ontario—*Taking Action! Political Action and Information Kit for RNs*	http://www.rnao.org/Page.asp?PageID=122&ContentID=1448&SiteNodeID=470&BL_ExpandID=

Online

REFLECTIONS on the Chapter...

❶ Nurses' policy roles and responsibilities may vary throughout their careers. As a senior student or new graduate, identify opportunities to enact a policy role in clinical practice, through student affairs, or in a professional association. Discuss ways in which you could fulfill the responsibilities of that policy role.

❷ One of the major challenges to nurses influencing the policy process is the invisibility of nursing as a political force. How might individual nurses and the nursing profession address this challenge?

❸ Identify a public policy—health or nursing—that has been developed at a government or professional association level. Determine how the policy process unfolded from issue identification to outcome evaluation.

❹ From your clinical or educational experience, identify and select an issue that concerns you and that you think requires a new or revised policy. Compose a letter or submission to an appropriate decision maker to propose a policy change.

❺ Review resolutions submitted to a recent annual meeting of your professional association. For one of the resolutions, critique the background, rationale, and recommendations for policy implications and the feasibility of developing a policy.

❻ Consider ways in which you have been influenced by a health or nursing policy—whether as a citizen, student nurse, or RN. Determine where in the policy process you could have been influential and what strategies you could have used to exert such influence.

References

Allemang, M.M. (2000). Development of community health nursing in Canada. In M.J. Stewart (Ed.), *Community nursing: Promoting Canadian's health* (2nd ed., pp. 4–32). Toronto: W.B. Saunders.

Anderson, J.E. (1990). *Public policymaking*. Boston: Houghton Mifflin.

Barnum, B.S. & Kerfoot, K.M. (1995). *The nurse as executive* (4th ed.). Gaithersburg, MD: Aspen.

Beck, C.T. (1982). The conceptualization of power. *Advances in Nursing Science, 8*, 1–2.

Brokering Program. (2004). Canadian Health Services Research Foundation. Retrieved October 19, 2008 from http://www.chsrf.ca/brokering/index_e.php.

Brooks, S. (1998). *Public policy in Canada: An introduction*. Toronto: Oxford University Press.

Brown, D.J. (2000). *The challenge of caring: A history of women and healthcare in British Columbia*. British Columbia: Ministry of Health and Ministry Responsible for Seniors, Women's Health Bureau.

Canadian Health Research Foundation. (2005). *A commitment to nursing, nursing leadership, organization, and policy theme*. Ottawa, ON. Canada: Author.

Canadian Nurses Association. (1980). *Putting "health" back into healthcare*. Submission to the Health Services Review '79. Ottawa, ON: Author.

_____. (2000a). Primary healthcare approach. Fact Sheet. Retrieved October 19, 2008 from http://www.cna-aiic.ca/CNA/documents/pdf/publications/FS02_Primary_Health_Care_Approach_June_2000_e.pdf.

_____. (2000b). Nursing is a political act: The bigger picture. *Nursing Now: Issues and Trends in Canadian Nursing, 8*, 1–5. Retrieved October 19, 2008 from http://www.cna-aiic.ca/CNA/documents/pdf/publications/Nursing_Political_Act_May_2000_e.pdf.

_____. (2003a). Primary healthcare—The time has come. *Nursing Now: Issues and Trends in Canadian Nursing, 16*. Retrieved October 19, 2008 from http://www.cna-aiic.ca/CNA/documents/pdf/publications/NN_Primary HealthCare_Sept_2003_e.pdf.

_____. (2005a). *Primary healthcare: A summary of the Issues*. CNA Backgrounder. Retrieved October 19, 2008 from http://cna-aiic.ca/CNA/documents/pdf/publications/BG7_Primary_Health_Care_e.pdf.

_____. (2005b). *Accountability: Regulatory framework*. CNA Position. Retrieved October 19, 2008 from http://www.cna-aiic.ca/CNA/documents/pdf/publications/PS80_Accountability_e.pdf.

_____. (2007a). *Canadian regulatory framework for registered nurses*. CNA Position. Retrieved October 19, 2008 from http://www.cna-aiic.ca/CNA/documents/pdf/publications/ PS90_Canadian_Regulatory_2008_e.pdf.

_____. (2007b). *Exercise your voice—your right, your responsibility*. Open letter from the CNA president. Retrieved October 19, 2008 from http://www.cna-aiic.ca/CNA/documents/pdf/publications/Open-Letter-Democratic-Process-e.pdf.

Canadian Nursing Advisory Committee. (2002). *Our health, our future: Creating quality workplaces for Canadian nurses*. Health Canada. Retrieved October 19, 2008 from http://www.hc-sc.gc.ca/hcs-sss/pubs/nurs-infirm/2002-cnac-cccsi-final/index_e.html.

Carper B. (1978). Fundamental patterns of knowing in nursing. *Advances in Nursing Science, 1*(1), 13–23.

Clarke, H.F., Lashinger, H.S., & Giovannett, P., et al. (2001). Nursing shortages: Workplace environments are essential to the solution. *Hospital Quarterly, 4*(4), 50–57.

Crowe C. (2000). My black bag. *Globe and Mail*. March 16:A20.

Decter, M. (2001). Who makes health policy? *Health Policy Forum, 3*(3), 2.

Dye, T. (1978). *Understanding public policy* (3rd ed.). Englewood Cliffs, NJ: Prentice-Hall.

Falk-Rafael, A. (2005). Speaking truth to power: Nursing's legacy and moral imperative. *Advances in Nursing Science, 28*(3), 212–223.

Ferguson, V.D. (1985). Power, politics and policy in nursing. In R.R. Wieczorek (Ed.), *Power, politics, and policy in nursing* (pp. 5–15). New York: Springer.

_____. (1993). Perspectives on power. In D.J. Mason, S. W. Talbott, & J.K. Leavitt (Eds.), *Policy and politics for nurses* (2nd ed., pp. 118–125). Philadelphia: W.B. Saunders.

Glass, H. & Hicks, S. (2000). Healthy public policy in health system reform. In M.J. Stewart. (Ed.), *Community nursing: Promoting Canadians' health* (2nd ed., pp. 156–170). Toronto: W.B. Saunders.

Grohar-Murray, M.E. & DiCroce, H.R. (1997). *Leadership and management in nursing*. Stamford, CT: Appleton & Lange.

Hart, C. (1994). *Behind the mask: Nurses, their unions and nursing policy*. London: Bailliere Tindall.

Jacobs-Kramer, M. & Chinn P. (1988). Perspectives on knowing: a model of nursing knowledge. *Scholarly Inquiry in Nursing Practice, 2*(2), 129–139.

Joel, L.A. (1993). Contemporary issues in nursing organisations. In D.J. Mason & S.W. Talbott (Eds.), *Policy and politics for nursing* (2nd ed., pp. 539–548). Menlo Park, CA: Addison-Wesley.

Krampitz, S.D. (1985). Historical overview of nursing and politics. In D.J. Mason & S.W. Talbott (Eds.), *Political action handbook for nurses* (pp. 10–22). Menlo Park, CA: Addison-Wesley.

Loveridge, C.E. & Cummings, S.H. (1996). *Nursing management in the new paradigm*. Gaithersburg, MD: Aspen.

Mason, D.J. & McCarthy, A.M. (1985). Politics of patient care. In D.J. Mason & S.W. Talbott (Eds.), *Political action handbook for nurses* (pp. 38–52). Menlo Park, CA: Addison-Wesley.

Mason, D.J., Talbott, S.W., & Leavitt J.K. (1993). *Policy and politics for nurses* (2nd ed.). Philadelphia: W.B. Saunders.

Moore, G. (2001). Advocates for culture, advocates for health. *Nursing BC, 33*(4), 18–22.

Nursing Sector Study Corporation. (2004). *Building the future: An integrated strategy for nursing human resources in Canada*. Retrieved October 19, 2008 from http://www.hc-sc.gc.ca/ahc-asc/media/nr-cp/2003/2003_67bk1_e.html.

Paulson, E., Zilm, G., & Warbinek, E. (2000). Pioneer government advisor: Laura Holland, RN, RRc, CBE, LLD (1883–1956). *Canadian Journal of Nursing Leadership, 13*(3), 36–39.

Primono, J. (2007). Changes in political astuteness after a health systems and policy course. *Nurse Educator, 32*(6), 260–264.

Pringle, D.M. & Roe, D.I. (1992). Voluntary community agencies: VON Canada as example. In A.J. Baumgart & J. Larsen (Eds.), *Canadian nursing faces the future* (2nd ed., pp. 611–626). St. Louis: Mosby Year Book.

Registered Nurses Association of Ontario. (2006). *Taking action! Political action and information kit for RNs*. Toronto, ON. Retrieved October 19, 2008 from http://www.rnao.org/Page.asp? PageID=122&ContentID=1448&Site NodeID=470&BL_ExpandID=.

Rodger, L.M. (1993). Nurses and the political process. *AARN Newsletter, 49*(2), 24–25.

Rodger, G.L. & Gallagher S.M. (2000). The move toward primary healthcare in Canada: Community health nursing from 1985 to 2000. In M.J. Stewart (Ed.), *Community nursing: Promoting Canadian's health* (2nd ed., pp. 33–55). Toronto: W.B. Saunders.

Romanow, R.J. (2002). *Building on values: The future of healthcare in Canada*. Retrieved October 19, 2008 from http://www.hc-sc.gc.ca/english/care/romanow/hcc0086.html.

Ross Kerr, J. & MacPhail, J. (1996). Political awareness in nursing. In J. Ross Kerr & J. MacPhail (Eds.), *Canadian nursing issues and perspectives* (pp. 208–215). St. Louis: Mosby.

Rowsell, G. (1982). Changing trends in labour relations: Effects on collecting bargaining for nurses. *International Nursing Review, 29*(5), 141–145.

Shamian, J. (2000). Office of Nursing Policy comes to Ottawa. *Registered Nurse, 12*(5), 5–6.

Shamian, J., Skelton-Green, J., & Villeneuve, M. (2003). Policy is the lever for effective change. In M. McIntyre & E. Thomlinson, (Eds.), *Realities of Canadian nursing–Professional, practice, and power issues* (pp. 83–104). Philadelphia: Lippincott Williams & Wilkins.

Solomon, S.B. & Roe, S.C. (1986). *Integrating public policy into the curriculum*. New York: National League for Nursing.

Splane, R.B. & Splane, V.H. (1994). *Chief nursing officer positions in national ministries of health: Focal points for nursing leadership*. San Francisco: University of California.

Titmus, R.M. (1974). *Social policy: An introduction* (p. 23). New York: Pantheon Books.

Vance, C. (1993). Politics: A humanistic process. In D.J. Mason, S.W. Talbott, & J.K. Leavitt (Eds.), *Policy and politics for nurses* (2nd ed., pp. 104–117). Philadelphia: W.B. Saunders.

White, J. (1995). Patterns of knowing: Review, critique, and update. *Advances in Nursing Science, 17*(4), 73–86.

World Health Organization. (1978, September 6–12). *Declaration of Alma-Ata International Conference on Primary Healthcare*, Alma-Ata, USSR. Retrieved October 19, 2008 from http://www.who.int/hpr/NPH/docs/declaration_almaata.pdf.

_____. (1986, November 17–21). *Ottawa Charter for Health Promotion: An International Conference on Health Promotion*. Retrieved October 19, 2008 from http://www.phac-aspc.gc.ca/ph-sp/phdd/pdf/charter.pdf.

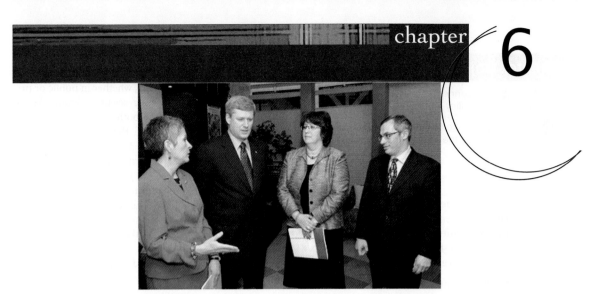

The power of representation is illustrated in political action. Here, Canadian Nurses Association president, Dr. Marlene Smadu (left), confers with the Right Honourable Stephen Harper, Prime Minister, Mary Jo Haddad, President and CEO of the Toronto Hospital for Sick Children, and the Honourable Tony Clement, Minister of Health, during a visit to the hospital in February 2008. (Photo by John Hryniuk. Used with permission of the Canadian Nurses Association.)

Policy: The Essential Link in Successful Transformations

Michael Villeneuve
Judith Shamian
Judith Skelton-Green

Critical Questions

As a way of engaging with the ideas in this chapter, consider the following:

1. What are your assumptions about what makes effective policy?

2. What do you assume to be the link between policy and research?

3. What do you already know about the influence of political agendas on policy development?

4. How do you understand the influence of policy on change?

Chapter Objectives

After completing this chapter, you will be able to:

1. Describe the relationship between research and policy.

2. Explain why credible research is insufficient to effect policy change on its own.

3. Identify and explain the key components of effective research–policy linkages.

4. Apply a basic-change formula to analyze and plan for change.

5. Identify the steps in the policy cycle and give examples of ways the various steps might play out with a real-world issue of concern to nurses.

Chapter Objectives (continued)

6 Describe the connection between political acumen and policy influence.

7 Identify ways in which political acumen may be leveraged in the advancement of nursing policy.

Policy "involves the application of reason and evidence to problem solving, whether in public or private settings. It connects basic scientific knowledge to practice . . . Policy incorporates both a process of decision-making and the product of that process" (Helms, Anderson, & Hanson, 1996, p. 32). In *Health Policy and Politics: A Nurse's Guide*, the term *public policy* is defined as the "directives that document government decisions . . . the process of taking problems to government agents and obtaining a decision or reply in the form of a program, law, or regulation" (Milstead, 1999, p. 1). *Health policy* has been defined as "the principles, plans and strategies for action guiding the behaviour of organizations, institutions and professions involved in the field of health, as well as their consequences for the healthcare system" (West & Scott, 2000, p. 818).

Policies exist as part of the everyday practice of nursing. They are found in many forms:

- governmental laws and regulations
- organizational policies
- union contracts
- nursing unit procedures.

At the most basic level, policies guide "the way things are done around here," particularly when they are explicitly stated. Policies are often equated with rules. And policies may even be found to be limiting, as in, "you can't do that for your patient because it is the policy here that we don't allow . . ." Indeed, Cheek and Gibson (1997) caution that the unrestrained generation of policy—particularly at the organizational level—can actually serve to limit and control negatively the practice of nursing.

Why should nurses be concerned with health policy? Clinical care can be improved either by focusing on the work of individual caregivers or by focusing on the systems in which they work. A clinical policy may guide nurses at the point of care, for example, by suggesting at what age a child should receive a certain vaccination or how often a tubing should be changed in a critical care unit. These "policies" really are examples of rules and guidelines. At the systems level, broader health policy will dictate how many hospital beds and community health centers will exist in the system to provide those services—and what will be the number and mix of caregivers employed to deliver them. The organization of healthcare services, the culture of healthcare organizations, and the quality of worklife are as important to quality patient care as the clinical policies that drive nurse–patient encounters (West & Scott, 2000). Health policy is an important vehicle for influencing and changing the environments in which nurses practise. As limiting as policy can be at times, it is certain that if ideas aren't translated into policy, they won't be translated into action.

This chapter illustrates the reasons that compelling research findings—often demonstrating clearly what nurses need in their work environments to optimize their contributions to society—may not be translated into changes that are needed in nursing practice environments. This chapter also proposes ways to overcome such barriers by recognizing that effective influence of policy occurs when five levers are utilized:

- high quality evidence or research
- effective research–policy linkages
- an understanding of change management
- an understanding of the policy cycle
- political acumen.

Ultimately, this chapter aims to help readers understand and use each lever, to provide examples of how others have done so, to examine lessons learned, and to encourage every nurse to think about and become involved, in some way, in influencing health policy.

THE CHALLENGE: AVOIDING CRITICAL SITUATIONS

North America is experiencing a nursing shortage that threatens to worsen considerably over the next 10 years. Given all the studies of nursing practice settings published over the past 25 years, it seems reasonable to expect that we would have learned lessons to help us avoid yet another crisis in recruitment and retention. For a number of reasons, this hasn't happened. First among those is the reality that, as health economist Robert Evans has said so simply, "policy is possible." Policy decisions taken in the 1990s to reduce the number of nursing graduates had their intended effect. Between 1990 and 2000, the number of registered nurse (RN) graduates dropped by some 40% at the same time as Canada's population increased by 15%. There were actually less RN graduates in 2000 than in the mid-1960s, and, of course, the existing nursing workforce continued to age and move toward retirement. Over just a decade, the balance has shifted such that the number of exits from nursing exceeds the number of new nurses coming into the profession even when we include nurses who migrate to work in Canada. So the appearance of shortages of nursing services in the early part of this century is a result of deliberate policy choices; it is not a mystery.

Shortages

So, what to do about shortages that are now before us? The actions taken to address historical "boom and bust" cycles of nursing shortages and surpluses have too often been short-sighted, providing interim relief but long-term residue. During the shortage of the 1980s, many organizations introduced unregulated healthcare workers to deliver some aspects of patient care. Research now shows that patient care outcomes may have been negatively affected by this decision (McGillis Hall et al., 2001). Alternately in Canada, during the period of fiscal restraint and healthcare system restructuring of the mid-1990s, thousands of nurses across the country were laid off or encouraged to accept offers of early retirement. Thousands more underwent job changes in the "bumping" that followed. In Quebec, the government-appointed Clair Commission concluded that these departures and changes contributed to weakening the level of expertise within the system and negatively affected team environments (Commission d'étude sur les services de santé et les services sociaux, 2000). The short-term solutions in both of these circumstances had long-range consequences that were not anticipated—and might have been avoided.

It is not a sufficient excuse that healthcare leaders and policymakers did not know, or could not have predicted, what the long-term consequences of these decisions might be. Research suggesting a correlation between levels of RN staffing and patient morbidity and mortality had begun to emerge well before many of the policy decisions impacting patients and nurses were taken in the 1990s (Aiken, Smith, & Lake, 1994; Hartz et al., 1989; Knaus et al., 1986; Prescott, 1993).

Second, policymakers, managers, and others have generally done an inconsistent job of translating research into actions. Despite increasingly robust research defining what nurses need to optimize the effectiveness of their work environments and to balance that with the demands of their personal lives, nurses have not always been very effective at influencing those who make the decisions that affect their practice.

Kimball and O'Neil (2001) suggest that several major developments have contributed to the unique and overwhelming nature of the current nursing crisis: a changing demography, a changing healthcare system, changing social values, and an alteration in the nature of work. They indicate that the size and complexity of these changes are so significant that strategies to deal with past nursing shortages will be inadequate for today's crisis. Recent evidence suggests that Canada's looming shortage threatens to rival only that of the United States as the worst of all the member nations of the Organization for Economic Cooperation and Development (OECD, 2004), and most of the member countries report worrying shortages. By about 2011 in the United States, for example, as the population continues to grow, the number of new RN licenses issued will, for the first time, be less than the number of retirees. By 2016, the RN shortage in Canada is predicted to be in the 30% range unless drastic countermeasures are taken immediately and are sustained over the next decade. Furthermore, the OECD work gives every indication that the demand for nursing services will continue to grow.

Actions to Ameliorate Shortages

Kimball and O'Neil (2001) describe a continuum of the kinds of actions needed to address shortages in the nursing workforce. They make a convincing case that for long-lasting, positive impact, solutions that use and respect the nurse as a valued asset and professional partner will be most effective. The four kinds, or stages, of actions follow.

STAGE 1: SCRAMBLE

In the early stage of a workforce shortage, there is a "scramble"—a flurry of short-term actions that are unilaterally initiated by providers of care. Examples include colorful recruitment brochures, international headhunting visits, sign-on bonuses, accelerated placement on the wage scale, and other activities focused on monetary incentives. These kinds of actions treat the nurse as a commodity that will respond to traditional market incentives. In the scramble stage, little attention is paid to changing nursing education, the nature of work, or the structure of the profession.

STAGE 2: IMPROVE

Once the reality and the seriousness of the shortage are clear, employers begin to recognize that nurses have particular wants and needs, after which the employers begin to approach nurses as customers. Interventions focus on increasing choice, reducing stress, and improving safety. Examples of improve-stage responses are improved clinical experiences in nursing programs, scholarships and loans, Internet-based distance learning, flexible benefits and scheduling, and preceptorship and mentorship programs—activities designed to make longer-term investments in people to cultivate their loyalty. In this stage, there is still minimal structural change to the professional aspects of nursing.

STAGE 3: REINVENT

As the challenge of providing high-quality care with fewer professional nurses continues to mount, it becomes clear that there is a need to rethink the ways professional nurses are recruited and trained, how they are integrated into the system, and how they are challenged and rewarded. In the reinvent stage, new roles are developed that blur the traditional boundaries between nursing roles. Examples of reinvent-stage responses include shared governance models, specialty internships, the adoption of magnet hospital values, and incentive rewards for sustained clinical outcomes improvement. The role of the professional nurse in the delivery of high-quality, patient-centered care is not only recognized but also leveraged by the employer as a valued asset. The employer, in turn, is rewarded with improved patient clinical outcomes and satisfaction.

STAGE 4: START OVER

At the far end of the response continuum are interventions in which nurses are viewed as professional partners practising at the upper limits of their professional licenses and respected by consumers as patient advocates, information resources, and teachers and supporters of self-care. Examples of start-over actions include new systems of care delivery and professional practice that cross traditional care boundaries such as academic nursing schools' establishment of community-based, primary-care clinics staffed by nurse practitioners.

Because this chapter is written in 2008, it would be difficult to say that nursing finds itself firmly in any of these stages. A decade into the shortage predicted by the late 1990s, we see mixed signals. Certainly there were indications of "scramble" and "improvement" actions over the past decade. For example, we have seen improvement mechanisms put into place that do make aspects of working life more tolerable for some nurses. But we have not moved to a serious rethinking of the way nurses are educated, integrated, and utilized. What evidence before us would indicate that the roles of professional nurses in the delivery of high-quality, patient-centered care "are not only recognized but also leveraged by the employer as a valued asset?" In fact, responding to the seriousness of the shortage and apparent inertia of response, some nurse leaders seem to have moved past Stage 3 altogether, suggesting that what is warranted is a revolutionary rethinking of the healthcare system and the ways the nurses in it will be educated, employed, deployed, and regulated (see, for example, Villeneuve & MacDonald, 2006).

Regardless of what theoretical stage of response we might be in, a key question is this: How can nursing recruitment and retention be managed in a more predictable, thoughtful, and stable fashion than in the past? In particular, how can policymakers move beyond short-term, knee-jerk scramble and improve strategies to longer-term reinvent and start-over strategies?

This shift will require more deliberate and more carefully managed approaches to the problem, with policy being the key that unlocks the door to these higher-level solutions; it is only with the introduction of significant, broad-based policy change that substantive solutions will have staying power. If nurses want to successfully influence the formulation of appropriate and relevant policy, they must learn to utilize the levers outlined on page 80.

 ## HIGH-QUALITY EVIDENCE

Evidence-informed decision making is a fact of life across the healthcare system in 2008—if not fully in practice, then at least in theory. No leader in the system today would admit to entering into decision making, whether for clinical aspects of healthcare, management, education or policy formulation, without first being informed by evidence and leading practices. Along with this expectation, funding for nursing research and related knowledge initiatives have increased significantly since the 1990s.

Essentially, two basic kinds of information or evidence are needed to make meaningful changes in nursing recruitment, retention, and role optimization:

1. *Information about nurses themselves.* What are the demographics of today's nurses? What will attract the right candidates into the profession? What is it that nurses need to perform their work most effectively? What is required to keep them in the workforce?

2. *Information about the context within which nursing is practised.* What are the health and healthcare needs of Canadians? What are the most significant determinants of health? What changes are occurring and anticipated in the Canadian healthcare system? What can be learned from what is happening elsewhere in the world? What are the plans, initiatives, and political agendas of those in power?

Progress is being made in both areas of research. The information to answer the first set of questions is becoming more plentiful and more robust. Provincial nurse registries now track the demographics of their members in a number of key dimensions. Numerous studies have been published that clearly point out the conditions that will attract, retain, and satisfy nurses. These studies have been cited in other parts of this chapter and in other chapters in this book. The Canadian Institute for Health Information (CIHI) regularly releases papers summarizing what we know and what we do not know about factors affecting the supply, demand, education, health, and worklives of the healthcare providers in Canada (e.g., Canadian Institute for Health Information [CIHI], 2005). Much of the information to answer the second set of questions is also available, although the data are somewhat more elusive and certainly less well known and less frequently accessed by nurses.

If the necessary evidence regarding nursing practice is growing, why is it that those in decision-making positions are not acting on the information? First, the timing may not be right. Policy windows open and close at their own pace, having more to do with election cycles, public opinion, and fiscal years than with the quality of research findings. Even when a study has been directly commissioned and competently performed, it will have to compete for attention with other priorities and influences at the time that it is completed.

Second, although some of the data may be in, the facts are not always clear. Jonathan Lomas, former executive director of the Canadian Health Services Research Foundation (CHSRF), cautions us that with recent increases in research funding come risks. Rather than research supporting and informing practice changes, a gap may emerge between researchers and decision makers (Lomas, 2000). On the one hand, researchers' bias for methodologic purity can limit the practical utility of their findings; on the other hand, managers' push for speed and output can compromise the quality of the research. The CHSRF has developed a unique linkage-and-exchange approach to its work, which it hopes will offset both risks. This approach is in keeping with Davis and Howden-Chapman's (1996) conclusions that research is more likely to be translated into policy if researchers, policy analysts, managers, and politicians negotiate the language and frame of reference before research is undertaken.

Finally, the pace at which evidence is being developed has surpassed our knowledge of how to most effectively use research findings to influence policy. As Canadian researcher Dr. Andrea Baumann observed during a personal communication, "We are data rich and information poor." Chunharas (2001) suggests that although high-quality research on policy-relevant issues with well-packaged and well-targeted products may succeed in informing decision-making processes, the linkages between policy and research will only be optimized through an understanding of the key components of their interface.

 # EFFECTIVE RESEARCH–POLICY LINKAGES

Chunharas (2001) identifies five key components of effective research–policy linkages:

- interface between the dual processes of research and policy development
- sensitivity to the context in which they both operate
- appreciation for the attitudes of the stakeholders involved
- astute use of the research outputs
- role of mediators.

Interface Between Research and Policy Development

Chunharas (2001) emphasizes the importance of building linkages between all steps of the research and decision-making processes, from the definition of research questions and policy priorities to the dissemination of research results and policy or program implementation. He argues that both processes will be richer for the interaction.

Sensitivity to Context

Chunharas uses the word *context* to mean the social, political, and economic environment surrounding the research and decision-making processes. He emphasizes the need to consider deep-seated values, practices, and traditions as well as prevailing decision-making climates and mechanisms and the influence of mass media.

Appreciation for Stakeholders' Attitudes

Chunharas identifies three main stakeholders in the research–policy interface: researchers, decision makers, and members of the community. He suggests that decision makers would be more likely to use research results if researchers involved them in formulating questions and problems. Researchers, on the other hand, may be more interested in conducting needed research if they were consulted about the appropriate approach and methodology, Finally, members of the community—the putative subjects and targets of research and decision making (and who are often intimidated by both researchers and decision makers and are forgotten in the processes)—can contribute much to both the issues that need investigating and the appropriate application of results.

Astute Use of Research Outputs

One of the critical requirements in using research outputs effectively is the ability to tease out from complex research methods and findings a limited number of clear, concise, and relevant messages.

West and Scott (2000) suggest that research ideas (and, we would suggest, messages) related to the "great themes of our times" and those that offer solutions to current problems are more likely to be taken up and implemented than ideas that are not currently high on the political agenda. This assertion emphasizes the importance of knowing the popular themes and priorities as well as the importance of making the connection between "our findings" and "their priorities." To ensure that important research comes to the attention of policymakers, West and Scott suggest publishing summaries of scientific papers in journals that policymakers are likely to read and including *health policy* as key words in academic publications.

Even more basic is the fact that the key policy-relevant messages in research papers are often difficult to locate. From their study of what got the attention of policymakers in presentations by tobacco control advocates, Montini and Bero (2001) advise that advocates present science in a format that is well organized and easily absorbed. Gebbie and associates (2000), in a study of 27 United States nurses active in health policy, suggest that researchers write findings in a style that can help policymakers draw conclusions and include in every study (including clinical studies) a clear and deliberate discussion of policy ramifications.

Role of Mediators

The differences between the priorities, time constraints, languages, and cultures of researchers and policy decision makers have been acknowledged, described, and likened to the existence of two communities that prohibit successful communication. A number of authorities (CIHI, 2001; Crosswaite & Curtice, 1994; Feldman, Nadash, & Gursen, 2001) argue the case for skilled mediators or research-knowledge brokers who can bridge the gaps. Research brokers have been described as individual specialists with effective communication skills, the ability to educate and report, and familiarity with differing approaches and research methods—a hybrid of journalist, teacher, and researcher (Crosswaite & Curtice, 1994). Although Chunharas (2001) recognizes that the mediator role can be critically important, he also emphasizes that researchers themselves must develop skills of communication and advocacy as well as an understanding of how decision makers make resource-allocation decisions and how policymakers develop, implement, and monitor policies. Nurses may argue that nurses and the nursing profession can act in a brokering role, strengthening the linkages among research, decision making, and policy formulation.

PLANNED CHANGE: WHY DOES IT HAPPEN ... OR NOT?

In a presentation to federal and provincial and territorial policymakers in Ottawa in 2001, Dr. Gina Browne, founder and director of the System-Linked Research Unit on Health and Social Service Utilization, stated, "I don't think we should ever fund another study on the efficacy of nurse practitioners. Every piece of research for 30 years has shown the effectiveness of the role. Why have we not been able to translate all those robust findings into action?" Browne went on to answer her own question this way: "I really don't think any more that we have a serious knowledge development problem. We have a serious research dissemination and transfer problem." In other words, leaders and policy-makers in the healthcare system generally haven't been very good at creating and managing change.

Dannemiller and Jacobs (1992) describe a basic change formula that is very useful for both diagnosing a situation and developing interventions in change situations. The formula is as follows:

$$D \times V \times F > R$$

Dannemiller and Jacobs state that change can and will only occur when the product of discomfort or dissatisfaction (D) with the present situation, a vision (V) of what is possible or desired, and the concrete first steps (F) toward reaching the vision are greater than the resistance (R) to the change. It is important to understand that it is the product of the factors on the left side of the equation with which one must be concerned. If any one of these variables (D, V, or F) is zero or near zero, the product of the three will also be zero or near zero, and the resistance cannot and will not be overcome.

Consider this example: Many hospitals have attempted to implement self-scheduling on their nursing units. The appeal (vision, V) of nurses managing their own schedules is clear, and it fits with their ideals of nursing autonomy and work–life balance (let's give the V a score of "1 out of 1"). The steps needed to implement self-scheduling are carefully thought out and put into place (first step, F, gets 0.8 out of 1). About a third of the staff is quite unhappy with the current scheduling system and keen to try the new system along with the manager. Some staff members are indifferent, and some are reluctant (let's say dissatisfaction, D, is initially 0.4, and resistance, R, is 0.2). At the outset of the change effort, the formula looks favorable, if not overwhelmingly so:

$$D\ (0.4) \times V\ (1.0) \times F\ (0.8) = 0.32$$

R, however, is only 0.2.

Nonetheless, implementing the new scheduling practices proves awkward; it creates tensions among staff members, and some individuals do not get as many of the "preferred" shifts as they had hoped. Grumbling breaks out, along with accusations of favoritism or breaking the rules. Some of the original proponents even become disillusioned (resistance, R, grows to 0.5; dissatisfaction, D, falls to 0.2). Eventually, those responsible for adequately staffing the ward (whether front-line staff volunteers or the manager) become discouraged, and the staff votes to discontinue the plan. This outcome can be explained by the fact that the change equation has shifted and now looks like this:

$$D\ (0.2) \times V\ (1.0) \times F\ (0.8) = 0.16$$

Here, R is 0.5.

What was missing in this change situation was that not enough staff members were unhappy enough with the old schedule to carry the change momentum through the difficult adjustment period. Spending more time at the outset getting people "on board" and really wanting to replace the "old, unsatisfactory" scheduling practices with new ones could have enhanced the likelihood of success.

The applications to the research–policy links are clear. One can think of examples of situations in which research data have been the primary drivers of health policy change—for instance, seatbelt and bicycle helmet legislation. In these cases, one might argue that the resistance to the policy change was low, and thus the dissatisfaction quotient did not play out as a large factor. On the other hand, there are other situations—like gun control and, in some cases, the right to smoke—in which organized resistance has been strong, and the absence of strong dissatisfaction with the status quo has hindered necessary policy change.

In summary, credible research may provide the data that underpin a vision of a better world for nurses. A robust and detailed plan may even be proposed to act on the research. However, if there is not sufficient dissatisfaction with the status quo to overcome resistance that may be encountered, desired policy changes may not occur.

POLICY CYCLE

Milstead (1999) elaborates on four major stages of the policy process: agenda setting, legislation and regulation, program implementation, and program evaluation. Agenda setting is concerned with identifying a problem and bringing it to the attention of government; legislation and regulation are the formal responses to the problem; program implementation is the execution of programs designed to enact the legislation; and program evaluation is the appraisal of the program's performance. Milstead emphasizes that "the policy process is not necessarily sequential or logical. The definition of a problem, which usually occurs in the agenda-setting phase, may change during legislation. Program design may be altered significantly during implementation. Evaluation of a policy or program (often considered the last phase of the process) may propel onto the national agenda (often considered the first phase of the process) a problem that differs from the original" (Milstead, 1999, p. 21).

Of particular concern in this chapter are the first two of Milstead's four stages. During the early part of this decade, the federal Office of Nursing Policy (ONP) organized some of its thinking based on a conceptual framework (adapted from Tarlov, 2000) that explains ways in which nurses can move matters onto the policy agenda and how they can move that agenda forward into action. Figure 6.1 illustrates the 8-step policy cycle of (1) values and cultural beliefs, (2) emergence of problems or issues, (3) knowledge and development of research, (4) public awareness, (5) political engagement, (6) interest group activation, (7) public policy deliberation and adoption, and (8) regulation, experience, and revision.

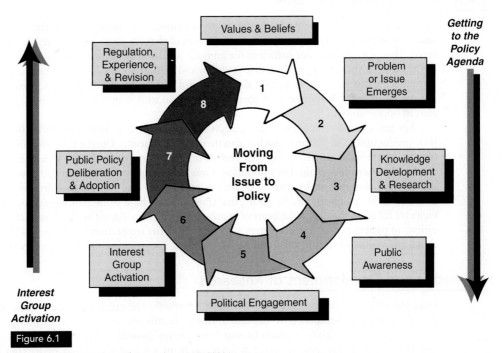

Figure 6.1

The policy cycle. (Adapted from Tarlov, 1999, 2000.)

The actions taken by the ONP to move the issues surrounding nurses' health and working conditions in the settings where nurses practise onto the country's policy tables serve to illustrate how the cycle works. Tarlov's policy cycle suggests two distinct phases, each of which is anchored by a particular step in the cycle. The first phase, *getting to the policy agenda*, is anchored by beliefs and values. If society and its representative structures do not value and believe in the issues that are put forth in the policy arena, the issues will have no oxygen to feed them and they will die on the floor.

The second phase, *moving into action*, is anchored by political engagement. To advance an issue to policy and then to action, political engagement is required. Without the engagement of political sponsors, policy issues can be "out there" and acknowledged by various stakeholders but they will not result in policy change.

Values and Cultural Beliefs

Action on any policy issue must be firmly grounded in a supportable set of values and cultural beliefs. In the case of the *Healthy Nurses, Healthy Workplaces* agenda, four basic—yet powerful—beliefs or values were dominant:

- Canadians are firmly in support of the principles of the Canada Health Act.
- Nurses are an essential part of the healthcare delivery system.
- To offer both access and quality, the healthcare system needs nurses.
- The public trusts nurses.

Identification, validation, and articulation of these basic values were important not only at the outset of the initiative (to ensure that the agenda was value based) but also in moving forward (to connect others who share those values).

Emergence of Problem or Issue

Kingdon (1995) makes the point that an issue can come from anywhere and that in some ways its source or origin does not matter. Rather, it is essential that the issue lands on fertile soil and is nurtured. That is to say, it is not sufficient for an issue just to exist; it must have some urgency. To have any traction, it must be a problem that is visible and important to others, not just to those immediately affected. Kingdon (1995, p. 167) also points out that "policy windows open infrequently and do not stay open long." It is important, therefore, for those who wish to advance policy initiatives to be alert to opportunities.

For years, nurses complained that aspects of their workplaces were negatively affecting not only their productivity and performance but also their personal health. During the 1990s and into this century, they were vocal in articulating the effects of organizational downsizing and restructuring on their workloads. They made plain that the situation was becoming intolerable and that it was contributing to increased absenteeism by driving down job satisfaction and morale and driving up illness and injury rates. Most importantly, by noting that shortages and high workloads were chipping away at the vigilance function that lies at the heart of excellent nursing care, nurses began to tie their working conditions to patient outcomes and patient safety. By 2000, the frustration boiled over, with highly emotional and visible job action surrounding labor contract negotiations in many provinces.

Knowledge and Development of Research

Once the issues are clear and pressing, one must ask whether research and solid evidence exist to support the anecdotal perceptions. In the case of nurses' health, the answer is a resounding "yes."

Data from the Statistics Canada Labour Force Survey showed that in 2002, the rate of RN illness- and injury-related absenteeism stood at 8.6%, up from 5.9% in 1987. That figure translated to the equivalent of paying 10,808 full-time nurses to stay off the job for a full year (Canadian Labour and

Business Centre, 2002). Although statistics were not available for licensed practical nurses (LPNs) or registered psychiatric nurses (RPNs), RNs had a rate of temporary absences due to illness and injury that was 83% higher than the Canadian average in 2002, exceeded only by the group that includes nurse-assisting occupations such as orderlies. That rate has climbed slowly and steadily each year since 1987, with no signs of slowing (Canadian Labour and Business Centre, 2002).

It is not only the absenteeism rate that is climbing. Looking again at 2002, 26% of RNs worked overtime *each week*—considerably higher than the rate of 15.3% working overtime in 1997 and higher than the average of 22.5% reported among all other workers. The Canadian Labour and Business Centre (2002) estimated then that the number of nurses working overtime more than doubled between 1997 and 2002. To fill that demand for nursing services, 8,643 full-time RNs would have had to be hired across Canada in 2002 alone.

Importantly during this time, the ONP team recognized that exisiting data on nursing absenteeism were proxy measures measured through the Labour Force Survey. While suggesting overall self-reported rates, the data did not adequately explain the reasons that might lie beneath the high rates of absenteeism in nursing. The ONP team pushed for the establishment of a national survey of nurses' health that would more fully explain the dynamics of absenteeism in nursing and would include all the regulated nursing groups, not just RNs.

The eventual result of years of lobbying work was the "2005 National Survey of the Work and Health of Nurses (NSWHN)"—a collaborative effort involving the CIHI, Health Canada, and Statistics Canada. The NSWHN examined links between the work environment and the health of nurses in Canada—the first nationally representative survey of its kind. With an 80% response rate, nearly 19,000 RNs, LPNs, and RPNs across the country were interviewed on topics including the conditions in which they practice, the challenges they face in doing their jobs, and their physical and mental well-being. The staggering absenteeism rates found in the study confirmed that earlier studies were underestimating the scope of the problem—and contributed importantly to the ongoing national nursing human resources dialogue.

Previously documented correlations between overtime and absenteeism seem to be borne out in the findings of these various studies. The impact of the RN overtime and absenteeism situation—not only on costs to the healthcare system but also on quality of patient care—is significant and unsustainable. It is especially a concern during a time of shortage to note that dropping the rate of RN absenteeism just to the Canadian average would return thousands of full-time job equivalents to the system.

The relationship between nursing and patient outcomes has also become increasingly well established, through, for example, the magnet hospital studies (Aiken et al., 1994) and the "International Study of Nurse Staffing and Patient Outcomes" (Aiken et al., 1998). Recent evidence suggests that, as a result of hospital-bed cuts in Ontario, more patients have to compete for both fewer beds and fewer nurses. Long wait times threaten patient health and safety, and growing demands on nurses and other caregivers still in the system play out as increased work pace and rising workloads. In light of these kinds of findings, it is even more compelling to note the growing body of research demonstrating that patient health outcomes are significantly better in settings that have more favorable nurse-to-patient ratios and higher proportions of RNs and LPNs on the care team. These studies have indicated that a higher number and proportion of RNs are associated with reduced risk-adjusted mortality, a lower risk of medical complications, a higher nurse-assessed quality of care, and a shorter length of stay (Organization for Economic Cooperation and Development, 2004).

And finally, multiple studies and reports—from the late 1970s (Slavitt et al., 1978), the 1980s (Blegen & Mueller, 1987; Price & Mueller, 1981), and the 1990s (Irvine & Evans, 1992), more than two decades of magnet hospital research (Scott, Sochalski, & Aiken, 1999), through to the most recent studies of Ontario's Nursing Health Services Research Unit (Clarke et al., 2001; O'Brien-Pallas & Shamian, 2003; O'Brien-Pallas et al., 2001; O'Brien-Pallas et al., 2004) and "Commitment and Care," a synthesis paper commissioned by the Canadian Health Services Research Foundation (Baumann et al., 2001)—have clearly, consistently, and repeatedly described the conditions that make a difference to nurses' satisfaction with the quality of their workplaces.

Although additional research might prove valuable, it was more important to make the messages about the existing results accessible and compelling. The ONP set out to do just that, creating tight, succinct, emotionally engaging messages (based on facts such as absenteeism statistics) that could be easily articulated, easily repeated, and easily reported. Speaking engagements for the executive director were used as opportunities to present these messages. To add emphasis and credibility to the case, the many sources supporting the key messages were cited.

Public Awareness

The next phase in the policy cycle is the creation of broad-based awareness—both of the issue and of the solution or strategy for addressing it, as identified in the research. In this quest, it is important to identify as many potential supportive audiences as possible and to customize the message for each audience. When customizing the message, one needs to think as the target group thinks, identifying how they would benefit from change. The various publics targeted by the ONP for the "Healthy Nurses, Healthy Workplaces" message included nurses and nursing organizations, other care providers, employers, unions, politicians (both government and opposition), and the general public. Of course, it was also important to include both the broadcast and print media: Radio, television, newspapers, and magazines such as *Chatelaine* and *Macleans* picked up articles about the health of nurses and the impact of healthy workplaces. That interest has only grown in the ensuing years, and now the working conditions and high absenteeism rates of nurses are common topics of discussion among many groups well beyond nursing and including the public.

Political Engagement

Kingdon (1995) says that for an issue to be placed on a political agenda, it must have been "softened up." The softening-up process refers to the fact that people have to get used to the idea so that support and acceptance for the proposed solution or strategy can be built. This process of political engagement should be designed to initiate a ripple effect that can grow into a wave of support for the proposed strategy. In planning for political engagement, it is critically important to accomplish the following:

- Know the government structure, committees, caucus, and key members of Parliament (those in power, those in opposition, and the nonelected players who have informal power).
- Target individuals with interest, information, passion, or influence regarding your topic.
- Utilize carefully considered, person-to-person contacts.
- Customize the message for each contact person.
- Keep these individuals regularly updated regarding your activities, your progress, and your specific needs for ongoing support.

Milstead (1999) emphasizes the importance of personal stories gained from professional nurses' experiences. These stories provide real-world anchors for altruistic conversations and forge an emotional link that is important in connecting the targets with the proposed strategies. In building support, it is also wise to encourage complementary initiatives that might be undertaken by other individuals or organizations. Our personal observations would be that assuming a "marathon, not a sprint" attitude is key; in most of these cases, nothing happens overnight and stamina over the long term is necessary.

Interest Group Activation

Once public awareness and political engagement have been sparked, it is important to exploit deliberately every opportunity to repeat the message and if possible, to build ripples of interest into a tidal wave. Actions taken by the ONP to engage other interest groups in the agenda included the following:

- direct mail from the office ("Here is the basic message; please spread and respond; please send input regarding any activities happening on the ground in your locale")
- publications (the ONP electronic newsletter, and editorials and columns in other nursing and health publications—both regular and by special request)
- word of mouth (speeches, regional visits, interviews, and formal and informal gatherings and meetings)
- bringing key people together (e.g., a National Policy Forum was hosted by the ONP in February 2003 immediately following the First Ministers' meeting and release of Health Accord 2003)
- direct dialogue with key nursing organizations (e.g., the Canadian Nurses Association, the Practical Nurses Canada, Registered Psychiatric Nurses of Canada, and the Canadian Federation of Nurses Unions) and other healthcare organizations (e.g., Canadian Council on Health Services Accreditation and the Canadian Healthcare Association).

Public Policy Deliberation and Adoption

When the wave of interest and support is great enough, the agenda needs to be deliberately moved to the tables where it can be debated and policy can be formulated. Kingdon (1995) says that once an issue is on the political agenda, it must meet five criteria if it is going to survive: *technical feasibility, value acceptability within the policy community, tolerable cost, anticipated public agreement,* and *a reasonable chance for elected officials to be receptive to it.*

The "Healthy Nurses, Healthy Workplaces" agenda has appeared on public and government agendas, including the First Ministers' meeting (February 2003), in the national level health system reviews conducted by Kirby and Romanow, and in similar reviews conducted in each of the provinces and territories. A final report of Nursing Strategy for Canada (2000) was released in 2003, and its offspring, the Canadian Nursing Advisory Committee (CNAC), issued its final report in 2002. The establishment of a national CNAC—the first recommendation of the Nursing Strategy for Canada—represented an important step forward in the policy cycle. The CNAC offered 51 recommendations to improve quality of nursing work life, further strengthening the positioning of nurses and nursing in the health and human resources policy agenda.

As a result of those cumulative efforts, including the ONP's strong relationship-building efforts within and across federal government departments, health human resources (HHR) was built into the federal, provincial, and territorial Health Accord 2003. Years of work had helped to position the idea of "healthy workplaces" as a key pillar of policy work underpinning national recruitment and retention efforts—and not just for nurses. As a result, the 2003 Health Accord included a specific focus on national HHR planning, recruitment, and retention; healthy workplaces; and interprofessional education for collaborative clinical practice. Nearly $90 million was targeted for 2004–2008 to strengthen Canada's HHR, and the ONP teams had a strong voice at the table when that aspect of the Health Accord was shaped and written.

The 2005 National Survey of the Work and Health of Nurses was an isolated study. Still ahead lie the challenges of putting mechanisms in place to provide accurate, ongoing information about nurses' health, absenteeism, and overtime to update the nursing and policy communities and to supplement—in greater detail—the annual Labour Force Survey.

Regulation, Experience, and Revision

In the final stage of the policy cycle, the proposed action becomes a formal policy, law, or regulation. This entity, in turn, becomes a new cultural value or norm, which is routinely experienced and revised until the next issue comes along. It is in this phase that the "Healthy Nurses, Healthy Workplaces" agenda finds itself in 2008—after nearly a decade of work. During this phase, program implementation and program evaluation take place, and these processes may, in turn, generate new information to continue the cycle.

With this agenda well on its way, by 2004 the ONP was able to move parts of it on to other important players. The CNA, for example, took on much of the leadership around development of quality worklife indicators by 2004–2005 and continues to play an important role in the agenda. Along with other partners, CNA was a founding member of the Quality Worklife Quality Healthcare Collaborative—a national interprofessional coalition of healthcare leaders "working together to develop an integrated action-oriented strategy to transform the quality of worklife for Canada's healthcare providers in order to improve patient care and system outcomes" (see http:// www2.cchsa.ca/qwqhc). The vision of the group is that all Canadian healthcare providers will work in healthcare settings that demonstrate leadership in healthy workplaces and management practices. Importantly the group states its belief that "it is unacceptable to work in, receive care in, govern, manage and fund unhealthy healthcare workplaces"—this was a key value when this whole agenda was first discussed in the late 1990s.

Currently, workplace quality indicators have been developed by the Canadian Council on Health Services Accreditation and are now being tested and integrated into *Qmentum*, the organization's new accreditation program. These indicators will become part of the standards used to assess accreditation of healthcare settings across the country and force employers to think about and address working conditions and their impact on employees and patients. Attention to these outcomes is critical given that outcome measures, such as absenteeism, continue to climb despite a decade of attention and 25 years of research focused on the practice settings of nurses.

Health Accord 2004 put in place accountability mechanisms that require provinces and territories to report on access to health professionals by the public to reduce waiting times and "lead to better care for patients, more efficient healthcare, and greater public confidence in Medicare" (Health Accord 2004). Putting that plan in place will continue to position the importance of HHR and the need to complete the work plan laid out in Health Accord 2003.

POLITICAL ACUMEN: THE DRIVE BEHIND POLICYMAKING

It is important to keep in mind that policymaking is not always—in fact, it is seldom—the rational, step-by-step process portrayed in the previous discussion. It *may* be driven by factual data or logical process, but it is more often a value-driven, dynamic, and at times chaotic cascade of influences and decision-making behaviors. The healthy workplaces agenda in Canada, for example, was enormously influenced by events such as the terrorist attacks of September 11, 2001 and later, the severe acute respiratory syndrome crisis of 2003. Since 2007, attention to health and the healthcare system has been distracted by an increasing interest in climate change and the environment.

Ultimately, policymaking is a process of social influence involving activities of persuasion, attitudinal change, decision making, and compromise (Mittelmark, 1999; Taylor, 1997), which is why the final requisite for influencing policy is political acumen. Florence Nightingale perhaps stands out as the ultimate role model for nurses' use of political skill to influence policy for the benefit of patients. Milstead (1999) traces the current recognition of the importance of the links among nursing, politics, and policy to the 1960s and 1970s, when the explosion of social programs and the raising of social consciousness alerted nurses to the value of political activity. Since that time, increasing numbers of nurses have realized that to control practice and to move the nursing profession forward as a major player in the healthcare arena, nursing and nurses need to become politically involved in influencing and formulating policy.

The CNA has a long history of targeted political activities. For example, CNA produced its first nursing human resources report—containing statistics, trends and issues, and concerns about recruitment and attrition and the need to better deploy nurses—in 1926. Its 1932 "Weir Report" influenced national policy in nursing education for a generation. And since the late 1930s, CNA has lobbied governments around issues such as the working hours and working conditions of nurses.

Recognizing that decisions affecting nurses and their patients were made in Washington, D.C., the American Nurses Association moved its national headquarters to that city in 1992. The CNA made its move to Canada's capital in 1954 to be at the heart of national policy decision making. During the 1980s, CNA would play such a significant role in shaping the Canada Health Act that its contributions were widely acknowledged by political leaders as being among the most significant influencers of the process.

Through the 1990s, initiatives, such as CNA's "Action 301," were aimed at ensuring that across Canada, nurses were actively engaging politicians on issues in each federal riding. And in this decade, CNA is leading the national discussion on the future of nursing and its place in the healthcare system of the 2020s. The CNA board and staff meet regularly with senior federal officials, including the health minister, and on some issues, collaborates strategically with partners, such as the Canadian Medical Association and the Canadian Healthcare Association, in its lobbying efforts.

Groups such as Practical Nurses Canada, the Academy of Canadian Executive Nurses, and the Canadian Federation of Nurses Unions (CFNU) have also widened their activities to include more education of their members around policy and politics. The CFNU has adopted a more evidence-informed approach to its lobbying efforts on behalf of nurses. In other words, evidence suggests that nurses and nurse leaders are rapidly awakening to the notion that the message and the timing really are as important as the content. According to Haylock (2000, p. 76), "for nurses to gain acceptance in health policy arenas, individual nurses and groups of nurses must become expert in assessing the environment, the interpretation of cues, and the development and implementation of realistic strategies targeting priority health policy and legislative issues." To these suggested areas of expertise may be added the use of social networks, rhetoric, and the media. This section of this chapter discusses these means to enhance nursing's political acumen.

Helms and colleagues (1996) emphasize the need to understand how the environment of policy-making shapes both the substance of policy change and the strategies needed for political adoption. They advise that both the healthcare sector and the healthcare policy agenda are large, complex, and profoundly affected by current organizational behavior. They offer a number of tips for nurses and nurse leaders to increase their chances of successfully influencing policy in this environment, three of which are offered here:

- Become "insiders" within the halls of policy formulation so you can identify and capitalize on opportunities of timing and design. This idea gets to a key principle in the world of policy—"you always want to be solving policy problems at the table, not a problem to be solved at the policy table."

- Learn to formulate policy options with greater potential for adoption within the range of available resources and controllable variables. Understand what can be done, not just what should be done.

- Do not try to formulate specific policy objectives too broadly. Rather, strive to nudge policy forward in smaller ways that can incrementally improve the health of the population and the role of nurses.

West and Scott (2000) highlight the importance of social relationships in the policymaking process. They describe *policy networks* as formal or informal groups of politicians, civil servants, policy analysts, experts, and professionals that use their relationships to influence the formation and implementation of policy. Boundaries around policy networks create "insider" and "outsider" roles, wherein insiders are needed by government for advice or cooperation to advance an item on the policy agenda. Nurses must maneuver to be included in policy networks as insiders; they can be successful in achieving this status on the basis of either their specialized knowledge or their ability to promote or thwart the aims and objectives of the policymakers.

Hewison (1999) argues that if nurses become skilled in the art of rhetoric and combine this with a thorough understanding of the policy process, they can be more effective in shaping policy. *Rhetoric* is defined as communication with the objective of persuading or identifying with an audience to influence attitudes and behavior. Hewison points out that language does more than simply reflect that which it attempts to describe; the act of labeling something plays a significant role in how that thing is perceived. Therefore, if nurses become skilled at using rhetoric, they will become more effective in influencing and modifying policy that never makes it onto the policy tables, even though there are people who feel and speak passionately about them. Rather, there exists a complex agenda-setting process, which is an ongoing competition among the proponents of a set of issues, to gain the attention of media professionals, the public, and policymakers. Problems, these authors suggest, require exposure—coverage in the mass media—before they will be considered public issues and thus of sufficient importance to be addressed through policy. The Centre for the Advancement of Health (2001) suggests the following tips for researchers in interacting with the media:

- Get their attention (be strategic!).
- Write an engaging news release.
- Think like a reporter.
- Prepare for and conduct successful interviews.

In 1996, several Centres of Excellence for Women's Health (CEWH) were established across Canada, with the goal to improve women's health. The CEWH research bulletin from the summer of 2001 investigates the influence that the centers have had on policy. Several of the articles describe mechanisms to "get the word out" and to ensure that research findings become part of policy debates. Processes used include media events, research symposia, Web sites, policy road shows, a dedicated research chair, and women's health awards. For example, the Montreal Centre hosted a symposium with caregivers' associations from various parts of the province of Quebec and then took this information, along with 5 years of research experience on women caregivers and a coalition of interested groups, into public consultations to change policy at the local community-health level.

The CNA has published several helpful documents for nurses wishing to enhance their knowledge and skills in the political arena, for example, "Getting Started: A Political Action Guide for Canada's Registered Nurses" (1997), "Nursing Is a Political Act: The Bigger Picture" (2000), and "Campaign 2008—CNA's Three Issues for the Next Election" (2008). CNA's Web site includes a number of companion documents encouraging nurses to engage in the policy and policical processes—and helping them anticipate what to expect. Similar publications are available from a number of provincial nursing associations as well as from unions and other bodies. A good example is the College and Association of Registered Nurses of Alberta's (CARNA's) *MLA Mentorship Program*, which encourages registered nurses to engage and interact with elected representatives to promote understanding of CARNA's positions and increase the individual nurse's understanding of ways that nurses can influence public health policy. And in 2007, CNA launched its new "Influencing Public Policy: Capacity Building Strategies and Tactics" workshop in South Africa. The Canadian program, beginning in 2008, provides nurses an intensive 2-day workshop exposing them to the theory and practice of a broad range of policy and political skills.

OVERCOMING BARRIERS: LESSONS FROM THOSE WHO HAVE WALKED BEFORE

In countless situations, nurses have been involved with change in general and the policy cycle in particular. Examples that illustrate many of the points made in this chapter follow.

Success Abroad

Aitken and coworkers (2001) describe the successful creation of a bill to fund a nurse home-visitation program for high-risk mothers in Arkansas. In summarizing what allowed them to be successful in this policy initiative, the authors noted six factors:

1. realistic time commitment
2. community needs assessment, data assimilation, and review of existing resources
3. identification and incorporation of stakeholders
4. narrow focus on the area of greatest need
5. backing of political partners
6. favorable opportunities to advance child health issues.

Valentine (2000, pp. 45–46) shares policymaking and political lessons learned in the course of a partially successful crusade to upgrade the chief nurse position in the U.S. Veterans Health Administration. Her insights and words of advice include the following:

1. Advocacy for a decision-making role in an organization requires stamina and commitment and takes time, effort, and passion.
2. Changing organizational culture takes time and requires the involvement of senior-level champions.
3. Never underestimate the value of non-nurse advocates.
4. Never underestimate the value of turnover among one's adversaries.
5. Nurses are right much of the time, but not all of the time—we need to listen to criticism more carefully.
6. Benchmarking is important, but it may not be sufficient to call the question.
7. There is no such thing as overnight success. The keys are hard work and never giving up.

Success at Home

Nurses do not have to look south of the border for examples. Professional nurses and nursing organizations across Canada have been successful in influencing policy change in several different venues. Take the following examples:

1. Across the country, provincial and territorial governments are putting in place regulatory mechanisms and legislation that will facilitate increased opportunities for the employment of nurse practitioners (NPs). New legislation will permit employers to engage the services of NPs wherever there is felt to be a need. That outcome reflects the culmination of a careful, collaborative process spearheaded by the CNA, its members, and its partners over many years. In 2004, CNA received $8 million in funding from Health Canada to integrate and sustain the role of the NP in primary healthcare by undertaking initiatives across the country in educational preparation, practice, policy, legislation, government and professional self-regulation, health human resource planning, change management, social marketing, and strategic communication. This project was given life within an environment of growing advocacy for primary healthcare—specifically, one in which the NP role in primary healthcare delivery was recognized as perhaps the most important initiative in health reform. For example, the College and Association of Registered Nurses of Alberta recognized the opportunity and timing and led the policy lobby in Alberta while governments worked collaboratively and enabled legislative changes, employers agreed to provide the actual employment and contractual arrangements, and nurse educators implemented the requisite NP programs—all serving as a prime example of nurse-led policy change that took perfect advantage of timing, stakeholder interest, and

political will. One of the outcomes of all this work is seen in the 60% increase in the number of NPs in Canada between 2003 and 2006.

2. In Quebec, the Ordre des infirmières et infirmiers du Québec (2000) actively used its political clout to obtain government adoption of a regulation enabling second-year nursing students to be hired as "externs" for summer and holiday season vacation relief work. This regulation, which benefits both the nursing students and employers, resulted in nearly 1,200 students being hired by 50 institutions in its second year of operation.

3. In the late 1980s, in response to research and lobbying by nursing associations for nurses to have greater participation in the decisions that affected them, the Ontario Minister of Health introduced a new regulation to the Public Hospitals Act, mandating the seating of elected staff nurses and (s)elected nurse managers on all hospital committees dealing with administrative, financial, operational, and planning matters (Skelton-Green, 1996).

4. In Saskatchewan, the "Band-Aid" campaign, led by student nurses and supported by the Saskatchewan Registered Nurses Association (SRNA), was significantly influential in forcing the provincial government to backtrack on an announced policy change that would have caused nursing education to revert from the baccalaureate degree to the diploma. In January 2000, the provincial government had said it could not support the SRNA's position on baccalaureate education as entry to practice for RNs and was going to look again at diploma programs. Backed by SRNA, the student nurses sent postcards to every member of the legislative assembly and to the premier and appeared in person on the steps of the legislature, asserting that reverting to diploma education was a "Band-Aid" solution that would do nothing for nursing recruitment and retention in the long term. Eventually, the government dropped its plan and has since supported the SRNA in its position on the minimal education for RNs.

5. In 1998, a nursing task force was established to address concerns regarding the future supply and retention of RNs and LPNs in Ontario. In 1999, in response to one of the two key recommendations of the task force, the Minister of Health and Long-Term Care (MOHLTC) created a $375 million Nursing Enhancement Fund (NEF). Over the next 2 years, the NEF supported more than 12,000 new nursing positions in the province (Joint Provincial Nursing Committee, 2001) and the rate of full-time work has increased (Joint Provincial Nursing Committee, 2004). As of June 2003, a total of 164 advanced clinical and practice fellowships had been awarded and 123 completed. Development of a broad slate of best practice guidelines is under way with funding through the MOHLTC, Health Canada, and the Registered Nurses Association of Ontario.

6. At the federal level, it was the successful lobbying of nurses, nursing organizations (such as the CNA), and individual nurse leaders that led to the creation of the ONP in 1999 and revival of the notion of a chief nurse for Canada. The same soon held true across the country as senior nurses were appointed in the governments of nearly every province.

These are just a few among dozens of success stories that continue to emerge, showing that clearly, Canadian nurses can make a difference in the development of healthy public policy!

OVERCOMING BARRIERS AND INITIATING ACTION

Nurses and the nursing profession are at the center of public health issues that are of tremendous and enduring importance—issues such as who has access to what providers and what makes a difference in quality and cost effectiveness of care. There are also issues crucial to the future of the nursing profession, such as who will be the gatekeeper in primary care and what is the appropriate scope of practice for RNs, LPNs, and RPNs across various service sectors. As Milstead (1999) says in *Health Policy and Politics: A Nurse's Guide:*

Nurses are articulate experts who can address both the rational shaping of policy and the emotional aspects of the process. Nurses cannot afford to limit their actions to monitoring bills; they must seize the initiative and use their considerable collective and individual influence to ensure the health, welfare, and protection of the public and healthcare professionals (p. 23).

She also says, "The opportunity to sustain an ongoing, meaningful dialogue with those who represent [us] . . . and those who administer public programs is ours to initiate. Nurses must become indispensable to elected and appointed officials (p. xi)."

Milstead contends that nurses who have been reluctant to become "political" cannot afford to do so any longer. She emphasizes that "each nurse counts, and collectively, nursing is a major actor in the effort to ensure the country's healthy future" (Milstead, 1999, p. 34). Gebbie and coauthors (2000) suggest several strategies that individual nurses can use to influence policy formulation:

- Cultivate and maintain relationships with knowledgeable and influential people.
- Become knowledgeable about current developments on policy-relevant issues.
- Join professional nursing organizations.
- Develop network strategies to mentor political neophytes.
- Share the "how to" success stories of individual nurses and nursing organizations in the policy arena.
- Create linkages between nursing research and political and policy-related activity.
- Develop clear, well-informed, jargon-free communication when interacting with policymakers.
- Capitalize on the positive views that communities have of the nursing profession by being visible at forums and other community meetings.

If individual nurses can do this much, organized nursing groups can accomplish even more. For example, Gebbie and coauthors (2000) suggest that representatives from nursing organizations could develop an annual national institute for policy to bring nurses' best research into the policy arena. Professional nursing organizations could set aside time at national meetings to allow nurses to converse about health policy strategies and activities and include planned discussions of ways that nurses can effectively influence health policy at individual and organizational levels. Individuals in these organizations should become experts in interacting with the media and positioning their work to draw media attention.

The perspective of nurses in shaping health policy is essential. Together, RNs, LPNs, and RPNs accounted for just under 50% of the Canadian health workforce in 2003 (CIHI, 2005). They exert an enormous influence on the health of this nation. Nurses know about health and healthcare; they know about communities and people. It is the knowledge and experience of nurses that shaped much of the public health history of this country and contributed significantly to the state of health that makes Canadians the envy of most of the world. It is the vigilance of nurses in hospitals, nursing homes, and long-term care facilities that continues to shepherd patients safely through their health challenges and transitions. The presence of nurses comforts, prevents disease, and improves health. And we know now that when the system creates conditions that result in too few nurses, the impact of work overload and fatigue on patients, families, and nurses themselves can be catastrophic. Nurses' voices must be heard and their knowledge integrated as health and social policy is developed. And so, this chapter concludes with a challenge to all nurses to think about ways in which they can positively influence health policy, both individually and collectively and wherever they practise.

SUMMARY

Effective policy is best linked with research findings. In healthcare, an example of what happens when policy does not factor in research is the recurrent cycle of nursing shortages.

Research indicates what nurses need in their work environments to optimize their contributions to healthcare, but these findings went unheeded when policymakers implemented workforce cutbacks.

A variety of levers can be used to effect change and influence healthcare policy. They include conducting credible research, making effective links between research and policy, understanding how to initiate and manage change, understanding the policy cycle, and being politically savvy.

Research is more likely to be translated into policy if researchers, policy analysts, managers, and politicians negotiate the language and frame of reference before any research is undertaken.

Keys to effecting change are having an appreciation and an understanding of the policy cycle, which includes agenda creation, legislation and regulation, program implementation, and program evaluation. Behind the development of policy are values and cultural beliefs from which certain problems or issues emerge. Ideally, interested parties then build knowledge and research related to the problems or issues; they bring the knowledge to the attention of the public, become politically active in various arenas, and participate in the activation of interest groups. Public deliberation and adoption of policy related to the issues ensue, and ongoing regulation, revision, and refinement of the policy follow. A component of most successful policies is political acumen, a process of social influence involving activities of persuasion, attitudinal change, decision making, and compromise.

Valuable tools and tactics for successful policymaking include maintaining ongoing positive relationships with knowledgeable and influential people, being interested in and understanding current developments in policy-relevant issues, promoting activity in professional nursing organizations, networking and mentoring, sharing success stories and previously successful strategies, creating links between nursing research and political and policy-related activity, communicating clearly and intelligently with policymakers, and capitalizing on nursing's positive aspects and image in the community.

Add to your knowledge of this issue:		Online
Canada Health Infoway	www.infoway-inforoute.ca	
Canadian Institute for Health Information	www.cihi.com	
Canadian Patient Safety Institute	www.cpsi-icsp.ca	
First Ministers' Accord on Healthcare Renewal (2003)	www.hc-sc.gc.ca/english/hca2003/accord.html	
First Ministers' Meeting on the Future of Healthcare (2004): A 10-year plan to strengthen healthcare	www.hc-sc.gc.ca/english/hca2003/fmm/index .html	
Health Council of Canada	www.hcc-ccs.ca	
Institute of Medicine (U.S.)	www.iom.edu	
National Forum for Healthcare Quality Measurement and Reporting	www.qualityforum.org	
The Organisation for Economic Co-operation & Development	www.oecd.org	
Patient Safety Institute (U.S.)	www.ptsafety.org	
QWQHC	http://www2.cchsa.ca/qwqhc/	
Statistics Canada	www.statcan.ca	
World Health Organization	www.who.int/en	

REFLECTIONS on the Chapter...

1 Think of an existing healthcare policy that you consider successful. What kind of research, if any, do you think is linked to this policy? What factors do you think make the policy successful?

2 Alone or with a group of classmates, select a problem or an issue that you have encountered in your own experience as a nursing student or in a related situation. What kind of action plan do you think would be effective in building a policy to address the issue(s)?

References

Aiken, L.H., Salmon, M., & Shamian, J., et al. (1998, April). *An international study of the effects of the organization and staffing of hospitals on patient outcomes.* Presentation at Outcomes/Indicators Session, WHO, CCNM, Korea.

Aiken, L.H., Smith, H.L., & Lake, E.T. (1994). Lower Medicare mortality among a set of hospitals known for good nursing care. *Medical Care, 32*(8), 771–787.

Aitken, M.E., Rowlands, L.A., & Wheeler, J.G. (2001). Advocating for children's health at the state level: Lessons learned. *Archives of Pediatrics and Adolescent Medicine, 155*(8), 877–880.

Baumann, A., O'Brien Pallas, L., & Armstrong-Stassen, M., et al. (2001). *Commitment and care: The benefits of a healthy workplace for nurses, their patients and the system. A policy synthesis.* Ottawa: Canadian Health Services Research Foundation & the Change Foundation.

Blegen, M.A. & Mueller, C.W. (1987). Nurses' job satisfaction: A longitudinal analysis. *Nursing and Health, 10,* 227–237.

Browne, G. (2001, October 24). *Key findings from the System-Linked Research Unit on Health and Social Service Utilization.* Presented to the Advisory Committee on Health Human Resources' Working Group on Nursing & Unregulated Healthcare Workers. Ottawa.

Canadian Institute for Health Information. (2001). An environmental scan of research transfer strategies. *Canadian Population Health Initiative,* February. Ottawa: Author.

_____. (2005). *Canada's healthcare providers: 2005 chartbook.* Ottawa: Author.

Canadian Labour and Business Centre. (2002). *Full-time equivalents and financial costs associated with absenteeism, overtime, and involuntary part-time employment in the nursing profession: A report prepared for the Canadian Nursing Advisory Committee.* Ottawa: Author.

Canadian Nurses Association. (1997). *Getting started: A political action guide for Canada's registered nurses.* Ottawa: Author.

_____. (2000). Nursing is a political act: The bigger picture. *Nursing Now. Issues and Trends in Canadian Nursing, 8.* Ottawa: Author.

_____. (2008). *Campaign 2008—CNA's three issues for the next election.* Ottawa: Author.

Centre for the Advancement of Health. (2001). *Communicating health behavior science in the media: Tips for researchers.* Washington, DC: Author.

Centres of Excellence for Women's Health. (2001, Summer). *Research Bulletin 2*(1).

Cheek, J. & Gibson, T. (1997). Policy matters: Critical policy analysis and nursing. *Journal of Advanced Nursing, 25*(4), 668–672.

Chunharas, S. (2001). Linking research to policy and action. In N. Neufeld & N. Johnson (Eds.), *Forging links for health research: Perspectives from the Council on Health Research for Development.* Ottawa: International Development Research Centre.

Clarke, H.F., Lashinger, H.S., & Giovannetti, P., et al. (2001). Nursing shortages: Workplace environments are essential to the solution. *Hospital Quarterly, 4*(3), 50–55.

Commission d'étude sur les services de santé et les services sociaux. (2000). *Les solutions émergentes: Rapport et recommendations*. Québec: Gouvernement du Québec. ISBN 2-550-36958-0.

Crosswaite, C. & Curtice, L. (1994). Disseminating research results: The challenge of bridging the gap between health research and health action. *Health Promotion International, 9*(4), 289–296.

Dannemiller, K.D. & Jacobs, R.W. (1992). Changing the way organizations change: A revolution of common sense. *Journal of Applied Behavioral Science, 28*(4), 480–498.

Davis, P. & Howden-Chapman, P. (1996). Translating research findings into health policy. *Social Science and Medicine, 43*, 865–872.

Feldman, P.H., Nadash, P., & Gursen, M. (2001). Improving communication between researchers and policy makers in long-term care: Or, researchers are from Mars; policy makers are from Venus. *The Gerontologist, 41*(3), 312–321.

Gebbie, K.M., Wakefield, M., & Kerfoot, K. (2000). Nursing and health policy. *Journal of Nursing Scholarship, 32*(3), 307–315.

Hartz, A.J., Krakauer, H., & Kuhn, E.M., et al. (1989). Hospital characteristics and mortality rates. *New England Journal of Medicine, 321*, 1720–1725.

Haylock, P.J. (2000). Health policy and legislation: Impact on cancer nursing and care. *Seminars in Oncology Nursing, 16*(1), 76–84.

Helms, L.B., Anderson, M.A., & Hanson, K. (1996). "Doin' politics": Linking policy and politics in nursing. *Nursing Administration Quarterly, 20*(3), 32–41.

Hewison, A. (1999). The new public management and the new nursing: Related by rhetoric. Some reflections on the policy process and nursing. *Journal of Advanced Nursing, 29*(6), 1377–1384.

Irvine, D. & Evans, M. (1992). *Job satisfaction and turnover among nurses: A review and meta-analysis.* Toronto: Quality of Worklife Research Unit, University of Toronto.

Joint Provincial Nursing Committee. (2001). *Good nursing, good health: A good investment. First progress report on the Nursing Task Force recommendations.* Toronto: Ministry of Health and Long-Term Care.

———. (2004). *Good nursing, good health: Progress report November 2003.* Toronto: Ministry of Health and Long-Term Care.

Kimball, B. & O'Neil, E. (2001). The evolution of a crisis: Nursing in America. *Policy, Politics, & Nursing Practice, 2*(3), 180–186.

Kingdon, J.W. (1995). *Agendas, alternatives, and public policies.* New York: HarperCollins College Publishers.

Knaus, W.A., Draper, E.A., & Wagner, D.P., et al. (1986). An evaluation of outcome from intensive care in major medical centers. *Annals of Internal Medicine, 104*, 410–418.

Lomas, J. (2000). Using "linkage and exchange" to move research into policy at a Canadian foundation. *Health Affairs (Chevy Chase), 19*(3), 236–240.

McGillis Hall, L., Irvine Doran, D., & Baker, G.R., et al. (2001). *A study of the impact of nursing staff mix models and organizational change strategies on patient, system and nurse outcomes.* Toronto: University of Toronto.

Milstead, J.A. (1999). *Health policy and politics: A nurse's guide.* Gaithersburg, MD: Aspen.

Mittelmark, M.B. (1999). The psychology of social influence and healthy public policy. *Preventive Medicine, 29*(6, Pt. 2), S24–S29.

Montini, T. & Bero, L.A. (2001). Policy makers' perspectives on tobacco control advocates' roles in regulation development. *Tobacco Control, 10*(3), 218–224.

O'Brien-Pallas, L., Duffield, C., & Alksnis, C. (2004). Who will be there to nurse: Retention of nurses nearing retirement. *Journal of Nursing Administration, 35*(6), 298–302.

O'Brien-Pallas, L. & Shamian, J. (with Buchan, J., Duffield, C., & Hughes, F., et al.). (2003, February 13). An international examination of the cost and impact of turnover on patient safety and nurse outcomes: Preliminary findings. *Fifth Joint National Conference on Quality in Healthcare,* Toronto.

O'Brien-Pallas, L., Thomson, D., & Alksnis, C., et al. (2001). The economic impact of nurse staffing decisions: Time to turn down another road? *Hospital Quarterly, 4*(2), 42–50.

Ordre des infirmiéres et infirmiers du Québec. (2000). *Le financement et l'organisation des services de santé et des services sociaux.* Mémoire présenté á la Commission d'étude sur les services de santé et les services sociaux. Montréal: Author.

Organization for Economic Cooperation and Development. (2004). *Resolving nurse shortages in OECD member countries.* Human Resources for Healthcare Nursing Project. Paris, France.

Prescott, P.A. (1993). Nursing: An important component of hospital survival under a reformed healthcare system. *Nursing Economics, 11,* 192–199.

Price, J.L. & Mueller, C.W. (1981). A causal model of turnover for nurses. *Academy of Management Journal, 24*(3), 543–565.

Scott, J.G., Sochalski, J., & Aiken, L. (1999). Review of magnet hospital research. *Journal of Nursing Administration, 29*(1), 9–19.

Skelton-Green, J.M. (1996). The perceived impact of committee participation on the job satisfaction and retention of staff nurses. *Canadian Journal of Nursing Administration, 9*(2), 7–35.

Slavitt, B.B., Stamps, P.L., & Piedmont, E.G., et al. (1978). Nurses' satisfaction with their work situation. *Nursing Research, 27,* 114–120.

Tarlov, A. (1999). Public policy frameworks for improving population health. *Annals of the New York Academy of Sciences, 896,* 281–293.

_____. (2000, August 10–13). *The future of health in Canada: "The art of the possible."* Proceedings of the 69th Annual Couchiching Summer Conference, Geneva Park, Orillia, Ontario.

Taylor, C. (1997). The ACIDD test: A framework for policy planning and decision-making. *Optimum, the Journal of Public Sector Management, 27*(4), 53–62.

Valentine, N.M. (2000). The evolving role of the chief nurse executive in the Veterans Health Administration: Policy and leadership lessons. *Policy, Politics, & Nursing Practice, 1*(1), 36–46.

West, E. & Scott, C. (2000). Nursing in the public sphere: Breaching the boundary between research and policy. *Journal of Advanced Nursing, 32*(4), 817–824.

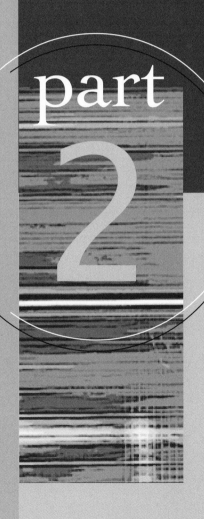

REGULATORY POWER

part 2

Canadian Nurses Centennial Logo. (Used with permission of the Canadian Nurses Association.)

The Canadian Nurses Association and the International Council of Nurses

Michael J. Villeneuve

With thanks to Ginette Lemire Rodger, Geertje Boschma, Barbara Brush, and Meryn Stuart who authored and contributed to earlier versions of the original chapters on the Canadian Nurses Association and the International Council of Nurses.

Critical Questions

As a way of engaging with the ideas in this chapter, consider the following:

1 What is the role, purpose, and relevance of national and international nursing organizations to 21st century nurses, students, citizens, and global health outcomes?

2 What are the roles of your own provincial and territorial nursing association(s) and how do they support, benefit from, and contrast with the work of the Canadian Nurses Association (CNA)?

3 How do national and international nursing organizations effectively bring the knowledge and experience of nurses to bear on population health outcomes and the development of healthy public policy?

4 How do national and international nursing organizations contribute effectively to global agendas in key areas impacting health outcomes, such as aging, gender, diversity, disease transmission, poverty, the environment, technology, system delivery innovations, and safety?

After completing this chapter, you will be able to:

1 Identify the types, roles, and purposes of professional and regulatory organizations and identify at least three leading pan-Canadian and international nursing organizations.

2 Describe four areas in which the power of representation of the CNA and the International Council of Nurses (ICN) have brought about changes to improve global health.

3 Differentiate the elements of the CNA's governance structure and describe three of its partnerships.

4 Identify five key issues, priorities, or challenges confronting CNA and ICN and their strategic responses as organizations.

This chapter provides an overview of the CNA and the ICN, and the contexts in which they exercise their respective roles and functions. Examples are used to highlight the complex kinds of issues confronting CNA and ICN, including the tensions and contradictions inherent in bringing about social change and improved health outcomes at national and international levels. The structure and governance of the CNA are described, examples of current priorities are discussed, and the challenges of balancing advocacy and regulatory functions are introduced. At the international level, the historical development of the ICN is highlighted to give context to its current objectives and the broader history of the evolution of organized nursing. The roles and influence of the ICN are discussed with regard to its contributions to global health and its initiatives to support the nursing profession within its member countries.

THE CANADIAN NURSES ASSOCIATION: THE NATIONAL VOICE OF NURSES IN CANADA SINCE 1908

The year 2008 marked the most significant milestone in the history of the CNA as the organization celebrated its 100th anniversary. Featuring a year of special events kicked off formally by the Prime Minister in February and overseen by an honourary leadership cabinet of distinguished Canadians, CNA celebrated the extraordinary achievements and impacts of individual canadian nurses, nursing associations and organizations, and its own century-long history of leadership within Canada and on the international stage. The centennial year themes led CNA's Board of Directors staff and partners, along with all Canadians and their nurses, to discuss, debate, and generate solutions in three key areas: *leadership, the future of nursing,* and *a healthy environment.* CNA is well positioned to move into its second century, but to understand the organization, its strengths, and likely future struggles, it is important to understand the foundation on which the centennial celebrations and themes were built.

Who and What Is CNA?

CNA is a federation of 11 provincial and territorial professional associations and regulatory colleges representing more than 133,700 Canadian registered nurses (RNs) and nurse practitioners—more than half of Canada's 253,000 employed RNs (Canadian Institute For Health Information [CIHI], 2007). With various mandates to protect the public, speak on behalf of the profession, or both, the federation includes the members named in Table 7.1.

ONTARIO AND QUEBEC

Missing from the CNA federation are *some* Ontario nurses and the nurses of Quebec. To practice in Ontario, its 90,000 employed RNs (CIHI, 2007) must register with the College of Nurses of Ontario (CNO), which has a mandate to protect the public. The CNO is *not* a member of CNA and, hence, those Ontario nurses are not members of CNA or ICN. However, the Registered Nurses Association of

Table 7.1	Provincial and Territorial Members of the Canadian Nurses Association

CANADIAN NURSES ASSOCIATION'S PROVINCIAL AND TERRITORIAL JURISDICTIONAL MEMBERS	WEB SITE	MANDATE REGULATORY	PROFESSIONAL
The Association of Registered Nurses of Newfoundland and Labrador	www.arnnl.ca	☐	☐
The Association of Registered Nurses of Prince Edward Island	www.arnpei.ca	☐	☐
The College of Registered Nurses of Nova Scotia	www.crnns.ca	☐	☐
The Nurses Association of New Brunswick	www.nanb.nb.ca	☐	☐
The Registered Nurses Association of Ontario	www.rnao.org	☐	☐
The College of Registered Nurses of Manitoba	www.crnm.mb.ca	☐	☐
The Saskatchewan Registered Nurses Association	www.srna.org	☐	☐
The College and Association of Registered Nurses of Alberta	www.nurses.ab.ca	☐	☐
The College of Registered Nurses of British Columbia	www.crnbc.ca	☐	☐
The Registered Nurses Association of the Northwest Territories and Nunavut	www.rnantnu.ca	☐	☐
The Yukon Registered Nurses Association	www.yrna.ca	☐	☐

Individual nurses who are members of their provincial and territorial nursing association automatically become full members of the Canadian Nurses Association and the International Council of Nurses.

Ontario (RNAO)—a professional association with *voluntary* membership—represents approximately 27,000 RNs and nursing students in Ontario and *is* a member of CNA. Therefore, Ontario nurses who voluntarily join RNAO become members of CNA and in turn, ICN. Ontario is the only Canadian jurisdiction having such a structure.

In Quebec, the Ordre des infirmières et infirmiers du Québec (OIIQ), which has both regulatory and professional mandates, withdrew from CNA in 1985 at the height of the political separatist movement. The OIIQ represents Quebec's 64,000 employed RNs (CIHI, 2007). Nurses in Quebec who wish to join CNA and ICN may do so by joining the Nurses Association of New Brunswick or the Yukon Registered Nurses Association, both of which offer associate-type memberships to non-resident nurses from other jurisdictions, who may then access membership in CNA and ICN.

STUDENT MEMBERS OF CNA: OUR FUTURE AMONG US
Delegates at the June 2006 annual meeting approved changes to CNA's bylaws so that students in nursing education programs can now become members of CNA. Nursing students are eligible to become individual members of CNA if they:

- are members in good standing of the Canadian Nursing Students' Association (CNSA)
- are members of a provincial and territorial jurisdictional association
- have paid the annual CNA membership fee.

Quebec nursing students may become CNA members through the CNSA and the Nurses Association of New Brunswick.

CNA's Vision, Mission and Goals

CNA is "the national professional voice of RNs, supporting them in their practice and advocating for healthy public policy and a quality, publicly funded, not-for-profit health system" (Canadian Nurses Association [CNA] Web site, 2008). Furthermore, CNA

speaks for Canadian nurses and represents Canadian nursing to other organizations and to governments nationally and internationally. It gives RNs a strong national association through which they can support each other and speak with a powerful, unified voice. It provides RNs with a core staff of nursing and health policy consultants, and experts in areas such as communication and testing. CNA's active role in legislative policy influences the healthcare decisions that affect nursing professionals every day (CNA Web site, 2008).

To accomplish its mission, CNA undertakes policy development and programs of work falling under six overarching goals; there is extensive information about related work in these areas on CNA's Web site:

1. CNA advances the discipline of nursing in the interest of the public.
2. CNA advocates public policy that incorporates the principles of primary healthcare (access; interdisciplinary practice; patient and community involvement); health promotion (including determinants of health and appropriate technology, roles, and models); and respects the principles, conditions, and spirit of the Canada Health Act.
3. CNA advances the regulation of RNs in the interest of the public.
4. CNA works in collaboration with nurses, other healthcare providers, health system stakeholders, and the public to achieve and sustain quality practice environments and positive client outcomes.
5. CNA advances international health policy and development in Canada and abroad to support global health and equity.
6. CNA promotes awareness of the nursing profession so that the roles and expertise of RNs are understood, respected, and optimized within the health system.

Governance Structure

An 18-member board of directors governs on behalf of the members and is accountable to them. During the June 2008 Centennial CNA Meeting held in Ottawa, the board presidency transferred from Dr. Marlene Smadu (Saskatchewan, 2006–2008) to Kaaren Neufeld (Manitoba), who will hold the post during the 2008–2010 biennium. The president elect, 2008–2010, is Dr. Judith Shamian (Ontario). The chief executive officer (CEO) of CNA is Lucille Auffrey, who retires from the position in 2009 after holding the post since 2001. CNA's presidents and executive directors over the past quarter century are listed in Box 7.1.

The 18 board members include the president, president-elect, presidents of the 11 provincial and territorial jurisdictional members, two representatives of CNA's 40 Associate and Affiliate Members and Emerging Groups (see Members, CNA Web site, 2008), two public representatives, and the CEO. The president of the CNSA also has an ex-officio (non-voting) seat at the CNA board table. The board's main role is to govern the organization, determine strategic directions, set goals, and monitor outcomes; in short, the board develops, sets, and monitors policy to help manage the CNA. The three major governance roles of the board currently are in the areas of *policy development, advocacy,* and *visioning.*

CNA's board meets quarterly and reports at each annual general meeting on the business transacted. At the annual general meeting, delegates from each jurisdiction meet to fulfill their fiduciary responsibilities, such as electing a president-elect (biannually), choosing an auditor, changing bylaws, and giving guidance to the board of directors through voting on resolutions regarding the policy areas that they believe should be pursued. Although the board of directors is not bound by the resolutions

BOX 7.1 Canadian Nurses Association Presidents and Executive Directors since 1980

CNA Presidents	CNA Executive Directors
Dr. Shirley Stinson, 1980–1982	Dr. Helen K. Mussallem, 1963–1981
Dr. Helen Glass, 1982–1984	Dr. Ginette Lemire Rodger, 1981–1989
Lorrine Bessel, 1984–1986	Judith Oulton, 1989–1995
Helen Evans, 1986–1988	Dr. Mary Ellen Jeans, 1995–2001
Dr. Judith Ritchie, 1988–1990	Lucille Auffrey, 2001–2009
Dr. Alice Baumgart, 1990–1992	
Fernande Harrison, 1992–1994	
Eleanor Ross, 1994–1996	
Rachel Bard, 1996–1998	
Lynda Kushnir Perkul, 1998–2000	
Dr. Ginette Lemire Rodger, 2000–2002	
Rob Calnan, 2002–2004	
Dr. Deborah Tamlyn, 2004–2006	
Dr. Marlene Smadu, 2006–2008	
Kaaren Neufeld, 2008–2010	
Dr. Judith Shamian, 2010–2012	

on policy directives, a review of annual reports submitted to membership confirms that almost all resolutions have guided the CNA and have been implemented.

CNA's board of directors decides on policy directions, priorities, and resources, ensuring that effective strategies are implemented by the CEO and staff. The board appoints the CEO, who has the authority and responsibility to implement the board policies, provide services to members, develop an appropriate network to fulfill the mandate, manage a team of staff members, and ensure linkage with CNA's subsidiary (i.e., Assessment Strategies, Inc.) and parallel organizations (i.e., the Canadian Nurses Foundation and the Canadian Nurses Protective Society).

The operational and staff structure complements the organization's goals, operating with a strong policy focus and programs in four areas: *International Policy and Development, Nursing Policy, Public Policy,* and *Regulatory Policy.* The entire organization is, of course, supported with experts and operational programs in the executive office, administration and finance, and communications and publications.

Partnerships

Nurses have always worked in partnership with others. However, recognizing that "stand-alone" organizations and initiatives truly are now considered things of the past, CNA actively engages in a broad range of formal partnerships to increase the influence of nurses and other health providers.

For example, the Health Action Lobby (HEAL) is a coalition of national health and consumer organizations dedicated to protecting and strengthening Canada's healthcare system. The CNA was a founding member in 1991 and co-chaired the coalition. HEAL now comprises 36 organizations representing more than 500,000 providers and consumers of healthcare (Health Action Lobby, 1992).

CNA is a partner in many other initiatives that bring the collective power of unified messages to bear in policy development. It is a founding member of the Canadian Health Leadership Network, the Quality Worklife—Quality Healthcare Collaborative, and the Canadian Consortium for Nursing Research and Innovation. It is an active partner in producing the annual "Healthcare in Canada" survey (led by Merck and POLLARA [see http://www.hcic-sssc.ca]). And, since the turn of the century, CNA has had a lead hand in rolling out broad, multistakeholder initiatives as diverse as the Canadian Nursing Advisory Committee, the Canadian Nurse Practitioner Initiative, and "Building the Future"—the National Occupational/Sector Study of Nursing. All of these national-level, multiyear projects were completed as a result of strategic collaboration and a rich matrix of trusted partnerships.

Multistakeholder partnerships also evolve around specific issues, such as patient safety or the need to have a strategy focused on healthcare human resources. In the latter case, CNA is part of a collective quietly called the "G-4", including CNA, the Canadian Medical Association, Canadian Healthcare Association, and Canadian Pharmacists Association. The group meets on an ad hoc basis with the federal minister and/or deputy minister, and CNA staff contributes information and evidence to inform policy decisions through links with the federal, provincial, and territorial Advisory Committee on Health Delivery and Human Resources and formal presentations to various federal committees.

CNA also maintains relationships through regular formal and informal meetings with key national *nursing* partners, including Health Canada's Office of Nursing Policy and, in turn, the group of federal, provincial, and territorial principal nursing officers. CNA's core nursing partners include such organizations as the Canadian Association of Schools of Nursing, CNSA, Academy of Canadian Executive Nurses, Canadian Federation of Nurses Unions, Practical Nurses of Canada, Canadian Council for Practical Nurse Regulators, and the Registered Psychiatric Nurses of Canada (the latter being an association in the four Western provinces where registered psychiatric nurses are regulated). Internationally, strategic bilateral and joint meetings with the American Nurses Association, Sigma Theta Tau, the Commission on Graduates of Foreign Nursing Schools, and other national nursing associations are ongoing. ICN's structure encourages national networking and collaboration among the diverse groups of nurses within the country (International Council of Nurses [ICN], 2001a).

The Power and Influence of CNA

Many national nursing organizations exist across the domains of nursing practice, representing interests in specific areas of practice and competence (e.g., clinical specialty groups, researchers, and educators). While some functions overlap, the main purposes of organizations are grounded in their *social roles*. In nursing, these could be conceptualized as a) primarily protecting the nurse or the individual practitioner (e.g., a union), b) primarily protecting the public or society (e.g., a regulatory college), or c) primarily speaking on behalf of the profession (e.g., a professional advocacy association).

Throughout the last decade Canada has seen the rise of nursing organizations in all these areas as well as *hybrid* organizations that hold mixed functions. With its complex membership and mandates, CNA in 2008 is a perfect example of such a hybrid organization and it is hardly alone; the ICN conducted a survey of its members in 1997 and found that 62% of its national nursing association members identified their major role as *representing the profession*; they did not have a specific regulatory role concerning protection of the public or protection of the nurse (i.e., a union or socioeconomic mandate). A total of 31% of national nursing associations were unions that negotiate for nurses, and just 7% had a solely regulatory mandate (ICN, 2001a).

WHERE IT ALL STARTED

In 1908, under the leadership of Mary Agnes Snively of Ontario, the first national nurses association was formed in Canada so that nurses could effectively and collectively exercise their professional responsibilities on behalf of the public and, secondly, to provide them with a vehicle by which to join the ICN (CNA, 1968). During that year, representatives of 16 organized nursing bodies met in Ottawa to form the Canadian National Association of Trained Nurses. By 1911, the association included 28 affiliated member societies, including alumni associations of hospital schools of nursing and local and regional groups of nurses. And, by 1924, with the existing nine member provinces each having a provincial nurses organization, the group changed its name to the *Canadian Nurses Association*.

Since its inception, CNA has been the national voice of nursing in Canada—influencing public policy, articulating the viewpoints of nurses on health and nursing issues, and playing a key role in the Canadian political process and in the development of nursing in Canada (CNA, 1958; CNA, 1968; MacPhail, 1996; Meilicke & Larsen, 1988). Over the past 20 years, the role of CNA has expanded considerably in the areas of advocacy, strengthening nursing and the broader health system, and protecting the public through its regulatory policy work.

While Florence Nightingale may be our most famous historical example of the impact of individual political activism and nursing advocacy, throughout history many social movements were spearheaded by nurse leaders even if many of them did not consider their role (either individually or collectively as professionals) to be *political activism*. The power of representation is exercised most of the time through *political action,* meaning "a systematic series of actions directed toward influencing others into conformity with a pursued goal" (Lemire Rodger, 1999, p. 281). Since the early 1980s, CNA has promoted political action by nurses at the pan-Canadian level as a means of exercising the power of representation.

CNA'S STRATEGIC RESPONSES TO PRIORITIES AND CHALLENGES CONFRONTING CANADIAN NURSING IN THE 21ST CENTURY

The national vision for nursing in Canada is that nurses, as a collective and with partners, work to advance health for all. Over the years, CNA has expressed its commitment to contribute to the health of the public in part through development of the profession. This vision has been reiterated in corporate objectives and in an ongoing legacy of position statements, studies, speeches, and briefs to governments, health committees, and commissions. CNA's six goals do not represent *all* of the pressing issues that a national association has to address, but they help focus the policy work and resources of the organization. The CNA board further refines the directions and priorities of its work after continually scanning the environment. These ongoing scanning exercises include surveys of national, provincial, and territorial organizations and the larger world around them to identify trends and emerging issues that might impact the CNA or the larger nursing agenda. Let's turn to consider examples of CNA's work and influence in its various policy priority areas.

Public Policy

> *CNA works with politicians and other health policymakers and national organizations working in the health sector. CNA's efforts are focused on public policy related to the nursing workforce, the functioning and financing of the health system and the determinants of health such as environment, child health development and personal health practices. CNA works with a grassroots network of nurses who actively lobby politicians and the media on nursing issues. CNA gathers and analyses data and participates in research related to the nursing workforce, workplace policies and practices and health system issues. It disseminates the results through its professional journal, Canadian Nurse. CNA also uses the research results as a basis for position statements and policies.*
>
> *(CNA Web site, 2008)*

CNA's public policy work is grounded in two sets of fundamental values. The first of these lies in the broad principles of primary healthcare (Box 7.2). They include health promotion and prevention of disease and injury, accessibility, public participation, multidisciplinary and intersectoral collaboration, and appropriate technology (World Health Organization, 1978). CNA would include within its

BOX 7.2 Primary Healthcare

The definition of *primary healthcare* approved at the 1978 Alma Ata conference of the World Health Organization (p. 21) stated that:

Primary healthcare is essential healthcare based on practical, scientifically sound and socially acceptable methods and technology made universally accessible to individuals and families in the community through their full participation and at a cost that the community and country can afford to maintain at every stage of their development in the spirit of self-reliance and self-determination. It forms an integral part both of the country's health system, of which it is the central function and main focus, and of the overall social and economic development of the community. It is the first level of contact of individuals, the family, and community with the national health system bringing healthcare as close as possible to where the people live and work, and constitutes the first element of a continuing healthcare process.

thinking about primary healthcare the notion that there are many determinants of health and that its policy work should reflect those values. Secondly, CNA's work is based on the principles of the Canada Health Act, including universality, portability, accessibility, comprehensiveness, and public administration (Government of Canada, 1984). All of these principles are central in the ongoing national debate about service delivery, funding, and system redesign—and are fundamental values grounding the work and thinking of CNA.

Nationally, a significant milestone for representation came in 1985, with the proclamation of the Canada Health Act. From coast to coast, many nurses participated for the first time in political lobbying that influenced changes in national legislation—changes that reflected nurses' values and beliefs about the future of the healthcare system. These beliefs were summarized in the brief, "Putting 'Health' Back Into Healthcare" (CNA, 1980) that has guided pursuant changes by the CNA since its publication. CNA's impact on legislative changes to the Canada Health Act of 1984 ensured that national and provincial plans for the future of the healthcare system were guided by the principles of primary healthcare and the Canada Health Act (Mhatre & Deber, 1992). The nursing voice was part of the review of the Canadian healthcare system by the National Health Forum in 1997 and, into this century, the national health system reviews undertaken by Commissioner Romanow and Senator Kirby.

ADVANCING LEADERSHIP IN HEALTH HUMAN RESOURCES PLANNING

An illuminating example of the impact of CNA's public policy work can be found in the area of leadership in health human resources planning. CNA's current position as the "go-to" place for nursing human resources data and information has been earned through a decade of purposeful planning and work, much of it in partnership with groups such as the Canadian Institute for Health Information and the Canadian Association of Schools of Nursing. Its 1997 report on the future supply of RNs in Canada (Ryten, 1997) predicted a serious shortage of nurses by 2011 if no strategic action was undertaken immediately. In the wake of that report, CNA made formal presentations to inform federal and provincial governments and associations of employers of the significant trend apparently unfolding (CNA, 1998; CNA, 1999; CNA, 2000; CNA, 2001) and undertook significant, informal political lobbying in Ottawa and nationally.

Further research (CIHI, 2005; Ryten, 2002) validated the projections, and attempts were made to engage governments in understanding that the situation was serious enough to undermine the very sustainability of the Canadian healthcare system. A concerted lobbying effort with the provincial jurisdictions and other nursing and health associations was also needed to persuade governments and employers that action was required immediately. The issues of recruitment and retention were addressed in these representations—and retention and the quality of the professional practice environment soon became priority policy areas for CNA.

CNA's formal presentations and effective behind-the-scenes lobbying played a key role in helping to build and launch a pan-Canadian agenda in the area of nursing and health human resources still playing out in 2008. Emerging from the chaos of 1990s system downsizing, CNA approached Canada's federal government in 1998 with its brief entitled, "The Quiet Crisis," in which it made plain the association's growing concern about a looming shortage of nurses and the need to bolster the academic and practice foundations of nursing for what looked like a rocky journey ahead. CNA's lobbying helped prompt the establishment of the new federal Office of Nursing Policy at Health Canada in 1999, mirrored in the following years by the appointment of "chief nurses" and senior nurse advisor positions in the provincial governments of Newfoundland, Prince Edward Island, Nova Scotia, New Brunswick, Ontario, Saskatchewan, and British Columbia. Other provincial governments also employed nurse advisors under various titles.

That agenda soon gave rise to a roster of pan-Canadian nursing initiatives unprecedented in number and scope, including the Nursing Strategy for Canada (Advisory Committee on Health Human Resources, 2000), Canadian Nursing Advisory Committee (2002), National Sector/Occupational Sector Study of Nursing (2006; "Phase II Final Report" is posted on CNA's Web site) and establishment of a decade-long, $25 million national nursing research fund. The Nursing Strategy for Canada and Canadian Nursing Advisory Committee prompted the governments of several provinces and territories to develop comprehensive plans to address nursing human resources—and the topic of nursing recruitment and retention was established as a regular item on the federal, provincial, and territorial policy agenda for health ministers.

The importance of the broader health human resources agenda, including the issue of healthy work environments, was reflected in the 2003 First Ministers' Accord on Healthcare Renewal wherein some $90 million in funding was directed to the issue of health human resources with particular attention to healthy workplaces, interprofessional education and collaborative practice, and recruitment and retention. CNA urged a principles-based HHR planning framework as outlined in "Toward a Pan-Canadian Framework for Health Human Resources: A Green Paper" and in its position statement, "National Planning for Human Resources in the Health Sector." CNA led the steering committee for the Diagnostic Phase for Internationally Educated Nurses national project. And to keep in close touch with policy decision makers and the larger healthcare community of key issues, CNA hosts the ongoing *Knowledge Series*, a monthly, multistakeholder policy discussion to examine specific issues related to health human resources. As a result of the ongoing leadership and collaborative actions of CNA, challenges related to the demand for nursing services and supply of nurses to provide them in 2008 are familiar not only to nurses but to employers, governments, other providers, and the public across the country.

Examples of other key areas of public policy work at the national level during this decade include:

- Primary Healthcare and Determinants of Health; Primary Healthcare Transition Fund Initiatives—Interprofessional Collaboration
  - Enhancing Interdisciplinary Collaboration in Primary Healthcare
  - Canadian Nurse Practitioner Initiative
- First Ministers' 10-Year Plan to Strengthen Healthcare
  - CNA was an active participant at the first ministers' meeting held in September 2004. In preparation for this meeting, CNA collaborated with the Canadian Healthcare Association, Canadian Medical Association, and Canadian Pharmacists Association on joint policy and media relations initiatives. This work included the preparation and dissemination of the document, "Common Vision for the Canadian Health System," media interviews, media statements, and media releases as well as on-site participation during the meeting.
- Emergency Preparedness (disasters, pandemics)
- Executive Training for Research Application (EXTRA) Program

- CNA has been a partner (with the Canadian Health Services Research Foundation [CHSRF], Canadian College of Health Service Executives, Canadian Medical Association, and a consortium of Quebec partners represented by the Agence d'évaluation des technologies et des modes d'intervention en santé) in the creation and promotion of the EXTRA Program—created to help Canadian healthcare executives from all backgrounds use existing research to make evidence-based decisions in their day-to-day decision making.

Nursing Policy

CNA encourages the integration of current knowledge into practice environments conducive to quality nursing care. Nursing policy develops national policies on nursing issues such as advanced nursing practice and the nurse practitioner and is involved in a number of initiatives on behalf of nurses. One such project is "Achieving Excellence in Professional Practice," a resource guide offering nurses and other professionals' assistance in developing or reviewing existing standards.

(CNA Web site, 2008)

PROVIDING LEADERSHIP TO PROMOTE QUALITY PROFESSIONAL PRACTICE ENVIRONMENTS

The power of representation was exercised with great determination by the CNA in recent years because issues related to the environments in which nursing is practiced have always been part of the CNA mandate. The socioeconomic environments of nurses were greatly transformed by the events of the 1990s, when major cutbacks in healthcare funding exerted a devastating effect on nursing education, the nursing workforce at large, and the settings where nurses practice. Thousands of nurses lost their positions when hospital and community services were curtailed by provincial governments across the country— and some 5,500 nursing leadership and administration positions disappeared. Workplaces saw increases in the number of patients or clients cared for by each nurse, and a loss of support structures for education and research. Since 2000, CNA has led and participated in a wide range of studies and projects contributing state-of-the-art knowledge to the growing understanding that quality practice environments, staffing, and staff mix are linked to outcomes. CNA has been a key participant and leader in the national Quality Worklife—Quality Healthcare Collaborative, which is building quality of worklife outcome indicators into the Accreditation Canada program—closing one part of a loop of work begun in partnership with the federal Office of Nursing Policy nearly a decade ago.

The National Nursing Research Agenda

A clear example of the power of representation can be seen in the overall progress and development of nursing research both nationally and provincially. Nursing has been recognized only recently as a "discipline" in Canada. In fact, most of the debate about the legitimacy of doctoral programs in nursing related to recognizing nursing as a discipline. Only in the 1980s did the Medical Research Council of Canada and some universities, such as McGill University and the University of Alberta, consider academic approval of doctoral programs in nursing and support for the research infrastructure.

CNA developed a national plan for the development of nursing research in Canada (CNA, 1984) and has lobbied government, universities, and foundations over the past 25 years. The power of representation of the CNA was effective even if some of the gains were not sustained (MacPhail, 1996). They include nursing representation at the policy level of the Medical Research Council of Canada in the 1980s and 1990s, and leadership at the National Health Research and Development Program of the Health Promotion Directorate of Health and Welfare Canada.

Funding for nursing science historically has been sparse—and was mirrored in the dearth of doctoral-level nurse researchers and leaders educated in Canada until the 1990s. The situation began to reverse during the 1990s and has significantly changed since establishment by the federal government of the $25 million Nursing Research Fund (1999–2009), advocated by CNA in its 1990s lobbying efforts. The fund has paid off; the production of nursing science and research capacity has similarly begun to grow. For example:

- Canada currently has 15 doctoral programs in nursing where there were none in 1990. Twelve nurses graduated from Canadian doctoral programs in nursing between 1990 and 1997—39 graduated in 2006 alone, and the number of enrolled candidates that year was more than 10 times the number of graduates.
- The research fund resulted in five nursing-specific CHSRF and Canadian Institutes of Health Research (CIHR) chairs and three nursing-related chairs of the 12 chair awards, 18 awards for nursing-related postdoctoral students, three Career Reorientation awards for nurses, and three Regional Training Centres.
- Training funds totalling $450,000 (including postdoctoral awards) were awarded in 2006, more than twice the amount seen in 1999.
- Forty-seven CHSRF Open Grants Competition have been awarded.
- Three full-scale nursing-related programs of research have been funded under the CHSRF Research, Exchange, and Impact for System Support competition between 2005 and 2007.
- *Nursing leadership, organization, and policy* has been the theme in the last 3 years of CIHR's Partnerships for Health System Improvement.
- CIHR operating grants to nurses as principal investigators increased from 38 grants in 2000–2001 to 130 in 2005–2006.
- Between 2003 and 2007 the Canadian Nurses Foundation provided more than $2.2 million to 160 nursing care research projects, leveraging $4.7 million from partners for a total investment of nearly $6.9 million.

Examples of other key areas of nursing policy work at the national level during this decade include:

- Leveraging technology to enhance nursing practice
  - CNA's e-nursing strategy guides the development of information and communication technology initiatives in nursing to improve nursing practice and client outcomes.
    - NurseONE—a personalized interactive Web-based portal providing Canadian nurses with reliable evidence-based resources to support their nursing practice through enhancing their decision-making process, managing their careers, and connecting with colleagues and healthcare experts. NurseONE offers up-to-date, accurate information on a wide range of topics fully vetted and reviewed by CNA and its editorial panel. Its extensive virtual Library houses more than 400 e-textbooks, 1,800 full-text journals, and 200 continuing education modules. Its reputation as a nurse's trusted online colleague is growing fast.
    - As a result of CNA's partnership with the ministries of health in Ontario, Prince Edward Island, and Saskatchewan, Canada Health Infoway has funded the Canadian Health Outcomes for Better Information and Care project to collect patient outcome information related to nursing care in the electronic health records of the partner provinces.
    - Publication of a strategy document to address the integration of information technology, Internet-based resources, and electronic health records into everyday nursing practice, "Supporting the Professional Practice of Canadian Nurses Through Information and Communications Technologies."
- Building evidence to support RN practice and new models of care
  - Evaluation framework to determine the impact of nursing staff mix decisions
  - Framework for the practice of RNs in Canada

- Advanced nursing practice
  - CNA played a central role in establishing the Canadian Nurse Practitioner Initiative to facilitate the sustained integration of nurse practitioners in the Canadian Health system, and created a national dialogue on the evolution of advanced nursing practice in Canada. "Advanced Nursing Practice: A National Framework" was published in 2008.
- Positioning nursing Leadership in the patient safety agenda
- Building leadership capacity through knowledge sharing and partnerships
  - Biannual National Nursing Leadership Conference
  - Healthcare Middle Management Conference
  - CNA Associate, Affiliate, and Emerging Groups
    - CNA has 40 associate and affiliate national nursing organizations representing over 430,000 nurses. CNA provides regular networking teleconferences to support and promote leadership development within these groups of expert and energetic nurses. Working with these organizations helps build CNA's capacity to respond to policy issues (such as an e-nursing strategy, nurse anesthetists, and unregulated healthcare workers) and, in turn, contributes to building capacity within these associations.

Regulatory Policy

To assure public safety, the CNA develops, manages and updates examinations for RNs and nurse practitioners, and administers certification exams in 17 specialties. CNA's "Code of Ethics for Registered Nurses" identifies principles to govern the ethical practice of nursing across the country. CNA has also articulated national regulatory frameworks for continuing competence and advanced nursing practice, as well as statements on regulatory matters such as educational requirements for entry into practice, telehealth and scope of practice.

(CNA Web site, 2008)

CNA has always played a supportive role in regulation and regulatory policy; however, its role has grown as regulation, licensing, ethics, and public protection are policy priorities that have experienced exponential growth in impact since the 1980s. Among its partnerships, the department works with the National Advisory Committee for Canadian English Language Benchmark Assessment for Nurses and the National Council of State Boards of Nursing in the United States and chairs the group of 19 organizations who make up the Canadian Network of National Associations of Regulators. Examples of CNA's regulatory policy work during this decade can be found in the following areas.

TESTING

By 1969 CNA had established a testing service to prepare and administer the national registration examination; that effort gave rise to the current Canadian Registered Nurse Examination (CRNE) we know today. One of CNA's flagship programs, the CRNE helps to protect the public by ensuring that entry-level RNs possess the competencies required to practice safely and effectively (CNA Web site 2008). As described by CNA, the level of competence of RNs in all provinces and territories (except Quebec) is measured in part by the CRNE. CNA develops and maintains the CRNE through its testing company, Assessment Strategies Inc., and in collaboration with the provincial and territorial nursing regulatory authorities who administer the exam and determine eligibility to write it. To assist nurses to write the CRNE successfully, CNA offers the popular "Canadian Registered Nurse Exam Prep Guide" (2005) and the "LeaRN CRNE Readiness Test" available online. Through its testing service, CNA also now provides the Canadian Nurse Practitioner Examination: Family/All Ages and the American Nurses Credentialling Center's Nurse Practitioner Examinations: Adult and Pediatric.

SPECIALTY CERTIFICATION

Recognizing the increasing specialization across the health system and demand for specialty recognition, CNA began developing specialty certification examinations during the mid 1980s. To date, more than 14,500 Canadian RNs have been certified in 17 nursing specialty certification programs (CNA, 2008). Soon to join the program are Enterostomal Therapy (2009) and Medical-Surgical Nursing (2010). The voluntary process requires periodic renewal and certifies that an RN has demonstrated competence in an area of nursing practice by having met predetermined standards. Certification is intended to:

- promote excellence in nursing care for the people of Canada through the establishment of national standards of practice in nursing specialty areas
- provide an opportunity for practitioners to confirm their competence in a specialty
- identify through a recognized credential those nurses meeting the national standards of their specialty.

The national nursing associations that are actively involved in, and endorse, the CNA Certification Program are listed in Table 7.2.

CODE OF ETHICS

CNA's "Code of Ethics for Registered Nurses" offers "guidance for decision-making concerning ethical matters, serves as a means for self-evaluation and reflection regarding ethical nursing practice and provides a basis for peer-review initiatives." Reflecting the impacts of changing social norms, constantly emerging health science, and new technologies on nurses and their practice settings, the code is reviewed on an ongoing basis and revised periodically. The most recent version of the code was released at the centennial meeting of CNA in June 2008. The code "not only educates nurses about their ethical responsibilities, but it also informs other healthcare professionals and members of the public about the moral commitments expected of nurses" (CNA Web site 2008). CNA also publishes "Ethical Research Guidelines."

MUTUAL RECOGNITION AGREEMENT

The 12 nursing regulatory authorities in Canada (including Ontario and Quebec) have developed a "Mutual Recognition Agreement" for RNs in Canada in compliance with the obligations of Chapter 7 of the *Agreement on Internal Trade*. This milestone signifies an historical moment in the history of nursing regulation in Canada. Since November 2006, the executive directors of all 12 provincial and territorial nursing regulatory authorities have met to develop an agreement that enables the unobstructed mobility of RNs in Canada. CNA serves as co-chair of that group, which has arrived at a pan-Canadian protocol that would facilitate mobility and be respected by all regulatory authority professionals.

NURSING EDUCATION: THE ENTRY-TO-PRACTICE STRUGGLE

In 1982, CNA members took the position that entry to the profession would be at a baccalaureate level. Today, reflecting the collective power of representation of CNA, baccalaureate education is required for entry to nursing practice in nearly every corner of the country. Quebec continues to offer diploma programs and Manitoba rolled back its entry-to-practice requirement by reopening one diploma school in 2000 as a response to shortages of nurses. However, all other jurisdictions have moved to university education, and college programs are now affiliated with *collaborative* university programs across Canada.

NURSING LEGISLATION

Nursing legislation has been substantially amended in most provinces and territories since 1980. With the exception of RNAO, all provincial and territorial nursing associations or colleges regulate the profession and approve educational programs. Internationally, a forum regrouping national nursing

Table 7.2	Canadian Nurses Association (CNA) Certification Programs	

SPECIALTY	DESIGNATION	NATIONAL ASSOCIATION AFFILIATED WITH CNA
Cardiovascular Nursing	CCN(C)	Canadian Council of Cardiovascular Nurses (CCCN)
Community Health Nursing	CCHN(C)	Community Health Nurses Association of Canada (CHNAC)
Critical Care Nursing	CNCC(C)	Canadian Association of Critical Care Nurses (CACCN)
Critical Care Pediatric Nursing	CNCCP(C)	Canadian Association of Critical Care Nurses (CACCN)
Emergency Nursing	ENC(C)	National Emergency Nurses' Affiliation (NENA)
Gastroenterology Nursing	CGN(C)	Canadian Society of Gastroenterology Nurses and Associates (CSGNA)
Enterostomal Therapy (2009)	tba	Canadian Association for Enterostomal Therapy (CAET)
Gerontology Nursing	GNC(C)	Canadian Gerontological Nursing Association (CGNA)
Hospice Palliative Care Nursing	CHPCN(C)	Canadian Hospice Palliative Care Association (CHPCA)
Medical-Surgical Nursing (2010)	tba	Canadian Association of Medical and Surgical Nurses (CAMSN)
Nephrology Nursing	CNeph(C)	Canadian Association of Nephrology Nurses and Technologists (CANNT)
Neuroscience Nursing	CNN(C)	Canadian Association of Neuroscience Nurses (CANN)
Occupational Health Nursing	COHN(C)	Canadian Occupational Health Nurses Association (COHNA)
Oncology Nursing	CON(C)	Canadian Association of Nurses in Oncology (CANO)
Orthopaedic Nursing	ONC(C)	Canadian Orthopaedic Nurses Association (CONA)
Perinatal Nursing	PNC(C)	Association of Women's Health, Obstetric and Neonatal Nurses—Canada (AWHONN—Canada)
Perioperative Nursing	CPN(C)	Operating Room Nurses Association of Canada (ORNAC)
Psychiatric/Mental Health Nursing	CPMHN(C)	Canadian Federation of Mental Health Nurses (CFMHN)
Rehabilitation Nursing	CRN(C)	Canadian Association of Rehabilitation Nurses (CARN)

associations involved in regulation was created. As a participant, CNA influences the agenda. An international framework for the development of credentialing (ICN, 2001b) and a registry for credentialing research have been developed to guide the evolution of credentialing in nursing (ICN, 2001c). In 2002, CNA hosted the third forum, which focused on credentialing in clinical practice. Credentialing indicates that an individual, program, institution, or product has met established standards; standards may be minimal and mandatory or above the minimum and voluntary (ICN, 2001b).

International Policy and Development (IPD)

In partnership with more than 30 national nursing associations from countries in Eastern Europe, Africa, Asia and Latin America, IPD works to advance the contribution of Canadian nurses to global health and equity. This is achieved through the development and implementation of international partnerships with international nursing associations and by working with Canadian nurses on international issues.

(CNA web site, 2008)

CNA houses a rich program of international policy, development, and partnerships that has a global reach. It maintains an active and formal relationship with the ICN and also links on an ad hoc basis with the World Health Organization (WHO) and its nursing office and a range of other international organizations. CNA's domestic priorities and challenges are reflected at the international level through these kinds of projects and partnerships.

FOSTERING CANADIAN LEADERSHIP WITHIN ICN

Through meetings such as the ICN Quadrennial Congress, Council of National Representatives, and ICN Socio-Economic Workforce Forum, CNA's membership in ICN provides the association and Canadian nurses with direct links to fellow nurses in 125 countries around the world. These links enable CNA to share nursing knowledge and best practices, collaborate on policy development, and contribute to strengthening the profession and the delivery of quality nursing care.

INTERNATIONAL HEALTH PARTNERSHIPS: CANADA'S PREMIER INTERNATIONAL NURSING DEVELOPMENT PROGRAM

In its development work, funded by the Canadian International Development Agency, CNA currently is involved with nine projects impacting partner nations on four continents, including the following examples:

- The *Strengthening Nurses, Nursing Networks, and Associations Program* (2007–2012) allows CNA to increase national nursing associations' capacity to build knowledge, influence and exercise leadership in health and nursing policies as well as legislative and regulatory development, and respond to the HIV/AIDS pandemic.
- The *Canada-South Africa Nurses HIV/AIDS Initiative* (2003–2008) works with the Democratic Nursing Organisation of South Africa to support its members through an awareness campaign called "Caring for the Caregiver." The campaign has involved 1,400 nurses, providing individual support for nurses, increasing understanding of health demographics, HIV care and treatment plans, and available services.
- The *Ethiopian Nurses and Needle Stick Injury Research Project* (2006–2008)
- The *Canada-Russia Initiative in Nursing* (2004–2008)

The spirit of partnership between CNA and the nursing associations of developing countries often extends beyond the funding of a project: more than 30 countries have been helped since 1970 and active relationships are maintained with many past partners and encouraged among partner countries (CNA Web site, 2008).

During this decade, the CNA's international policy and development work has also included:

- Responding to emergencies
- Contributing to gender equality
- Reinforcing institutional capacity
- Engaging Canadian nurses
  - Canadian RNs share knowledge and skills with international national nursing associations to support nursing capacity building in global health and development.
- International liaison: Sharing knowledge, leadership in action

- National HIV/AIDS Forum and International Nurses' Forum (Nurses at the Forefront of HIV/AIDS: Prevention, Care and Treatment—pre-conference international nurses' forum prior to the International AIDS Conference in Toronto, August 2006)
- WHO—CNA has contributed to the consultation and report of the WHO strategic and technical advisory committee for HIV/AIDS and CNA has a seat on this WHO advisory committee.
- Contributing to global health and equity
  - Social Justice Initiative
  - Make Poverty History Campaign
  - International Research Internship Strategy
  - International Policy and Research Initiative (Teasdale-Corti Global Health Research Partnership Program in collaboration with the University of Ottawa and the University of Alberta)
- Building policy capacity—an intensive 2-day workshop to build understanding of public policy, how it is developed and influenced, and strategies for success. This program has been offered on the international stage and will be offered to domestic audiences beginning in 2008.

Communication, Publications, and Administration

In support of its priority policy programs, CNA offers sophisticated communications, translation, and publications services. These teams provide and support programs such as the annual Media Awards (in partnership with the CMA), National Nursing Week events and materials, CNA's own annual general meeting and biennial national convention, the biennial National Nursing Leadership Conference (along with partners), and the editing, translation, and publication of dozens of position statements, papers, studies, and pamphlets every year. They are also responsible for CNA's leading communication vehicles, *Canadian Nurse*, Canada's oldest peer-reviewed nursing journal; CNA's Web site; and the nurseONE portal. To manage all these many staff and activities, CNA has a respected financial and administration team that oversees the physical plant, finances, information and communication technology, and human resources.

Toward 2020: Navigating CNA's Journey Forward

In the spring of 2006, CNA published "Toward 2020: Visions for Nursing" (Villeneuve & MacDonald, 2006) with the intention of laying out evidence about global and health system trends and to provoke dialogue and debate about scenarios that could shape nursing in the future. And *provoke* it did: The organization perhaps underestimated the national, and even global, appetite among nurses for the discussion it led. In less than 2 years, the report and its summary snapshot were downloaded from CNA's Web site more than 240,000 times, and more than 11,000 nurses and other health leaders across the country had participated in workshops, lectures, and seminars focused on the futures document and its scenarios.

That level of uptake and interest sends an interesting signal to CNA from its members and to all of Canada's leaders from the country's nurses. Many of the messages in the futures dialogue mirror those of nurses, who for years have advocated, for example, for more and better services for Canadians in their communities, schools, homes, and non-acute institutional settings. They know that their practice can and should be expanded and elevated to provide better and faster access to care for the Canadians they serve. They are dissatisfied with working conditions in many practice settings and tired of *study* usurping *action* on the ground at real points of care and service delivery. Despite the plethora of the best-intended, high-level responses, many working nurses and other care providers see little relief in sight after years of climbing absenteeism, overtime, and soaring workloads. Nurses also expect a modern curriculum and education system that capitalizes on their education and prior learning, enabling them to move seamlessly to new and different levels of education. And they want to be able to move just as seamlessly around the country and even beyond, within and across jurisdictional borders. The futures document captured some of that same spirit.

CNA's futures work since 2004 has identified worrying global, health, and nursing trends and accompanying opportunities for nursing, on many fronts. The interest of nurses in CNA's thinking—and their consequent expectations of "next steps" leadership by CNA—are clear. Going forward, CNA faces major challenges in both its own membership and business roles and in its *de facto* stewardship of Canadian nursing at large. How will CNA balance this complex matrix of variables and competing priorities? What are the activities in which CNA must be engaged in the interests of its own members and for the nursing and the health system at large?

PRIORITIES AND ISSUES IMPACTING CNA AS AN ORGANIZATION AND BUSINESS

To be sustainable and relevant in this new century, there are key policy issues CNA will need to address on several fronts. A smart and proactive association is sensitive to the members it represents and the issues they and the profession are likely to face in the future. The future focus and high-level nature of an effective national association is likely to create at least some tensions within the membership who live in the "here and now." Some member discontent is, in fact, a positive indicator of an organization fulfilling its role for the public, the profession, and the members. Too much discontent makes an organization dysfunctional and paralyzes action. CNA will need to continually seek balance and keep an eye on the tipping point.

A proactive nursing organization also seeks opportunities in the sociopolitical environment to pursue its objectives and takes advantage of these opportunities to inform and influence through a nursing lens. The ability to mobilize quickly is critical. At the same time, the finite resources, the challenge of information sharing in a vast country, the membership base represented, and the effectiveness of its spokespersons are part and parcel of this complexity and of CNA's ability to respond and influence.

Influencing policy and shaping change are required skills of professional associations like CNA. In a complex environment where many agendas compete for attention, finding points of access to influence change and understanding the right policy levers and timing to do so is a very challenging endeavor. Nurses understand the importance of being prepared to take on this work: Among the most popular themes of conferences and meetings of provincial and territorial, national, and international specialty groups are political action, power and influence, strategies, managing change, and leadership. The topic of political action is also becoming increasingly visible in the curriculum of many nursing education programs. Nurses will never speak with "one voice," but CNA could provide a valuable intervention by continuing to seek partnerships and mechanisms that allow the multitude of nursing voices to speak some common messages.

Key business and organizational challenges CNA faces internally include:

- maximizing success within a competitive federated model
- sustaining and growing membership in an era of slow (or even stagnant) overall growth of the nursing workforce
- attracting new members—Canadian nursing and its political positions would be greatly strengthened if *all* Canadian nurses were represented at federal and pan-Canadian tables together within one collective federation and association
- generating strategies to both balance and take advantage of the strong and growing regulatory policy agenda on the one hand, and the equally strong need for professional representation and advocacy on the other.

PRIORITIES AND ISSUES IMPACTING NURSING AND THE HEALTHCARE SYSTEM

As well as a strong professional nursing association, Canadians and their governments need a strong nursing *profession* to improve population health and ensure sustainability of the healthcare system. The challenge is likely only to grow in light of economic uncertainty in the United States spilling over to Canada and globally; the pressure to again rein in costs across the healthcare system will grow. To support an effective workforce and health system, CNA will need to be closely involved in the following kinds of issues over the short and medium term:

- *Credentialing and regulation*—The road ahead will include phenomenal growth in the areas of credentialing and regulation from provincial and territorial to international levels. The ICN framework will guide the need to pursue credentialing of individuals, programs, and products. In Canada, credentialing mechanisms have been developed for individuals in regard to registration for entry to practice and certification in a specialty, for example. We have credentialing for some programs, such as accreditation of a school of nursing or nursing services, but we have not developed credentialing for all products. CNA must continue to forge a leadership role in this environment, especially as pressure continues to mount to dismantle traditional regulatory structures that are seen by some as unjustified barriers to practice and mobility.

- *Leadership*—In the wake of dismantling of the professional infrastructure in healthcare in the late 1990s, we are long past thinking of leadership as solely something positional. The profession needs to continue to move toward a model of leadership and influence by all professionals so nursing values can be present in all disciplinary and multidisciplinary networks in healthcare. CNA's leadership continues to be sought; its ability to boost leadership across all roles and domains of practice (e.g., by linking nurses to educational offerings or perhaps providing some of them directly) would be added value for Canadian nurses.

Still largely unresolved and meriting the leadership and intervention of CNA include:

- building work environments that support the health of those who deliver and those who receive nursing services—including putting in place an effective number and mix of staff, adequate supervisory and professional development supports, appropriate levels of productivity, maximized scopes of practice for all providers, and workloads commensurate with the demands and resources in the environment

- development of a next-generation base of support for Canadian nursing science

- expansion of public policy responses and programs to address broad determinants of health, including climate and the environment, housing, poverty, age, race, and gender

- working with governments to shift the focus of care away from tertiary and acute care to include funding for reasonable, universal access to community, home, long-term, and palliative care

- working with governments, employers, educators, and other partners to reduce the mismatch between demand for nursing services and the supply of them—with strategies to include more seats in schools of nursing, determining the best possible deployment and utilization of nurses in the future, and developing education models to address new demands, new roles, and new competencies

- preparing for emergencies and pandemic communicable diseases at home and abroad

- working with international partners to plan appropriate and ethical migration programs and finding ways to weave the recruitment and retention, migration, and international development agendas

- working with partners in nursing education and governments to maximize enrollment in nursing education programs and develop the models of learning, teaching, curriculum, and professional development needed to move nursing forward in the 21st century.

All of these issues merit the attention and expertise of the CNA as it builds on an enviable record of success and sets a course forward into a vibrant second century at the helm of Canadian nursing.

THE INTERNATIONAL COUNCIL OF NURSES: A HISTORICAL PERSPECTIVE

In 1999, at its Centennial Conference in London, the ICN celebrated its 100th year as an international organization for nurses. For more than a century, the ICN has sustained its place as an important and meaningful organization for nurses around the world. The overall goal of the ICN is to unite nurses worldwide by forming a confederation of national nursing organizations, while supporting national nursing organizations in their efforts to influence national health and nursing policy. Throughout the years, motivation, commitment, and enthusiasm banded nurses together despite turbulent social and economic changes, hardships of war, and profound cultural differences. Currently, the ICN represents national nursing organizations from more than 120 countries and has more than one million members. However the ICN started out as a small organization within the broader context of the women's movement. It was founded in 1899 on the initiative of the British nurse and suffragist Ethel Gordon Manson, later Mrs. Bedford Fenwick, a prominent leader of the British Nurses Association.

Early Goals

From the outset, the professional welfare of nurses, the interests of women, and the improvement of human health were intertwined goals for the founders of the ICN. A small group consisting primarily of British, American, Canadian, Scandinavian, and German nurses, the ICN intended to unite nurses worldwide through an international organization. Nursing as a respected, paid, professional occupation for middle-class women was a new phenomenon at the end of the 19th century.

Healthcare profoundly changed as a result of industrialization and urbanization. Hospital reform and modern hospital development were important goals throughout Europe and North America at the time, and the foundation of hospital schools to train nurses followed in their wake. The women's movement sprung in part from the desire of middle-class women to make themselves more socially

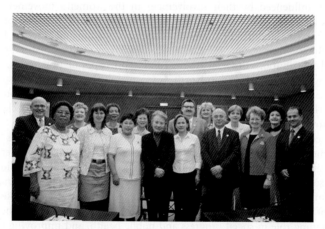

The International Council of Nurses Board of Directors (2005–2009) numbers 15 and comprises the President (Dr. Hiroko Minami, center front row), three Vice Presidents, and 11 members (elected on the basis of ICN voting areas). (Used with permission.)

useful and to carve out respectable work opportunities in areas deemed appropriate for women—thereby extending women's traditional roles in the family, such as caring for the sick, teaching, and performing social work. The founding members of the ICN were part of the growing number of women who were active in social and healthcare reform and who simultaneously sought to improve women's social position and to obtain the right to vote.

On July 1, 1899, Fenwick attended the Annual Conference of the Matron's Council of Great Britain and Ireland in London, where 200 women and nurses from around the world had gathered. At this meeting she proposed organizing an international council of nurses, modeled after the International Council of Women. The next day, she instituted a provisional committee to draft a constitution. Among the founders were Lavinia L. Dock, a nurse and activist in the women's movement from the United States and Mary Agnes Snively, an influential Canadian nurse, along with representatives from Australia, Denmark, the Netherlands, New Zealand, and the Union of South Africa. A year later, the constitution was approved, with Fenwick elected as president, Dock as secretary, and Snively as treasurer.

The ICN held its first meeting in 1901 in Buffalo, New York, at the Pan-American Exposition, and met again 3 years later in Berlin in conjunction with the congress of the International Council of Women. Aware of the need to establish their independence as a predominantly female professional group and to run their own affairs free from hospital, medical, or state control, the early leaders envisioned the ICN as a federation of national nurses' organizations, headed by a nurse, representing nurses only. However, at that time, nurses in most countries had not organized on a national level. At the 1904 meeting, only Germany, Great Britain, and the United States were ready for confederation.

In many ways, the ICN requirement that only *self-regulated bodies of nurses* could join stimulated the formation of independent national nursing organizations. For example, Canadian nurse leaders were organized jointly with their United States colleagues until that time. After the Berlin meeting however, Snively, who served as director of the influential Toronto General Hospital School of Nursing from 1884 until 1910, helped form the Canadian National Association of Trained Nurses, later the Canadian Nurses Association (CNA, 1968). Canada joined the ICN at its next congress, held in 1909 in London, as did the Netherlands, Finland, and Denmark.

As nurses organized, their commitment to creating an international body of nurses became evident. Indeed, influenced by their involvement in the women's movement, the founding leaders believed that an international organization of nurses would improve their professional standing and unite their efforts to develop a firm basis for nursing education and practice. They argued that if nursing practice met *universal standards* and was protected by state regulation, nurses, as women, could make crucial contributions to social progress and improve population health. The examples of professional nursing already developed in North America and western Europe inspired the founding leaders. In a sense, their ideas reflected Western cultural dominance typical of international politics at the time. The early ICN leaders—all from American and western European backgrounds—were strongly committed to spreading the international idea of nursing.

At the second quinquennial ICN Congress (London, 1909), Germany's Agnes Karll was elected president. The congress strongly supported women's suffrage and recommended that each national group advocate for state regulation of nursing practice. Although the ICN did not retain a regulatory function, it supported the establishment of state regulation through its member organizations. That early activism continued through the Cologne congress of 1912 where the keynote speech addressed the effects of physical strain and fatigue on nurses' health. In addition, the objectives of suffrage, nurses' expanding role in social progress and public health, and improving nurses' work conditions were paramount. Delegates also discussed the need for common standards of nursing and for clear ICN admission criteria.

By 1922, ICN represented 15 countries. Christiane Reimann (Denmark) became secretary, replacing Lavinia Dock, who had been in the position for 22 years. Reimann pushed publication of the *ICN Bulletin*—the small newsletter that evolved to become the *International Nursing Review,* the official journal of the ICN (published quarterly).

The ICN and World Health During the War Years and the Great Depression

From its founding, ICN was strongly committed to the improvement of world health. In the early decades of the 20th century, contagious diseases and high infant mortality exerted a devastating impact in the rapidly industrializing Western world. The years following World War I saw the expansion of public health services, especially in child welfare and tuberculosis care, and set a new public health agenda. The Red Cross and the League of Nations facilitated the preparation of qualified nurses for public health activities, but philanthropic foundations, such as the Rockefeller Foundation, also funded the training of public health nurses. The Rockefeller Foundation considered nurses essential for public health service. Through their International Health Commission, the Rockefeller Foundation supported public health programs throughout the world, either by founding or by cooperating with existing medical and nursing schools. Foundational support often involved and facilitated linkages with the ICN because American and European nurses led most of the foundation's projects.

During the 1929 ICN meeting in Montreal, massive changes in public health nursing dominated the agenda. Acceptable standards and conditions for general and public health nursing education provoked much debate. The powerful presence of Columbia University's Teacher's College graduates in the ICN influenced its position that science and research in nursing should be promoted as a way to strengthen the nursing profession. For most membership countries, this novel idea had limited immediate relevance, although the issue would never disappear from the ICN agenda.

By the 1930s, the worldwide economic depression had exerted a significant impact on nursing and health systems, and soon the threat of war once again shaped the actions of ICN's leaders. The rise of national socialism in Germany ended the independence of the German Nurses Association, which dissolved into the Reich's Union of German Nurses and Nursing Assistants in 1939, and World War II (WWII) began the same year. The disruption, destruction, and political realignments of the two World Wars resulted in profound social change and ultimately changed the identity of the ICN. The organization struggled to regain normalcy as many member associations had changed, others no longer existed, and some rejoined under new circumstances. After WWII, international initiatives to make healthcare "accessible for all" gained momentum. The momentous advent of antibiotics and innovative medical technology on a wider scale generally increased confidence that world health could be improved and should be considered a basic human right.

In 1948, the newly established WHO declared health to be "a state of complete physical, mental and social well-being and not merely the absence of disease or infirmity" (Howard-Jones, 1981, p. 472). In many ways, the 50th anniversary meeting (1949) in Stockholm truly introduced the ICN's voice—and thus nurses' voices—on the international stage with other players all working toward the common goal of world health. Gradually, the ICN carved out the right to speak for nursing in an ever-wider sphere of influence, assuming more activist stances and linking with international organizations, such as the United Nations and WHO. The ICN implemented a new global agenda, addressing economic, racial, religious, and gender issues that continued to complicate the professional development of nursing in many countries.

The ICN's "official relationship" status with the WHO gave it new privileges and responsibilities. In 1949, Olive Baggallay, formerly the secretary of the Florence Nightingale International Fund, became the first nursing consultant to WHO. During the 1950s, ICN also strengthened its relationship with the International Labour Organization and began to officially represent nurses on employment issues. During this time, the ICN developed the "International Code of Nursing Ethics" (1973) and translated it into numerous languages. It still provides national nurses associations with a valuable resource to address ethical nursing issues; up until the 1980s, CNA for example, relied on the ICN ethical standards for its own code of ethics.

The powerful statement on the unique function of the nurse formulated by Virginia Henderson became the basis for the ICN's vision statement on nursing. Henderson's influence was largely due to her leadership status in U.S. nursing. A longtime faculty member of the department of nursing at

Teachers' College, Columbia University, Henderson moved away from detailed descriptions of separate nursing tasks to a comprehensive perspective on the goals of nursing: "The unique function of the nurse is to assist the individual, sick or well, in the performance of those activities contributing to health or its recovery (or to a peaceful death) that he would perform unaided if he had the necessary strength, will or knowledge" (Lynaugh & Brush, 1999). At its 60th anniversary meeting in Helsinki in 1959, the ICN board approved Henderson's *Basic Principles of Nursing Care* as a core publication on behalf of the ICN Nursing Service Division. Within five years, the booklet had been translated into 12 languages, eventually becoming a classic nursing text translated into more than 30 languages.

In 1966, ICN relocated its headquarters to Geneva, reflecting the importance of the ICN's growing external relationships. At that time, Canadian Alice Girard was president (1965–1969). She was the founding dean of the Faculty of Nursing Education at the Université de Montreal, and the first bilingual president of the CNA (1958–1960). She is still the only Canadian ever elected to the presidency of the ICN, although many other distinguished Canadian nurse leaders—including Mary Agnes Snively, Jean Gunn, Grace Fairley, Helen Evans, Helen Glass, Alice Baumgart, Eleanor Ross, and Verna Huffman Splane—have served as ICN vice presidents. All except Huffman Splane also served as presidents of CNA. Dr. Huffman Splane's vice presidency (1973–1977 and 1977–1981) followed with her tenure as Canada's first federal government *principal nursing officer* (1968–1972).

Increasing Activism: Position Statements

During the 1980s, the ICN and the League of Red Cross and Red Crescent Societies collaborated in preparing a teaching kit on human rights and the Geneva Convention. The increasingly activist role of the ICN impacted its political course. At the international meetings, the ICN began to adopt position statements that publicly articulated the membership's point of view on nursing and health matters, such as "the nurse's role in family planning" or "smoking and health." Also, more political statements were accepted on topics, such as "activities of war and their influence on personality development of children and adolescents" (ICN, 2004a). Position statements had political implications; the aim was that national nursing organizations would strive to implement the suggestions made in the statements within their countries. In doing so, nurses at the national level would be better able to influence national health policy and to develop strategies for nursing action.

However, an increasingly political course created new dilemmas. Although the ICN claimed neutrality in the national affairs of its member countries, a profound internal conflict arose within the ICN over the membership of South Africa. The South African Nurses Association adhered to its country's apartheid directives, inhibiting non-White membership into the organization. Faithful to the ICN standpoint on racial matters, some member organizations insisted that South Africa open up membership to all nurses irrespective of racial background or national law. Eventually the Dutch and Swedish national organizations moved that the ICN accept a resolution to expel South Africa from membership; the resolution passed in 1974. By declaring itself against racism, the ICN also disapproved of the internal politics of one of its member associations. As a consequence, the ICN lost one of its earliest members (Rafferty & Brush, 1995). Today, a newly integrated South African national nursing organization, the Democratic Nursing Organisation of South Africa, is an active ICN member and close partner of the CNA.

By 1985, the ICN represented 97 countries, and national nurses associations paid dues based on their number of individual members. "ICN membership grew 18% between 1980 and 1985, from 862,123 to 1,056,066 members" (Brush et al., 1999, p. 169). Despite the ICN's increasing diversity however, 11 countries (Japan, United States, Canada, United Kingdom, Sweden, Denmark, Australia, Spain, Finland, Norway, and Switzerland) alone accounted for 86% of its members. As such, the agendas of industrialized countries disproportionately influenced policy directions within the ICN. However, the political point of view of the ICN changed from the past and now represented a more multinational vision. During the 1970s and 1980s, the ICN clearly spoke out against human rights violations and political suppression; the ICN considered health a basic human right for all.

Current Thinking: Issues for the ICN and the International Community

Many concerns facing the ICN in the 1990s had been issues throughout the organization's history, including professional service issues, economic stability, international relations, and global nurse representation. During the 1990s, the ICN sought new ways to address old and familiar problems. As the century drew to a close, more than 4,500 nurses from every region of the world gathered at the ICN Centennial Conference in London, where they accepted a new vision to lead the ICN and nursing into the 21st century.

REGULATING NURSING

With the many new national nurses associations joining the ICN in the 1970s and 1980s, regulation of nursing again became an agenda of the ICN. Many national associations facing difficult legal and cultural circumstances often called on the ICN for help in dealing with these complex matters. To assist leaders of national nurses associations to develop and implement national nursing regulatory systems that would meet international ICN guidelines, the ICN held six "Nursing Regulation: Moving Ahead" project workshops between 1988 and 1991. Through this project, the ICN helped prepare 161 nurses from 99 national nursing associations and 62 governments to take an active role in assessing and revising national regulations and laws controlling nursing practice and care delivery in their countries. At its 1995 meeting, the Council of National Representatives approved continued international examination of national nurse regulation and the W.K. Kellogg Foundation provided the ICN with funding for a 3-year nursing regulation study.

Korean Mo-Im Kim, elected ICN president in 1989, played an essential role in increasing political activities in regard to nursing regulation. Dr. Kim, who had previously served as the president of the Korean Nurses Association and as a member of the Korean Parliament (1981–1985), was keenly aware of the urgency for all nurses to become more politically involved in defining nursing's place in their countries' healthcare systems. Without an official position on international regulation of nursing practice, she argued, the ICN and its member associations were vulnerable to the ad hoc decisions of local government officials. Nurse education and practice varied widely among nations, which enhanced opportunities for politicians to create nurse practice acts based on their own political agendas rather than on professional nursing standards. Dr. Kim was followed as president by Margretta ("Gretta") Madden Styles (United States), elected at the Madrid, Spain meeting in June 1993, and then by Kirsten Stallnecht (Denmark), elected at the Vancouver, Canada meeting in 1997.

STANDARDIZATION AND CREDENTIALING

At the Centennial Conference in 1999, the Council of National Representatives proposed to expand nursing's role in professional standard setting and quality assurance in healthcare. It believed the time was right to develop a framework and criteria for international standardization and credentialing procedures for nursing and healthcare as a way to assure healthcare recipients of the competency of nurses and other health professionals.

Regulation became one of the key program areas of the ICN in addition to professional practice issues and the socioeconomic welfare of nurses. The ICN's long-standing goal to enforce standards for nursing education and practice provoked a renewed effort to develop universal guidelines for basic and specialty practice. In this way, the ICN sought to assist National Nurses Association

(NNAs) dealing with expanding roles of nurses, new educational standards, and the evolution of nursing specialties.

After WWII, membership countries faced the increased use of auxiliary and unlicensed personnel in a rapidly expanding healthcare system, making clear definitions and explication of boundaries of nursing practice all the more urgent. The ICN's recent involvement in an advisory and supporting role in credentialing is part of its strategy to respond to changing practice demands. The ICN's position on these issues and its effort to collect reliable data on nursing help NNAs to effectively represent nursing within national health policy debates and governmental politics (ICN, 2004b). The ICN has established the Web-based Registry of Credentialing Research, to make research findings on credentialing available to researchers and nurses, thereby assisting NNAs with their credentialing processes (ICN, 2004c).

THE GLOBAL SHORTAGE OF NURSES

The urgency of addressing issues related to regulation, credentialing, and classification of nursing care in the 1990s provoked a range of responses and strategies within ICN. However, critical nursing shortages emerging around the world compromised these initiatives at the same time. In its 1989 report to the 42nd World Health Assembly, the ICN urged WHO member states to develop strategies to:

- recruit, retain, and educate nurses and midwives
- elevate nurses to senior leadership and management positions
- support nursing research
- adopt policies to include nurses in primary care activities.

Factors that influenced decreasing numbers of nurses in many industrialized nations included declining lengths of hospital stays, increased nursing workloads through the use of technology and higher patient acuity, shift work, and attrition through marriage and childbirth. Low wages and layoffs resulting from health reform in the 1990s also played a role. Facing severe budget cuts in healthcare and consequent layoffs in nursing during the early 1990s, Canada, for example, saw many of its qualified nurses have their hours reduced or positions eliminated, and some crossed borders to nations like the United States. Simultaneously, nurses from developing countries were attracted to Canada. To balance their demand for nurses, many wealthier nations recruited nurses from developing countries: Higher salaries and better working conditions, coupled with high-powered recruitment strategies, attracted nurses to the United States, Canada, Great Britain, Australia, Israel, and other industrialized nations.

A case in point is the Philippines, which faced a severe "brain drain" of its qualified nurses during the 1980s. In 1989, about 65% of the country's 13,000 new nurse graduates emigrated abroad, mostly to the United States and Middle Eastern countries, leaving many healthcare facilities in the Philippines short of staff (Brush, 1999a). Among many other worried voices on the world stage, Beverly Malone, then general secretary of the United Kingdom's Royal College of Nurses, commented on the ethical dimensions of international recruitment, emphasizing the importance for governments, employers, and nurses alike of maintaining responsible recruitment and hiring strategies (Malone, 2003).

African nations have suffered severe shortages of nurses because of the increased demand for nursing and preventive care in the face of a rapidly spreading AIDS epidemic—set against the reality that so many nurses, doctors, and other providers were themselves infected. As of 2007, an estimated 33.2 million people are living with HIV globally—68% of them in sub-Saharan Africa (77% of all cases in women). Largely as a result of HIV/AIDS and its related complications, among the 25 nations having the lowest life expectancies on earth, only two—Haiti and Afghanistan—lie outside Africa. With economic prosperity directly correlated with spending on healthcare and, in turn, nurse density, it is no surprise that despite the widespread need for nursing care, African nations fall far short of the supply they need. Nurse density varies as much as a hundredfold across the members states of WHO.

WHO noted in 2006 that "57 countries, 36 of which are in sub-Saharan Africa, have severe shortages of health workers. More than four million additional doctors, nurses, midwives, managers and public health workers are urgently needed to fill this gap" (2006). In Europe, reports on nursing shortages are varied. The Netherlands and Norway, for example, had more than 2.5 times as many nurses per capita as did Canada in 2000, but their nursing workforces, too, were aging and not being adequately replenished with new graduates. Other members of the European community also reported increasing national shortages of nurses. The United States and Canada reported similar, and sometimes even worse, current and looming shortages.

Nurse migration compromises local and international efforts to improve short-term nurse recruitment and retention as well as long-term personnel planning. The ICN seeks to assist member associations in studying nursing personnel needs and resources, sharing information pertaining to nursing's worldwide employment status, and continuing discussions of the international impact of nurse shortages (Brush, 1999a). A new global partnership, the Global Health Workforce Alliance, was launched by the WHO in 2006 to address the worldwide shortage of nurses, doctors, midwives, and other health workers. It was created to "draw together and mobilize key stakeholders engaged in global health to help countries improve the way they plan for, educate and employ health workers" (World Health Organization, 2006). Despite a decade of attention, worrying global shortages, migration, and recruitment challenges remain far from resolved in 2008, and, in many nations, demand for nursing services continues to far outpace an adequate supply of nurses to provide them.

ADVANCING NURSING PRACTICE

A key problem with global nurse regulation is the dearth of data about *what* constitutes nurses' work and *how* it is shaped by healthcare service payments. In response, in 1989, the American Nurses Association (ANA) proposed a council resolution urging national nurses associations to develop nation-specific classification systems for nursing care. The initiative may have been triggered by a difficult situation with which the ANA was confronted when the American Medical Association proposed introducing a new healthcare worker in the United States. The ANA, which successfully lobbied against such a decision, argued that the nursing profession must name its distinct contribution to healthcare to be recognized in worldwide healthcare planning and financing. The ANA offered to collect, document, and share data on nursing practice across countries, clinical settings, and patient populations to assist national associations in planning types and amounts of nursing needed, in determining skill mixes for various care settings and patient groups, and in evaluating clinical efficacy and cost.

Responding to the ANA resolution in 1990, the ICN board of directors invited June Clark (United Kingdom) and Norma Lang (United States) to develop a feasibility study for an International Classification for Nursing Practice (ICNP). Gretta Styles, who was chair of the Professional Services Committee, nurse consultant Fadwa Affara, and Denmark's Randi Mortenson and Gunnar Nelson completed the team. From 1990 to 1997, they consulted with nurses and classification experts to collect, group, and rank nursing phenomena, interventions, and outcomes, with the ultimate goal of creating a universal nursing language (Brush, 1999a). In 2000, the ICN made ICNP an official program and continued to update and revise the classification system (ICN, 2004d). In that same year, the ICN published an updated version of its "Code of Ethics for Nurses" to provide nurses with a continuous resource to help maintain ethical practices worldwide (Fry, 2002).

Another pertinent issue arising through the 1990s was advancing nursing practice to respond to expanding primary healthcare demands and changing conditions of specialty nursing care. The ICN established an International Nurse Practitioner/Advanced Practice Nursing Network with the view to provide international resources for nurses practising in these roles and to alert policymakers and health planners to the essential function of these roles in enhancing healthcare services. Again, the ICN sees it as a major responsibility to provide relevant data and to support nurses and countries in the process of expanding nurses' roles (ICN, 2004e).

THE ICN IN THE 21ST CENTURY

During the 1990s, the ICN prepared various policy decisions and initiated planning to lead nursing into the 21st century. In 1993, at the Council of National Representatives meeting in Madrid, the ICN adopted Toward the 21st Century: A Strategic Plan, 1994–1999. The plan addressed the issues the ICN considered crucial to health planning for the new century, including formulating health and social policy, establishing professional standardization and socioeconomic equity, collaborating with other international bodies, disseminating nursing knowledge, and developing frameworks for identifying and measuring nurses' work. The strategic plan clearly laid out the ICN's goals for the future, which realistically could be accomplished considering available resources.

Two years later, at the 1995 Council meeting in Harare, Zimbabwe, the ICN endorsed several key position statements, emphasizing its expansionist agenda. Revisiting its 1981 Resolution of Female Excision, Circumcision and Mutilation, the ICN resolved to work with local, national, and international groups opposed to the practice. Position statements related to psychiatric mental health nursing and to the costs and value of nursing were also endorsed. Other resolutions specifically addressed issues of nurse titling, health policy participation, nursing school accreditation, and nursing students' roles in national nursing associations (Brush, 1999a; ICN, 2004a).

In 1997, Canadian Judith Oulton, formerly executive director of the CNA, assumed the post of CEO of the ICN. She brought with her the belief that it is critical for nurses in all countries to participate in shaping health policy and to have their work backed up by accurate data demonstrating nursing's contributions to health outcomes. During that year, some 5,000 nurses from 120 countries convened in Vancouver, Canada, to "Share the Health Challenge" at the ICN's 21st Quadrennial Congress. It was the first time Canada had hosted an ICN congress since the 1929 meeting in Montreal. Enhancement of nurses' political influence was a persistent theme: "We must raise our social status as a profession to our level of social contribution and our influence to the level of our strength," said outgoing ICN President Gretta Styles. "We must raise the intensity of our politics to the intensity of our ethics" (Brush, 1999a, p. 155).

At the 1999 Centennial Conference in London, the white heart was adopted as a symbol to commemorate a century of ICN nurses caring for and contributing to world health and welfare. ICN President Kirsten Stallknecht (Denmark) addressed the audience at the opening ceremony of the conference, urging nurses to "forge a renewed vision for nurses and nursing" that emphasized "high-touch" over "high-tech." At the end of her speech, she unveiled the ICN's vision statement for the 21st century, which opens as follows: "United within ICN, the nurses of all nations speak with one voice. We speak as advocates for all those we serve and for all the unserved, insisting that prevention, care, and cure be the right of every human being" (Brush, 1999a, p. 155).

Reflecting the demands and priorities of the world around it in a new century, ICN's diverse activities include human rights (including a focus on the rights of women and girls), the issue of task-shifting and its impacts on nursing, patient safety, and disaster preparedness. In 2006 it established the International Centre for Human Resources in Nursing in partnership with the Florence Nightingale International Foundation. Billed as a unique online service serving anyone involved in nursing human resources, the Centre is dedicated to "strengthening the nursing workforce globally through the development, ongoing monitoring and dissemination of comprehensive information, standards and tools on nursing human resources policy, management, research and practice" (ICN Web site, 2008). The companion International Centre on Nurse Migration serves as "a global resource for the development, promotion and dissemination of research, policy and information on nurse migration" (ICN Web site, 2008). It occupies a key role in establishing effective global and national migration policies and practices to facilitate safe patient care and positive practice environments for nurse migrants. And in line with both of these initiatives, ICN also hosts the International Socio-Economic Workforce Forum where interested member nations meet to hammer out these vexing human resources issues. Partnering with the Canadian Federation of Nurses Unions, CNA is always a participant in the forum, both providing information to the forum and sharing in it.

Judith Oulton completed her term as CEO in the fall of 2008, turning over the reins to David Benton, formerly a senior consultant at ICN. The year 2009 will find thousands of nurses from some 130 member countries meeting in Durban, South Africa, for the 110th anniversary Congress of the ICN, taking yet another step forward in ICNs illustrious journey of international leadership of nurses and nursing.

SUMMARY

This chapter has reviewed the evolution and major roles, priorities, and challenges of the CNA and the ICN. In Canada, the CNA's role is to protect the public, speak on behalf of the profession, and put strategies in place to strengthen the healthcare system. As the national voice of nursing, it focuses on the power of representation and regulatory policy. CNA's regulatory policy work is reflected in the educational field and in the evolution of credentialing in nursing. Examples of the power of representation include the CNA's influence on the initial Canada Health Act, and in the rich tapestry of work now being carried out by its policy departments. For example, during this decade CNA has developed significant expertise and leadership in health and human resources planning, quality nursing practice environments, and international development. Current priorities for the CNA include leading the "futures" agenda by developing visions for a redesigned health system strongly based in principles of primary healthcare, quality practice environments, development of information and communication technologies, leadership, international development, and environmental health. Future challenges for Canadian nursing include maintaining strong and united voices and messages, with increased representation in Quebec and Ontario; development of appropriate leadership models to promote nursing values in and across multidisciplinary healthcare networks and delivery models; and growth and influence in the areas of credentialing and regulation.

The ICN's vision for nursing in the 21st century reflects the organization's century-long involvement in the politics of healthcare. The new century will undoubtedly present many challenges and opportunities, including the internationalization of markets, which may create an unknown effect on the process of reworking and redefining nursing. Tensions between generations of nurses and philosophical differences among ICN member associations also may pose new challenges to the ICN in the 21st century. However, throughout the past 100 years, the ICN has proven its ability to respond to change, making it likely that the ICN will maintain its enduring meaning for many nurses around the world in the new century.

Add to your knowledge of this issue:

Online

Canadian Resources

Canadian Nurses Association	**www.cna-aiic.ca**
CNA's nurseONE Portal	**www.nurseone.ca**
Academy of Canadian Executive Nurses	**www.acen.ca**
Canadian Association for the History of Nursing	**www.ualberta.ca/~jhibberd/cahn_achn**
Canadian Association of Schools of Nursing	**www.casn.ca**
Canadian Council on Health Services Accreditation	**www.cchsa.ca**
Canadian Federation of Nurses Unions	**www.cfnu.ca**
Canadian Healthcare Association	**www.cha.ca**
Canadian Medical Association	**www.cma.ca**
Canadian Nursing Students' Association	**www.cnsa.ca**
Health Action Lobby	**www.heal.ca**
The Margaret M. Allemang Centre for the History of Nursing	**www.allemang.on.ca**

International Resources

International Council of Nurses	**www.icn.ch**
Organization for Economic Cooperation and Development	**www.oecd.org**
United Nations	**www.un.org**
United Nations Educational, Scientific, and Cultural Organization	**www.unesco.org**
World Health Organization	**www.who.int/en**

REFLECTIONS on the Chapter...

❶ Describe a professional association you are familiar with and explain what role it fulfills in society.

❷ Over the past 20 years, what issues have been affected by the power of representation of the CNA? Select one and describe how the influence of the CNA changed the course of action.

❸ What are two current policy priorities for the CNA and ICN? Discuss one priority and its progress at both the national and international levels.

❹ Having read this chapter, in what ways are CNA's Web site (http://www.cna-nurses.ca) and nurseONE portal (http://www.nurseone.ca/) and ICN's Web site (http://www.icn.ch) useful to you as a student and a beginning practitioner? If you have suggestions, how would you communicate them to CNA and ICN?

5 Discuss the impact of organized international nursing on changing healthcare demands and world health. Identify three political strategies nurses developed to change healthcare and health.

6 Identify three important issues that the ICN has faced throughout its history and discuss strategies it developed in response.

7 What roles does the ICN play in issues of regulation of nursing practice? How do they interrelate with CNA's roles?

8 Select a position statement from the CNA Web site (http://www.cna-aiic.ca) or the ICN Web site (http://www.icn.ch) and discuss its potential impact on health policy. How could the position statement contribute to informing or resolving the issue at the local level or in your nursing practice?

References

Advisory Committee on Health Human Resources (2000). *The nursing strategy for Canada.* Ottawa: Author.

Boschma, G. & Stuart, M. (1999). ICN during wartime: 1912–1947. *International Nursing Review, 46*(2), 41–46.

Brush, B.L. (1999a). Leading nurses to a new century: ICN during the 1990s. *International Nursing Review, 46*(5), 151–155.

_____. (1999b). Turmoil and transformation: ICN during the postwar years. *International Nursing Review, 46*(3), 75–79.

Brush, B.L., Lynaugh, J.E., Boschma, et al. (1999). *Nurses of all nations: A history of the International Council of Nurses, 1899–1999.* Philadelphia: Lippincott Williams & Wilkins.

Canadian Institute for Health Information. (2005). *Registered nurses database.* Retrieved March 2005 from http://www.secure.cihi.ca.

_____. (2007). *Workforce trends of registered nurses in Canada 2006.* Ottawa: Author.

Canadian Nurses Association. (1958). *The first fifty years.* Ottawa: Author.

_____. (1968). *The leaf and the lamp.* Ottawa: Author.

_____. (1980). *Putting 'health' back into healthcare: Submission to the Health Services Review.* Ottawa: Author.

_____. (1984). *The research imperative for nursing in Canada: A 5-year plan towards the year 2000.* Ottawa: Author.

_____. (1998). *The quiet crisis in healthcare.* Ottawa: Author.

_____. (1999). *Repair, realign, and resource healthcare.* Ottawa: Author.

_____. (2000). *Rebuilding Canada's health system starts with renewing the nursing workforce.* Ottawa: Author.

_____. (2001). *Revitalizing the nursing workforce and strengthening Medicare.* Ottawa: Author.

_____. (2006). *Operational report of the Chief Executive Officer.* Ottawa: Author.

Canadian Nursing Advisory Committee. (2002). *Our health, our future: Creating quality workplaces for Canadian nurses.* Ottawa: Health Canada.

Fry, S. (2002). Guest editorial: Defining nurses' ethical practices in the 21st century. *International Nursing Review, 49*(1), 1–3.

Government of Canada. (1984). *Canada Health Act of 1984—Bill C-3.* Ottawa: House of Commons, Government of Canada.

Health Action Lobby. (1992). *Medicare: A value worth keeping.* Ottawa: Author.

Howard-Jones, N. (1981). The World Health Organization in historical perspective. *Perspectives in Biology and Medicine, 24*(3), 467–482.

International Council of Nurses. (1973). *ICN code for nurses: Ethical concepts applied to nursing.* Geneva: Author.

_____. (2001a). *From vision to action: ICN in the 21st century* (revised February 2001). Geneva, Switzerland: Author.

_____. (2001b). *The ICN credentialing framework.* Unpublished manuscript. Geneva, Switzerland: Author.

_____. (2001c). *The ICN credentialing research registry—Draft 1.* Unpublished manuscript. Geneva, Switzerland: Author.

_____. (2004a). *ICN position statements* [Online]. Retrieved on October 20, 2008 from http://www.icn.ch/policy.htm.

_____. (2004b). *Regulation: Regulation programme area overview* [Online]. Retrieved on October 20, 2008 from http://www.icn.ch/regulation.htm.

_____. (2004c). *About the International Council of Nurses' registry of credentialing research.* [Online]. Retrieved on October 20, 2008 from http://www.icn.ch/rcrhome.htm.

_____. (2004d). *International classification for nursing practice (ICNP).* [Online]. Retrieved on October 20, 2008 from http://www.icn.ch/icnp.htm.

_____. (2004e). Nurse practitioner/advanced practice network [Online]. Retrieved on October 20, 2008 from http://icn-apnetwork.org/.

Lemire Rodger, G. (1999). Intraorganizational politics. In J.M. Hibberd & D.L. Smith (Eds.), *Nursing management in Canada* (2nd ed., pp. 279–295). Toronto: Saunders.

Lynaugh, J.E. & Brush, B. (1999). The ICN story 1899–1999. *International Nursing Review, 46*(1), 3–8.

MacPhail, J. (1996). The role of the Canadian Nurses Association in the development of nursing in Canada. In J. Ross Kerr & J. MacPhail (Eds.), *Canadian nursing issues and perspectives* (3rd ed., pp. 31–54). St. Louis: Mosby.

Malone, B. (2003). Guest editorial: Promoting the value of nursing in the context of a global nursing shortage. *International Nursing Review, 50*(3), 129–130.

Meilicke, D. & Larsen, J. (1988). Leadership and the leaders of the Canadian Nurses Association. In A.J. Baumgart & J. Larsen (Eds.), *Canadian nursing faces the future* (pp. 421–459). St. Louis: Mosby.

Mhatre, S.L. & Deber, R. (1992). From equal access to healthcare to equitable access to health: Review of Canadian provincial commissions and reports. *International Journal of Health Services, 22*(4), 645–668.

Rafferty, A.M. & Brush, B.L. (1995). Conflict and consensus: The International Council of Nurses and international nursing. *International History of Nursing Journal, 1*, 4–16.

Ryten, E. (1997). *A statistical picture of the past, present, and future of registered nurses in Canada.* Ottawa: Canadian Nurses Association.

Ryten, E. (2002). *Planning for the future: Nursing human resource projections.* Ottawa: Canadian Nurses Association.

Villeneuve, M. & MacDonald, J. (2006). *Toward 2020: Visions for nursing.* Ottawa: Canadian Nurses Association.

World Health Organization. (1978). *Primary healthcare: Report on the International Conference on Primary Healthcare,* Alma Ata, USSR, September 6–12, 1978. Geneva, Switzerland: Author.

World Health Organization. (2006). *New global alliance seeks to address worldwide shortage of doctors, nurses and other health workers.* Retrieved April, 2008 from http://www.who.int/ mediacentre/news/releases/2006/pr26/en/ index.html.

Acknowledgments

The CNA section of this chapter could not have been completed without the personal communications of CNA's executive leaders, policy directors and staff, the extensive information contained in CNA's Web site (2008), and in the "2006 Operational Report of the Chief Executive Officer" (CNA, 2006). The ICN section of this chapter is based largely on research conducted by Barbara L. Brush, Joan E. Lynaugh, Geertje Boschma, Anne Marie Rafferty, Meryn Stuart, and Nancy J. Tomes for *Nurses of All Nations: A History of the International Council of Nurses, 1899–1999* (Philadelphia: Lippincott Williams & Wilkins, 1999), used in this chapter with permission from the publisher. A series of articles on the history of the ICN, published by the same authors, have also been used with permission. They include:

Lynaugh, J.E. & Brush, B. (1999). The ICN story 1899–1999. *International Nursing Review, 46*(1), 3–8

Boschma, G. & Stuart, M. (1999). ICN during wartime: 1912–1947. *International Nursing Review, 46*(2), 41–46.

Sections of the ICN discussion were adapted with permission from:

Brush, B.L. (1999a). Leading nurses to a new century: ICN during the 1990s. *International Nursing Review, 46*(5), 151–155.

Brush, B.L. (1999b). Turmoil and transformation: ICN during the postwar years. *International Nursing Review, 46*(3), 75–79.

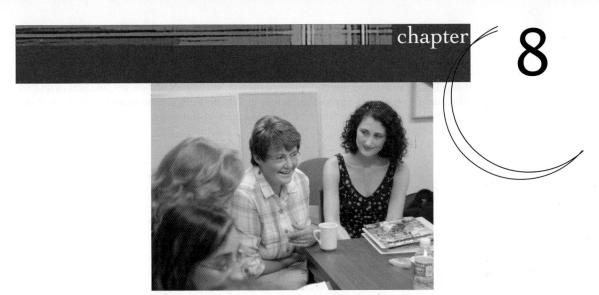

chapter 8

Students discuss issues of provincial and territorial regulation of nurse practitioners with Dr. Mary Ellen Purkis at the University of Victoria.

Canadian Provincial and Territorial Professional Associations and Colleges

Laurel Brunke

Critical Questions

As a way of engaging with the ideas in this chapter, consider the following:

1 Are you aware of which groups of workers in the healthcare system are regulated and which are not? Who do you imagine is responsible for the regulation of healthcare workers?

2 In reflecting on what you know about the structure of the Canadian healthcare system and the tensions between national and territorial and provincial political priorities, what would you anticipate as tensions arising in the regulation of registered nurses (RNs)?

3 Given the mandate of the International Council of Nurses (ICN) and the Canadian Nurses Association (CNA), what role do you imagine they might play in the regulation of RNs?

Chapter Objectives

After completing this chapter, you will be able to:

1 Describe the evolution of nursing regulation in Canada.

2 Recognize how differences in legislation have resulted in different approaches to nursing regulation.

3 Identify differences in the roles and responsibilities of provincial and territorial associations and colleges.

4 Understand issues associated with registration mobility and trends in regulation.

5 Discuss potential implications of current issues facing provincial and territorial colleges and associations.

This chapter will assist the reader in understanding and appreciating the value of nursing self-regulation. To achieve this end, the evolution of nursing regulation in Canada is described, as are differences in regulatory approaches across jurisdictions, issues associated with these differences, and considerations for the future of the regulation of nursing by provincial and territorial nursing associations and colleges.

REGULATION

The purpose of regulating the nursing profession is straightforward: to protect the public, which makes regulation itself a most complex issue.

The What and Why of Regulation

What is regulation? Simply, regulation is the "forms and processes whereby order, consistency, and control are brought to an occupation and its practices" (International Council of Nurses [ICN], 1985, p. 7). The ICN states the following goals of regulation:

- Define the profession and its members.
- Determine the scope of practice.
- Set standards of education and competent and ethical practice.
- Establish systems of accountability and credentialing processes (Styles & Affara, 1997).

Finocchio and colleagues, with the Taskforce on Healthcare Workforce Regulation (1995), take a broader view of regulation. They believe that regulation of the healthcare workforce best serves the public's interest if it promotes effective health outcomes and protects the public from harm; ensures accountability to the public; respects consumers' rights to choose their healthcare providers from a range of safe options; encourages a healthcare system that is flexible, rational, and cost effective and that facilitates effective working relationships among healthcare providers; and provides for professional and geographic mobility of competent providers.

Evolution of Regulation

Regulation of professions really began with the formation of crafts and guilds. There was, and always has been, competition among tradespeople in relation to the goods they sold and the services they provided. The crafts and guilds were made up of the people who were known to provide quality products and services, in part because they developed standards for these products and services. Of course, with increased quality came increased costs and, in some circumstances, a monopoly on the products and services the guilds were providing. From these guilds and crafts arose licensing laws intended to protect the public and ensure that only members of the crafts or guilds could provide the specified services and products (Cutshall, 1998). These traditional licensing laws provided for exclusive scope of practice, or what is sometimes referred to as *turf protection*. Today, there is a shift away from this approach to regulation, a topic discussed later in the chapter.

The nature of regulation has changed in other ways over the years. Historically, professional regulation focused essentially on gatekeeping, that is, setting the requirements for those who can enter the profession and disciplining those who fail to meet the standards of the profession. Finocchio and colleagues (1995, p. vii) have said, in relation to healthcare workforce regulation in the United States, "Though it has served us well in the past, healthcare regulation is out of step with today's healthcare needs and expectations." However, nursing regulatory bodies in Canada have for some time embraced a more contemporary approach to regulation. This approach recognizes that there is more to regulation than gatekeeping.

The CNA (2007a, p. 1) believes that:

Public protection is promoted when regulatory frameworks strengthen nursing practice and leadership in all domains of practice, including clinical practice, administration, education and research; when they provide supports to correct and improve practice; and when they focus not only on individual nurses but also on practice environments that support nurses in providing safe, competent and ethical care.

Some nursing regulatory bodies in Canada have adopted a regulatory framework of promoting good practice, preventing poor practice, and intervening when practice is unacceptable. The benefits of promotion and prevention strategies—the quality improvement approach—mean that intervention with unacceptable practice can be kept at a minimum.

REGULATION OF NURSING

Many nurses take it for granted that nursing is a profession and that, like other professions, nurses are entitled to collective professional autonomy, that is, the self-regulation of the profession as a whole. Professional autonomy means that, with appropriate public input, professional groups govern themselves. Canada has a tradition that communities of people within society take responsibility for meeting their obligations, both to themselves and the community at large. They do this by managing their affairs in a way that respects and furthers the good of society while recognizing the legitimate interests of their members. This is the essence of self-regulation (Registered Nurses Association of British Columbia [RNABC], 2000). However, self-regulation is a privilege of a profession, not a right. In Canada, self-regulation of nursing is less than a century old.

History of Nursing Regulation in Canada

The move to obtain registration for nurses began in 1893 with the formation of the American Society of Superintendents of Training Schools for Nursing of the United States and Canada. This was followed by the development of the Associated Alumnae of the United States and Canada in 1896. Securing legislation to "differentiate the trained from the untrained" (Canadian Nurses Association [CNA], 1968, p. 35) was the purpose of the Associated Alumnae. When it was recognized that the fight for the nursing legislation had to be fought separately in each country, the Canadian and American groups separated. Consequently, the Canadian Society of Superintendents of Training Schools for Nurses was formed in 1907, with formation of the Provisional Society of the Canadian Nurses Association of Trained Nurses following in 1908 (CNA, 1968).

The development of provincial graduate nurses associations was due in large part to the increase in the number of nursing personnel that occurred at the end of the 19th century. Competition between trained professional nurses and nurses with little or no professional training was evident in the areas of wages and status. Moreover, no mechanisms for ensuring uniformity in nursing service standards were in place (CNA, 1968). Kerr (1996) identified two powerful social forces that affected the pursuit of legislation for the registration of nurses: first, consciousness raising regarding women's rights that was part of the effort to obtain the vote for women, and second, the increased valuing of nurses and nurses' services that occurred during World War I. Kerr speculated that these factors, as well as a general recognition that a mechanism was needed to ensure that nurses were qualified, led to the passage of legislation in all provinces over a 12-year period—a relatively brief time.

In 1910, the nurses of Nova Scotia became the first to have nursing legislation. Registration was voluntary, and nongraduate nurses could still practise. The Registered Nurses Act, which incorporated the Graduate Nurses Association of Nova Scotia, set out, among other things, the powers of the association and the duty of officers, admission of nurses as members, discipline of members, and appointment of examiners. Legislation proclaimed in Manitoba in 1913 was more in keeping with current legislation, as it set out minimum standards for admission, curriculum in schools of nursing, and the registration and discipline of practicing nurses. By 1914, all provinces except Prince Edward Island had a provincial nurses association.

Work to achieve legislation was not easy, as can be seen in the following example from British Columbia, where efforts to achieve legislation began in 1912. In 1914, the government decided that the nurses' bill could not be accepted as a government measure, and the association was advised to have the bill presented as a public measure introduced by a private member.

When the bill was reintroduced in 1916, it was suggested that the president and secretary of the College of Physicians and Surgeons should be members of the council of the nurses association and that the orders, regulations, fees, and bylaws should be subject to the approval of the College of Physicians and Surgeons. The nurses association decided to withdraw the bill rather than include these amendments. A letter was sent to the College of Physicians and Surgeons asking if these amendments met with their approval and if they wished to have graduate nurses under their control. This suggestion was unanimously opposed by the college. A revised bill was passed in 1918, and, interestingly enough, the first council was named by the College of Physicians and Surgeons (Kerr, 1944).

Ontario was the last province to achieve legislation for nursing because of objections from nurses who believed they could not meet the qualifications and because some hospital administrators feared that they could not meet education standards. However, by 1922, all nine provinces had some form of nurse registration.

The first act concerning nursing in Newfoundland came into effect in 1931, and the Newfoundland Graduate Nurses Association was incorporated in 1935. Newfoundland formed as a province in 1949 and enacted legislation for nurses, with mandatory registration, in 1953. Legislation regulating nurses in the Northwest Territories and the Yukon was enacted in 1988 and 1994, respectively. Membership in the Northwest Territories Registered Nurses Association, formed in 1975, was initially voluntary. Before the legislation enacted in 1994 in the Yukon, RNs working there had to be registered in another Canadian jurisdiction.

Mandatory Registration

Initial legislation for nursing varied across provinces, and, in some instances, aspects of the legislation were inconsistent with the primary purpose of the regulation of the profession, (i.e., protection of the public). Initially, not all nurses had to be registered to practise nursing. In some jurisdictions, these nonregistered individuals were permitted to use the title "registered nurse" even if they did not meet the requirements for entry to the profession or uphold the profession's standards. In 1922, the Nova Scotia Act was amended to the effect that a register be kept "in which shall be entered the name of every member of the Association" and "only those persons whose names are entered in the register shall be deemed qualified to hold themselves out to the public as registered nurses" (S. Farouse, personal communication, 2002). Although not the same as mandatory registration, it was a first step toward this important mechanism for public protection.

Quebec was the first province to have mandatory licensing with the passing of the Quebec Nurses' Act in 1946 (CNA, 1968). The achievement of mandatory registration took considerably longer in other provinces, with British Columbia and Saskatchewan being the last to make this change to existing legislation. Mandatory registration was a requirement in the first acts for nursing enacted in the Yukon and Northwest Territories.

Authority of Nursing Regulatory Bodies

In Canada, authority to regulate the profession comes from legislation enacted by provincial and territorial governments. The nature of the legislation varies across Canada, although there is increasing interest from governments in enacting uniform legislation for all professions in a province or territory. Regardless of the form of the legislation, nursing regulatory bodies in Canada generally have authority for the following:

- standards of education and qualifications for registrants
- standards of practice and professional ethics
- use of title
- scope of practice
- professional discipline
- approval or recognition of education programs for entry to the profession
- continuing competence requirements for registrants.

Responsibility for regulation of registered nursing rests with a provincial and territorial professional association or college. In Ontario, this authority rests with the College of Nurses of Ontario (CNO), which also has responsibility for regulating registered practical nurses. In other provinces, this group of professionals, also known as licensed practical nurses or certified nursing assistants, is regulated by separate organizations. Ontario is the only jurisdiction in Canada to have both a regulatory organization and professional association, the Registered Nurses Association of Ontario (RNAO). The RNAO's mission is to pursue healthy public policy and to promote the full participation of RNs in shaping and delivering health services now and in the future. Contrast this with the mission of the CNO to protect the public's right to quality nursing services by providing leadership to the nursing profession in self-regulation. Risk (1992, p. 368) identifies that the uniqueness in Ontario "is based on the philosophical premise that there is an inherent conflict (real or perceived) between professional self-interest and public interest, and that regulatory decisions must be separate from professional advancement." At the heart of this issue is the question of whether an association that has as one of its goals the promotion of the profession can do this in a way that does not interfere with meeting its public interest mandate. In Alberta, the College and Association of Registered Nurses, has, as can be seen by its name, both a regulatory and association mandate.

There is no evidence to suggest that this combined role has affected the ability of the other Canadian nursing regulatory bodies to meet their public protection mandate. Perhaps that is why the Ontario model is unique, not only in Canada but in many other countries as well.

Other differences between jurisdictional authorities relate to approval of nursing education programs, requirements for continuing competence for registration renewal, requirements for re-entry into practice, language requirements for registration, and approaches to regulation of nurse practitioners (NPs).

APPROVAL OF NURSING EDUCATION PROGRAMS

Of particular interest is the authority for approval or recognition of nursing education programs for entry to the profession. This authority typically includes establishing the criteria for approval of the nursing education program as well as actually approving the program. Essentially, this gives the profession the authority to establish the education, that is, the competency requirements for entry to the profession. In most instances, approval is limited to education programs for entry to the profession. However, the College of Registered Nurses of British Columbia (CRNBC) and the Association of Registered Nurses of Newfoundland and Labrador have authority to approve and recognize education programs for NPs. Until recently, the responsibility and authority for approving nursing education programs resided with the nursing regulatory body, except in Ontario and Quebec. Until 2005 in Ontario, authority for approval and monitoring of university programs was vested in the Council of University Programs in Nursing and the university senate or governing council. Effective January 1, 2005, changes to the Nursing Act in Ontario provide for nursing education programs to be approved by a body or bodies designated by the council or by the council itself. This is a very significant change because, before this, the CNO had no formal role in the approval of schools. The CNO has selected the Canadian Association of Schools of Nursing as the agency to conduct the approval process. In Quebec, the Ministère de l'Éducation, du Loisor et du Sport has responsibility for nursing programs. In 2001, the Ordre des Infirmières et Infirmiers du Quebec was invited to participate in the consultation process for nursing curriculum for the first time. This consultation resulted in a revised nursing education program. In British Columbia, with the transition to regulating RNs under the Health Professions Act, the British Columbia Cabinet must approve any changes to the schedule listing education programs recognized by the CRNBC. Many consider this new requirement to be an erosion of the profession's authority to self-regulate.

Regulation of Nurse Practitioners

Another area of notable difference among jurisdictions is in the current or intended approaches to the regulation of NPs. RNs have been working in extended or expanded roles, predominantly in rural or remote settings, for many years. Although these roles are considered by some to parallel those of the NP, authority to carry out functions such as diagnosing, prescribing, and managing labor and delivery comes through delegated medical acts rather than legislation that authorizes RNs to carry out these functions autonomously. Pressures related to physician shortages, particularly in underserviced areas, and increasing pressures on health budgets have resulted in renewed interest in implementing the NP role. The current status of NPs across Canada can be seen in Table 8.1, which demonstrates that use of NPs varies considerably across the country, as does the way in which the role is enacted. In some jurisdictions, collaborative relationships with physicians are mandated; in others, they are not. In some jurisdictions, such as Newfoundland, the title "nurse practitioner" is, or will be, protected; in others, there are no plans to protect the title. In some provinces, these nurses are identified in different ways; in Ontario, for example, they are registered as RN/Extended Class.

This variation raises questions as to how the public can be easily informed about which RNs have authority for some of the functions commonly associated with the NP role. Another significant difference is that, in some jurisdictions, the NP has authority for a "package" of functions, such as in Ontario and Newfoundland, whereas in others, such as Manitoba, authority will be given for each individual function.

The evolution of the regulation of NPs provides a good example of how differences in regulatory approaches can have implications for the consumer of healthcare. Consider how much easier it would be for consumers and other healthcare providers to understand the role and the responsibilities of NPs if the regulatory framework was the same in all jurisdictions. It also provides an example of how differing approaches to regulation can affect the mobility of nurses across the country because the requirements for recognition as an NP are beginning to vary across jurisdictions.

 ## ISSUES IN REGULATION

As demonstrated in earlier sections of this chapter, there is a need for regulation to evolve to respond to the changing world and the needs of the healthcare system. Emerging issues in regulation are related to a variety of factors.

Impact of Globalization

Globalization of the economy presents significant challenges to countries to remain competitive in world markets. In this context, policies are being adopted that favor deregulation, decentralization, and, in some instances, a reduced role for government. Advances in technology are already affecting how healthcare is delivered, with increasing use of video and data communications. At the same time, trade agreements, such as the General Agreement on Trade in Services, the North American Free Trade

Table 8.1	Regulation of Nurse Practitioners in Canada
JURISDICTION	**STATUS OF NURSE PRACTITIONER LEGISLATION**

Alberta	• The Health Professions Act—Registered Nurses Profession Regulation (AR 232/2005) provides for the regulation of nurse practitioners ([NPs] passed in November 2005).
	
	 • The NP title is protected.
	
	 • NPs may perform the following restricted activities:
	
	   • prescribe a Schedule I drug within the meaning of the Pharmaceutical Profession Act
	
	   • prescribe parenteral nutrition
	
	   • prescribe blood products
	
	   • order and apply any form of ionizing radiation in medical radiography
	
	   • order any form of ionizing radiation in nuclear medicine
	
	   • order non-ionizing radiation in magnetic resonance imaging
	
	   • order or apply non-ionizing radiation in ultrasound imaging, including any application of ultrasound to a fetus
	
	   • prescribe diagnostic imaging contrast agents
	
	   • prescribe radiopharmaceuticals, radiolabelled substances, radioactive gases, and radioaerosols.
	
	 • NPs can also diagnose as it is not a restricted activity.

British Columbia	• The Health Professions Amendment Act passed in the fall of 2003 provides for the regulation of NPs.
	
	 • An NP may carry out the reserved actions authorized to registered nurses and may also, in accordance with standards, limits, and conditions established by the College
	
	   • set or cast a closed simple fracture of a bone, or reduce a dislocation of a joint
	
	   • apply X-ray for diagnostic or imaging purposes, except X-ray for computerized axial tomography
	
	   • give an order to apply one or more of the following forms of energy:
	
	     • ultrasound for diagnostic or imaging purposes, including any application of ultrasound to a fetus
	
	     • X-ray for computerized axial tomography
	
	     • prescribe or give an order to compound, dispense or administer by any method a drug that is specified in Schedule I or II of the Drug Schedules Regulation, B.C. Reg. 9/98.

(Continued)

Table 8.1	Regulation of Nurse Practitioners in Canada *(Continued)*
JURISDICTION	**STATUS OF NURSE PRACTITIONER LEGISLATION**
	• make a diagnosis identifying a disease, disorder, or condition as the cause of the signs or symptoms of the individual • manage normal labour in an institutional setting if the primary maternal care provider is absent or unavailable • give an order to apply X-ray for diagnostic or imaging purposes, except X-ray for computerized axial tomography. • The title NP is protected.

Manitoba	• The Extended Practice Regulation came into effect on June 15, 2005. This regulation, made under the Registered Nurses Act, provides the regulatory framework for registration on the extended practice register at the College of Registered Nurses of Manitoba.
	
	• Once registered on the extended practice register, the individual uses the designation registered nurse (extended practice), RN(EP). Work has begun on protecting the title NP by amending the Extended Practice Regulation.
	
	• RN(EP)s are expected to practise in accordance with the "Standards of Practice for Registered Nurses on the Extended Practice Register" and the "Competencies for the Registered Nurse (Extended Practice) Register."
	
	• In addition to the scope of practice of a registered nurse, RN(EP)s have the legislated authority to include the following services in their scope of practice:
	
	  • Ordering and receiving results of screening and diagnostic tests specified in Schedule A of the Extended Practice Regulation (Additional tests may be ordered if the RN[EP] is employed by a facility or regional health authority that has established written policies permitting this)
	
	  • Prescribing drugs and devices identified in Schedule B of the Extended Practice Regulation (RN[EP]s may renew prescriptions for drugs other than those identified in Schedule A but only for those patients who are being managed collaboratively with another healthcare provider who has the authority to prescribe the drugs. Additionally, drugs and devices other than those identified in Schedule A may be prescribed if the RN[EP] is employed by a facility or regional health authority that has established written policies permitting this. RN[EP]s may also prescribe any nonprescription drug in order to permit a patient to access a drug plan that covers nonprescription drugs)
	
	  • Performing minor surgical and invasive procedures in accordance with the parameters outlined in the Extended Practice Regulation.

New Brunswick	• In 2002, the Nurses Act and other relevant acts were amended to enable the practice of NPs in New Brunswick. The Nurses Act sets out the NP definition and practice, while amendments to the other relevant acts provide the authority for NPs to do their work.
Newfoundland and Labrador	• An NP may diagnose or assess a disease, disorder, or condition; communicate the diagnosis or assessment to the client order; interpret screening and diagnostic tests; select, prescribe, and monitor the effectiveness of drugs; and order the application of forms of energy. Schedules establish the screening and diagnostic tests that may be ordered and interpreted, the drugs that may be selected or prescribed, and the forms of energy that may be ordered by the NP. • The NP title is protected.
Northwest Territories/Nunavut	• The Nursing Profession Act of the Northwest Territories came into effect in 2003 and amendments to the Nunavut Nursing Profession Act were proclaimed in January 2004. Language to include NPs was established through subsequent amendments to other acts (e.g., Pharmacy Act). • The NP is entitled to apply advanced nursing knowledge, skills, and judgment to make a diagnosis identifying a disease, disorder, or condition; communicate a diagnosis to a patient; order and interpret screening and diagnostic tests authorized in guidelines; select, recommend, supply, prescribe, and monitor the effectiveness of drugs authorized in the guideline; and perform other procedures authorized in the guidelines. • The NP title is protected in both territories. • NPs are authorized to make diagnoses of diseases, disorders, or conditions and communicate those diagnoses to clients; order and interpret selected screening and diagnostic tests; select, recommend, prescribe, and monitor the effectiveness of certain drugs and treatments; and perform other procedures.

Ontario	• The primary healthcare NP role was regulated in the extended class in 1998.
	
	• In August 2007, three new NP specialties were added to the extended class:
	  • NP—Adult
	  • NP—Paediatrics
	  • NP—Anesthesia[a].
	
	• The NP title is protected.
	
	• NPs can communicate a diagnosis of a disease or disorder; order certain laboratory tests, diagnostic ultrasounds, and X-rays; and prescribe drugs, or categories of drugs, designated in regulations.

(Continued)

Table 8.1	Regulation of Nurse Practitioners in Canada *(Continued)*
JURISDICTION	**STATUS OF NURSE PRACTITIONER LEGISLATION**
Prince Edward Island	• Prince Edward Island's NP regulations were approved in February 2006. The Registered Nurse Act defines NP and practice of an NP as follows: (1) "nurse practitioner" means a registered nurse who holds a license[b] that is endorsed with an NP's endorsement; (2) "practice of a nurse practitioner" means the practice in which an NP may, in accordance with any standards of practice for NPs established or adopted in the bylaws, (i) diagnose or assess a disease, disorder, or condition and communicate the diagnosis or assessment to the client; (ii) order and interpret screening and diagnostic tests; (iii) select, prescribe, and monitor the effectiveness of drugs, subject to subsection 12(3)[c]; and (iv) order the application of forms of energy.
Quebec	• Legislation was amended in January 2003 to regulate NP practice. • Four specialties have been established: neonatology, cardiology, primary healthcare, and nephrology. • NPs are authorized to engage in prescribing diagnostics examinations, using diagnostic techniques that are invasive or entail risks of injury, prescribing medications and other substances, prescribing medical treatments, and using techniques or applying medical techniques that are invasive or entail risks of injury. • There are two conditions for nurses to do the above. The nurse must hold a specialist's certificate from the Ordre des Infirmières et Infirmiers du Quebec and the nurse must be authorized to perform one or more of the acts according to a College of Physicians regulation that defines the specific conditions for the nurse to perform the act. • The NP title is protected.
Saskatchewan	• Amendments to the Registered Nurses Act in 2003 authorize NPs to order, perform, receive, and interpret tests; prescribe and dispense drugs; perform minor surgical and invasive procedures; and diagnose and treat common medical disorders. • The RN title is protected.
Yukon	• Amendments to the Registered Nurses Profession Act are currently being prepared in order to regulate practice of NPs. • The NP title will be protected.

[a]In developmental stages
[b]The license referred to in the NP definition is the RN license.
[c]Subsection 12 (3) refers to the Diagnostic and Therapeutic schedule for drugs.

Agreement, and the Treaty on European Union, are facilitating the movement of goods, people, and services across national boundaries. These agreements have significant implications for regulated professions because they promote uniform standards and reduce bureaucratic and regulatory barriers to mobility.

MOBILITY IN CANADA

In Canada, the Agreement on Internal Trade (AIT) requires governments to recognize mutually the occupational qualifications of workers who are qualified in any other province or territory and to reconcile differences in occupational standards. Standards, criteria, and indicators to support the registration process are developed by jurisdictions to ensure that practitioners are able to provide safe, competent, and ethical nursing care. RN regulatory bodies are committed to registration processes that are efficient, transparent, and fair and that are guided by the following principles:

1. *Public interest*—Nursing is regulated in the public interest. The purpose of regulation is to protect the public from incompetent or unethical practitioners, to promote efficient and high-quality provision of services, and to strike a balance between the rights and responsibilities of members and those of the public.
2. *Flexibility*—Processes must evolve to allow for growth, change, and innovation.
3. *Fairness and equity*—Demonstration of fairness and equity in all regulatory processes is essential to maintaining the public's trust that the profession should retain the privilege of self-regulation.
4. *Administrative efficiency*—The interests of the public, members, and applicants are best served when regulatory bodies operate in a cost-effective and efficient manner.
5. *Mobility*—Mobility of nurses means that nurses wishing to register in another Canadian jurisdiction encounter only those registration processes necessary to ensure that quality care for the public is not compromised (RNABC, 2001).

Work to achieve registration by endorsement in Canada began in the early 1980s with a series of resolutions passed at the CNA's annual meeting. Initially, discussions centered on developing standards for reciprocity of registration, which implied that a nurse registered in one Canadian jurisdiction could become registered in another jurisdiction simply by showing his or her registration card. Because of concerns that reciprocity, interpreted in this way, did not allow for jurisdictional differences in legislation and might not fully protect the public, it was agreed to work toward endorsement as the mechanism to support mobility.

Endorsement means that once a nurse has established registration in a Canadian province or territory, that nurse should be granted registration on the basis of having been registered in another Canadian province or territory, provided that the nurse's registration is in good standing and that the nurse has met the requirements regarding current practice in the province in which she or he is making application. Standards and criteria, with indicators for each criterion, are used as the basis for endorsement and the identification of differences in requirements between jurisdictions. Four concepts form the basis for the standards: initial competence, continuing competence and capacity to practise, satisfactory professional conduct and character, and confirmed identity (Box 8.1). These standards form the basis of the Mutual Recognition Agreement (MRA) developed by Canadian RN regulatory bodies in response to the requirements of AIT. Substantial work has been done to ensure that all RN regulatory bodies can sign this agreement. At the time of writing all but one jurisdiction had indicated its intent to sign the 2008 version of the MRA. Work is beginning to develop a similar agreement for NPs.

In April 2006, the British Columbia and Alberta governments signed the British Columbia–Alberta Trade, Investment, and Labour Mobility Agreement (TILMA). One of the requirements of the agreement is that, by April 2009, workers certified for an occupation will have their qualifications recognized in both provinces. The CRNBC and the College and Association of Registered Nurses of

BOX 8.1 Standards for Endorsement of Registration

Standard 1: The applicant has acquired the competencies (knowledge, skills, attitudes, abilities, and judgment) required for entry to practice as a registered nurse in a Canadian jurisdiction.

Standard 2: The applicant has met the continuing competence requirements imposed by the jurisdiction in which the nurse is registered/licensed or was most recently registered to practise.

Standard 3: The applicant demonstrates the capacity to practise as a registered nurse.

Standard 4: The applicant demonstrates the good character and ethical professional conduct necessary to practise as a registered nurse.

Standard 5: The applicant establishes and confirms identity for entry on the register.

Alberta (CARNA) have determined that additional work is required in several areas to reconcile registration and practice requirements for NPs. These areas include the conceptualization of the streams of NP practice as well as entry-level education, examination, and continuing competence and quality assurance requirements; prior learning assessment; and lapsed practice and re-entry processes. Options for reconciling these differences will undoubtedly result in one or both regulators requesting government support and perhaps intervention if legislation or regulations require amendment. If legislative changes are required, compliance with the April 2009 deadline will be difficult. Of concern to both regulators is the possibility that they will be required to lower standards in order to achieve compliance.

A similar agreement has been signed by federal, provincial, and territorial governments. The work that CRNBC and CARNA are doing to achieve compliance with the TILMA requirements will serve all nursing regulators well as work is undertaken to achieve the requirements under this agreement.

COMPETENCIES OR CREDENTIALS AS THE BASIS FOR REGISTRATION

Because of government agreements about trade and mobility, such as AIT, there is increasing emphasis on competencies rather than credentials as the basis for registration. The challenge is twofold: first, how to achieve consensus across Canada regarding the competencies required for RNs' practice and second, how to develop an efficient, affordable approach to competence assessment.

Consensus on the competencies required for entry-level practice in 1996 and projected for 2001 for RNs, registered psychiatric nurses, and licensed/registered practical nurses was reached in 1997 through the National Nursing Competency Project (CNA, 1997). In addition, the project identified contexts for entry-level practice in 1996 and 2001 for these three nursing groups as well as entry-level competencies that are shared and those that are unique. The competency statements developed were intended to provide information for decision making regarding registration of new graduates, equivalence of out-of-province graduates, requirements for entry examinations, and curricula for basic nursing education programs. It was cautioned that the competency statements would need to be considered in the context of a healthcare system characterized by constant and rapid change. The report further cautioned that the competency statements are not at a level of specificity that would be required for measurement or assessment, and further work would be required to refine the results (CNA, 1997).

In 2004, a joint project was initiated by several regulatory bodies to revise the entry-level competencies with the aim of enhancing their consistency among the participating jurisdictions. The goal is, over time, to develop one set of competencies that are used at the jurisdictional level. By 2007, all RN regulatory bodies in Canada, with the exception of Quebec, had used the revised competencies document (Jurisdictional Collaborative Project for Entry-level Competencies, in press). Plans are in place to revise these competencies during 2010–2012 with the goal of having them used by all RN regulatory bodies in Canada. The competencies for the Canadian Registered Nurse Examination (CRNE) draw on these entry-level competencies. The CRNE is a significant means of reducing barriers to mobility of the nursing workforce across Canada as required by the AIT.

Development of an efficient, affordable approach to competence assessment presents considerable challenge. The reality is that affordable assessment technology is not readily available. If competence assessment is to substitute for credentials as a mechanism for ensuring assessment for practice, the tools must be valid and reliable, and development of these takes both time and money. For example, estimates of the individual cost for assessment of competencies required for certification as a NP range as high as $4,000, not including developmental costs for the process. The question is who should pay—the practitioner, the profession through the regulatory body, or the governments driving this change? This is a significant question because competence assessment processes must evolve as practice evolves and therefore do not represent a one-time cost. Mount Royal College (MRC) in Calgary received funding from Health Canada to develop a competence-assessment process. The College now hosts the Internationally Educated Nurse (IEN) Assessment Centre, which is dedicated to assisting nurses educated in other countries to prepare for the RN credentialing process. MRC assesses the professional knowledge, judgement, and skills of internationally educated nurses and supports them in completing their registration requirements in Alberta. The Western and Northern Health Human Resource Forum, with funding from Health Canada's Internationally Educated Health Professional Initiative, is now implementing, in collaboration with MRC, the Capacity Building for IEN Assessment Project in the western and northern provinces. Nova Scotia is also working with MRC, creating the possibility that, over time, a consistent pan-Canadian approach to the assessment of internationally educated nurses will be possible.

REGISTRATION ACROSS BORDERS

As technology increases, the geographic borders of practice begin to disappear. RNs working in call centers, as well as those providing consultation or education services over the Internet, may be providing services to patients in other provinces, territories, or even countries. Canadian nursing regulatory bodies have agreed in principle that, when the nurse and the patient are in two different jurisdictions, the nurse is considered to be practising in the jurisdiction in which he or she is located. As such, the expectation is that RNs provide these services in a manner consistent with the code of ethics, standards for nursing practice, practice guidelines, and relevant legal authority of the province or territory in which they are registered and practising. Under this model, RNs must ensure that patients are aware of the nurse's name, professional designation, provincial or territorial regulatory body, and place of work to ensure that the patient has the information required to follow-up with the nurse if needed or make a complaint regarding the nurse's practice, if needed (CNA, 2007b).

This approach differs from that being implemented in the United States, where the National Council of State Boards of Nursing agreed to establish a model for multistate recognition of the basic entry-level nursing license for RNs, licensed practical nurses (LPNs), vocational nurses (VNs), and advanced practice nurses. The model, based on the driver's license model, provides for one license only to be issued by the state of the nurse's residence and allows the nurse to practise in other states (remote states) under the authority of the state of residence but the practice requirements of the remote states. Individual states are required to enter into interstate compacts that supersede state laws and may be amended by all party states agreeing and then changing individual state laws. As of October 2007, 23 states had enacted the RN and LPN/VN Licensure Compact with two others pending. To date, only Utah, Iowa, and Texas have passed the Advanced Practice Registered Nurse (APRN) Compact legislation. The rule writing between participating states has not yet begun, no date has been set for the implementation of the APRN Compact, and therefore no nurses are yet participating in this APRN Compact.

Advantages of the one-license concept include reducing barriers to interstate practice, improving tracking for professional conduct purposes, and facilitating interstate commerce (National Council of State Boards of Nursing, 1996–2001). Nurses will be held accountable to the nursing practice laws and other regulations in the state in which the patient is located at the time care is given.

Remaining to be seen are what differences, if any, emerge in implementing the Canadian versus the U.S. model. Of more relevance is that these models signal that regulation must continue to evolve in response to globalization and increased use of technology in healthcare. "End Provincial Lock on Professional Licenses," was the title of an editorial printed in a large Canadian newspaper in 2001 (The Vancouver Sun). Its author maintained that national licensing is the only way to ensure that skilled professionals do not have to "jump through hoops" when they wish to practise their profession in another province or territory. It further suggested that provincial licensing is a waste of time and money. The system of provincial licensing evolved because health, under the Canadian constitution, is a provincial and territorial responsibility, and we continue to see the federal, provincial, and territorial governments struggle with this issue. Is it likely that registered nursing in Canada will move to a national registration system? Perhaps. In April 2007, representatives of all but one Canadian nursing regulatory organization met in Vancouver to explore the concept of a national assessment service for IENs and achieve consensus on what such a service would include, identify the criteria to be met by a national assessment service in order to ensure use by a critical number of regulatory organizations, and determine the next steps to be taken to establish a national assessment service. At the end of the meeting, it was agreed to develop a National Assessment Service Steering Committee with representatives from the RN, registered psychiatric nurse, and LPN groups. The Committee was charged with developing funding proposals for researching and making recommendations towards harmonization of registration requirements and evidence required to demonstrate that the requirements have been met, developing a model for a database of international educational programs to be used in determining education equivalence, and developing a business case for a national assessment service. That work is still underway and the possibility of a national approach to the assessment of internationally educated nurses is closer than ever.

Is it also likely that the day will come when there will be agreement for nurses to move between countries with licensure or registration only from their home countries? Certainly, there is increasing pressure from the federal government to streamline the process of registration for out-of-country applicants. Significant funds are being directed by the federal government to this issue. If the day does come when nurses move between countries with licensure only from their home countries, as is happening in the European Union, care must be taken to ensure that regulatory responsibilities for activities such as monitoring the competence and conduct of members are not diluted.

Changing Approaches to Regulation

Governments across Canada have been exploring and, in some jurisdictions, implementing new approaches to the regulation of health professions. Driving these changes to legislative frameworks are concerns regarding accountability of professions to the public, turf protection, creation of economic monopolies by self-interested occupational groups, and lack of uniformity in legislation regulating health professions causing confusion for consumers.

SCOPE OF PRACTICE LEGISLATION

Traditional licensing laws provide for exclusive scope of practice, or turf protection. As identified earlier in the chapter, governments are beginning to move away from this approach to regulation and toward a model that is the same for all regulated health professions in the jurisdiction. This model includes a broad, nonexclusive scope of practice statement describing what the profession does, the list of reserved acts (also called *controlled acts* or *restricted actions*) that practitioners are authorized to carry out, and protected titles.

Use of broad, nonexclusive scope of practice statements is intended to break down unnecessary practice monopolies that limit a consumer's right to choose a health provider, inhibit access to healthcare through limiting consumer choice, and increase the cost of healthcare. Although some may consider that this approach serves the interests of powerful groups such as physicians, employers, and government because of the overlapping roles and the potential to use health professionals differently, others argue that this approach will result in new and exciting roles for RNs.

An example of a nonexclusive scope statement comes from the Ontario Nursing Act (2004) in which the practice of nursing is established as "the promotion of health and the assessment of, the provision of care for and the treatment of health conditions by supportive, preventive, therapeutic, palliative and rehabilitative means in order to attain or maintain optimal function" (p. 3).

The Ontario Nursing Act does not differentiate the scope of practice of RNs and registered LPNs. In other jurisdictions, the scope of practice of these two nursing groups differs significantly, which poses the following question: Is there one scope of practice for the profession of nursing or is the scope different for each of the three nursing groups?

Within the new regulatory framework being implemented, differentiation of practice occurs primarily through the reserved acts that practitioners are authorized to carry out. Reserved acts are tasks or services performed by a health professional that carry such a significant risk for harm to the health, safety, or well-being of the public that they should be reserved to a particular profession or shared among qualified professions (Health Professions Council, 2001). The intended outcome of reserving only those acts that present a significant risk for harm is to ensure that the focus of professional regulation remains public protection and not the enhancement of professional status or control. The Manitoba Law Reform Commission (1994) identified three factors to evaluate in considering the seriousness of a threatened harm:

- likelihood of its occurrence
- significance of its consequences on individual victims
- number of people it threatens.

Examples of controlled acts that RNs in Ontario are authorized to carry out include performing a prescribed procedure below the dermis or a mucous membrane; administering a substance by injection or inhalation; and putting an instrument, hand, or finger beyond the external ear canal, beyond the point in the nasal passages where they normally narrow, and beyond the larynx.

Procedures below the dermis include cleaning, soaking, irrigating, probing, debriding, packing, dressing, and performing venipuncture to establish peripheral intravenous access and maintain patency of the vessel using a solution of normal saline (0.9%), in circumstances in which the individual requires medical attention and delaying venipuncture is likely to be harmful to the individual.

Regulations under the Ontario Nursing Act set out the conditions under which RNs may initiate and carry out these acts. Legislation in British Columbia and Alberta is similar in its specificity. Important questions for consideration are: What impact will this specificity have on the ability of RNs to practise to the full scope of their competence? Can regulations be revised with sufficient frequency to reflect changes in practice? Does legislation such as this reduce nursing to a list of tasks and procedures? Will this approach to regulation ensure public safety while enhancing consumer choice? These questions remain unanswered.

UMBRELLA LEGISLATION

The changing regulatory approach brings with it a changing legislative framework. Historically, every profession has had its own act that developed over time in response to the needs of the profession and the public it served. The British Columbia Royal Commission on Healthcare and Costs (1991) concluded that, in British Columbia, lack of consistency in professional acts contributes to insufficient accountability to the public and that lack of uniformity in the structure, organization, and language of statutes results in confusion for the public. The same conclusions can be drawn from a review of health professions legislation across Canada. For example, in some jurisdictions, some regulatory bodies are called colleges while others are called associations. In Alberta, Alberta Association of Registered Nurses, in coming under the Health Professions Act, became CARNA. Processes related to managing complaints from the public vary among professions, as do the legislated responsibilities of regulatory bodies.

Umbrella legislation, seen by some as a mechanism to address these issues, has been implemented in Ontario, Alberta, and British Columbia. Different approaches to umbrella legislation range from one act for all professions to individual acts for each profession with parallel legislative language. The Ontario model relies on the Regulated Health Professions Act to set out the overall guidelines for the health professions, with each profession having its own satellite act. In British Columbia and Alberta, there is no provision for satellite acts. Instead, the requirements unique to each profession are set out in regulations under the act. It remains to be seen what differences in regulatory outcomes, if any, emerge from these differing models. On one hand, there may be more consistency in public policy as it relates to governance of health professions, and the public may be better able to understand how to get assistance with problems. On the other hand, the one-size-fits-all approach may be ineffective in addressing the differing issues of new and established professions and considering how differences in clinical practice should be reflected in regulation of the professions.

PUBLIC PARTICIPATION IN REGULATION

It should come as no surprise that the public wants to play an increasingly active role in the regulation of health professions. Consumers believe that their complaints about the healthcare system are not heard, and the increased focus on "customers" in the private sector is beginning to spill over into the government and not-for-profit sector. In the 1970s, the Registered Nurses Association of British Columbia became one of the first to appoint public representatives to its board of directors. Today, most nursing regulatory bodies have, on their boards or councils, public representatives appointed by government. In Ontario, public representatives make up just fewer than 50% of board members.

Public representation on the boards of regulatory bodies is an important public accountability mechanism as well as a means of ensuring that the public interest is served by the boards' decisions. For a profession to be truly self-regulating, public representatives should not exceed 50% of the membership of the board of directors. Even in this situation, an issue that polarizes the nurse representatives on the board can result in the public representatives being the decision makers on a significant nursing practice policy issue. In March 2001, the Ontario Health Professions Regulatory Advisory Committee (HPRAC) completed a review of the Regulated Health Professions Act and concluded that self-governance should be maintained by keeping professional members on boards in the majority. The HPRAC maintained that increased accountability for governing professions in the public interest "can be achieved through methods other than changing the mix of elected and appointed members and moving away from self-regulation" (HPRAC, 2001, p. 45). Contrast this with the view from the United Kingdom that "The Government is convinced that in order to establish and sustain confidence in the independence of regulators, all councils should be constituted to ensure that professionals do not form a majority" (The Secretary of State for Health, 2007).

Essential to the success of public representation is that public representatives can meaningfully articulate the public perspective. Of concern is the practice noted in some jurisdictions of board appointments being based on political affiliation rather than on criteria, such as knowledge, abilities, and commitment to fulfill the public role as well as criteria that will ensure geographic, cultural, and demographic diversity. Also of concern is the orientation received by public representatives. Typically, the regulatory bodies assume responsibility for orientation. Although the regulatory bodies are best positioned to do this in relation to regulatory and profession specific issues, government must play a role in ensuring that public representatives are knowledgeable about their roles on boards and have access to information and other supports.

Challenges to Regulatory Authority

Challenges to the authority of regulatory bodies come from many sources. At the time of labor strife, governments and the public may question whether leaving decisions regarding the standards for entry to the profession has implications for the potential size of the labor pool and hence the wages that can be demanded. Others suggest that allowing regulatory bodies to establish education requirements can result in "credential creep," or increasing the academic credentials required for entry to a profession, which serves only to improve the status of the profession and has no direct impact on the outcome of care service provided by the profession. In 2003, the Conference of Federal/Provincial/Territorial Deputy Ministers of Health put in place a process to establish principles and policies to assist government to determine whether a change for a request in an entry to practice education credentials is based on a comprehensive, impartial process that would serve the interest of patient care and the effectiveness of healthcare delivery in the jurisdiction.

Some suggest that regulatory bodies entrench barriers to registration to ensure the required need for the regulatory body itself. The truth is that regulation does pose barriers—barriers that are intended to protect the public served by the regulatory body. The question that must always be asked is whether the regulatory body has achieved the appropriate balance in safeguarding the interests of the public and those of the profession.

SUMMARY

This chapter addresses the purpose of and issues associated with the regulation of nursing in Canada. Nursing regulation has evolved significantly since first set in motion in the early 1900s. The impact of globalization, evolving regulatory frameworks, and new roles for RNs will ensure that regulation in nursing is dynamic in meeting the healthcare needs of Canadians. The great unknown is how regulation will evolve and whether in its evolution it will serve to not only protect the public interest but also contribute to the advancement of the profession.

Add to your knowledge of this issue:	
The Canadian Nurses Association	**www.cna-nurses.ca**
The International Council of Nurses	**www.icn.ch**
Provincial and Territorial Organizations	
Association of Registered Nurses of Prince Edward Island	**www.arnpei.ca**
Association of Registered Nurses of Newfoundland and Labrador	**www.arnnl.nf.ca**
College and Association of Registered Nurses of Alberta	**www.nurses.ab.ca**
College of Nurses of Ontario	**www.cno.org**
College of Registered Nurses of British Columbia	**www.crnbc.ca**
College of Registered Nurses of Manitoba	**www.crnm.mb.ca**
College of Registered Nurses of Nova Scotia	**www.crnns.ca**
Nurses Association of New Brunswick	**www.nanb.nb.ca**
Ordre des Infirmières et Infirmiers du Québec	**www.oiiq.org**
Registered Nurses Association of the Northwest Territories and Nunavut	**www.rnantnu.ca**
Registered Nurses Association of Ontario	**www.rnao.org**
Saskatchewan Registered Nurses Association	**www.srna.org**
Yukon Registered Nurses Association	**www.yrna.ca**

Online

REFLECTIONS on the Chapter...

① Examine the legislation that regulates nursing practice and education in your province or territory and highlight the similarities and differences you note with other provinces and territories.

② Identify at least one issue in nursing practice that you would describe as a regulatory issue. What strategies would you formulate to address this issue?

③ What are some of the viewpoints you have heard from practicing nurses regarding regulation? What is your analysis of the differences in opinions?

④ What are the advantages and disadvantages of regulation of nursing practice and the registration of nurses?

⑤ How does the regulation of nursing practice compare to the regulation of healthcare professionals and other professionals?

⑥ Formulate and support a stance regarding the use of umbrella legislation to regulate health professions.

References

British Columbia Royal Commission on Healthcare and Costs. (1991). *Closer to home.* Victoria: Province of British Columbia.

Canadian Nurses Association. (1968). *The leaf and the lamp.* Ottawa: Author.

_____. (1997). *National nursing competency project.* Ottawa: Author.

_____. (2007a). *Position statement: Canadian regulatory framework for registered nurses.* Ottawa: Author.

_____. (2007b). *Position statement: Telehealth: The role of the nurse.* Ottawa: Author.

College of Nurses of Ontario. (2004). *Legislation and regulation. RHPA: Scope of practice, controlled acts model.* Toronto: Author.

Cutshall, P. (1998). Regulating nursing: A new chapter begins. *Nursing BC, 30*(3), 35–38.

End provincial lock on professional licenses. (2001, January 18). *The Vancouver Sun,* p. A14.

Finocchio, L.J., Dower, C.M., McMahon, T., et al. (1995). *Reforming healthcare workforce regulation: Policy considerations for the 21st century.* San Francisco: Pew Health Professions Commission.

Health Professions Council. (2001). Shared scope of practice working paper [Online]. Retrieved on October 20, 2008 from http://www.hlth.gov.bc.ca/leg/hpc/review/shascope.html.

Health Professions Regulatory Advisory Committee. (2001). Adjusting the balance: A review of the Regulated Health Professions Act [Online]. Retrieved on October 20, 2008 from http://www.hprac.org/downloads/fyr/RHPAReport.pdf.

International Council of Nurses. (1985). *Report on the regulation of nursing: A report on the present, a position for the future.* Geneva, Switzerland: Author.

Jurisdictional Collaborative Project for Entry-level Competencies, Black, et. al (in press). Competencies in the Context of Entry-level Registered Nurse Practice: A Collaborative Project in Canada. International Nursing Review.

Kerr, J.R. (1996). Credentialing in nursing. In J.R. Kerr & J. MacPhail (Eds.), *Canadian nursing: Issues and perspectives* (3rd ed., pp. 363–372). New York: Mosby.

Kerr, M. (1944). *Brief history of the Registered Nurses' Association of British Columbia.* Vancouver: Author.

Manitoba Law Reform Commission. (1994). *Regulating professions and occupations.* Winnipeg: Author.

National Council of State Boards of Nursing. (1996–2001). Nursing regulation: Mutual recognition: FAQ [Online]. Retrieved on October 20, 2008 from http://www.ncsbn.org/public/regulation/mutual_regulation_faq.htm.

Registered Nurses Association of British Columbia. (2000). *The regulation of nursing: Statement of principles.* Vancouver: Author.

_____. (2001). *Canadian registered nurse endorsement document.* Vancouver: Author.

Risk, M. (1992). Regulatory issues. In A.J. Baumgart & J. Larsen (Eds.), *Canadian nursing faces the future* (2nd ed., pp. 365–379). Toronto: Mosby.

Styles, M.M. & Affara, A.A. (1997). *ICN on regulation: Towards 21st century models.* Geneva, Switzerland: International Council of Nurses.

Secretary of State for Health. (2007). *Trust, assurance and safety—The regulation of health professionals in the 21st century.* London, England: The Stationary Office.

Way, L. (2001). Nursing education program approval board: An update. *Alberta RN, 57*(4), 15.

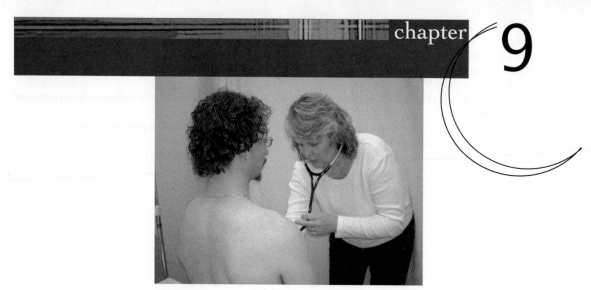

chapter 9

Nurse practitioner students practice assessment skills at the University of Victoria. (Used with permission of University of Victoria, School of Nursing. Phtographer Carolyn Hammond.)

The NP Movement: Recurring Issues

Carol McDonald
Marjorie McIntyre

The authors would like to acknowledge the contribution of Ester Sangster-Gormley, University of Victoria School of Nursing, whose comments assisted us in updating this chapter.

Critical Questions

As a way of engaging with the ideas in this chapter, consider the following:

1 What do you already know about nurse practitioner (NP) practice and education in Canada?

2 On the surface, what appeals to you about pursuing a career as an NP?

3 What do you imagine would be the benefits of graduate education for NPs?

Chapter Objectives

After completing this chapter, you will be able to:

1 Identify relevant issues in relation to the NP movement.

2 Articulate selected ways of understanding the issue.

3 Understand different interpretations of the recurring issues in the NP movement.

4 Identify past and current barriers to the resolution of issues affecting the movement.

5 Identify strategies that might facilitate resolution of issues surrounding the NP movement.

All across Canada in the offices of ministries of education and health, at curriculum meetings in schools and faculties of nursing, and on boards of national and provincial professional nursing associations and colleges, plans are underway to implement educational programs and to standardize and regulate the work of NPs. Although it is not entirely clear what or who initiated this movement or what directs and sustains it, what is clear is that plans, big plans, are underway. One could speculate that a movement of such a grand scale would have only been undertaken after careful consideration of the current strengths, limitations, and resources of our current healthcare system. A closer look, however, suggests that no such consideration has occurred and that the current situation is based on the belief that NPs variously conceptualized can do many things—not the least of which is to address Canada's need for reform in primary healthcare delivery.

SITUATING THE TOPIC: THE NATURE OF THE ISSUE

This chapter opens by making explicit those assumptions that for us, as authors and professional nurses, make this a topic worthy of study. Our first assumption is that the current interest in NPs is a response primarily to a political rather than a health agenda. Historically, the evolution of NP practice in Canada has been sporadic and inconsistent—often created to address short-term problems such as physician shortages (Pringle, 2007). Second, despite the numerous studies exploring the benefits of NPs in primary or acute care settings in Canada, the United States, and the United Kingdom over the past several decades, the evidence supporting these benefits is inconclusive (Horrocks et al., 2002; Martin-Misener et al., 2004; Sidani et al., 2000; Spitzer et al., 1974; Spitzer, 1984). Third, the history of NP practice and employment in Canada has been irregular and uncertain (Chambers & West, 1978; LeFort & Kergin, 1978; Spitzer, 1984). "As of March 2006, legislation exists in all provinces and two territories in Canada that allows NPs to implement their expanded nursing role" (Dicenso et al., 2007, p.104); however, a lack of definitive information about NP employment (where they will work) continues to be a major concern for employers and practitioners alike.

ARTICULATING THE TOPIC AS AN ISSUE

Although there has been significant progress to standardize NP education and regulation at a graduate level across Canada, there continue to be unresolved and seemingly unresolvable issues for this group of nurses. While it is the case that positions have been created, in many cases it is the employer rather than the NP scope of practice, developed by regulatory bodies, that shapes NP practice. In these situations not only is NP practice limited but other graduate-prepared nurses, such as those in clinical nurse specialist positions, are negatively impacted by an infringment on their scope of practice. Perhaps the most enduring issue has been the absence of infastructure to support NPs employment. In part, the delay of this needed infastructure can be understood as resistance on the part of employers or a lack of political will on the part of government bodies. In addition, the cooperation of physicians' professional bodies is needed to create space, resources, and renumeration for the realization of NP practice.

ANALYZING THE ISSUE: WAYS OF UNDERSTANDING

An analysis of the NP movement opens us to understandings of what makes this a significant issue for nurses, for nursing, and for Canadians seeking healthcare. In part, the complexity of the issue lies with the discordance between the imagined benefits from the installation of NPs in Canada's healthcare system and the realities of what is really possible or probable within the context of our current political, educational, and regulatory worlds. On the surface, we have the impression that the realization of the NP movement could address significant gaps in the system of healthcare delivery, benefiting the healthcare of Canadians; facilitate the autonomous functioning of nurses in practice, expanding the professional practice of individual NPs; and provide an opportunity for the discipline of nursing to support and enact the Canada Health Act by improving access to the provision of primary healthcare. The intention of the analysis and, we would suggest, the reason behind the urgency of such an analysis is to move below the surface impressions of the NP movement and to open to questioning and understanding the conditions and realities that will shape the future of NP practice in Canada.

Understanding the Issue Historically

The point is to write about and to render historical what has hitherto been hidden from history.

Joan Scott, 1992

A historical analysis raises questions for consideration in relation to the origin and evolution of the issue. In the case of the NP movement, this includes the conditions surrounding the issue and, importantly, how those conditions have changed over time. The significance of this analysis is that rather than merely recounting history as it has been recorded, a historical analysis opens to question our taken-for-granted understandings of the issue. If we draw on the work of feminist historians, such as Scott (1992), we come to realize that histories are written from particular perspectives. A historical analysis reminds us that the issues of advanced nursing practice that we are currently facing have their origins in the past and have continued salience for the future of NP practice.

The way a topic such as the NP movement is understood historically contributes to the way issues on that topic get articulated. For example, the history of nurses practising beyond their scope of practice (i.e., in addition to what they have been educated and authorized to perform) has been fraught with problems for nurses.

Part of Canada's nursing history includes the reality that nurses have acted in an NP-like role, often in rural and remote regions, and commonly where physicians were unavailable or unwilling to practice. The expanded scope of practice for these nurses evolved in response to conditions where physician-delivered healthcare was unavailable. Despite the significant contribution these nurses have made to the health of Canadians, the formal recognition of such a role has "historically been sporadic and inconsistent, especially with respect to role title, scope of practice, licensure requirements or continuing competence requirements. Over time, different provinces and territories have developed a hodgepodge of approaches to these key concerns" (Canadian Nurses Association, 2003b, p. 2).

The 1970s was a time of great promise and excitement in the NP movement in Canada. Pilot projects were underway in several Canadian provinces. In Newfoundland, a nine-month, expanded-role nursing education program was offered jointly by the School of Nursing and the Faculty of Medicine at Memorial University (Chambers & West, 1978). Graduates of this program were engaged as family practice nurses (FPNs) attached to urban medical practices. Although this pilot project was deemed to be successful, "when federal government project funding terminated, hesitation by the provincial government and the fee-for-service physicians to plan for the future of the FPNs led to the dissolution of the urban attachments after the initial one year period" (Chambers & West, 1978, p. 459). Similarly, a pilot project for NPs in rural areas of Saskatchewan was announced in 1973. One of the purposes of this pilot project was to evaluate how a nurse–physician team would be accepted by physicians and by community members seeking care (Cardenas, 1975). Although 302 door-to-door interviews with community members were held, in which individuals were reportedly "enthusiastic about the arrival of nurse practitioners in their towns" and indicated "that they would make use of any healthcare services the nurse could provide" (p. 715), "as has been reported in many other projects, physicians vary widely in their ability to accept with confidence the competence of nurse practitioners" (p. 719). In her analysis, Cardenas further points out that "where the physician has seen the practitioner role as an extension instead of a complement of his [sic] own, episodic medical care has resulted in place of more comprehensive individual care" (p. 719). The NPs found over time that they had "a unique dimension to add to healthcare services" (p. 719).

During this same era, nurses were being prepared as NPs at McMaster University. The reflective article "The Nurse Practitioner—What Happened?" documents an interview held with Dorothy Kergin, who was instrumental in founding this first family NP program in Canada in 1970. Kergin (LeFort & Kergin, 1978, p. 15) reports that the Ontario Ministry of Health, like many governments,

> was convinced that demonstration projects and research in the primary care field were worth doing. A big factor too was the number of what they termed medically underserviced areas. The Ministry was interested in having nurses as providers of primary care in some of those underserviced areas. Our provincial funding for 1970 and subsequent federal funding centered on providing care in these underserviced areas.

In the same published interview (LeFort & Kergin, 1978, p. 16), Mona Callan, director of the Educational Program for Nurses in Primary Care, relates the following:

> In 1970 there was a shortage of physicians . . . so the nurse practitioner wasn't a threat, she was an asset. Now, there is a surplus of physicians and people are perceiving the situation in a different way. Some physicians acknowledge that nurse practitioners make important contributions to primary care but they are unable to employ them because of the lack of reimbursement for their services under provincial health insurance plans.

The landmark research from this era, "The Burlington Randomized Trial of the NP" (Spitzer et al., 1974), was undertaken by a team of nurses and physicians. Although the results of this randomized control study, conducted to assess the effects of substituting NPs for physicians in primary care, found "that a nurse practitioner can provide first-contact primary care safely and effectively, with as much satisfaction to patients, as a family physician" (p. 255) and is "cost effective from society's point of view, the new method of primary care was not financially profitable to doctors because of current restrictions on reimbursement for the nurse-practitioner services" (p. 251).

A decade later, in the article "The Nurse Practitioner Revisited: Slow Death of a Good Idea," Spitzer laments, "The promise that the nurse-practitioner movement held in the early 1970s for better quality and more balanced primary care, better access for the disadvantaged, containment of health-service costs and a more rational deployment of health manpower is largely unfulfilled" (1984, p. 1050). In this article, a year after the closure of the last educational program for NPs in Canada at McMaster University, Spitzer reflects on his earlier optimism for the NP movement in Canada. "In 1978, I wrote that the experiment with nurse practitioners seemed to be off to a promising start, but the final verdict was not yet in. I [now] judge the verdict to be clear in Canada. The programs, the opportunities for practice, and concrete plans for the future are dead" (1984, p. 1050). Although Spitzer goes on to say that the future for NPs in the United States is less clear, he points out that "the most important factor in the economic viability of the nurse practitioners in the United States will be the level of their remuneration," citing two studies where NPs are "increasingly disillusioned with their role because of low pay and their inefficient use as a resource" (1984, p. 1050).

It is important to point out that for several decades nurses have been participating in educational programs to prepare themselves to practice beyond the scope of a registered nurse, and these nurses have faced problems that we have yet to resolve. Historically, nurses have faced the reality that, after completing very challenging and expensive educational programs, the positions open to them through pilot projects have been discontinued and many of the opportunities to work in primary care have been located in very rural and remote parts of the country (Pringle, 2007; Spitzer, 1984).

Although the closure of the McMaster Family Practice Nurse Program (later called Educational Program for Nurses in Primary Care) may have marked the end of an era of the NP movement in primary care, the recurrence of a physician shortage less than a decade later led to yet another strategy for the use of NPs, this time with an acute-care focus:

> In the 1990s, acute care hospitals in Ontario witnessed a reduction in the number of medical residents and an increase in the number of admissions for patients who were acutely ill, and required complex and comprehensive care. The hospitals introduced Acute Care Nurse Practitioners (ACNPs) as qualified healthcare providers to effectively and efficiently meet these changes (Sidani et al., 2000, p. 6).

However, these practitioners were different from their earlier counterparts in primary care in that "they do not work in isolation and do not replace physicians or residents; they are an integral member of the healthcare team" (Sidani et al., 2000, p. 12).

Although the barriers to the implementation of the role of ACNPs are significant and include a lack of knowledge of and a perceived lack of support for the role by other healthcare team members and absence of mentorship for new ACNPs in clinical practice (van Soeren & Micevski, 2001), their contribution to "*outcome* achievement is yet to be determined" (Sidani et al., 2000, p. 12; italics added).

As the emerging role for NPs in acute-care settings continues, we see once again the re-emergence of educational and practice initiatives for NPs in primary healthcare. For example, the Strengthening Primary Care Initiative in Nova Scotia, launched in 2000, was funded by the provincial and federal governments and included the introduction of primary healthcare NPs working in collaboration with one or more family physicians. The project findings suggest that some of the difficulties with this initiative rest with the realities that "not only were the NPs new and unfamiliar in the province, [but that] the nature of the practice configuration historically was not based on a collaborative practice model" (Martin-Misener et al., 2004, p. 42). In commenting on this report, Gallagher identifies structured, unstructured, and policy-driven barriers for collaborative interdisciplinary projects. Among these barriers are legislation, fee-for-service frameworks, and dated policies that privilege physician authority (2004). Added to these structural barriers are relational issues, intolerance for the unpredictable and the unknown, and "insufficient political will for change" (Gallagher, 2004, p. 46).

More recently, the Canadian Nurse Practitioner Initiaitve (CNPI) "consulted with over 5,000 individuals and groups to develop a pan-Canadian framework to facilitate the sustained integration of the [NP] role" (2006, p.17). While the intent of the "sweeping recommendations" is impressive, the reality of an enactment of a pan-Canadian approach to lisencing and regulation seems remote given that we have been not been able to achieve such a goal even at the level of RNs across the provinces and territories.

Understanding the Political Nature of the Issue

Politics is often talked about as the art of influencing another person. Although some nurses claim they are not political, others insist that there is no escaping politics. In the history of the NP movement, one can identify multiple decisions that have been politically motivated and influenced by the multiple stakeholders, including governments, nurses, and other healthcare provider groups. A political analysis asks about the relationship of knowledge and power in a particular situation, including who gets to decide what counts as knowledge and whose knowledge counts as important. When individuals and groups with disparate values enter into decision making, politics shapes the content of what is discussed and the decision-making process itself. In this analysis, we raise the questions about how important decisions related to the NP movement get made, who makes these decisions, and by what authority; this analysis is not to establish whether the NP movement is good or bad.

One of the central questions in this analysis is who has the authority to decide what NP practice will look like (Canadian Nurses Association [CNA], 2003a). Multiple groups want to influence the decisions of what constitutes NP practice, including nurse educators, provincial and territorial regulatory powers, government bodies, and the medical community. In the case where the provision of NP practice responds to a political agenda, the interests of particular governments will be served.

Typically, the medical community has more influence on governmental decision making than other healthcare providers. This imbalance implies that those seeking to influence governmental decisions will have to lobby and gain the support of other groups that hold power and influence with the government. What is perhaps most surprising is that the recipients of healthcare have such little influence on governmental decisions.

Closely linked to the topic of power and influence, and to the circumstance that underpins the questions of who has the authority to decide, is the allocation of economic resources. Educational institutions, in particular, are inextricably tied to governmental agendas as they negotiate for funds for NP educational programs.

Economic Understandings

An economic analysis of this issue is complex, in part because it explores the allocation of resources in the lives of individuals, educational institutions, and governments. In many situations, an economic analysis looks at ideas of supply and demand. In the case of the NP movement, however, governments are providing considerable funds to increase the supply of NPs across the country, without any clear indication of whether these positions will be funded federally or provincially and territorially. In other words, there is a supply being generated that is driven by something other than a demand for these positions. We would suggest that the economics that underpin the NP movement are motivated by the government desire to please the public in the short term—for example, by reducing wait lists—rather than by putting in place a comprehensive plan for healthcare provision that incorporates NPs as fully integrated and supported members of the healthcare team.

Throughout the history of the NP movement, questions have been raised about the economic benefits of use of NPs in Canadian healthcare delivery. Although there is research evidence over a 25-year period that indicates "patients are more satisfied with nurse practitioner care than physician care and that there are no differences in terms of patient health status in the two types of care" (Shortt, 2004, p. 8), the research exploring the economic benefits of NPs is merely speculative. In a systematic review of research literature conducted in 2002, Horrocks and associates found that "it was not possible to conduct a robust economic analysis of the costs of care from nurse practitioners compared with doctors . . . the lack of good evidence about the economic impact of substituting nurse practitioners for doctors needs to be addressed in future research, otherwise changes may be introduced that are thought to be efficient when they may not be so" (Horrocks, Anderson, & Salisbury, 2002, p. 822). It would seem that the most significant barrier to a comprehensive economic analysis of the use of NPs is the disparity between the methods of remuneration; for example, the majority of NPs would be in salaried positions, whereas most physicians work on a fee-for-service payment schedule.

We have some sense from this analysis of what underlies the political agenda to expand the NP movement. The resounding question, however, is, given the historical and political realities, what compels individual nurses to pursue NP practice and education? Is it the belief of nurses that, given the opportunity and resources, NPs might offer a different healthcare service leading to improved health for Canadians?

Social and Cultural Understandings

Cultural ideas about gender are inherent in claims about what constitutes skill or what counts as knowledge, and these often unexamined assumptions create boundaries shaping what we are able to see and perhaps more importantly, what we don't see when we look to understand nursing.

Ronnie Steinberg, 1990

Important questions that contribute to our understandings of the social and cultural context explore the prevailing attitudes, the values and priorities, and the privileging of the dominant culture and the influences of these on a particular issue. Given the uncertainty that surrounds this movement, and the question we have raised of what compels individual nurses to pursue NP practice and education, we look to social and cultural attitudes and values to extend our understanding. We would like to suggest several possibilities that underlie nurses' participation in the NP movement, drawing on nurses' position as members of society as well as on their informed access to the realities of the current healthcare system. As members of society, many nurses internalize the prevailing attitudes of society that highlight the value of medical practice over nursing practice. Nurses are understandably influenced by the status ascribed to the expanded scope of NP practice, which includes diagnosing, ordering investigative procedures, and prescribing a full range of pharmaceuticals and treatments. It is not surprising that many nurses who have been carrying out these functions with varying degrees of supervision or autonomy under the cover of physicians' orders would welcome the opportunity to extend their knowledge base and practice independently.

In addition to being members of society, many nurses have a particular view of the inadequacies of the current healthcare system and a vision of how an NP might attend to the healthcare needs of the significant portion of society whose needs are not well addressed in the current system. It is important to say that, in embracing the NP movement, nurses envision improved healthcare not only for people who are living in rural and remote regions of the country but also for underserved people in urban settings as well as for countless Canadians whose needs are poorly served in the current physician-driven model of healthcare. Nurses, as informed consumers of healthcare, are in a position to see the current reality and how it could be otherwise. Also, nurses working in the current system experience the daily frustrations of a system moving away from addressing healthcare toward a business model of healthcare delivery that makes nursing practice as they originally envisioned it almost impossible. Thus, it is easy to see why nurses would respond to an opportunity to practice differently.

Critical Feminist Understandings

A feminist analysis helps us to understand the views and the effects of the views that others hold about nurses' abilities and realities. It also makes us more aware of how we as nurses—most of us women—participate in perpetuating these views. Put another way, a feminist analysis helps us to understand our own complicity in sustaining structures and ideologies that foster misinterpretation of women's and nurses' experiences. A feminist analysis of a nursing issue is useful because it increases our knowledge and awareness of relevant power structures and, thereby, positions us effectively to participate in changing them. The discourses that define nurses are more than merely "ways of thinking"; they are ways of constituting the knowledge, practices, subjectivities, and relations of power that together make up the meanings of nursing (Weedon, 1999). The term *discourse* as it is used here pertains to "the social practices, values and cultural beliefs that prevail in a given culture or subculture at a specified historical moment, and shape the collective view of what is right, proper, worthwhile and valuable" (Thorne, McCormick, & Carty, 1997, p. 2).

In the situation of the NP, a critical feminist analysis asks how this issue is influenced by power inequities and the hierarchical structures within the healthcare system. For example, we might consider the power inequities in remuneration between NPs and physicians. On the one hand, it would seem plausible, even reasonable, that NPs and medical practitioners performing the same work would be compensated similarly. The reality to date, however, is that it appears unlikely that NPs will receive the same model of remuneration as physicians. Another question that this inequity raises is whether governments and employers, who may see NPs performing the same work as physicians for less remuneration, expect a savings to the system. It could be said that the argument for NPs as "cost effective" to the system really means that (1) the expectation is that nurses would do the same work for less and that (2) NPs will take up the care of less prestigious populations and carry out that work in less than ideal conditions.

Ethical and Legal Understandings

An ethical-legal analysis of the NP movement considers questions of regulation and who will have the authority to define the scope of NP practice. Like the healthcare system itself, tensions generated by differences between national and provincial/territorial legislation result in significant and important distinctions in what constitutes NP practice across the country. An in-depth discussion of these difference can be found in Chapter 8. Although it is the case that the CNPI (2006) was intended to decrease differences in NP education and regulation between provinces and territories, it should be noted that there are still significant differences regarding what NPs can do and the degree of autonomy NPs can have.

 # BARRIERS TO RESOLUTION

One of the most important strategies for moving an issue toward resolution is identifying barriers that may impede the resolution process. Once the barriers are identified, chances for resolution through mediation, collaboration, or negotiation increase. What makes identifying barriers so useful in issue resolution is that we may lack awareness of the taken-for-granted assumptions that sustain an issue and obstruct its resolution. Nowhere is this truer than for the issues surrounding the NP movement.

The first barrier is that, despite a well-developed theory base dating back to the 1960s that distinguishes the professional practice of nurses from that of other disciplines, many educational programs and NPs themselves have been hesitant to make the theory base central to their professional practice. Instead, the dominant conceptualization has been that of NP practice as roles and competencies rather than as a dimension of professional nursing practice that is informed by the advanced nursing knowledge that graduate-level education provides. Competencies and roles make clear what it is that NPs are able to do, which accounts in part for professional practice. However, this conceptualization fails to account for the need for an articulation of advanced knowledge that underpins the competencies. The appeal of conceptualizing NP practice as roles, competencies, and standards lies in the ease with which they can be demonstrated, measured, and tested. Although this model appeals to the provincial and territorial professional organizations whose concern it is to regulate practice, a tension is created for educators, employers, and nurses in that it accounts for part but not all of professional NP practice. For example, Baer (2003, p. 51), in her chapter on the philosophical and historical bases of advanced practice nursing, states that "nursing's focus on people: its blend of medical, behavioral and social science expertise; and its commitment to caring, teaching and counseling and supporting patients are the characteristics of nursing that make nurses so uniquely qualified to provide advanced practice and primary healthcare services to the public." Baer (2003, p. 47) also draws on the classic work of Donaldson and Crowley in their discussion of the discipline, noting:

> nursing's recurrent themes and focus on the wholeness of people, the interaction between people and their environment, and nursing's management of people and environment to enhance comfort, quality of life, and general well being during, and beyond, illness. In fact, and with irony, it must be noted that this very breadth of background is what makes nursing so clearly suited to the primary healthcare provider role.

With a move toward graduate education for NPs across the country (Pringle, 2007), we can expect to see an increase in the theoretical and research knowledge in the curricula of nursing practitioner programs informing their understanding of advanced practice nursing in addition to the dominant framework of competencies and roles. And further, it is possible that locating NP education within graduate education in schools of nursing will raise our collective awareness regarding the question of who or what should determine NP practice and its place within the discpline.

While there has been increased consensus between provinces and territories regarding educational preparation and entry to practice, there remains significant differences in the scope of practice for NPs across the country (see Chapter 8). In some locations, NPs will have the autonomy to diagnose, treat, and prescribe a full range of pharmaceuticals. In other provinces and territories, NPs can perform the same functions but only in collaboration with or under the supervision of medical practitioners. Some jurisdictions set limits on the types of pharmaceuticals that NPs can prescribe. The consequences of this high degree of variability between provinces and territories include limiting the mobility of NPs between provinces and interfering with the understanding of NP practice by both other healthcare practitioners and healthcare consumers.

An additional barrier is the political nature of the designation of funds to support nursing education—put another way, the connection between educational institutions and government funding. Regardless of the programs that educators might imagine would benefit the healthcare system, they rely on government funding, which is directly linked to political agendas. That is, governments faced with primary care physician shortages are willing to fund NP programs to alleviate this shortage, whereas nursing programs not linked to political agendas are underfunded. In this way, political agendas serve as barriers to healthcare agendas. We might also add that the teaching resources in educational institutions are likely to follow the funding, meaning that teaching resources are diverted to the politically motivated NP agenda. As a consequence, other nursing programs within faculties and schools of nursing have been put aside while the NP agenda takes precedence. The NP movement, an initiative in response to a political agenda, has been instituted at a time when graduate programs across the country have been concerned with the long-term goals of preparing nurse leaders to participate in and direct healthcare reform.

There is a lack of definitive information about NP employment across the country. If governments would have educational institutions graduate increasing numbers of NPs, it would seem reasonable that governments would also allocate sufficient funding within healthcare budgets for institutions to be able to hire these graduates. However, anecdotal evidence suggests that employers cannot foresee hiring new NP graduates until they receive funds to cover the additional costs that remuneration to NPs would require. In some provinces this leaves nurses in the position of entering an NP program with limited prospects for employment. In some cases where positions have been created or plans for positions are underway, employers, when asked, were unable to say what a fair remuneration for an NP position would be. Given that at least part of what these nurses would be doing has, until now, been considered medical practice, it seems clear that the fee-for-service remuneration model, which applies to most physicians, is not being considered for NPs. An additional complexity with the barrier of remuneration centers on the inclusion or exclusion of NPs from the collective bargaining process, also varying between provinces and territories. The argument for inclusion of NPs in the collective bargaining process suggests that NPs would benefit from protection against changing political agendas and shifting "solutions" put forth by employers. On the other hand, some suggest that professional NP practice would benefit from being outside the agenda of nursing unions. This difference may arise, in part, from the inherent contradiction in a role that includes the functions of both medical practice and nursing practice, a notion that could be problematic for union supporters.

A related barrier is that, regardless of what we imagine nurses might be able to do in "collaborative practice," NP practice relies on the good will and tolerance of individual medical practitioners. The CNA document titled "Helping to Sustain Canada's Health System: Nurse Practitioners in Primary Healthcare" reports that there are "concerns about collaborative practice expressed by the medical community" (2003b, p. 2). On the one hand, it would seem that unless we have the full cooperation of the medical community, the NP movement will not be able to progress in the way that has been imagined. On the other hand, the cost of obtaining that cooperation might mean less autonomy than we had first imagined for NP practice or, even more disturbing, that NP autonomy would be at the discretion of individual medical practitioners.

STRATEGIES

After the articulation, analysis, and discussion of barriers to resolution of a nursing issue, strategies for resolution must be generated. Although there are a wide variety of effective strategies to choose from, a complex issue such as the NP movement calls for particular strategies for resolution. As the analysis of issues surrounding the NP movement in this chapter has clearly shown, long-term strategies are most important in moving this issue toward resolution. Given the political nature of this issue, the strategies will be directed toward uncovering the political agenda of the NP movement and will challenge those points that might suggest the agenda is other than political.

The first strategy, then, is for us to acknowledge the political nature of this movement and that, as such, many of the strategies that will need to be in place to move these issues to resolution depend on political agendas and political power. This acknowledgment includes the reality that we are working amidst diverse provincial and territorial political agendas. This is not to say that we are powerless in addressing these issues but to suggest that much of the energy that is driving these issues lies outside of nursing. Thus, our strategies as nurses must include a vocal critique of the political nature of the movement so that what does unfold across the country serves not the political agenda but professional nursing practice and, thereby, the health of Canadians.

Although no one can argue about the differences across provinces and territories and the influences those differences must have on the way the NP movement is unfolding, deans and directors of educational institutions and presidents and executive directors of professional nursing organizations and colleges have worked to support the development of national standards for professional NP practice. A Core Competency Framework developed in June, 2004, to direct the development of a national blueprint for a Canadian Nurse Practitioner Examination was approved by all provinces except British Columbia and Ontario at the CNA Forum on Nurse Practitioner Assessment. In 2004, the CNA Forum on Nurse Practitioners completed a blueprint for the first national examination; the first offering of the examination was in 2005. Unfortunately, this examination has not been taken up across the country as Ontario and British Columbia again did not endorse the national examination. As positive as the sense of accomplishment around this development is, we cannot underestimate the need for continued strategies to move all of the provinces and territories toward a shared agreement that requires their NPs qualify to take—and pass—this examination. The CNA, funded by the federal government, formed CNPI, whose overall goal was to "collaboratively develop mechanisms and processes to support the implementation of the NP role in Canada"(2006, p.17). The CNPI is organized around five broad mandates:

1. *Educational preparation*—Develop recommendations for educational preparation of NPs, including prior learning assessment, continuing education, and re-entry.

2. *Practice and evaluation*—Articulate appropriate and consistent practice guidelines, and develop a framework to support full integration of NPs into primary care health settings.

3. *Government legislation and professional self-regulation*—Develop recommendations related to legislative framework, including a common definition of the role(s), and related to professional regulation of NPs, including a national examination.

4. *Change management, social marketing, and strategic communications*—Foster a collaborative environment in which governments, health professionals, employers, and academics integrate the NP role into Canada's healthcare system. This integration will also require gaining public acceptance of a new model of care that includes the NP role as well as promoting the role as a desirable nursing career choice.

5. *Health human resource planning and primary healthcare*—Develop usable models so that provinces and territories can determine current and future demands for NPs as well as develop recommendations to increase the nationwide pool of NPs.

SUMMARY

The issues surrounding the NP movement are complex and multilayered. This chapter highlights some of the issues that the NP movement presents for educators, regulators, and potential employers, not to mention the dilemmas posed for potential NPs.

In our analysis, in which we open the issues to multiple understandings, a number of barriers to the resolution of the issues emerge. The potential implementation of the NP movement will have to negotiate significant obstacles created through the variability and inconsistency across the country regarding scope of NP practice, entrance to practice requirements, entry requirements, and the absence of definitive employment opportunities and a commitment on the part of physicians to practice collaboratively with NPs. Because of the complexity and the breadth of these barriers, it is neither possible nor desirable to move to a position of resolving them. To bow to a political agenda that views these issues as merely problems to be solved obscures both the historical contribution that nurses have made and the potential for the development of a viable, sound, nationally coherent NP practice.

The CNPI (2006) has made some important recommendations and has developed a number of useful tools that, if they are endorsed and acted on by *all* provinces and territories—at the time of this writing British Columbia and Ontario have yet to endorse them—would go a long way toward addressing the issues that have historically plagued NP practice in Cananda and still do.

Add to your knowledge of this issue:	
Canadian Health Services Research Foundation	www.chsrf.ca
Canadian Nurses Association	www.cna-aiic.ca
Canadian Nurse Practitioner Initiative	www.cnpi.ca
Canadian Provinces and Territories Links	www.canada.gc.ca/ othergov/prov_e.html
Centre for Health Services and Policy Research	www.chspr.ubc.ca
Government of Canada	www.gc.ca
Health Canada	www.hc-sc.gc.ca
Parliament of Canada	www.parl.gc.ca

Online

REFLECTIONS on the Chapter...

1. What information would influence your decision to pursue NP education and practice?

2. Locate the Web site for the professional nursing organization within your province or territory and answer the following questions: What is the scope of practice for NPs in your area? Are NPs regulated in your province or territory? What is the educational requirement for NP licensure in your province or territory?

3. What are the strengths and the limitations of national competencies, exams, and standards for NP practice?

4. What other barriers to and strategies for resolving this issue can you identify?

5. What other readings or resources have assisted you in understanding this complex issue?

GLOSSARY OF TERMS

Adapted from the Canadian Nurses Association (2002, April). *Advanced nursing practice: A national framework*. Ottawa: Author.

ADVANCED NURSING PRACTICE (ANP)

ANP is an umbrella term. It describes an advanced level of nursing practice that maximizes the use of in-depth nursing knowledge and skill in meeting the health needs of clients (individuals, families, groups, populations, and entire communities). In this way, ANP extends the boundaries of nursing's scope of practice and contributes to nursing knowledge and the development and advancement of the profession.

BASIC EDUCATION

Education required for entry into the profession; this may be a diploma or a baccalaureate degree in nursing, depending on the requirements of the provincial or territorial registering body.

CERTIFICATION

A voluntary and periodic process (recertification) by which an organized professional body confirms that a registered nurse has demonstrated competence in a nursing specialty by having met predetermined standards of that specialty.

CLIENTS

Individuals, families, groups, populations, or entire communities.

CLINICAL NURSE SPECIALIST (CNS)

A CNS is a registered nurse who holds a master's or doctoral degree in nursing and has expertise in a clinical nursing specialty. An expert practitioner, the CNS provides direct care, education, and consultation to clients as well as education and consultation to the healthcare team.

COMPETENCIES

The specific knowledge, skills, judgment, and personal attributes required for a registered nurse to practise safely and ethically in a designated role and setting.

EXPERT PRACTICE

Expert practice is characterized by the ability to assess and understand complex client response in a particular practice area; to have a significant depth of knowledge and intervention skills, often acquired informally; and to possess strong intuitive skills in the practice area.

GRADUATE EDUCATION

Education beyond a baccalaureate degree level, extending from the master's to the doctoral and post-doctoral levels.

NURSE PRACTITIONER (NP)

An NP is an advanced practice nurse whose practice is focused on providing services to manage the healthcare needs of individuals, families, groups, and communities. The NP role is grounded in the nursing profession's values, knowledge, theories, and practice and is a role that complements rather than replaces other healthcare providers. NPs have the potential to contribute significantly to new models of healthcare based on the principles of primary healthcare.

PROTECTED TITLE

A title protected by legislation and, therefore, not to be used by others.

SCOPE OF NURSING PRACTICE

The activities nurses are educated and authorized to perform, as established through legislated definitions of nursing practice and as complemented by standards, guidelines, and policy positions issued by professional nursing bodies.

STANDARD

A desirable and achievable level of performance against which actual performance can be compared.

References

Baer, E. (2003). Philosophical and historical bases of advance practice nursing roles. In M. Mezey, D. McGiven, & E. Sullivan-Marx (Eds.). *Nurse practitioners: Evolution of advanced practice* (4th ed., pp. 37–53). New York: Springer.

Canadian Nurses Association. (2000). *Position statement: The nurse practitioner.* Ottawa: Author.

_____. (2002a). *Fact sheet: Cost effectiveness of the nurse practitioner role.* Ottawa: Author.

_____. (2002b). *Fact sheet: Financing nurse practitioner services.* Ottawa: Author.

_____. (2003a) *Fact sheet: Legislation, regulation, and education of the nurse practitioner in Canada.* Ottawa: Author.

_____. (2003b). *Helping to sustain Canada's health system: Nurse practitioners in primary healthcare.* Ottawa: Author.

Canadian Nurse Practitioner Initiative. (2006). Canadian nurse practitioner initiative: Final report urges consistency in licensing nurse practitioners. *Canadian Nurse, 102*(7), 17.

Cardenas, B.D. (1975). The independent NP: Alive and well and living in rural Saskatchewan. *Nursing Clinics of North America, 10*(4), 711–719.

Chambers, L.W. & West, A.E. (1978). Assessment of the role of the family practice nurse in urban medical practice. *Canadian Journal of Public Health, 69*(6), 459–468.

Dicenso, A., Auffrey, L., & Bryant-Luksoius, D., et al. (2007). Nurse practitioner practice in Canada. *Contemporary Nurse, 26*(1), 104–115.

Donaldson, S. K. & Crowley, D.M. (1978). The discipline of nursing. *Nursing Outlook, (26)*2, 113–120.

Fagin, C. (2003). Primary care as an academic discipline. In M. Mezey, D. McGiven, & E. Sullivan-Marx (Eds.), *Nurse practitioners: Evolution of advanced practice* (4th ed., pp. 65–83). New York: Springer.

Gallagher, S. (2004). Commentary: Nurses lead the way . . . *Canadian Journal of Nursing Leadership, 17*(2), 45–46.

Horrocks, S. Anderson, E., & Salisbury, C. (2002). Systemic review of whether nurse practitioners working in primary care can provide the equivalent care to doctors. *British Medical Journal, 324,* 819–823.

LeFort, S. & Kergin, D. (1978). The nurse practitioner—What happened? An interview. Part I. *Canadian Nurse, 74*(4), 14–17.

Martin-Misener, R., McNab, J., & Sketris, I.S., et al. (2004). Collaborative practice in health systems change: The Nova Scotia experience with the Strengthening Primary Care Initiative. *Canadian Journal of Nursing Leadership, 17*(2), 33–45.

Pringle, D. (2007). Editorial: Nurse practitioner role: Nursing needs it. *Canadian Journal of Nursing Leadership, 20*(2), 1–5.

Scott, J. (1992). Experience. In J. Butler & J. Scott (Eds.), *Feminists theorize the political* (pp. 22–40). London: Routledge.

Shortt, S. (2004). Reflection on continuity in contemporary Canadian primary care. *Canadian Journal of Nursing Research, 36*(2), 7–10.

Sidani, S., Irvine, D., Porter, H., et al. (2000). Practice patterns of acute care nurse practitioners. *Canadian Journal of Nursing Leadership, 13*(3), 6–12.

Spitzer, W., Sackett, D., Sibley, J., et al. (1974). The Burlington randomized trial of the nurse practitioner. *New England Journal of Medicine, 290*(5), 251–256.

Spitzer, W.O. (1984). The nurse practitioner revisited: Slow death of a good idea. *New England Journal of Medicine, 310*(16), 1049–1051.

Steinberg, R. (1990). Social construction of skill: Gender, power and comparable worth. *Work and Occupations, 17*(4), 449–482.

Thorne, S., McCormick, J., & Carty, E. (1997). Deconstructing the gender neutrality of chronic illness and disability. *Healthcare for Women International, 18*(1), 1–16.

van Soeren, M.H. & Micevski, V. (2001). Success indicators and barriers to acute nurse practitioner role implementation in four Ontario hospitals. *AACN Clinical Issues: Advanced Practice in Acute and Critical Care, 12*(3), 424–437.

Weedon, C. (1999). *Feminism, theory and the politics of difference.* Malden, MA: Blackwell.

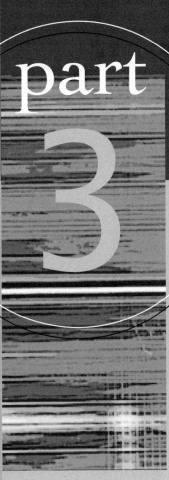

NURSING KNOWLEDGE:
How We Come to Know What We Know

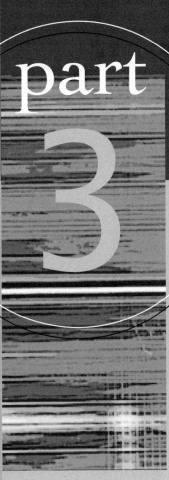part

3

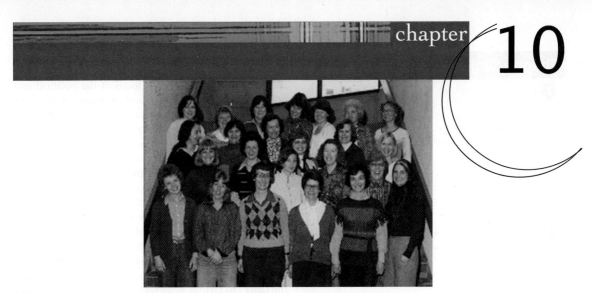

First graduating class in the Baccalaureate Degree in Nursing, University of Victoria, 1978. (Used with permission from University of Victoria Archives.)

Challenges and Change in Undergraduate Nursing Education

Margaret Scaia
Kathryn McPherson

Critical Questions

As a way of engaging with the ideas in this chapter, consider the following:

1 What are the social, cultural, and educational factors that influence nurses' power over their practice and how are these reflected in the history of nursing and nursing education?

2 How do global and national issues in health-care shape nursing practice and nursing education?

3 Nurses are educated to "care." In a health-care system that increasingly values efficiency and measurable outcomes, what are the tensions for new nurses as they achieve their credentials and assume the role of the professional nurse?

4 The baccalaureate degree as entry to practice for nurses in Canada suggests that a homogeneous certification in nursing is both desirable and possible. What are the present and historical tensions around this assumption?

5 How does undergraduate nursing education fit within the creation of a nursing workforce?

Chapter Objectives

After completing this chapter, you will be able to:

1 Provide a critical overview of significant events in Canadian nursing history and understand their relationship to current issues in undergraduate nursing education.

Chapter Objectives (continued)

2 Locate past, present, and future concerns in nursing related to changing national and international healthcare environments and understand how nursing education is challenged to meet these complex demands.

3 Identify the rationale behind changing approaches to undergraduate nursing education and credentialing of nurses in Canada.

4 Identify key issues for the future of undergraduate nursing education and envision future directions for nursing.

For more than 100 years, undergraduate education has been a major focus of the political and policy initiatives of organized nursing in Canada. Preparation of the next generation of registered nurses (RNs) determines the viability of the profession and its ability to influence and respond to national and global health concerns. In advocating for change in undergraduate education, leaders in nursing have struggled to come to terms with tensions around the nature of nurses' work, who identifies themselves as nurses, and the demands for nursing care within a healthcare system dominated by the medical paradigm. As a result of these internal and external forces, nurses continue to struggle for recognition of their unique body of knowledge and to determine their own standards of practice. Initiatives to change undergraduate education in order to better meet current and future challenges in healthcare provides examples of the barriers, innovations, and successes nurses have experienced in shaping and defining their profession. The knowledge of what nursing is about has changed over time and reflects changes in the theory and scholarship that supports nursing practice. The baccalaureate degree as entry to practice for RNs demonstrates how the profession has responded to a more complex healthcare system that requires greater depth and breadth in nursing knowledge than was previously required. At the same time, as nursing education has responded to the expectation that nurses will work in increasingly diverse and independent roles, the shortage of Canadian-trained nurses, retirement within the profession, and the relatively high attrition rate in the first year of entry into the profession has created an urgency within government departments and within the profession to produce more nurses within a shorter period of time (International Council of Nurses; Florence Nightingale International Foundation, 2006). Other issues of concern regarding the shortage of nurses include opportunities for career development that offer better working conditions and better pay while demanding similar levels of training and education. While some may believe that "current" issues in nursing and nursing education are new, history reveals many recurring themes.

This chapter addresses some of the key challenges facing contemporary nursing students and suggests some ways that history helps us understand those challenges. In a profession like nursing, historical knowledge shapes everyday work life in a variety of ways. Individual practitioners, for example, accumulate experiences over the course of their careers. Those personal histories inform how nurses see their profession and respond to workplace issues, sometimes causing conflict or misunderstanding between nurses of different ages, with different experiences, and different personal histories. History is also reflected in nursing's legislative and regulatory frameworks: Laws determining who should be considered a nurse and what constitutes nursing continue to exert powerful influences on the profession long after they are passed. Nursing organizations and institutions—like our own nursing schools—are invested in knowing about their pasts. They collect and preserve information about their own histories because they see how specific events and decisions in the past explain current practices. Nursing's past is also represented in popular culture and public opinion, where traditional images of nurses—however old-fashioned and outdated—are reproduced in film, television, and mass media. Throughout work life, then, nurses will encounter a range of ways that history is used—personal, legal, institutional, and popular. In these contexts, scholarly histories of nursing written by nurse-historians can offer some benchmarks from which to evaluate these sometimes competing versions of nursing's past, while also offering perspective on challenges for the future.

ROOTS AND WINGS: ISSUES IN UNDERGRADUATE NURSING EDUCATION

How well prepared are nurses to work within the complex demands in healthcare today as they take on the title, role, and responsibility of the "RN?" What are some of the historical issues in nursing that have shaped the role, the profession, and the education of nurses? And what does the future hold? While nurses are educated to work within the current healthcare setting, nurse leaders are charged with anticipating future trends in healthcare and providing guidance for nurses as they face new and perhaps unimagined professional challenges. When you look at the photo on the cover page of this chapter taken only 30 years ago—how well prepared do you think nurses graduating from this class felt as they entered the social, political, and healthcare climate of the 1980s? Do you think that these graduates could have anticipated the coming of computer-generated charting, telehealth nursing, and evidence-informed practice? The nurses who graduated in this picture—the first graduating class at the University of Victoria in the 1978 Bachelor of Science in Nursing program—are now senior members of the profession and have helped shape the knowledge of the discipline, create the curricula that inform nursing education today, and conduct the research that guides current nursing practice and policy. Thus, in acknowledging that change is a constant factor in the healthcare system, the preparation of nurses must be broad enough to include knowledge about the discipline that will enable them to respond to change in a way that reflects the history and integrity of the discipline. Each age has new challenges and each graduating class faces unknown demands for nursing knowledge and skill. Grounding in the discipline's knowledge and history are important tools in facing current and future challenges. The knowledge of the discipline evolves through the process of theory building, research, and practice and this iterative process has been part of nursing education for over two centuries.

How do we come to know what the knowledge of nursing is about? How are standards of practice established and how does this translate into nursing curricula and the credentialing of RNs in Canada? What social, political, and cultural influences inform our understanding about issues in undergraduate nursing education? In the spring of 2007, third-year nursing student Tanya Barnard wrote:

My ideas of nursing have changed dramatically since I've started nursing school. When I first started, I was unaware of what the nursing scope of practice is and just how often nurses practice autonomously. Furthermore, I was under the impression that physicians' knowledge was the be all and end all. I was under the impression that physicians' orders were orders that nurses dutifully performed. Being in practice has made me realize that my own views, coupled with social views, have shaped this thinking (personal communication, July 2007).

We can see from nursing student Barnard's observation that nurses are not passive bystanders in the transmission of cultural norms related to nursing. Indeed, nurses are increasingly challenged to not only understand the culture of nursing and the ways in which working conditions support or create barriers for practice but must also be concerned about understanding the culture of other professional healthcare providers. To understand other professional cultures, we must come to understand our own social and historical influences.

Allen (2006) comments that the interpretation of what nurses are being educated for changes over time and differs within practice contexts. He states that a particular "interpretation reflects the perspective, the cultural location, from which it is undertaken" (p. 66). For example, the way that nurses understand their role in communicating with families over discharge planning may be very different than the way that social workers understand the role of nursing in this patient-care process. Indeed, nursing students today are expected to work within complex professional cultures often called "interdisciplinary," "multidisciplinary," or "interprofessional" teams. In this environment, acute-care nurses will find themselves collaborating with occupational therapists, physical therapists, internists, spiritual guides, physicians, social workers, and mental health workers. Each of these disciplines has its own scope of practice, its own history of professional development, and its own body of knowledge and philosophical orientation. According to Hebert (2005), cooperation between disciplines is supported by Commissioner Roy romanow's report (2002) on the future of health care in Canada. Effective and efficient healthcare delivery within Canada that is multidisciplinary in nature is also mandated by the 2003 Canadian Federal Budget (Hebert, 2005).

Hebert (2005) explores the initiative toward greater interdisciplinary education from a historical perspective and observes that, "Over the past forty years, there has been much discussion in Canada of the healthcare team concept and of the need to have 'the right health professional doing the right job in the right place,' if we are to sustain our healthcare system" (p. 1).

Hebert observes that in nursing, "we have not succeeded in shifting from a culture of healthcare silos to a system of cooperating independent equals who contribute to a common vision of health" (p. 1). In order to make this cultural shift, Hebert (2005) claims we must work together to create a new collaborative multidisciplinary culture. Resistance to letting go of individual professional identities is understandable given the rich history of each profession. Each healthcare discipline has strongly held traditions and beliefs about the unique contribution it makes to society and to serving the public. For example, think about the traditions of nursing, such as the capping and pinning ceremony, or the way that nursing students once identified seniority by the number and color of the stripes on their caps. Many nurses still regret the passing of ceremonies and traditions that marked their entry into the profession. In the classroom and in the workplace, individual nurses may differ significantly in what they believe are the core values and central role of nursing in society, depending on their personal and professional experience.

Resistance to creating a "new" tradition of interprofessional practice that includes and represents many professions in healthcare on an equal basis also comes from historical tensions around the relationship of each discipline to the other. Traditions of conduct and behaviour, such as the relationship of nurses to doctors with its unequal distribution of decision-making power, are examples of how the influence of gender, class, and culture continue to create barriers to change. Even within nursing, tension exists today in some settings, such as where licensed practical nurses (LPNs) implement their full scope of practice and are perceived by some RNs to be infringing on "their" traditional areas of practice—medication administration, for example.

Tensions within the workplace environment impact the quality of nurses' work-life and the quality of the practice education experience for students. In a report on nurses' workplace issues, the Canadian Federation of Nurses Unions (CFNU) held focus groups across the country with members of the nursing profession, including LPNs, RNs, and registered psychiatric nurses (RPNs). One observation that members of the profession reported was that "Lack of respect among nurses, particularly between RNs and [LPNs], has decreased morale and overall team functioning . . . LPNs expressed that they do not have equal opportunity to attend . . . [education] sessions, since RNs are often given priority for continuing clinical education" (http://www. nursesunions.ca/content.php?doc=90).

Tensions among categories of nurses may require the kinds of educational initiatives designed by Health Canada to promote collaboration and cooperation between health professionals (http://www.hc-sc.gc.ca/hcs-sss/hhr-rhs/strateg/interprof/index_e.html). At the University of Manitoba, for example, a Health Canada–funded program called the Interprofessional Education for Geriatric Care (IEGC) Program is a two-year, nine-month project researching interprofessional education for collaborative patient-centered practice (http://www.umanitoba.ca/outreach/iegc/). At Memorial University in Newfoundland and Labrador, the Faculty of Medicine has developed the Centre for Collaborative Health Professional Education whose mission statement is "to initiate, facilitate and coordinate activities to enhance the education of health professionals—social workers, pharmacists, nurses, and physicians" (http://www.med.mun.ca/cchpe/default.asp). While many nurses today would probably identify themselves as nurses before they would identify themselves as "healthcare providers," the culture of nursing is indeed changing. This change is reflected in third-year nursing student Tanya Barnard's observations during her third-year practicum on an acute medical ward. Tanya observed that,

> *Interdisciplinary team work is slowing but steadily emerging in the current healthcare setting. Last week I had the opportunity to sit with a first-year resident physician who was part of the CTU (Collaborative Teaching Unit) team. We sat at a table and discussed the patient in a manner that*

was respectful and informative to one another. I was able to contribute the results of my assess-
ments and from that she was able to prescribe care that was patient focused. We both had questions
for each other specific to our perspective disciplines. Together, as two members of the same team we
developed a care plan suited for this particular patient. This experience taught me the value that
nursing brings to the healthcare setting and that by meeting each discipline with openness and an
understanding of their specific scope of practice that true team work is possible and works best
within the healthcare setting . . . not the degree of criticalness like I have felt in the past (personal
communication, June 2007).

PREPARED TO CARE?

Nursing students today must learn how to work in multidisciplinary, team-oriented healthcare set-tings. But at the same time, they must come to know what distinctive skills nurses bring to those mul-tidisciplinary teams. Sometimes this means coming to terms with popular views about nursing that are embedded in historical attitudes and societal beliefs about women, in which decision-making power is located within the medically dominated healthcare system. Traditionally, nurses have been taught to carry out physicians' orders without a great deal of critical questioning. However, particu-larly since World War II (WWII), nursing has evolved to include more specialized knowledge and, thus, more independent and critical thinking skills. For example, the increasing use of complex med-ical technology, including the Internet, computers, and robotics as well as artificial intelligence, means that nurses are expected to make complex decisions that include understanding how to use and inter-pret patient information from a number of diagnostic and monitoring technologies. Training in and use of this equipment has been seen as a challenge by some to traditional nursing skills. Historically, nursing has identified its position in healthcare as the profession most responsible for direct patient care. Tensions and challenges to this identity are constantly being expressed as new technologies emerge that are perceived as "foreign" or antagonistic to what is considered the basic relationship of nursing to patient care. The "official" position on nursing and technology does not always ring true with front-line nurses or nursing students. Lucille Aufrey, chief executive officer of the Canadian Nurses Association (CNA) said in a 2006 news release that nurses have embraced technology innova-tions and challenges. She describes this as an advance in nursing:

Today, nurses work in a variety of e-health programs such as tele-triage. They access online libraries
and databases of clinical practice guidelines in their workplaces and interact with their peers in dis-
cussion groups over the Internet. Nurses are also involved in developing standards to implement elec-
tronic health records, and many nursing educational programs are now offered online.

In contrast, Sandelowski (2000) claims that the discussion about nursing and technology is broader in scope and reflects the ways that nursing is constantly challenged to reframe its location within healthcare and society. Sandelowski claims that changes in the use of technology in nursing as a result of new developments in medicine—for example, the use of IV therapy and blood transfusion in WWII—continue to create tensions in nursing. She states that following WWII, nurses were con-cerned that "technical procedures were becoming synonymous with nursing and thereby eroding the essence of nursing." Box 10.1 contains reflective questions on this issue.

CONSTRUCTING BODIES: WHO BECOMES A NURSE?

Understanding how students become acculturated into the profession also includes an examination of the history of the profession and the ways that the discipline has been shaped by normative values around gender, class, culture, and ethnicity. That nursing and nursing education in Canada has largely reflected social norms of white, working, and middle-class Canadian society needs to be examined in

BOX 10.1 Reflecting on Technology and Nursing

World War II introduced new knowledge and skills to nurses working in army hospitals overseas. Toman (2003) states "although the majority of Nursing Sisters did not return to the hospitals, many medical technologies did become part of the hospital practice, such as penicillin, transfusions, and intravenous therapy" (p. 268).

What are some the new technologies in healthcare that you see emerging and how does this "fit" with your understanding and philosophy of nursing care?

What do you see as the relationship between technology and bedside nursing?

What ethical or moral issues arise in the increased use of technology in recording and documenting patient care?

How has technology changed in regard to nursing care since you entered your undergraduate education?

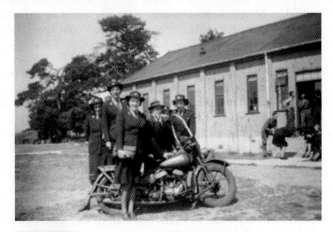

Figure 10.1

World War II Nursing Sisters, England, 1944. Nursing Sister Alice Read Bird seated on a motorbike. (From the William Bird Collection.)

terms of the challenges facing nursing today (Melchior, 2004; McPherson 1996). These values are reflected in the processes of induction into the culture of the discipline.

Membership in the culture of nursing has historically included a process of "proving" oneself as a nurse in terms of what one knows about providing patient care and how one performs the act of nursing in accordance with social, cultural, and historical norms. Taking on the identity of a nurse and being accepted as a member of the nursing profession includes becoming aware of and accepting the values, beliefs, and assumptions of that culture. To a great extent, nursing students come to know how nurses think, act, and respond through their educational process. But this is not the only influence. Although the majority of nursing students in Canada come to their educational experience with knowledge of and membership in the dominant culture, the demographic profile of nursing students and RNs is changing. So, too, is the assumption that nursing students understand and accept one particular view of the profession.

Change is often accompanied by tension and viewed with suspicion. Internationally educated nurses (IENs) are an example of a population within the nursing community that struggles with acceptance and integration into the Canadian healthcare system. Identifying the issues and challenges that these nurses face is a topic of research that has come to the forefront in recent years. This research challenges previous assumptions about homogeneity in nursing education and nursing practice. McGuire and Murphy (2005), for example, state that "the diversity of IENs can be seen as both a strength and a challenge. At the same time, the profession must ensure that it makes available the tools for this population of nurses to integrate successfully into the healthcare system. Again, because they are not a homogeneous group, IENs have unique educational needs" (p. 29). Box 10.2 examines the impact of IENs on the workforce.

How do nurses and nursing students from nondominant cultures and orientations experience nursing? How has the body of knowledge about nursing been influenced and shaped by those who have shaped the culture of the profession?

The experience of nursing students working with senior nurses in practice settings is a significant way in which nurses begin to convey the acceptance or rejection of behaviours and characteristics appropriate to a nurse and transmit that knowledge to students. When individuals do not understand subtle assumptions about the traditional role of nursing in healthcare or do not accept common behavioral practices within the profession, they may feel isolated and excluded by the profession. Finding ways to include students who traditionally have not been recruited into the profession is essential if we are to address the current and projected nursing shortage and open up the profession to those who would enrich and broaden our horizons.

In this regard, there is a perception that at present there are many foreign-trained nurses working in Canada. This perception is false. According to the Canadian Institute for Health Information (2004), and Statistics Canada (2005), numbers of IENs have increased slightly, but the overall number remains steady over the past five years at 6%. In addition, in 2004, according to Statistics Canada , only 2% of seats in healthcare programs at Canadian universities were occupied by non-Canadian students, compared with an overall average of 6% for all university programs" (p. 69). Barriers for bridging educational differences among IENs also include the ability to navigate a maze of bureaucratic systems related to education, licensure, language, and other types of competency assessments. Coffey (2005, as cited in Jeans, Hadley, Green & Da Prat, 2005) also states that while 4,000 IENs applied for licensure in Canada in 2004, only 1,400 of those applicants met the language and education requirements to practice. According to the Jeans, Hadley, Green and Da Prat (2005) report, "we claim to welcome immigrants but have established a complex bureaucratic process which is anything but welcoming" (p. 44).

Recruiting international nurses as a solution to Canada's nursing shortage also raises questions about the impact on the home countries of foreign-trained nurses. The nursing shortage is a global issue, and as Aiken et al. (2004) report, importing nurses "will deplete the supply of qualified Nurses in less developed countries, thus crippling their healthcare systems" (p. 69). Providing Canadian funds to educate nurses in foreign countries or improving immigration procedures so as to

BOX 10.2 The Impact of IENs on the Nursing Workforce in Canada

The global nursing labor market is experiencing a general human resources shortage in all but a small number of Asian and European countries, with Canada being no exception. It has been predicted that Canada will experience a shortfall of 78,000 RNs by 2011 and 113,000 RNs by 2016. Fifty percent of nurses employed in Canada will retire in the next 15 years, whereas annual graduation levels from Canadian nursing programs are one third of the required 18,000 graduates each year needed to meet the projected demand. To sustain the nursing workforce beyond this period, there have been calls for development of creative and innovative nursing education models. A bachelor of science in nursing (BScN) bridging program designed specifically for internationally IENs is one such innovation (Coffey, 2005, as cited in Jeans, Hadley, Green & Da Prat, 2005).

expedite the immigration of nurses or nursing students into Canada may address the nursing short-age in Canada but raises issues for feminist postcolonialists who examine heath issues in relation to race, gender, and social class (Racine, 2003). Indeed, critical social theory is becoming increasingly important in nursing research and nursing education as nurses today are challenged to better understand issues of power, inequity, and social change within nursing and within healthcare more generally.

 ## ACTIVE EDUCATION: CONNECTING THE GLOBAL AND THE LOCAL

How can we become aware, as emerging practitioners, of the political, historical, and social issues that have shaped the profession in particular ways? A postcolonial feminist analysis of who is included and excluded from nursing practice and education provides a way of understanding some of the ways exclusionary practices have evolved in nursing and nursing education. Postcolonial feminism seeks to understand the ways gender roles, identities, and experiences are produced or challenged in the context of global relations of power. What is the relationship between postcolonial feminism and other feminisms? In all its forms, feminism provides a critical analysis of how societies define gender identities, how power is allocated according to gender (usually unevenly), and which political strategies can produce equality between genders. Many feminists also seek to understand how gender intersects with other forms of social inequality, especially class, race, ethnicity, sexuality, and ability. Because of the intersection of these social categories, feminists argue, women living in the same neighborhood might experience discrimination or inequality very differently, with some women enjoying a fair degree of privilege (based on their race or class or sexual orientation) even while they experience gender inequality (receiving less pay than their male peers do, for example). Postcolonial feminism has further complicated this analysis, arguing that European colonialism of past centuries and the global economic structures of this century combine to unevenly distribute economic and political power between the affluent Western societies—now termed the "global north"—and the struggling economies of the "global south." Postcolonial feminism critiques any characterization of women in the global south as passive victims in need of rescue—the "Third-World woman"—and insists that instead we need to listen carefully to what women in the global south say about their day-to-day struggles with economic and political instability. Postcolonial feminism also challenges women living in the global north to interrogate how colonialism also defines their societies and their lives. In Canada, this means acknowledging the ongoing effects of colonialism on Aboriginal Canadians. It means seeing how divisions of race, ethnicity, class, and sexuality have been created through state policies such as immigration regulations. And it means recognizing the racially produced privilege that White Canadians enjoy.

Racine (2003) encourages a feminist postcolonial view of nursing, which "accounts for the multiple contextual layers that shape culture" (p. 92). She suggests that the popular view of Canadian society as "multicultural" has implications for nursing practice and education and that this view serves to exclude those who do not fit the dominant profile. Learning how to interrogate the "dominant profile" of nursing is complicated. Certainly, gender has defined nursing work in significant ways. As a female-dominated occupation, nursing has often reflected (or been expected to reflect) societal beliefs about the gendered roles of women. Additionally, nursing historically occupied a subordinate place in the hierarchy of the male physician–dominated medical system. But nurses have also commanded substantial social power. Most Canadian nurses are white; all are educated, skilled practitioners on whom patients, families, communities, and government agencies rely. As the demographic profile of nursing students gets more diverse and as nurses are asked to understand varied culturally specific needs of patients and communities, gender, race, and class will continue to intersect in uneven and untidy ways. Critical social theory like postcolonial feminism helps nursing students better understand these complex social relations. Nursing students today are educated to understand the political processes that have shaped nursing and healthcare in Canada and globally. Engaging actively in the politics and processes of healthcare delivery creates the potential within nursing to influence change in that political process at the local, national, and international level.

The development of nursing courses, such as those offered at the University of British Columbia (UBC), are examples of how nursing is responding to current issues such as cultural diversity as well as intra- and interprofessional collaboration. Two such courses at UBC are "Nursing Care of Individuals Within the Context of Community" and "The Sociocultural Construction of Health and Illness" (http://www.nursing.ubc.ca/). University schools of nursing also consider issues around cultural diversity through programs such as Dalhousie University's initiative to recruit and retain African Nova Scotian students (http://nursing.dal.ca/) and the University of Victoria's (UVic's) initiative to recruit and retain Aboriginal students. According to the school's Web site, the UVic School of Nursing has numerous initiatives underway related to indigenous nursing (http://nursing.uvic.ca/). Also, the School of Nursing at UVic is currently partnered with Tsawout First Nation in Saanich, British Columbia on the Reciprocal Partnership Model in Nursing Education Project, funded by the British Columbia Ministry of Advanced Education, Aboriginal Special Projects for 2007–2008 (http://nursing.uvic.ca/IndigenouseInitiatives.php). A final example of how nursing educators are responding to current Canadian and global health care issues is reflected in the Mission Statement of the School of Nursing at the University of Western Ontario: "The mission of the School of Nursing is to educate nurses who are reflective practitioners, and to develop and disseminate knowledge related to nursing practice, promotion of health and healing, and equitable and innovative health care delivery"(http://www.uwo.ca/fhs/PDFs/brochures/Nursing_Research_2004.pdf).

ADVOCATING FOR NURSING: CHANGE IS POLITICAL

Policy and political issues about nursing education in the 20th century included the need for registration to recognize nurses who met educational standards, thus protecting the public from those with inadequate nursing preparation. The competencies that demonstrate these standards include "the knowledge, skills, attitudes and judgment expected of practitioners" (Canadian Nurses Association [CNA], 1997, p. 42) as described by nursing regulatory bodies. Another issue was which kind of institution (service or educational) should educate undergraduate nurses. A consequential issue is the level at which nurses needed to be educated to meet the competencies required by the bodies that regulate nursing practice and register beginning practitioners.

Since their earliest days, Canadian nursing organizations, such as the CNA and the Canadian Association of Schools of Nursing (CASN), have made recommendations about undergraduate nursing education designed to ensure that graduates have the competencies to meet the needs of the patient or population and the increasingly complex demands of healthcare systems. Implementation of such recommendations usually depended on legislation and funding. Nursing, like law, medicine, and engineering, for example, is a self-regulating profession. The regulators of nursing concluded, therefore, that to provide nursing care to meet the needs of the Canadian public, educational standards for entry to practice would have to change. Persuading provincial governments to make the required changes to legislation or regulations, despite the strong evidence for the need for change, has proved to be a major challenge. Nurses have thus mobilized and used political processes to create political will. Commonly, in seeking changes for the profession to meet the changing needs of the healthcare system and the needs of the public, nurses have met opposition from governments, other health professions, other professions, and other nurses.

An important example of the power of nurses to influence change in response to changing demands for nursing care and nursing knowledge is the introduction of the baccalaureate degree as entry to practice in Canada in the 1980s. By 1989, all provincial professional associations had passed resolutions to promote the university degree as the basic qualification for nursing practice (Bajnok, 1992). However, there was resistance from many provincial governments, from members of other professions, and from a number of nurses. The need for increased education of nurses was questioned on the grounds that existing nurses were adequately prepared, concerns that baccalaureate-prepared nurses would be more expensive to educate and hire, and an implied fear that more educated nurses would be less compliant. Concerns on the part of diploma-prepared nurses that they would lose their jobs if the entry standard were changed were reduced by grand-parenting provisions in all provinces and by the realities of a nursing shortage. Many governments have been slow to support the new entry-level requirement and some, such as in Saskatchewan and Manitoba, have attempted to move away from baccalaureate as entry to practice after it was established as public policy. A key question to ask is whether these governments would consider reversing support of educational requirements viewed as necessary by the members of the profession for any profession other than nursing. Political action by nurses, nursing students, and other healthcare providers has been pivotal in persuading provincial governments that nurses do need the content of the baccalaureate curriculum (Buresh & Gordon, 2000). While there are benefits from this increased educational preparation, the four-year degree has also created barriers for those who do not have the time or money to invest in this educational requirement.

The CNA report, "20/20 Visions for the Future" (Villeneuve & MacDonald, 2006) suggests that the sometimes confusing educational pathways on the route to obtaining the designation "RN" acts as a deterrent to entering the profession. One suggestion in the CNA report is a laddering process whereby experience and education at one level of nursing builds toward the next. For example, the experience and education behind the designation of resident care aide and LPN or RPN could contribute to obtaining the title and credential of RN, which, in turn, could build toward a master's of nursing or Ph.D. (Villeneuve & MacDonald, 2006).

Obtaining the appropriate credentialing for nursing is only one step in the process of assuming the role and identify of an RN. As undergraduate students, nurses are exposed to particular ways of conceptualizing the discipline and particular ways of viewing their role. This knowledge includes ethics, skills, relational practice, politics, history, and the culture of nursing practice. Entering the workplace may present challenges and dilemmas about how to enact those standards of practice when they come into conflict with the culture of a particular practice setting. Understanding the history of nursing education and how the social construction of nursing is shaped by gender, class, politics, and culture will increase their understanding and appreciation of the complexity of the sometimes troubled interface between the "theory" and the "practice" of nursing.

WORKPLACE BLUES

For students, the tension between the theory of nursing, learned in the classroom setting, and the realities of the workplace is experienced during that first clinical practice placement. According to a Statistics Canada report (2005), the top three reasons that students withdraw from baccalaureate programs are a poor "fit" with nursing, negative feedback from practicing nurses, and the treatment of students in clinical settings. In her reflective practice narrative written toward the end of her nursing degree, third-year nursing student Tanya Barnard wrote:

> There have been times during this practicum that I've been the victim of horizontal violence. There is a staff member that has repeatedly said things to me that were inappropriate and rude. One time I was sitting down in the report room, looking over charts and talking with a coworker and this person walked into the room and said "I guess we get what we pay for" (personal communication, July 2007).

Longo and Sherman (2007) write that horizontal violence is an aggressive act that one colleague exhibits towards another colleague or student. It can be verbal, emotional, or physical and overt or subvert. The authors suggest that this behaviour results from feelings of oppression, low self-esteem, and lack of respect from others. Furthermore, they state that horizontal violence is a response to the situation the individual is in and is not necessarily directly related to the coworker. In coming to understand the culture of nursing from a student perspective, third-year nursing student Tanya Barnard observed that,

> While researching this topic, I have begun to understand why this nurse said these things to me. I realized that it wasn't a direct personal attack but a way that this nurse was getting frustrations out. Now I don't think that this excuses this type of behaviours, and I don't condone or agree with it, but I do look at it from a more sympathetic approach (personal communication, July 2007).

Some of these frustrations stem from staffing models that reflect the emergence of business-systems models of healthcare. Allen (2006) emphasizes that institutions of nursing education strive to inculcate students with high ethical standards of practice but fail to recognize that in some practice settings these standards become eroded by pressures to work faster and with fewer hands to provide high-quality nursing care. Allen (2006) states, " in various forms, most professional educational and clinical models employ 'system' or cybernetic assumptions that regard students as raw material to be shaped into products, to have competencies instilled in them" (p. 67). Another study by Thorpe and Loo (2003), recommended that in order for nurses to experience satisfaction and enjoyment of their work, they need "adequate resources, training and development as well as supportive work environments. Adequate resources speak to the need for more registered and licensed practical nurses to meet reasonable staffing requirements" (p. 329). Having adequate available nursing staff resources means that students have the attention and expertise of an RN available to them when they need it at this critical time in their professional development. Thorpe and Loo (2003) claim that lack of fiscal resources results in the hiring of casual rather than full-time staff, which means that highly skilled and experienced nurses are difficult to find and retain and, thus, not available as mentors for students and new nurses.

The impact of this seemingly chronic shortage is revealed in a statement on the Registered Nurses Association of Ontario Web site in a discussion about the increasingly complex health and social issues faced by nurses today:

> Although nurses provide vital services and nursing is an exciting career option, we are in a serious situation provincially, nationally and internationally. As the need for nurses increases, the pool of available nurses continues to decline. Funding cuts have resulted in unbearable working conditions and unhealthy work environments. Poor staffing patterns resulting in heavy workloads, and the lack of professional development opportunities, have led to an emotionally and physically exhausted nursing workforce . . . furthermore, boom and bust cycles of nursing employment, in the context of widening career opportunities for women, do not contribute to the recruitment of women and men into the profession (http://www.rnaoknowledgedepot.ca/ strengthening_nursing/rar_the_ nursing_shortage.asp).

Staff shortages are not new. The Romanow Commission (2002, p. 94) documented the fluctuating supply of nurses from 1980 to 2000, showing a decline in nurse–patient ratio throughout the 1990s. Other scholars point to even longer histories of nursing shortages. During WWII nurse leaders became concerned as many existing nurses enrolled in military service and created an urgency to produce more nurses in less time for the civilian population (Toman, 2007). The history of poor working conditions for nurses is also documented by Toman (2007) in her discussion an Ottawa Civic Hospital report in 1949 that discusses the impact of changing technology, reduced nursing staff and a novice student workforce on the care of patients at that hospital.

Nurses have not been silent about how staff shortages have compromised their working conditions. Following wage and price controls implemented in 1975 by the Trudeau government, nurses

BOX 10.3 Workplace Issues From the Union Perspective

In recent cross-Canada focus groups, front-line nurses in hospital and non-hospital settings reported workloads that exceeded the capacity of the staff, resulting in undue time constraints and decreased quality of care and lack of job satisfaction. The detrimental effects of poor working conditions on recruitment and retention contribute to high rates of turnover that, in turn, lead to decreased morale and further deterioration in the work environment. Participants indicated that resources were inadequate to address current healthcare demands. The number of hospital beds has decreased without increasing community-based services, despite the requirements for higher complexity of care in the community because of shorter hospital stays. Nurses need to become politically active because the numbers threaten our very existence unless immediate action is taken to enhance enrollments and to retain senior nurses in the workforce. We also need to ensure that new graduates are able to find full-time employment if we want to retain them in Canada (Hayes, McGrath, & O'Brien-Pallas, 2004, as cited on Canadian Federation of Nurses Unions, http://www.nursesunions.ca/content.php?doc=90

Source: The Canadian Federation of Nurses Unions. http://www.nursesunions.ca/ content.php?doc=90)

mobilized at the political level. When, in 1978, the CNA drafted a code of ethics that implied that it would be unethical for nurses to strike, nursing unions from across the country laid the groundwork for a national voice for nursing to address workplace issues. The result was the formation in 1981 of the National Federation of Unions, renamed in 1999 to the Canadian Federation of Nurses Unions. Since then, nursing unions have worked at the provincial and federal levels to improve the quality of the workplace for nurses.

Box 10.3, adapted from information provided by the Canadian Federation of Nurses Unions Web site (http://www.nursesunions.ca/content.php?doc=90), links past to present concerns about working conditions.

LOOKING FORWARD; LOOKING BACK

Nursing historians maintain that understanding past and current issues in nursing and nursing education involves more than delineating what nursing is and is not or streamlining the various credentialing pathways. The history of nursing, they claim, is very much tied to wider social trends, well beyond the specific curricula of particular educational programs. These social trends include the history of women's changing roles in society, the history of oppression of women by the patriarchal society, and the ongoing struggle within nursing to establish itself as a profession within a largely physician-controlled system as well as issues like colonialism, immigration, and the emergence of the welfare state. Toman and Stuart (2004) observe that 20 years ago, scholars attempted to create an image and history of nursing as one "unified" profession. Since that time, the history of nursing has been shown to be much more diverse—with many historical paths being recognized as leading to the designation of "nurse." To suggest that there is some emerging virtue in standardizing nursing practice and education seems to deny the complexities of nursing history as an important conduit for women's entry into the paid and professional workforce. Toman and Stuart (2004) suggest that, "rather than clearly delineated boundaries, there have been continuing practice shifts and ongoing negotiations among practitioners, strongly suggesting there is something more to the art and science of nursing than specific tasks and who performs them" (p. 224).

Now, let us look more closely at the history of undergraduate nursing education in view of these past and current issues and try to envision a future for nursing that honors our past but also acknowledges the power of nursing to promote change within nursing and within society.

HISTORICAL ISSUES IN UNDERGRADUATE NURSING EDUCATION

Over the past two centuries, the ways in which nurses were educated has fundamentally shaped the work nurses performed, the conditions in which nurses worked, and even who was considered a nurse. Indeed, nursing education has changed significantly since the early 19th century and examining some of those shifts helps illuminate how the definition of nursing is itself produced socially and historically. A historical overview of these shifts reveals that although the term "nurse" seems to represent a singular category of work and practitioners, historically it has contained a range of practitioners with a range of training and experience. Since at least 1800, when the British colonies of North America were expanding geographically and politically, there have been many paths to nursing, many routes to claim status as a nurse.

Diversity and Difference in the Early 19th Century

In the early 19th century, the particular combination of education, experience, and personal attributes varied widely among kinds of attendants and kinds of nursing care. Some, like the nuns of Catholic orders, acquired substantial expertise as healers by apprenticing under the senior members of the order and then working with the European-trained physicians and surgeons who returned to British North America to practice. In an era when physical health was directly linked to spiritual health and salvations, nuns combined religious ministry with more material services like bedside care, preparing pharmaceuticals, assisting with—and sometimes performing—surgery, and even midwifery. Because religious orders were responsible for Catholic institutions, many nuns were also skilled healthcare administrators, running large hospitals like Hotel Dieu. Aboriginal societies, too, relied on midwives and female caregivers who were sanctioned by the community and might even have been selected at early ages to apprentice as midwives.

Lay nurses rarely boasted such extensive formal instruction and sanctioned status. True, lay midwives—whose practice was not made illegal until later in the 19th century—might well have trained at one of the many lying-in hospitals in England, Scotland, and Ireland. Of course, many midwives gained their experience at a more personal level, giving birth to their own children and perhaps helping family members before becoming known in their community as "grannies" or "aunties" who could be relied upon for their experience, if not their formal education. Regardless of their training, midwives often combined managing a delivery with work as a "monthly nurse," staying with mothers and their newborns in the weeks following the birth. In the mid-1860s, when midwifery was deemed illegal in most jurisdictions of Canada, the number of midwives formally recorded in business directories or census returns declined, but monthly nurses continued to advertise their services. So, too, were "sick nurses" and "children's nurses" available for hire to tend the sick, injured, or infirm in the family home. In an era before the advent of nursing schools, all these practitioners would have blended personal experience caring for family members with experience working with local physicians and surgeons and maybe also with knowledge gained from reading medical and nursing manuals to carve out particular combinations of expertise for which they were known. These practitioners would have sought to distinguish themselves from domestic servants, nannies, or even governesses, all of whom would have been hired by middle-class and upper-class families.

Caregivers working in 19th-century hospitals would have had a harder time distinguishing themselves from the servant class. Lay hospitals inherited from the 18th century an uncomfortable alliance with poorhouses, and the women and men who staffed 19th-century hospitals were understood to provide custodial and domestic cleaning functions as much as any direct patient care. With the growth of hospitals in the later 19th century, what was expected of hospital staff began to expand, especially with respect to treating children and to performing surgeries. Hospitals thus began to mobilize to recruit a more respectable class of women to work as nurses and to retain those nurses who acquired specific skills as a result of working directly with staff doctors. This skilled staff coexisted with the older style nurse.

Nineteenth-century nurses claimed personal experience, informal apprenticeship with a doctor or pharmacist, structured apprenticeship with a religious order, formal midwifery certification, or knowledge derived from published manuals, and more of these kinds of training as the basis of their expertise. As a result, those who might call themselves nurse was also varied: Every ethnic or racialized community contributed to its local nursing workforce, though the degree to which nurses of one ethnic group could work in another depended very much on the specific politics of ethnocentrism and the economies of need that prevailed. As Kristin Burnett's research on prairie women shows, women living in white settler communities often relied on Aboriginal women for skilled attendance during childbirth or illness in the early years of agricultural settlement.

Uniformed and Unified 1880–1950

Changes in the nature of scientific medicine and the structure of Canadian society changed all this variability. By the 1880s, hospitals were becoming increasingly important sites of new medical procedures, and local medical associations started to more carefully control not only their own memberships but also which allied healthcare providers could practice and on what terms. Midwifery was made illegal, as was homeopathy and chiropractics. Medical authorities saw hospital nurses as particularly in need of reform, and, in 1874, a St. Catherine's Ontario hospital instituted what would become the first of a long line of hospital-based nursing schools. Over the next 50 years, more than 70 hospital schools of nursing had opened across Canada. Initially organized around a two-year curriculum, the three-year program soon became the norm. Young, single women, between the ages of 18 and 35, with at least one year of high school to their credit, lived and worked in their institution, learning through some direct instruction and through extensive "on-the-ward" experience. When they graduated, they could call themselves "graduate nurses" and advertise their services on the private healthcare market, attending patients in their own homes or in private hospital wards and charging the family directly for services rendered.

The advent of the hospital-prepared nurse did not immediately eradicate the presence of the older style. informally trained nurse of the 19th century. Indeed, nursing registries, established in urban centers to help families locate and hire nurses, continued to list "graduate nurses" alongside "other nurses" throughout the first decades of the 20th century. But a clear hierarchy was being produced, and, by the 1920s, graduates of hospital schools held significant prestige in the healthcare market. Meeting the entry requirements of hospital programs demanded that prospective students had completed at least some high school, a firm command of either English or French, and enough family resources such that their families could afford to live without their daughters' incomes for the three years of the nursing education program. Whatever their education, language, or financial status, non-white women and men of all ancestries were denied entry to most hospital schools of nursing. Thus, although early 20th-century graduate nurses hailed from rural and urban households and from a range of occupational backgrounds (including farming communities, working class communities, and middle-class communities), the graduate nursing workforce was predominantly single, female, white, English-speaking (or French-speaking in parts of Quebec and New Brunswick), and had completed some high school. Graduate nurses thus held significant social prestige, even if they had to work to earn their living. Nursing was, then, a popular and prestigious occupational choice for young women seeking respectable work that would permit them economic independence and the ability to move across Canada and internationally. Their unique social position was physically represented in their uniform—despite the unique design elements that each hospital school gave to the uniforms of its students and graduates. To the general public, the white uniform, cap, and perhaps darker cloak or coat symbolized the education and expertise that a graduate nurse brought to the bedside.

Working in hospitals with scientifically trained physicians and surgeons, student nurses gained invaluable skills performing a range of procedures. This skill set included a solid theoretical knowledge of the germ theory and of disease and infection, including the symptoms of the most prevalent diseases of the day, such as diphtheria and tuberculosis, as well as sophisticated applied knowledge of how to maintain aseptic conditions, create a sterile field, assist in often-complicated surgical and medical procedures, and prepare and administer medications, including intramuscular injections. This skilled workforce was instrumental in making hospitals safe and efficient institutions for the delivery of scientific medicine.

In spite of the skills student nurses acquired and in spite of the relative privilege of membership in nursing, not everyone was satisfied with this model of nursing education. Nursing was too important to the hospital, and thus improvements in the conditions of work or the structure of education was too hard for nursing educators to achieve. Nursing leaders and educators grew increasingly frustrated with what they saw as flaws in this system. Hospitals were so reliant on student labour that too much learning was being done "on the job" and not enough time was set aside for classroom instruction and theoretical preparation. Classes were often held before and after students worked 12-hour shifts on the ward. As a result, nursing was not, in the eyes of some educators, attracting a "better class" of student: too many applicants to nursing programs held the bare minimum educational requirements. All nursing educators agreed that the proliferation of hospital nursing programs had resulted in an overproduction of graduate nurses, many of whom were having trouble finding work in private duty work.

With these concerns in mind, the CNA commissioned a study to investigate the crisis of employment. The 1932 "Weir Report on Nursing Education" recommended a significant increase in educational standards and a dramatic decrease in the number of hospital schools. The report also endorsed the efforts of dynamic nursing leaders like Kathleen Russell who were working to establish university nursing programs.

But radical change was hard to achieve during the Great Depression. In the 1930s, neither hospitals nor universities could afford to put money into a new system of educating nurses—nor was change possible during WWII when mobilization for war diverted graduate nurses into military work. But at war's end, new scientific and technological advances in healthcare, combined with new state funding programs for hospital construction and growth, provoked significant changes in nursing education.

Specialization and the Emergence of the Canadian Welfare State 1950–2000

The 1950s ushered in a very different set of educational structures and the definition of who was a "nurse" again changed. Between 1950 and 2000, the internal coherence and homogeneity of nursing was again transformed as new programs for educating nurses, new interest in recruiting a wider range of women and men from Canada and internationally, and the need to introduce new levels of subsidiary attendants combined to create a more heterogeneous workforce of nurses.

Many of these changes were sparked by the continued growth in hospitals after WWII and by new biomedical knowledge that accelerated Canadians' demand for scientific medicine. Put bluntly, during the second half of the 20th century, Canadians wanted and needed more health services, and the Canadian healthcare system wanted and needed more front-line attendants. The combination of new scientific knowledge and constant shortage of nurses facilitated three kinds of changes to occur within nursing education. First, hospital administrators began to hire RNs to staff the wards: Student nurses didn't always have the advanced skills needed for some of the new procedures and many of the new procedures simply couldn't be learned "on the ward." As a result, hospital-based nursing programs began to devote more resources to classroom-based learning but still could not meet the constant demand for more graduates. In this context, community colleges initiated two-year diploma courses in nursing. Meanwhile, the struggle to establish university-based baccalaureate programs in nursing had been won. By 1950, 10 Canadian universities offered Bachelor of Nursing or Bachelor of Science in Nursing degrees, and another dozen were established in the 1960s through 1980s. Some universities offered four-year "integrated" degree programs, whereby students combined their basic sciences, liberal arts courses, and nursing-specific curriculum throughout the four years. Other universities offered two-year "post RN" degrees that had to be completed once students had graduated from a hospital or community college diploma program. In 1982, the CNA endorsed the position that the entry to practice for nurses should be a bachelor's degree and set the year 2000 to reach that goal, but the reality for the 1950–2000 era was that the nursing workforce boasted a range of educational credentials.

If the postwar nursing workforce was characterized by the diversity of educational background, it was equally diverse in terms of the ethnic, racial, and national origin of its members. Few non-white women had been admitted to Canadian nursing schools before WWII. In 1944 and again in 1947, the CNA passed resolutions advocating nondiscrimination in student admission policies, but breaking racist barriers was a slow process. African-Canadian women and First Nations women were first admitted to Canadian nursing schools in the late 1940s, joining the small number of Chinese and Japanese-Canadian women who were enrolled. Despite the eradication of formal racist barriers, and reflecting the ethnic make-up of Canada at mid-century, nursing remained dominated by women of European ancestry until well into the 1960s and 1970s when immigration laws and patterns changed (Flynn, 2002). In those decades, foreign-born and foreign-trained nurses began to hold a greater presence in Canadian healthcare, reaching 13% of the RNs employed in 1971. The integration of male nurses was a slower process, with men representing less than 10% of the nursing workforce throughout the post-war era. In fact, the most pronounced change in the demographic composition of Canada's nursing workforce in this era was the marked increase in the presence of married women and of women with children—and, as a result, the age profile of nurses has grown older as nurses remain active longer throughout their life course.

Older, more ethnically diverse, including a larger number of men, and boasting a wide range of educational backgrounds, the workforce of RNs changed dramatically after 1950. Yet, in spite of these efforts to widen the pool of recruits, shortages within Canadian hospitals continued throughout the postwar era. Hospitals responded by introducing new levels of subsidiary workers to take up particular duties that had once been the domain of RNs or student nurses. Some, like LPNs, received formal training and certification; others were trained on the job. In some provinces, RPNs received distinctive education and licensing. In all provinces, university schools began graduating nurses with master's and doctorates in nursing or in related disciplines (such as education or administrative studies.) The homogeneity that had once characterized the largest workforce in the Canadian healthcare system—the "nurse"—was gone. As in the 19th century, there were many paths to working at the bedside and many ways to become a nurse.

THE FUTURE: NEW OLD ISSUES?

No one can tell what will happen in the Canadian healthcare system in the next 20 years. However, an understanding of historical developments related to nursing education helps us see how past events influence current and future directions in undergraduate nursing education. Nursing curricula across Canada reflect trends related to beliefs and values about health and illness and how health needs should be met. In writing about nursing education in 1989, Bramadat and Chalmers (1989) observed that nursing needed to unify education streams within nursing programs as well as bring some consistency to credentialing processes. Bramadat and Chalmers (1989) identified central issues in nursing practice and nursing education that remain relevant today. The authors concluded that, "earlier educational pathways have not always represented progress. The persistence of alternate routes for the preparation of registered nurses, and the continuing divisiveness among nurses with differing educational backgrounds are problem areas that still require resolution" (p. 719). The authors also claim that multiple entry points to nursing and multiple credentialing serve to confuse and to detract from a clear understanding of exactly what nurses are educated for and what skills they offer healthcare. Their view is that, "we can no longer afford to proceed along the divergent and often divisive pathways of the past. It is vital that we re-examine the assumptions underlying our educational system to ensure that we chart clear pathways for future progress" (p. 725). What these authors seemed to suggest 20 years ago is that differing streams of nursing education serve to divide the profession. But, considering the interdisciplinary nature of today's healthcare and the expectation to provide "the right person for the right healthcare job," how can this division be avoided? What potential is there for nursing to chart its own course, given the public funding of undergraduate nursing education and the funding of hospitals through government and public funding?

SUMMARY

There are more than 251,675 nurses (five for every doctor) in Canada today (CNA, 2006). Nursing students today are entering a profession that they might imagine is very powerful and very influential. However, as Manojlovich (2007) argues, nursing has historically been viewed as women's work where "a lot of nursing work is done in private, behind drawn curtains" (Wolf, 1989, as cited in Manojlovich, 2007). Nurses form the backbone of the Canadian healthcare system and are valued by the Canadian public. Nursing plays a vital role in maintaining the integrity of the publicly funded healthcare system, and nurses are a symbol to many of the "heart" of healthcare. Educational changes, such as the baccalaureate degree as entry to practice, demonstrate how nurses have been able to mobilize the members of their profession, the larger society, and government to advocate for a higher standard of care for patients and communities. According to Buresh and Gordon (2000), in order to understand and influence change in healthcare, nursing education must include awareness about the political process, social justice, feminism, and critical social theory. Fortunately, CNA is celebrating 100 years of representing the voice of nursing in Canada, and the organization has developed as a powerful ally of nursing and nursing education. This professional regulating body serves to promote health-related interests that are dearly held by nurses. They also act to promote and regulate excellence and standards of nursing education and practice. CNA and CASN confirm that nursing curricula, standards of practice, and the processes of regulation have evolved to place greater emphasis on collaboration within and between healthcare disciplines. According to the CNA "Canadian Regulatory Framework for Registered Nurses" (2006), most provincial and territorial governments grant regulatory privileges to the separate professional bodies that define the scope of practice for RNs and other healthcare workers, including LPNs and RPNs.

In her 2005 "Marion Woodward Lecture," Dr. Cynthia Toman talks about the value of understanding the history of nursing in terms of understanding today's nursing concerns. She states, "I believe that nurses develop both 'roots' and 'wings' when they know more about their profession . . . Roots that ground them in the knowledge of events that have shaped current practice, and wings that empower them to address current practice from more fully informed perspectives (http://www.nursing.ubc.ca/About_Us/History/Marion_Woodward_Lecture.htm).

Add to your knowledge of this issue:		Online
Canadian Association of Schools of Nursing	http://www.casn.ca/	
Canadian Federation of Nurses Unions	http://www.nursesunions.ca/content.php?doc=90	
Canadian Nurse	http://www.canadian-nurse.com/	
Canadian Nurses Association	http://www.cna-nurses.ca/CNA/default_e.aspx	
Health Canada—Interprofessional Education for Collaborative Patient-Centred Practice	http://www.hc-sc.gc.ca/hcs-sss/hhr-rhs/strateg/interprof/index-eng.php	
Memorial University—Centre for Collaborative Health Professional Education	http://www.med.mun.ca/cchpe/default.asp	

Continued

Add to your knowledge of this issue: (Continued)	
Registered Nurses Association of Ontario	http://www.rnaoknowledgedepot.ca/ strengthening_nursing/rar_the_nursing_ shortage.asp
Romanow Commission—Health Human Resources Planning	http://www.hc-sc.gc.ca/hcs-sss/hhr-rhs/ strateg/romanow-eng.php
Statistics Canada: Health Reports	http://www.statcan.ca/english/ads/ 82-003-XPE/index.htm
University of British Columbia School of Nursing	http://www.nursing.ubc.ca/
Univeristy of Dalhousie, School of Nursing	http://nursing.dal.ca/
University of Manitoba—Interprofessional Education of Geriatric Care	http://www.umanitoba.ca/outreach/iegc/
University of Victoria School of Nursing	http://nursing.uvic.ca/
University of Western Ontario School of Nursing	http://www.uwo.ca/fhs/nursing/

Online

REFLECTIONS on the Chapter...

1 What strategies would you use to attract members of other underrepresented groups and nurses who have come to Canada but have difficulty accessing licensure in Canada?

2 How could educational and service organizations work together to improve the clinical education of undergraduate students, which strengthens the nursing student's understanding of social justice? What policies would need to be in place for students and for faculty?

3 What is the regulatory body in your province or territory? Has the policy of the baccalaureate as the minimum educational requirement for entry to practice been implemented in your province or territory?

4 Discuss the established domains of nursing (practice, education, research, and administration). What would be the likely impact of adding leadership and policy as two additional domains of nursing?

5 What are the ways that gender, class, and culture impact your view of nursing, and how do you carry that awareness into practice as a nurse?

6 How has understanding the social and historical factors that have shaped undergraduate nursing education changed your view of today's issues in undergraduate nursing education?

References

Advisory Committee on Health Human Resources. (2000). *The nursing strategy for Canada* [Online]. Ottawa: Health Canada. Retrieved October 21, 2008 from http://www.hc-sc.gc.ca/english/pdf/media/nursing_strategy.pdf.

Aiken, L., Buchan, J., Sochalski, J., Nichols, B., & Powell, M. (2004). Trends in international nurse migration. *Health Affairs, 23*(3), 69–75.

Allen, D. (2006). Whiteness and difference in nursing. *Nursing Philosophy, 7*, 65–78.

Bajnok, I. (1992). Entry-level educational preparation for nursing. In A.J. Baumgart & J. Larsen (Eds.), *Canadian nursing faces the future* (2nd ed., pp. 401–419). Toronto: Mosby Year Book.

Baker, G., Norton, P., Flintoft, V., et al. (2004). The Canadian adverse events study: The incidence of adverse events among hospital patients in Canada. *Canadian Medical Association Journal, 170*(11), 1678–1686.

Benner, P. (1984). *From novice to expert: Excellence and power in clinical nursing practice.* Menlo Park, CA: Addison-Wesley.

_____. (2000). Forward. In B. Buresh & S. Gordon (Eds.). *From silence to voice* (p. ix). Ottawa: Canadian Nurses Association.

Boychuk Duchscher, J.E. (2001). Out in the real world: Newly graduated nurses in acute-care speak out. *Journal of Nursing Administration, 31*(9), 426–438.

Bramadat, I.J. & Chalmers, K.I. (1989). Nursing education in Canada: historical 'progress'—-contemporary issues. *Journal of Advanced Nursing, 14*(9), 719–726.

Buresh, B. & Gordon, S. (2000). *From silence to voice: What nurses know and must communicate to the public.* Ottawa: Canadian Nurses Association.

Canadian Association of University Schools of Nursing. (1995). *Accreditation guidelines.* Ottawa: Author.

Canadian Institute for Health Information. (2001). *Canadian Institute for Health Information reports moderate rise in registered nurses workforce, fewer RNs working on casual basis, more working full-time* [Executive Summary, Online]. Retrieved October 21, 2008 from http://secure.cihi.ca/cihiweb/dispPage.jsp?cw_page=media_23may2001_e.

_____. (2004). Canada's nursing workforce in 2003. News Release, Dec. 14, 2004.

Canadian Nurses Association. (1997). *National nursing competency project final report.* Ottawa: Author.

_____. (1998). The quiet crisis in health care: A proposal for a federal government investment in quality health care [Brief, Online]. Retrieved 2002 from http://www.cna-nurses.ca/pages/qcrisis/frames/qcframe.htm

_____. (2000). Cultural diversity: Changes and challenges. *Nursing Now, 7*(1–4).

_____. (2006). Canadian regulatory framework for registered nurses. Canadian Nurses Association, Ontario, Canada.

Carpenter, H.M. (1970). The University of Toronto School of Nursing: An agent of change. In M.Q. Innis (Ed.), *Nursing education in a changing society* (pp. 86–108). Toronto: University of Toronto Press.

Coburn, J. (1981). "I see and am silent": A short history of nursing in Ontario. In D. Coburn, C. D'Arcy, P. New, et al. (Eds.), *Health and Canadian society* (pp. 182–201). Toronto: Fitzhenry & Whiteside.

Davidson Dick, D. (2004, March). Designing a safer health care system: What it means for nursing education (excerpt, Message from the dean, SIAST Nursing Division News). *Canadian Nurse, 100*(3), 32–33.

Davidson Dick, D. & Hoffman, C. (2004, October). *Designing a safer system: Nursing education embraces partnerships.* Paper presented at the meeting of the Registered Nurses Association of Ontario, International Nursing Education Conference, Toronto.

Dick, D.D. (1985). *Politics, power and the political process.* Tel Aviv, Israel: ICN Quadrennial Congress.

Duchscher. J.E.B. (2004). Transition to professional nursing practice: Emerging issues and initiatives. In M.H. Oermann & K.T. Heinrich, *Annual review of nursing education* (Vol. 2, pp. 283–303). New York: Springer.

Errington, J. (1990). Pioneers and suffragists. In S. Burt, L. Code, & L. Dorey (Eds.), *Changing patterns: Women in Canada* (pp. 51–78). Toronto: McClelland & Stewart.

Flynn, K. "Race, class and gender: Black nurses in Ontario 1950–1980." Ph.D. dissertation, Women's Studies, York University, 2002.

Garey, D. & Hott, L.R. (Producers). (1988). Sentimental women need not apply: A history of the American nurse [videorecording by Florentine Films]. Willowdale, ON: McNabb & Connolly.

Gibbon, J.M. & Mathewson, M.S. (1947). *Three centuries of Canadian nursing.* Toronto: MacMillan.

Government of Canada. (1964–1965). Royal commission on health services [E. Hall, Chairman]. Ottawa: Queen's Printer.

Hebert, M. (2000). A national education strategy to develop nursing informatics competencies. *Canadian Journal of Nursing Leadership, 13*(2), 11–14.

The History of Nursing Society, School for Graduate Nurses, McGill University. (1929). *Pioneers of nursing in Canada.* Montreal: Canadian Nurses Association.

Horsburgh, M.E., Stamler, L.L., Snowdon, A.W., et al. (1998, July). The role of the professional nurse mentor and staff nurse outcomes in the clinical education unit. In *Proceedings of the workgroup of European Nurse Researchers, 9th Biennial Conference* (Vol. 1, pp. 342–348). Helsinki, Finland: International Council of Nurses.

Jeans, M.E., Hadley, F. Green, J., & Da Prat, C. (2005). *Navigating to become a nurse in Canada: Assessment of international nursing applicants.* Ottawa: Canadian Nurses Association.

King, M.K. (1970). The development of university nursing education. In M.Q. Innis (Ed.), *Nursing education in a changing society* (pp. 67–85). Toronto: University of Toronto Press.

Kirby, M.J.L. (2002). *The health of Canadians—The federal role.* Ottawa: The Standing Senate Committee on Social Affairs, Science and Technology, Government of Canada. Retrieved October 21, 2008 from http://www.hc-sc.gc.ca/english/hhr/1

Kirkwood, R.A., & Bouchard, J.L. (1992). *Take counsel with one another: A beginning history of the Canadian Association of University Schools of Nursing, 1942–1992.* Ottawa: Canadian Association of University Schools of Nursing.

Kramer, M. (1974). *Reality shock: Why nurses leave nursing.* St. Louis: Mosby.

Lasswell, H.D. (1958). *Politics: Who gets what, when, how.* New York: World Publishing.

Longo, J. & Sherman, R. (2007). Leveling horizontal violence. *Journal of Advanced Nursing, 42*(1), 90–96.

Manojlovich, M. (2007). Power and empowerment in nursing: Looking backward to inform the future. *Online Journal of Issues in Nursing, 12*(1), 15-15. Retrieved March 20, 2008, from Academic Search Premier database.

McPherson, K. (1996). *Bedside matters: The transformation of Canadian nursing 1900–1990.* Toronto: Oxford University Press.

McGuire, M. & Murphy, S. (2005). The internationally educated nurse. *Canadian Nurse, 101*(1), 25–29.

Melchoir, F. (2004). Feminist approaches to nursing history. *Western Journal of Nursing Research, 26*(3), 340–355.

Mussallem, H.K. (1965). Nursing education in Canada [submission to Royal Commission on Health Services]. Ottawa: Queen's Printer.

Nelson, S. (1999). Entering the professional domain: The making of the modern nurse in 17th century France. *Nursing History Review, 7,* 171–187.

Paul, P. (1998). Nursing education becomes synonymous with nursing service. In J.C. Ross-Kerr (Ed.), *Prepared to care: Nurses and nursing in Alberta 1859–1996* (pp. 129–153). Edmonton: University of Alberta Press.

Racine, L. (2003). Implementing a postcolonial feminist perspective in nursing research related to non-Western populations. *Nursing Inquiry 10*(2), 91–102.

Reverby, S. (1987). A caring dilemma: Womanhood and nursing in historical perspective. *Nursing Research, 36,* 5–11.

Rogers, M.E. (1970). *An introduction to the theoretical basis of nursing.* Philadelphia: F. A. Davis.

Romanow, R.J. (2002). *Building on values: The future of health care in Canada—Final report.* Ottawa: Government of Canada. Retrieved September 27, 2004 from http://www.hc-sc.gc.ca/english/pdf/care/romanow_e.pdf.

Ross-Kerr, J.C. (1998). *Prepared to care: Nurses and nursing in Alberta, 1859 to 1996.* Edmonton: University of Alberta Press.

Sandelowski, M. (2000). *Devices and Desires: Gender, Technology and American Nursing.* Chapel Hill: UNC Press.

Sullivan, B. (2000, September/October). Gender diversity vs cultural diversity. *Journal of Professional Nursing, 6*(5), 253–254.

Therrien, L. (1992). *CUNSA & CNSA: A beginning history* [Online]. Retrieved October 21, 2008 from http://www.cnsa.ca/publications/history/.

Thorpe, K. & Loo, R. (2003). Balancing professional and personal satisfaction of nurse managers: Current and future perspectives in a changing health care system. *Journal of Nursing Management, 11,* 321–330.

Toman, C. & Stuart, M. (2004). Emerging scholarship in nursing history. *CBMH/BCHM, 21*(2), 223-227.

Toman, C. (2007). *An officer and a lady: Canadian military nursing and the Second World War.* Vancouver: UBC Press.

Villeneuve, M. & MacDonald, J. (2006). Towards 2020: Visions for nursing [Electronic version]. *Canadian Nursing Association.* Ottawa, ON.

Weir, G.M. (1932). *Survey of nursing education in Canada.* Toronto: University of Toronto Press.

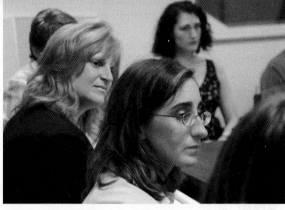

chapter 11

University of Victoria School of Nursing faculty and graduate students.

Graduate Education

Sally Thorne

This chapter focuses on the contributions made to the healthcare system by nurses educated at the graduate level. A special emphasis is placed on the contributions of nurses prepared at the master's level, whose focus is advanced practice, and those prepared at the doctoral and post-doctoral levels, whose focus is research.

Building on a historical overview of the evolution within graduate education in Canada, this chapter examines the impact of graduate education in general as well as some of the specific contributions made by Canadian nurses with graduate level education. Within this discussion, the reader will find a further exploration of some of the realities of graduate-prepared nurses in their places of work, the issues that arise for these nurses in practice, and the barriers that need to be addressed if the full potential of these nurses is to be realized.

HISTORY OF GRADUATE NURSING EDUCATION IN CANADA

The second half of the 20th century brought graduate nursing education into the mainstream for the profession in Canada. In 1959, the first master's program in the country was launched at the University of Western Ontario, followed quickly by the inauguration of three more within the next decade, at McGill, Montréal, and the University of British Columbia (UBC). With a handful of new programs becoming available each decade, 25 universities were offering master's degrees in nursing by 2007 (Association of the Universities and Colleges of Canada [AUCC], 2007). The first doctoral program in the country, at the University of Alberta, admitted students in 1991, and within the next 15 years, the country boasted 11 established doctoral programs in nursing (AUCC, 2007; Canadian Association of Schools of Nursing, 2006). The history of the evolution of graduate programs in Canada explains something of the shape that graduate nursing education has taken in comparison to that of other jurisdictions and provides a foundation for understanding some of the issues that nurses face with graduate preparation in the current academic, scientific, and social context.

Evolution of Master's Degree Programs

Although graduate degrees in other disciplines have been available to nurses for a much longer time, the history of master's programming in the country is one of under 50 years. As can be seen in Table 11.1, there has been a relatively stable proliferation of new master's degree programs in nursing every decade. However, graduate programs designated as *nursing* degree programs still compete with a range of other options open to nurses in Canada, and nursing programs remain only one of several routes by which Canadian nurses obtain graduate education.

Before the local availability of master's nursing programs in Canada, many nurses obtained their graduate preparation in other countries, particularly in the United States. Others undertook graduate work at Canadian universities in such fields as public health, education, medical science, social science, or business administration (Field, Stinson, & Thibaudeau, 1992). Although some of these degree programs drew nurses away from the main focus of their discipline for much of their academic development, others were quite sensitive to the special needs of nurse leaders and produced graduates with specialization in the study of problems directly relevant to their profession. In some instances, nursing faculty members with cross-appointments augmented the learning opportunities for nurses in those disciplines. In other instances, some nurses managed to retain their disciplinary focus within academic environments that were not entirely supportive.

For reasons of proximity and preference, many Canadian nurses continue to obtain graduate education outside of the discipline, and, for the most part, the profession has enjoyed the healthy skill-set

Table 11.1	Proliferation of Graduate Nursing Programs in Canada	

UNIVERSITY	MASTER'S PROGRAM	DOCTORAL PROGRAM
Athabasca University	2003	
Dalhousie University	1975	2003
Laurentian University	2004	
L'université de Laval	1991	
L'université de Moncton	1997	
L'université de Montréal	1965	1993
McGill University	1961	1993
McMaster University	1994	1994
Memorial University	1982	
Queens University	1994	
Université du Québec	2001	
University of Alberta	1975	1991
University of British Columbia	1968	1991
University of British Columbia-Okanagan	2006	
University of Calgary	1981	1999
University of Manitoba	1979	
University of New Brunswick	1995	
University of Northern British Columbia	2005	
University of Ottawa	1993	2004
University of Saskatchewan	1986	2007
University of Toronto	1970	1993
University of Victoria	2003	2006
University of Western Ontario	1959	2003
University of Windsor	1994	
York University	2005	

Note: Data compiled from most recent Canadian statistics AUCC (2007) and CASN (2004). Not listed above are graduate programs leading to a degree other than nursing (such as the Master of Health Sciences, Master of Science in Community Health, Maîtrise en sciences cliniques, interdisciplinary PhD, Doctorat en sciences cliniques) or graduate nursing degrees occurring outside of an approved program, such as doctoral degrees by special arrangement.

mix that can derive from an interdisciplinary perspective. In the early years, however, nurses tended to be less confident that their discipline would produce the highest quality graduate-level preparation for their advancement within such fields as nursing education and health administration (Beaton, 1990;

Field et al., 1992; Ford & Wertenberger, 1993); hence, consciousness raising about the relevance of graduate preparation within nursing has been an ongoing challenge.

A continuing complication has been the availability of graduate programs designed specifically with nurses in mind but located somewhat outside of the disciplinary core such as Master of Health Science programs. In some universities, these programs have evolved collaboratively with the involvement of other disciplines as an evolutionary step toward more comprehensive nursing master's degree offerings (McBride, 1995).

In recognition of the urgent need for augmented graduate educational opportunities for nurses to advance the general academic level of professional nursing in Canada (Mussalem, 1965), nursing leaders creatively pursued a variety of strategies and mechanisms in developing master's programs. Among the strongest supporters of this initiative was the Kellogg Foundation. This foundation was a major presence in Canadian nursing education from 1949 through 1981 (Wood & Ross-Kerr, 2002). The foundation's fellowships to individual nurses helped Canadians obtain graduate degrees elsewhere, and its development grants helped many Canadian universities to support initial programs in their early phases. Approvals to deliver graduate programs were accomplished individually by each university's senate and, in most instances, were explicitly built on a foundational history of high-quality undergraduate programming (McBride, 1995).

Within the Canadian nursing master's programs, the initial focus was primarily on filling the articulated needs within nursing education or nursing administration (McBride, 1995). Since the mid-1970s, that focus has shifted from these functional areas toward clinical specialization and leadership (Allen, 1986; McBride, 1995). Although nursing theory and science are still integral to the curriculum, the primary role of master's degree programs in preparing nurse researchers has gradually shifted since the 1980s as more Canadian nurses have had access to doctoral programs. Although rigorous research preparation was the standard within Canadian nursing master's programs until the advent of doctoral programs in 1991 (Kerr & McPhail, 1996), the master's thesis has become increasingly controversial since then. Some master's programs in nursing continue to require a research-based thesis or include a thesis option; others no longer provide direct research training at this level (Gein, 1994; Kerr & McPhail, 1996; McBride, 1995).

Over its history, master's education in Canadian nursing has also experienced the effects of other trends and innovations. Because Canada's geography makes proximity to learning experiences a significant barrier for many nurses, and because the dominantly female constitution of the profession implies multiple demands upon learners, accessibility and flexibility of graduate education have been important aspects of the ongoing discussion (Broughton & Hoot, 1995; Kerr, 1988). Over the years, a number of innovations in distance learning have been noted (Kerr, 1988), and some components of many of the existing programs are available by distance delivery or Web-based format. Beyond those now delivered entirely by distance format, alternative-format master's programs are likely to proliferate across the country as the technology becomes available to ensure high-quality interactive learning experiences (Canadian Nurses Association [CNA], 2004). Two early innovations in the formatting of master's degree programs were the clinical training master's program available at the Family Nursing Unit in Calgary (Wright, Watson, & Duhamel, 1985) and the generic master's program at McGill (Ezer, MacDonald, & Gros, 1991). More recently, nurse practitioner training opportunities are being delivered at the master's level across the country (Rutherford, 2005). Although the dominant language of master's instruction in the country has remained English, the University of Ottawa was the first to offer a bilingual program, in 1993 (Kerr & McPhail, 1996).

Although master's programs have rapidly proliferated and produced a generation of leaders for nursing practice, administration, education, and research, this evolution has not resolved the leadership shortage, let alone addressed the projected future demand at this point in our history (Mass et al., 2006). It is well recognized that, in the early 21st century, Canada has insufficient numbers of adequately prepared nurse educators and that a significant percentage of the current cadre of nurse educators is within sight of retirement age (Canadian Institute for Health Information, 2007; May, 2000; Nursing Education Council of British Columbia, 2001). In addition, almost 20 years after Beaton

(1990) raised the alarm about the issue, consensus remains elusive as to what constitutes graduate education in nursing, how it ought to be funded and delivered, and whether academic or professional jurisdictions ought to take the lead in shaping the direction of future developments in master's preparation for Canadian nurses.

Evolution of Doctoral Degree Programs

The evolutionary process for doctoral nursing education in Canada has been much more recent and strategic than the development of master's degree programs. In 1978, the Canadian Nurses Association (CNA) sponsored a national seminar in which nursing leaders endorsed the value of working toward making doctoral nursing education possible in Canada (Zilm, Larose, & Stinson, 1979). From that, the Canadian Nurses Foundation (CNF) and the Canadian Association of University Schools of Nursing developed a proposal dubbed "Operation Bootstrap" to obtain funding for the infrastructure on which doctoral programs in nursing might be established (Kerr & McPhail, 1996). Although that proposal was never funded, the cooperative efforts involved in its development stimulated nursing educational leaders across the country to engage in sufficient strategic dialogue to create the basis on which explicit program proposals became successful a decade later. Through this process, Canadian nursing leaders developed a consensus with regard to the general conditions under which doctoral programs ought to be established, including the following:

- universities with a successful track record in undergraduate and master's programming in nursing
- close proximity to a full range of interdisciplinary doctoral and medical degree programs
- sufficient number of doctorally prepared faculty members
- explicit research development resources (such as programs of research or research units)
- sufficient levels of research funding and a high degree of scholarly productivity shared among a range of faculty members (Field et al., 1992).

Although the first Canadian nurse to obtain a doctoral degree was Sister Denise Lefebre, SQM, Ph.D. (Docteur de Pédagogie) from l'université de Montréal in 1955, the first to graduate with a doctoral degree in nursing on a special-case basis was Francine Ducharme from McGill in 1990 (Banning, 1990). Such special arrangement programs, allowing nurses to obtain doctoral degrees with a substantial nursing component, developed in a number of universities before the launching of actual nursing doctoral programs (Field et al., 1992; Wood & Ross-Kerr, 2002) and have continued in some universities to the present. They differ from interdisciplinary doctoral degrees or degrees taken in another discipline in their explicitly nursing focus but lack the programmatic core disciplinary component that the established nursing programs offer (Kerr & McPhail, 1996).

In 1991, the University of Alberta was the first in the country to launch a fully funded doctoral program in nursing, and its first graduate was Joan Bottorff in 1992, having begun her studies as a special-case student. The political negotiating involved in obtaining funding for that program and admitting the first group of students attracted considerable excitement across the country and was recognized as a landmark achievement (Brink, 1991; Field et al., 1992; Godkin & Bottorff, 1991; Rodger, 1991; Trojan et al., 1996). A second program, at UBC, admitted its first students later that same year (1991), and, in rapid succession, programs were launched at the University of Toronto and by collaborative arrangement at McGill and Montréal in 1993 and at McMaster a year later (Kerr & McPhail, 1996).

Because of the commitment to dialogue and strategic planning throughout the developmental phase of advancing graduate education for the country, the character and shape of the Canadian doctoral nursing programs evolved in a somewhat distinct manner from those in other parts of the globe. A forum on doctoral education in Canada, which was held in late 1990 in Edmonton just before the country launched its first programs, compared the history of doctoral nursing education in the United Kingdom, the United States, and Europe and took advice from such international leaders as Rozella Schlotfeldt and Lisbeth Hocky. By unanimous agreement, the Canadian leaders who were present concluded that doctoral preparation in Canada should lead to a doctorate of philosophy in nursing, rather than a professional doctorate (Jeans, 1990).

A second invitational conference, held in Toronto in April 1995, brought together student and faculty representatives from the five doctoral programs in existence at that time, as well as from universities in which special-case opportunities were available for doctoral degrees in nursing, to examine the substantive context of Canadian Ph.D. nursing programs as they were evolving and developing (Wood, 1997). It was noted that the Canadian programs all had a rather similar structure, requiring an average of four or five courses in core disciplinary knowledge. On that foundation, both coursework and research training were individualized in conjunction with a carefully matched faculty supervisor for each student. Led by Ada Sue Hinshaw, who drew on American examples to point out the quality and resource challenges that a rapid proliferation of doctoral programs could create, participants at that meeting also grappled with such challenging questions as how many doctoral programs Canada ought to support.

As doctoral programs took hold within the profession's national consciousness, it became apparent that they provide nursing not only with high-quality research training but also, and perhaps more importantly, with the following:

- the capacity to study the clinical phenomena pertinent to the discipline
- the conceptual leadership to direct the development of scholarly practice
- the grounded analytic skills to design systems of nursing practice and healthcare delivery (Field et al., 1992).

In so doing, these programs create a cadre of future leaders with expertise in both the art and science of nursing.

The ongoing development of doctoral nursing education in Canada remains a challenge. Among the most pressing concerns has been the difficulty in obtaining funding for student support. In contrast to the academic trajectory in nonclinical disciplines in which doctoral degrees are pursued before the establishment of family and professional responsibilities, most Canadian nursing doctoral students to date have been mid-career professional women, for whom full-time study is often problematic and expensive. Financial support exclusive to nursing has been scarce, with the CNF able to provide only small numbers of graduate fellowships (Wood & Ross-Kerr, 2002). Further, many of the substantive problems relative to nursing-care delivery and its outcomes that nurses wish to investigate do not fit neatly into competitive clinical (medical) and social science funding priorities. The CNA (2003) has called on partners within government, healthcare agencies, universities, and nursing associations to plan cooperatively and share resources to support doctoral education for nurses.

With the advent of the Canadian Institutes of Health Research in 2000, nursing leaders played an active role in shifting the traditionally narrow direction of research support beyond basic and biomedical science to include such concerns as the social determinants of health, the psychosocial experience of illness, and the impact of health service delivery models. On the basis of this effort, there is considerable optimism for the profession's continued progress in the funding of doctoral nursing education (Wood & Ross-Kerr, 2002). Without doubt, the exceptional calibre and productivity of Canada's first generation of nursing doctoral program graduates bodes well for the profession's continuing success in this regard.

 ## PRACTICE REALITIES AND CHALLENGES FOR GRADUATE-PREPARED NURSES

In the early years of graduate nursing education in Canada, advanced preparation was generally understood to be a route away from the bedside and into teaching or administration. However, as the percentage of Canadian nurses prepared at the master's level has risen, it has become increasingly apparent that a significant proportion of nursing's professional leadership and scholarship ought to be in the clinical practice arena. Although all aspects of nursing scholarship play a significant role in advancing nursing knowledge and influence, the unique contribution of the discipline to the Canadian healthcare system inherently depends on the application of knowledge in the practice arena.

Thus, since the early 1980s, a number of master's programs have explicitly shifted their emphasis to professional and clinical leadership as a primary objective. Moreover, they have expanded the opportunities for a range of clinical leadership learning options. Similarly, when doctoral programs came on board in the 1990s, most nurses assumed that their primary goal would be to produce the next generation of academic nurse researchers. Although many graduates have gone on to faculty positions, the potential for developing clinical scholarship leaders at that level has also been recognized. Thus, the practice reality for nurses with graduate preparation in the discipline is a moving target, in keeping with the rapid changes in the population, the healthcare system, and knowledge proliferation within society.

Among the more subtle but challenging practice realities for nurses at the graduate level has been the general level of skepticism and distrust within the mainstream nursing population for the value that advanced education brings to the profession. In preparing this chapter, a wide range of students and recent graduates were interviewed for the purpose of clarifying the issues that might be included in the discussion. Many of them pointed out that, although attitudes are slowly shifting, it is not uncommon for nurses "coming back to do their master's work" to report the absence of endorsement or support from their colleagues. Even those who remain active in their clinical roles for the duration of their studies may find it an ongoing challenge to convince their practice colleagues that the university has anything relevant to provide to the practice setting.

Expertise and professional leadership within the practice setting are often attributed to the special qualities of an individual nurse, rather than to knowledge and skills that graduate education can bring to the effectiveness of nursing practice.[1] Perhaps because nurses have had long-standing debates about entry-to-practice levels and scope of responsibility, some remain reluctant to recognize the value of diversifying to achieve collective aims. Pressures from union ideologies, an inherent democratizing ideal, and a reluctance for self-promotion have made nurses more comfortable with the general notion that "a nurse is a nurse is a nurse" than with the ramifications of leveling and specializing nursing contributions. By packing extreme amounts of content and experience into tightly crafted curricula, and by sending new graduates out into a healthcare system that is exceedingly complex and strained, nurses sometimes feel that their educational programs have set them up for failure (Griffiths, 2000). This pressure may be felt particularly strongly by diploma-level graduates in the context of the current climate of health reform and instability.

Sadly, however, nurses have not always provided one another with a mechanism for understanding how their practice reality is shaped by the prominent forces of the day. Many simply fail to appreciate that the profession is advantaged, not disadvantaged, by an increasingly educated majority. Thus, nurses as a group have not always been supportive of the continuing educational advancement of their peers and may interpret "going back to school" as abandonment rather than as adding ammunition for their collective battles. Certainly, an emphasis on increasing social awareness and political analysis among the mainstream of practicing nurses will continue to be an important element in the general experience of graduate education and the practice reality of nurses prepared with graduate degrees.

A somewhat similar climate of misunderstanding can occur for doctorally prepared nurses with primary appointments in a clinical practice setting. Although the profession has had a generally high

---

[1] As a teacher of graduate students, I have been fascinated by how prominent and resistant to change these negative attitudes can be within nursing. Increasingly, graduate students take seriously the "ambassador" role that they can play in showing their colleagues the value of their graduate education. New learning is made manifest not simply in the wearing of a new degree but, more importantly, in the new levels of confidence, critical thinking skills, and "big-picture" thinking that they begin to apply to their practice. –Sally Thorne

level of collective comfort with the traditional model of the academic researcher-educator, it seems much less comfortable with how to apply the skills of doctorally prepared nurses in the clinical context. Nurses in clinical leadership and scholar positions may find, for example, that the research component of their role is less valued than is the administrative aspect. As a result, although nursing has made great strides in cultivating a generation of accomplished researchers, this may have been at the expense of other critically important leadership roles. For example, many of the recent dean and director searches for Canadian nursing schools have been long and protracted, and it is generally understood that the available applicant pool has been diminished by other opportunities in research and scholarship as well as by an extended period of time in which nursing administrative scholarship was relatively unsupported. Thus, in contrast to the situation that faces the master's prepared nurse attempting to re-enter the practice domain, doctorally prepared nurses graduate into a professional culture characterized by an inordinate valuing of specialized research training and acquiring protected time away from distractions to attain the highest level of research funding possible. In its own way, this attitudinal climate is as problematic and counterproductive as that of the academically resistant mainstream.

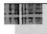 ## ISSUES AND CONTROVERSIES IN GRADUATE EDUCATION

In contrast to the career paths typical of many professions, nurses still perceive the option to take their graduate education in nursing or consider advanced study in other disciplines. Although the proliferation of programs at the graduate level across the country and the increased availability of distance offerings have made higher degrees in nursing a viable option for all Canadian nurses, many still decide to look elsewhere for their academic advancement. Certainly, the history of the nursing profession in Canada has been well served by many noted leaders who returned to the fold after completing their master's or doctoral degrees in such fields as education, psychology, business administration, public health, anthropology, medical sciences, or sociology. From those disciplines, we have derived benefits in theoretical diversity, methodology, and analytic processes. We also recognize that the world in which nursing is practised is inherently interdisciplinary and, therefore, that nurses have a natural affinity for the models, methods, and substantive knowledge of a range of disciplines.

At the same time, despite individual exceptions, leaders who lack an in-depth understanding of the complex theoretical, historical, and philosophical grounding of the nursing discipline can be considerably disadvantaged when they attempt to articulate a nursing perspective. Even more problematic may be that they do not even know they lack this understanding. Nursing is difficult to describe, delineate, and encapsulate in language due to its ineffable nature and complexity. Canada needs a cadre of leaders who are adept at conceptualizing the discipline and its contributions within an ever-changing context. Thus, although graduate preparation in nursing will remain a high priority for the discipline's development in this country, there are many opinions on how best to achieve it.

Theoretical Debates

An explicit concern for issues of a theoretical nature evolved in the second half of the 20th century in response to the explosion of new knowledge in the physical and social sciences and the availability of new theoretical challenges arising from the core projects of a variety of academic disciplines. Nursing theory emerged as a mechanism for organizing and making sense of "this infinitely dynamic and complex body of information" so that nurses could use knowledge in a "professional, accountable, and defensible manner" (Beckstrand, 1978).

As the influence of physicians and the medical model on healthcare delivery systems expanded, new species of healthcare professionals and technicians proliferated and nursing curricula evolved away from the more traditional medical science and apprenticeship structure. As such, nurses began to recognize an urgent need to articulate the uniqueness and distinctiveness of their profession among others in the healthcare system (Chinn & Kramer, 1999; Engebretson, 1997). To do this, they began to create conceptual maps that would depict the manner in which nursing informational and decisional processes might relate to a theoretically infinite range of clinical situations (Ellis, 1968; Johnson, 1974; McKay, 1969; Wald & Leonard, 1964). In calling such conceptual frameworks "nursing theory," they located nursing thought within the rather rigid academic and scientific community of the era and, thereby, created a context within which nursing science could be legitimized and acknowledged (Cull-Wilby & Peppin, 1987; Jones, 1997).

The conceptual model-building era that lasted from the mid-1960s through the mid-1980s was remarkable in its optimism and enthusiasm for extending the boundaries of existing scientific and philosophical thinking. In a context in which theory development in science was understood to follow a reductionist linear causation model, the nursing theorists were essentially attempting to capture complexity and infinite variation within a rigorous and systematic scientific matrix.

Considering some of the philosophical and scientific innovations with which we can now reflect on the project, some aspects of their efforts may seem naïve in retrospect. However, it can also be said that their efforts to develop a science accounting for both the generalities of substantive knowledge and theory as well as the particularities of an infinite range of new applications was impressive in its capacity to recognize the complexities inherent in excellent clinical nursing reasoning and to respect the diversities of expanding knowledge within which nursing operates (Barnum, 1994; Benner, Tanner, & Chesla, 1996; Meleis, 1987; Raudonis & Acton, 1997; Thorne & Perry, 2001).

However, the model-building enterprise was not well understood within the dominant mainstream of nursing and, for the most part, remained a distinct enterprise from the research scholarship that developed through the latter decades of the century. As the theorists themselves became embroiled in debates about whose conceptual structure should dominate the discipline, much of academic nursing tired of the discourse and began to consider the theoretical debates a minor embarrassment in nursing's history (Engebretson, 1997). Indeed, where comparative analysis of the theoretical models had been a prominent aspect of graduate education in nursing, many programs eliminated the issue from their curricula in favor of a shift toward what Meleis (1987) termed the *substance* of nursing theory.

Because it is arguable that mainstream nursing theorizing was evolving toward embracing aspects of those directions anyway, the "revolution" in nursing thinking became something of a turf war in which ideologic claims about the inherent intentionality of theoretical positions took the form of abject generalizations about the beliefs and motives of those who did and did not sit on the same side of the paradigm fence (Thorne, Reimer Kirkham, & Henderson, 1999). Further, instead of welcoming debate, some proponents of simultaneity theory have elected to interpret challenges to the inherent value of simultaneity theories within the discipline as nothing more substantive than a "vicious diatribe" (Cody, 2000) or an intentional "mis-take"(Pilkington & Mitchell, 2003) and have even suggested that criticism from outside of that paradigm cannot be taken seriously because it is inherently misguided (Parse, 1998). Perhaps one fortunate consequence of this turn of theorizing is that it brought the relevance of theoretical thinking back into the forefront of academic nursing and stimulated many nurse scholars to pay attention to the debates. Because of this, critical analysis of the implications of theoretical positioning has come back into favor in graduate nursing education as a relevant and entirely necessary body of scholarship. Further, the explosion of misunderstanding and accusation among the discipline's theorists has forced academic nursing to recognize the imperative of understanding more fully its philosophical underpinnings.

Philosophical Challenges

Among the most overt and easily recognized philosophical challenges facing nursing scholarship from the 1980s to the present has been the qualitative–quantitative methodologic debate. Although research methodology has technical aspects, much of this debate underscores a number of much deeper and more complex philosophical schisms within the scientific and academic communities of which nursing is a member. Overt attention to the philosophy of science was at one time rare in nursing curricula at any level but it is now well recognized as a hallmark of a credible graduate program in the discipline, and this recognition has crept downward into most undergraduate curricula as well. Thus, an appreciation for the philosophical positioning of the ideas of the discipline has emerged as a critically important element in professional leadership.

As a result of the popularization of Kuhn's (1962) treatise on scientific revolution, academic discourse is no longer characterized by indisputable facts and truths, but rather by claims and positions. In a climate in which postmodern thinking permeates society, knowledge previously considered immutable by virtue of its scientific grounding has become fodder for deconstruction and revisioning (Haack, 1998; Hacking, 1999). The evolution of scientific knowledge is no longer understood as linear and rational, but rather as an entirely human enterprise, subject to ideational and political pressures over time (Van Doren, 1991). What we knew to be true yesterday is disputable today and may be considered reactionary tomorrow. For a discipline such as nursing, the dramatic shift from a realistic ontologic orientation, in which factual truths exist, toward consideration of knowledge as social construction, in which there may be different ways of understanding truth, has had tremendous appeal. For example, nurses know that every practice principle must have its legitimate variations and that every theoretical claim one might make about human health and illness experience will break down in the face of individual human uniqueness. To some degree, one might argue that theoretical relativism has always been philosophically consistent with the kind of flexibility and adaptability that are the hallmarks of excellent nursing practice. Because of this, nursing scholarship has enthusiastically embraced qualitative methods, subjective knowledge, and critical-emancipatory inquiry as consistent with its general moral underpinnings.

In a climate in which theoretical truths are no longer as comfortable as they once were, however, many nurse scholars now find themselves struggling to find purchase on an increasingly slippery platform of disciplinary knowledge. For the profession to have a social mandate, certain basic philosophical truths or positions seem to be prerequisites. For example, although it might be interesting to philosophize about whether human pain and suffering exist apart from our ability to apprehend them subjectively, nursing is solidly morally bound to an assumption that they do and that nurses have an obligation to ameliorate them when possible, despite the individual variations they might manifest and the possibilities that they might simply be profound subjective constructions within the minds of those afflicted. Thus, in reaction to the notion that qualitative methods were more true to human subjective experience and, therefore, more relevant to the knowledge required for nursing practice, many scholars now recognize the inherent limits of any singular methodologic approach for generating knowledge suitable to a practice science. To develop useful knowledge in relation to a substantive field, for example, nursing might require population-based surveys, linear-regression modelling, phenomenologic interpretation, and emancipatory-action research. Thus, members of the nursing academy are scrambling to expand beyond their traditional methodologic expertise and develop the more rounded philosophical and methodologic buttressing that scholars of the future will require. For doctoral programs in nursing, this means that skill within a range of inquiry methods, including qualitative research, quantitative research, and philosophical analysis, will be foundational to producing a new generation of excellent scholars.

Although traditional doctoral training has relied heavily on mentorship models, the scholarship of the future will inevitably require a shift in student and supervisor relationships. The postmodern challenge within academia has raised awareness that traditional science recreates itself, such that genuine innovation must inevitably resist and react against the dictates of older models and authorities. Of course, in the extreme version, the notion of expertise is rejected entirely (Thorne, 1999). However, although that extreme version clearly exists within the academic community in Canada (Good, 2001), nursing's professional practice mandates seem to have kept it somewhat more grounded in a perspective in which the ideas one holds have meaningful implications for the society we live in and the individuals who constitute it. However, it also seems quite common for Canadian nursing graduate students, especially those at the doctoral level, to view the scholarship forms of their mentors with a critical lens, to envision combinations of methodologic and philosophical approaches that extend beyond the specific expertise of their supervisors, and to chafe under academic regulations that create barriers to building their own programs of scholarship in a less rigid and bounded science than did their predecessors.

Practical Challenges

Although many of these debates underscore the challenge of understanding the theoretical and philosophical nature of the discipline, there are also a number of somewhat technical and practical issues that relate centrally to the question of core disciplinary knowledge. Historically and currently, Canada has little dedicated source of funding for the development of nursing knowledge (the relatively minor amounts available from the CNF notwithstanding). The issue of a separate nursing fund was hotly debated during the developmental phase of transforming Canada's research infrastructure into the Canadian Institutes for Health Research. Although nurses have clearly demonstrated the capacity to successfully compete with other health disciplines for research dollars within the mandates of the specific institutes, the career opportunities within the more fundable substantive fields may be at the expense of sustained inquiry into the core knowledge of the discipline.

For those whose graduate preparation was outside the discipline, the problems associated with core nursing knowledge may seem tangential to the larger enterprise. Given the contentious nature of the nursing theoretical debates, reluctance to engage in these issues is understandable. However, this tension between allegiance to "substantive" knowledge (such as children's health or family health) and "disciplinary" knowledge (such as the nature of nursing or the dynamics of clinical nursing reasoning) has played itself out in graduate nursing curricula, with some nursing scholars advocating immersion in the substance and others pressing for the disciplinary competence within which to ground it. Ongoing debates with regard to the optimal balance between such topics as the nature of nursing knowledge and interdisciplinary knowledge associated with distinct fields of nursing specialization are likely to continue and to complicate curricular planning for the foreseeable future.

A related practical challenge derives from the applied and practical nature of the science of nursing. Although graduate education has not always been understood as an inherent adjunct to the practice of nursing, increasing numbers of master's and doctoral students seek advanced degrees for the explicit purpose of enhancing and strengthening their practice effectiveness. Although it has been natural for the discipline to consider the conduct and dissemination of research as a scholarly enterprise, the notion of practice scholarship has been much more difficult to articulate. Although many Canadian universities continue to support and encourage advancement of practice knowledge using a variety of strategies, the continuous pressure to evaluate the quality of academic units on the basis of the research dollars they attract and the publications they produce is unavoidable. Thus, particularly at the doctoral level, there has generally been less overt support for scholarship in the practice tradition than for more conventional health research scholarship, and students seeking to create clinical scientist careers may find themselves seduced by the apparent credibility afforded the more usual career track strategies.

As graduate education continues to proliferate in this country, nursing is confronting many permutations of these theoretical, philosophical, and practical challenges. As graduate education becomes the norm rather than the exception, increasing pressure toward flexibility and access will inevitably occur, and smaller academic nursing units will start to feel left behind if they are not offering graduate degree programs.

CHALLENGES FOR GRADUATE-PREPARED NURSES

Nurses prepared at the graduate level are the current and future leaders of the profession in Canada. In that capacity, they are vulnerable to the effects of the current healthcare climate. Various health reforms in Canada since the 1990s have reflected attempts to control health spending by shifting resources from the acute-care sector to the community sector, mechanisms to rationalize resource allocation decision making, and efforts to bring healthcare system–decision making closer to home within national regions (CNA, 2000). The strongly held principles articulated in the Canada Health Act, and traditionally embraced by nurses, have been challenged as never before in the context of this conflictual health reform climate (May & Ferguson-Pare, 1997). Nursing shortages and the "graying" of the profession (Bradley, 1999) occur in a climate in which nursing leadership is increasingly scarce (King, 2000; Mass et al., 2006).

The weight of navigating the discipline's journey through the health reform process over the next several decades will undoubtedly sit squarely on the shoulders of practice leaders, many of them prepared at the master's level. Clearly, their capacity to make nimble adjustments in health human resource planning, economic accountability, health policy processes, and professional practice leadership will determine the shape of professional nursing for the next generation. Because these fields of inquiry have not been dominant within nursing's disciplinary scholarship over the most recent decades, there is a recognized shortage in scholarship related to nursing work, nursing service, and the delivery of nursing care. Because formal research scholarship has eclipsed academic and administrative leadership as a priority since the 1980s, it will take some time before graduate nursing programs can take a sufficient shift in course to cultivate a new generation of professional leaders. Meanwhile, collaborative partnerships between practice settings and universities will be essential to resolve the challenges inherent in the shortage of nursing personnel at all levels and in the conditions of nursing work. Thus, we can expect issues of the workplace to take an increasingly prominent position among the scholarship arenas of graduate education, such that issues traditionally considered the domain of the functional specialization of nursing administration will become mainstream and foundational expectations of nursing in any leadership role.

Although the number of nurses entering graduate programs continues to increase at all levels, the pressures on nurses to extend their academic commitment have also exponentially increased. First-rate graduates of master's programs are quickly seduced into doctoral programs, doctoral graduates are encouraged to shift immediately into postdoctoral training, and postdocs are expected to seek career award funding to protect their research investment. Although each of these progressions is laudable and necessary, it is also important for the profession to remain vigilant to the continuing need for nursing scholarship and leadership throughout the system. University (and college) programs will increasingly be hungry for new faculty members to teach the next generation of nursing students, and clinical agencies will be desperate for nurses capable of combining practice knowledge with policy work, administrative strength, evidence-based practice development, and corporate leadership. As the current generation of faculty and administrators retires from the active roster, the demand for the next generation to fill the gaps will clearly exceed the current capacity of the profession to train and groom appropriate numbers. Thus, we can anticipate that the global effects of Canada's nursing shortage have only just begun (Canadian Institute for Health Information, 2007).

In the current climate, the healthcare community will more urgently demand that the university play a strong role in resolving the critical human and material resource challenges that Canada will face in its development and delivery of health services to an increasingly diverse and complex population. Pressure to meet the emergent needs of the system will take the form of new professional practice roles, increasingly specialized training expectations, and greater numbers of excellently prepared graduates. Without dialogue and debate to create a national consensus on our shared beliefs, role definitions, and disciplinary core values, nursing may well experience discord and organizational disarray. And with the urgent demands on the system insinuating themselves on our education and practice contexts as well as on our research, it may be difficult in the next few decades to take the time we require to reflect on our past and direct our future.

STRATEGIES FOR ADVANCING GRADUATE EDUCATION

Canadian nurses have been strong advocates for the principles embedded in the Canada Health Act, and they have also been consistently proud of a national tradition of high-quality professional education and service delivery. As the pressures to increase the number of graduates inevitably lead to more programs and more diverse program delivery modes, it will be increasingly imperative for Canadian nursing to attend to the quality of the educational opportunities on which its leaders build their professional careers.

Canadian nursing has no quality-monitoring mechanism at the graduate level. Programs preparatory to professional licensure are all regulated by provincial statute and professional organizations, and there is a voluntary accreditation system by which the quality of baccalaureate nursing programs is well supported. Although the Canadian Association of Schools of Nursing has created position statements on master's and doctoral level education (Box 11.1), graduate program approval tends to be entirely within the authority of the individual university senate. The approval is typically based on the market demands of the specific institution as well as on the degree to which it considers conventional academic quality criteria in its program decisions.

Because university administrators tend to assume that graduate programs, especially at the doctoral level, attract fellowship dollars, increase the rate of faculty publication, and expand the research capacity of the organizational unit, some may be unconcerned that there is insufficient support within a nursing department for core disciplinary knowledge, research training, or scholarly mentorship. Thus, preserving the quality of doctoral education in Canada within the context of pressure for rapid program proliferation has been recognized as an urgent priority (Wood, Giovanetti, & Ross-Kerr, 2004).

Similarly, there is continuing pressure to expand the flexibility and accessibility of master's programs (CNA, 2004). A review of the CNA's current program listings suggests that most Canadian nursing master's programs have some courses available by distance delivery mode or are working toward complete program delivery online or using modern information technology. Although there is no doubt that these fulfill an identified need, the implications of responding to the pressure *en masse* should be an important agenda for national discussion and deliberation. Some of the less objective attributes of a high-quality master's program, such as developing the skills of collegial networking, challenging one's own concepts and core values, and being mentored by knowledge brokers and generators within the discipline, all become experiences of a different nature when conducted in intellectual isolation. Thus, it seems more important than ever for Canadian nurses to remain vigilant to the question of quality monitoring of graduate education and to take ownership of the standards by which excellence (and mediocrity) can be judged.

Because the financial imperatives of universities will undoubtedly continue to create the conditions under which scholarship is evaluated in the external academic community, nursing academics and their leaders will have to find strategies by which a balance between lucrative and meaningful inquiry can be supported. At present in Canada, there is an influx of opportunity for funding research projects, programs, and training centers within the national agenda of health system and health service demands. To the extent that nurses can align their scholarship with those national agendas as they unfold, they will be increasingly successful in attracting additional resources to their academic units. Unfettered adherence to these agendas, however, would have predictable and unacceptable effects on the culture and nature of nursing academic departments. Within any department offering graduate degree programs, it will remain important to have faculty who teach as well as do research, who engage

BOX 11.1 Canadian Association of Schools of Nursing (CASN) Position Statements on Graduate Education (2006)

CASN Position Statement on Master's Level of Nursing

Background

The purposes and nature of master's education are based on the following assumptions:

- Nursing practice is an inclusive term that incorporates care of individuals, families, and communities as well as involvement in nursing education, administration, research, and policy development.
- Many nursing practices are founded on rationales that have not been critically validated or critically examined.
- Nursing practice is enhanced by nursing-related research, scholarship, and theory.
- The Canadian healthcare system needs advanced practice nurses with the knowledge and skills necessary for appraising the "state of nursing science" in areas relevant to nursing practice, and transferring this to the practice setting.
- Master's level education is the minimum requirement for advanced nursing practice, leadership positions, and faculty positions in nursing education programs.

Position

At the master's level, students build upon the knowledge and skills acquired at the baccalaureate level. Emphasis is placed on developing the ability to analyze, critique, and use research and theory to further nursing practice. Provision should also be made for examination of current issues in healthcare and the ethical values that influence decision making. The master's curriculum should include a definitive component designed to enable students to synthesize research, theory, and practice at an advanced level. The focus of master's study may include the preparation of nurses with advanced skills in the practice of nursing (e.g., nurse practitioner). Master's programs encompass a *program continuum* that includes programs that require a master's thesis, programs that require a major project or practicum, and programs that are course based. Individual master's programs may include both required and elective courses designed to prepare graduates to assume positions in advanced nursing practice, teaching, administration, and policy development and to provide a foundation for Ph.D. study.

Doctoral Education in Nursing in Canada

Background

Canada will require significant increases in the number of nurses with doctoral preparation in order to:

- build the faculty base necessary to educate sufficient numbers of new graduates to meet the healthcare system workforce needs,
- generate the evidence required to address the health problems of Canadians, and
- advance the knowledge base within which the practice of nursing is grounded.

Since 1991, a small number of Canadian universities have produced excellent graduates from nursing doctoral programs characterized by research intensivity, core disciplinary knowledge, and expertise within a substantive field. However, the production of new graduates has not kept pace with the country's requirements.

Position

Quality Standards

Because the traditional on-site, full-time Ph.D. training program model fails to reach some groups of talented and qualified potential students, CASN anticipates that innovative and creative delivery models will emerge and new programs will be developed. In order to ensure that this process occurs in an effective and constructive manner, explicit articulation of the quality criteria to which Canadian programs should be held is an imperative.

Among the criteria required for effective Ph.D. programs in nursing are the following:

- Research-intensive academic nursing units, housed within universities with well-established graduate program infrastructure and access to high-quality interdisciplinary interactions
- A critical mass of active faculty researchers capable of supporting the mentorship, research training, and socialization required to engage in the full complement of roles associated with success in the competitive Canadian health research context

- Learning experiences related to at least three core components: 1) research training, 2) core disciplinary knowledge related to the history, context, and theoretical underpinnings of nursing, and 3) knowledge of the current state of science and scholarship within a substantive field within the discipline
- A combination of a modest amount of coursework, comprehensive examinations, and completion of a dissertation
- Opportunities for active engagement in a scholarly learning environment
- Evidence of a rigorous external evaluation benchmarking research effectiveness and productivity, infrastructure and resources, and outcomes.

The critical attributes of graduates of Canadian programs include the capacity for:

- obtaining competitive research funding
- conducting research that is both rigorous and original to address a problem of concern to the discipline
- articulating and establishing a program of research
- communicating effectively through peer-reviewed journal publication, presentation at scholarly meetings, and in professional and scientific interactions.

CASN proposes to undertake further work to more fully articulate necessary and expected attributes of Ph.D. in Nursing programs in Canada and implement processes whereby high-level quality standards can be assured.

Professional or Practice Doctorates

The Ph.D. in Nursing in Canada is a research-focused degree program. CASN does not support, at this time, the concept of the professional or practice doctorate, such as has been adopted in some other jurisdictions, and remains the subject of considerable controversy as an appropriate focus for Canadian universities at this time.

Accessibility

Strategies to increase accessibility to appropriate doctoral education must be multiple and creative. Recognizing that there are legitimate geographic and demographic barriers to access, creative strategies are required by which Canada's research-intensive programs can be made more accessible to the target audience, and thoughtful articulation of quality standards will assist with this process. In addition, CASN recognizes that some nurses who seek doctoral-level education will not be ideally served by a research-intensive Ph.D. in Nursing model. However, to address the particular needs of nurses who do not select to do research-intensive Ph.D.s, CASN encourages creative and collaborative mechanisms whereby these nurses may be appropriately accommodated through such means as interdisciplinary doctoral programs, special-case doctoral initiatives, or collaborative distance delivery mechanisms by which potential mentors from universities not currently delivering Ph.D. programs may become involved. CASN believes that active support of such creative options is an appropriate mechanism whereby researchers and scholars in the discipline can indirectly assist with this aspect of capacity building.

CASN believes that the future needs of Canada will be appropriately served by placing the current emphasis on the research-intensive Ph.D. in Nursing, and anticipates that this degree will become the expected basis for leadership roles across a variety of settings over the course of time. In this context, CASN recognizes the need for a clear and coherent communication mechanism whereby the explicit outcome criteria associated with the Ph.D. in Nursing are clearly articulated to potential students, potential employers, and others.

Students

In order to address the future needs of the Canadian healthcare system, ensure the development of an adequate professoriate to prepare the next generation of nurses, and to sustain the momentum that has been established within the nursing research community, Canadian nursing doctoral programs must target potential students at earlier points in their academic programs and in their careers and actively support their continuing development through to senior research and academic leadership roles. This focus requires efforts to actively engage students in research at an undergraduate level, to ensure the development of a strong base of master's prepared nurses, and to create the context in which excellent nurses anticipate and plan for doctoral education as a natural progression at an early stage within their career development.

(continued)

BOX 11.1 Canadian Association of Schools of Nursing (CASN) Position Statements on Graduate Education (2006) (continued)

Targets

In order to meet the needs of the Canadian healthcare system, explicit predictions are needed of the number of doctorally prepared nurses that will be required so that coherent strategies to meet those targets can be established.

Funding

In order to reach these goals, significant increases in funding will be required for doctoral students, for nursing research infrastructure, and for the infrastructures for graduate programs within schools of nursing. Because CASN recognizes that this will require concerted effort at all levels, including institutional, regional, and provincial, it strongly supports the development and implementation of a unified nursing voice to address this challenge at a national level.

Approved November, 2004, **Revised** June, 2006. Canadian Association of Schools of Nursing. (2008). Retrieved from http://www.casn.ca/media.php?mid=205&xwm=true

in practice scholarship as well as traditional research, and who examine the philosophical and theoretical problems of the discipline as well as respond to the immediate expressed needs of the society around them.

Among the more complex challenges for academic nursing will be enacting strategies and processes that reward a range of professional leadership and scholarship (Boyer, 1990; Glassick, Huber, & Maeroff, 1997) and creating the kinds of graduate learning environments that are both grounded strongly within the discipline and credible within the larger arena. The nursing profession will require the capacity for healthy dialogue and consensus-building on matters relevant to a national strategy for graduate education if it is to remain the exemplar of world-class quality that we enjoy today. In the coming years, we will undoubtedly have to wrestle with new challenges, such as pressure toward the practice doctorate that has been endorsed in the United States amid protracted contentious debate (American Association of Colleges of Nursing, 2006; Parse, 2008) and a campaign toward a separate and distinct graduate degree option in psychiatric nursing on the part of registered psychiatric nurses in Western Canada (Ryan-Nicholls, 2004).

Nurses in Canada have made great strides toward developing professional scholarship and academic credibility during an era in which the pressing problems of society have demanded unprecedented attention. They have attempted to stay true to a vision of professional integrity as they flow with the changing tides of acceptable inquiry methods and theoretical locations. In an increasingly interdisciplinary world in which truth is never static and credibility is always open for discussion, nurses have collectively assumed a rightful place in the academy, in the healthcare delivery and policy arenas, and in society. And, as Florence Nightingale might have reminded us, the worth of a society can be measured by the quality of its nursing.

SUMMARY

Graduate education in nursing has advanced rapidly in Canada over the past half century. Today it serves to advance leadership within the profession in two distinct ways: professional scholarship at the master's level and research-intensive training at the doctoral and postdoctoral levels.

Canada needs a cadre of nursing leaders who are adept at conceptualizing the discipline and its contributions in an ever-changing context of diverse theories and structures. A vibrant infrastructure of graduate education in nursing will serve to ensure that Canada sustains a knowledgeable nursing workforce in the years to come and that our discipline has the capacity to retain its ownership of the standards by which its excellence (or mediocrity) can be judged. Graduate education serves as the primary vehicle through which the nursing discipline maintains a philosophical grounding within its social mandate and its science, ensuring that a nursing angle of vision is brought to bear upon the challenges that confront the Canadian healthcare system of the future.

Add to your knowledge of this issue:	
Association of Universities and Colleges of Canada	http://www.aucc.ca/index_e.html
Canadian Association of Nursing Research	www.canr.ca
Canadian Association of Schools of Nursing	www.casn.ca
Canadian Health Services Research Foundation	www.chsrf.ca
Canadian Institute for Health Information	www.cihi.ca
Canadian Nurses Association	http://www.cna-nurses.ca/cna/

Online

REFLECTIONS on the Chapter...

1 What priorities and trends have most influenced the changes in Canadian master's and doctoral nursing degree curricula since the 1960s?

2 Attitudes toward graduate education within the mainstream practicing nurse population may not have consistently supported nurses in their efforts to obtain master's or doctoral nursing education. Why do such attitudes exist? What social, political, and economic forces within nursing might contribute to their continuation?

3 It can be argued that many nurses with graduate degrees in the discipline are ambivalent about the value of studying "nursing theory" or the theoretical debates within the discipline. What characteristics of the theories or the understanding of them may have created this climate of misunderstanding?

4 As academic nursing evolves over the next two decades, how can it appropriately attend to a balance between core disciplinary knowledge and the substantive knowledge that will drive advances in clinical practice?

5 Should Canadian nursing leaders engage in formal dialogue about the future direction of graduate education in this country? If so, who should lead that discussion, and what should be the primary objective?

References

Allen, M. (1986). The relationship between graduate teaching and research in nursing. In S.M. Stinson & J.C. Kerr (Eds.), *International issues in nursing research* (pp. 151–167). London: Croom Helm.

American Association of Colleges of Nursing. (2006). *The essentials of doctoral education for advanced nursing practice.* Retrieved January 22, 2008 from http://www.aacn.nche.edu/DNP/ pdf/Essentials.pdf.

Association of the Universities and Colleges of Canada. (2007). *Directory of Canadian universities searchable database.* Retrieved January 22, 2008 from http://www.aucc.ca/can_uni/ index_e.html.

Banning, J.A. (1990). Nursing PhD comes to Canada [Editorial]. *The Canadian Nurse, 86*(11), 3.

Barnum, B.J.S. (1994). *Nursing theory: Analysis, application, evaluation* (4th ed.). Philadelphia: J. B. Lippincott.

Beaton, J. (1990). Crises in graduate nursing education. *The Canadian Nurse, 86*(1), 29–32.

Beckstrand, J. (1978). The notion of a practice theory and the relationship of scientific and ethical knowledge to practice. *Research in Nursing & Health, 1,* 131–136.

Benner, P., Tanner, C.A. & Chesla, C.A. (1996). *Expertise in nursing practice: Caring, clinical judgement, and ethics.* New York: Springer.

Boyer, E. (1990). *Scholarship reconsidered: Priorities of the professoriate.* Princeton, NJ: Carnegie Foundation for the Advancement of Teaching.

Bradley, C. (1999). Doing more with less in nursing work: A review of the literature. *Contemporary Nurse, 8*(3), 57–64.

Brink, P.J. (1991). Editorial: The first Canadian Ph.D. in nursing. *Western Journal of Nursing Research, 13*(4), 432–433.

Broughton, K. & Hoot, T. (1995). Commentary: Canada needs accessible masters' programs. *The Canadian Nurse, 91*(10), 55.

_____. (2006). *Member programs.* Retrieved January 22, 2008 from http://www.casn.ca/Education/members_programs.htm.

Canadian Institute for Health Information. (2007). *Workforce trends of registered nurses in Canada, 2006.* Retrieved January 22, 2008 from http://www.icis.ca/cihiweb/dispPage.jsp?cw_page=AR_20_E.

Canadian Nurses Association. (2000). *Framework for Canada's health system.* Ottawa: Author.

_____. (2003). *Joint Canadian Nurses Association and Canadian Association of Schools of Nursing position statement on doctoral preparation in nursing.* Retrieved January 22, 2008 from http://www.cna-nurses.ca/CNA/documents/pdf/ publications/PS75_doctoral_preparation_e.pdf.

_____. (2004). *Joint Canadian Nurses Association and Canadian Association of Schools of Nursing position statement on flexible delivery of nursing education programs.* Retrieved January 22, 2008 from http://www.cna-nurses.ca/CNA/ documents/pdf/publications/PS74_flexible_delivery_e.pdf.

Chinn, P.L. & Kramer, M.K. (1999). *Theory and nursing: Integrated knowledge development* (5th ed.). St. Louis: Mosby.

Cody, W.K. (2000). Paradigm shift or paradigm drift? A meditation on commitment and transcendence. *Nursing Science Quarterly, 13*(2), 93–102.

Cull-Wilby, B.L. & Peppin, J.C. (1987). Toward a coexistence of paradigms in nursing knowledge development. *Journal of Advanced Nursing, 12,* 515–521.

Ellis, R. (1968). Characteristics of significant theories. *Nursing Research, 17*(3), 217–222.

Engebretson, J. (1997). A multiparadigm approach to nursing. *Advances in Nursing Science, 20*(1), 21–33.

Ezer, H., MacDonald, J., & Gros, C.P. (1991). Follow-up of generic master's graduates: Viability of a model of nursing in practice. *Canadian Journal of Nursing Research, 23*(3), 9–20.

Field, P.A., Stinson, S.M., & Thibaudeau, M.F. (1992). Graduate education in nursing in Canada. In A.J. Baumgart & J. Larsen (Eds.). *Canadian nursing faces the future* (2nd ed., pp. 421–445). St. Louis: Mosby.

Ford, J.S. & Wertenberger, D.H. (1993). Nursing education content in master's in nursing programs. *Canadian Journal of Nursing Research, 25*(2), 53–61.

Gein, L. (1994). Defending the master's thesis in nursing graduate programs: The Canadian context. *Journal of Nursing Education, 33*(7), 330–332.

Glassick, C., Huber, M., & Maeroff, G. (1997). *Scholarship assessed: Evaluation on the professoriate.* San Francisco: Jossey-Bass.

Godkin, M.D. & Bottorff, J.L. (1991). Doctorate in nursing: Idea to reality. *The Canadian Nurse, 87*(11), 31–34.

Good, G. (2001). *Humanism betrayed: Theory, ideology, and culture in the contemporary university.* Montreal & Kingston: McGill & Queens University Press.

Griffiths, H. (2000). Nursing education at the crossroads. *Nursing BC, 32*(2), 21–23.

Haack, S. (1998). *Manifesto of a passionate moderate.* Chicago: University of Chicago Press.

Hacking, I. (1999). *The social construction of what?* Cambridge, MA: Harvard University Press.

Jeans, M.E. (1990). Advancing doctoral preparation for nurses. *Canadian Journal of Nursing Research, 22*(2), 1–2.

Johnson, D.E. (1974). Development of theory: A requisite for nursing as a primary health profession. *Nursing Research, 23*(5), 372–377.

Jones, M. (1997). Thinking nursing. In S.E. Thorne & V.E. Hayes (Eds.). *Nursing praxis: Knowledge and action* (pp. 125–139). Thousand Oaks, CA: Sage.

Kerr, J.R. (1988). Nursing education at a distance: Using technology to advantage in undergraduate and graduate degree programs in Alberta, Canada. *International Journal of Nursing Studies, 25,* 301–306.

Kerr, J.R. & McPhail, J. (1996). *Concepts in Canadian nursing.* St. Louis: Mosby.

King, T. (2000). Paradigms of Canadian nurse managers: Lenses for viewing leadership and management. *Canadian Journal of Nursing Leadership, 13*(1), 15–20.

Kuhn, T.S. (1962). *The structure of scientific revolutions.* Chicago: University of Chicago Press.

Mass, H., Brunke, L., Thorne, S., & Parslow, H. (2006). Preparing the next generation of senior nursing leaders in Canada: Perceptions of role competencies and barriers from the perspectives of inhabitants and aspirants. *Canadian Journal of Nursing Leadership, 19*(2), 75–91.

May, K.A. (2000). *Ensuring the future of Canadian nursing: A framework for a national nursing education strategy.* Ottawa: Canadian Association for University Schools of Nursing.

May, K.A. & Ferguson-Pare, M. (1997). Preparing nurse leaders for the future: Views from Canada. *Seminars for Nurse Managers, 5*(2), 97–105.

McBride, W. (1995, October 10–12). *State of the art and trends in graduate nursing programs in Canada.* Converging Educational Perspectives: An Anthology from the Pan American Conference on Graduate Nursing Education, Bogatá, Colombia (pp. 255–257). NLN Pub. #19-6894.

McKay, R. (1969). Theories, models, and systems for nursing. *Nursing Research, 18*(5), 393–399.

Meleis, A.I. (1987). ReVisions in knowledge development: A passion for substance. *Scholarly Inquiry for Nursing Practice, 1*(1), 5–19.

Mussalem, H.K. (1965). *Nursing education in Canada.* Ottawa: Queens University Printer.

Nursing Education Council of British Columbia. (2001). *Who will prepare the next generation of nurses?* Vancouver: Author.

Parse, R.R. (1998). The art of criticism. *Nursing Science Quarterly, 11*(2), 43.

_____. (2008). Proliferation of degrees in nursing: A call for clarity (Editorial). *Nursing Science Quarterly, 21*(1), 5.

Pilkington, F.B. & Mitchell, G.J. (2003). Mis-takes across paradigms. *Nursing Science Quarterly, 16*(2), 102–108.

Raudonis, B.M. & Acton, G.J. (1997). Theory-based nursing practice. *Journal of Advanced Nursing, 26*(2/1), 138–145.

Rodger, G.L. (1991). Canadian nurses succeed again! The launch of Canada's first doctoral degree in nursing. *Journal of Advanced Nursing, 16,* 1395–1396.

Rutherford, G. (2005). *Education component: Literature review report.* Canadian Nurse Practitioner Initiative. Retrieved January 22, 2008 from http://www.cnpi.ca/documents/pdf/ Education_Literature_Review_Report_e.pdf.

Ryan-Nicholls, K.D. (2004). Impact of health reform on registered psychiatric nursing practice. *Journal of Psychiatric and Mental Health Nursing, 11,* 644–653.

Thorne, S. (1999). Are egalitarian relationships a desirable ideal for nursing? *Western Journal of Nursing Research, 21*(1), 16–34.

Thorne, S.E. & Perry, J.A. (2001). Theoretical foundations of nursing. In P.A. Potter, A.J. Perry, J.C. Ross-Kerr, et al. (Eds.). *Canadian fundamentals of nursing* (2nd ed., pp. 86–100). Toronto: Mosby.

Thorne, S.E., Reimer Kirkham, S., & Henderson, A. (1999). Ideological implications of paradigm discourse. *Nursing Inquiry, 6,* 123–131.

Trojan, L., Marck, P., Gray, C., et al. (1996). A framework for planned change: Achieving a funded PhD program in nursing. *Canadian Journal of Nursing Administration, 9*(1), 71–86.

Van Doren, C. (1991). *A history of knowledge: Past, present, and future.* New York: Ballantine.

Wald, F.S. & Leonard, R.C. (1964). Toward development of nursing practice theory. *American Journal of Nursing, 13*(4), 309–313.

Wood, M.J. (1997). Canadian Ph.D. in nursing programs: A new age. *Clinical Nursing Research, 6,* 307–309.

Wood, M.J., Giovanetti, P., & Ross-Kerr, J.C. (2004). *The Canadian PhD in nursing: A discussion paper.* Canadian Association of Schools of Nursing. Retrieved January 22, 2008 from http://www.casn.ca/media.php?mid=60.

Wood, M.J. & Ross-Kerr, J.C. (2002). The growth of graduate education in nursing in Canada. In J.C. Ross-Kerr & M.J. Wood (Eds.). *Canadian nursing: Issues and perspectives* (4th ed., pp. 466–488). Toronto: Mosby.

Wright, L.M., Watson, W.L., & Duhamel, F. (1985). The family nursing unit: Clinical preparation at the master's level. *The Canadian Nurse, 81*(5), 26–29.

Zilm, G., Larose, O., & Stinson, S. (1979). *PhD (nursing).* Ottawa: Canadian Nurses Association.

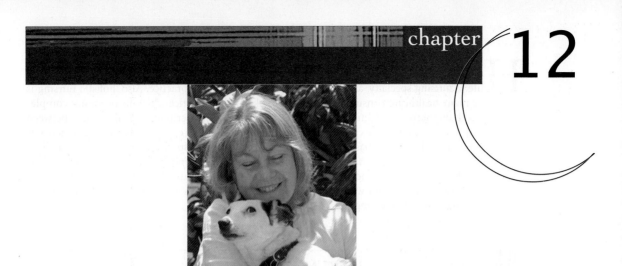

chapter 12

Katie the terrier shares experiences of holistic healing with Noreen Frisch of the University of Victoria School of Nursing. (Photography by Larry Frisch. Used with permission.)

The Challenges of Holistic Nursing Practice

Noreen Frisch

Critical Questions

As a way of engaging with the ideas in this chapter, consider the following:

1. What comes to mind when you think of holistic nursing practice?

2. Do you assume that all nursing practice has the potential to be holistic in nature?

3. Have you thought about how you might look after yourself as the "instrument of your practice" during your nursing career?

4. What are your assumptions about an electronic patient care record and the ways in which holistic care might be documented on this record?

Chapter Objectives

After completing this chapter, you will be able to:

1. Describe the development of holistic thought in the discipline of nursing.

2. Explore the influences of holistic philosophy and nursing theory on holistic practice.

3. Compare and contrast holistic nursing movements internationally.

4. Examine the challenges to implementation of broadly defined holistic care.

5. Define holistic nursing within your own nursing practice.

Holistic nursing has been defined as an approach to care, a theory of practice, a philosophy of life, a nursing specialty, and an integral part of all nursing practice. Also, holistic nursing is viewed by many healthcare consumers and nurses alike as that practice which incorporates complementary and alternative modalities. Nursing literature includes descriptions of differences between holistic care and comprehensive care; technical care and professional care, with holistic approaches as the distinguishing difference; basic nursing practice; and holistic specialty practice. There is little doubt that the term *holistic nursing* will lead to confusion and misunderstanding among many. The purpose of this chapter is to review the development of holism in nursing and to provide the reader with enough background from which to make informed judgments about the personal and professional meaning of holistic nursing.

WHAT IS HOLISTIC NURSING?

While there are competing definitions of holistic nursing, there seems to be general agreement that the practice of holistic nursing has to do with an understanding of the person as a whole. Nurses have long been taught that one does not care for the disease or illness, but rather must give care to the *person* with the condition. Most nurses remember the instructions to "address the patient by name," "individualize care," "put yourself in the bed," "understand your patient as a person," and the like. Any approach that calls for nurses to individualize care and to see each client as a unique person calls for some understanding of the person as a whole being. At its very basic level, holistic nursing means addressing more than the client's disease state or physical needs and requires nurses to give care to the client as a unique individual.

Introductory nursing texts offer differing perspectives on holistic care. Authors of a popular fundamentals of nursing book state that, "when applied to nursing, the concept of holism emphasizes that nurses must keep the whole person in mind and strive to understand how one area of concern relates to the whole person" (Berman, Synder, Kozier & Erb, 2008, p. 271). These authors go on to state that nursing interventions aim to restore harmony and serve a client's sense of meaning and purpose in life. To define holistic nursing, these authors simply state, "holistic nursing is nursing practice that has as its goal the healing of the whole person" (p. 1546), taking their definition from that of the American Holistic Nurses Association (AHNA). In contrast, another introductory nursing text states that holism in nursing means "that individuals function as complete units that cannot be reduced to the sum of their parts" (Daniels, 2004, p. 1546). The words *whole, complete,* and *harmony* provide descriptors that assist in understanding a broad approach to care that can be called holistic.

At a more advanced level, holistic nursing is the embodiment of the role of "nurse healer." In 1992, Quinn, in her effort to bring clarity to the concept of holism in nursing, noted that our word *heal* stems from the Greek word *hael* "to make sound or whole," Thus, Quinn encouraged nurses to conceptualize a relationship between nursing the whole and healing. She stated, "wholeness as it relates to human beings is much too big, too comprehensive, and too encompassing to be constrained by/in the physical . . . healing and health are about body-mind-spirit" (p. 553). She went on to present a perspective that wholeness requires people to be in relationship with others. Further, she states that healing is about becoming whole and the locus of healing is within each person. Quinn believed the holistic nurse becomes one who assists innate healing to occur, perhaps reflecting on nursing heritage and the Nightingale directive to "put the patient in a place where nature can act upon him" (Nightingale, 1946, p. 79).

Understanding the concept of holistic nursing requires knowledge of the development of holistic nursing thought in the discipline. Though, since the time of Nightingale, nursing has addressed aspects of holism, there were events in the 20th century that called attention to holism and affirmed nursing's role in holistic care. These developments will be summarized in the following section.

HOLISM IN NURSING: 20TH CENTURY DEVELOPMENTS

Nurse-theorist Myra Levine is credited with being the first person to use the words "holistic nursing" in her writings. In 1971 she wrote: "The logic of all human experience tells us that we are *whole*, and yet the concept of *holism* is labeled esoteric, elusive and even impractical" (Levine, 253). She was presenting work on her developing nursing theory and recognized that modern scientific thought brought a reductionistic view of all phenomena. Research, scientific findings, and technological advances provided many startling benefits to people, but also suggested a view that people could be "reduced" to a series of physiochemical equations. Science brought explanations about disease, molecules, and treatment but could not bring explanations about cure, recovery, and endurance that accounted for individual differences Levine focused on concepts of integration, interdependence with the environment, change, and adaptation and believed that nursing care should assist to establish or re-establish individual integrity (Levine, 1969, 1971).

Levine, however, was not the only nurse scholar of her time who expressed concern over the real or potential dehumanization of care that modern technology could bring. Nor was she alone in calling attention to a holistic paradigm that refused to define nursing as a science of sickness and disease. In 1970, Martha Rogers stated that "human beings are more than and different from the sum of their parts" (p. 46). Others, most notably Jean Watson, developed and expanded the idea that nursing involved caring and was grounded in an important person-to-person relationship between client and nurse. These nursing theorists took a clearly holistic view different from the prevailing scientific view held by many nurses, physicians, and scientists of the time. Reflecting on nursing's past, Erickson (2007) describes the developments this way: One group of nurses was advocating for the advancement of the profession through the specialization of nurses in the care of specific organs or disease conditions (i.e., medical-surgical nurses, neurology nurses, and nephrology nurses). This group believed that people were *"wholistic"*—that people had parts such as a psychosocial part, a biological part, or a cognitive part—but also believed that nursing care could be delivered to one part of the person in isolation from the others. Thus, *"wholistic"* came to mean the view that the whole is the sum of the parts and that the parts are independent. Erickson reports that those skilled in this view became experts in technology, objectivity, and scientific treatments. The other group of nurses, represented by the theorists mentioned above as well as others, argued for a *"holistic"* paradigm that understood the whole as greater than the sum of the parts. This view guided nurses to become concerned with the client's perceptions. These nurses focused on the caring and comforting aspects of nursing (those aspects that the profession inherited from Florence Nightingale) and developed into the true *art* of nursing practice. Erickson describes the work of these early holistic nurses:

> *[They] . . . recognized the importance of stimulating the five senses as a way of facilitating balance and harmony in themselves and their clients. They used touch, music, massage, soft voice tones, quiet, and other nursing techniques and strategies that helped people regain balance in body, mind, and spirit. They talked about the person, their perceived needs, and what nurses could do to help the person feel connected and comfortable (2007, p. 144).*

The 1970s and 1980s marked a dramatic turning point in the development of nursing as a discipline, as there were four simultaneous movements that later would have huge impacts on holistic nursing. These developments were: 1) presentation of holistically oriented nursing theories, 2) development of nursing language and classification systems, 3) writings by practitioners that guided holistic nursing interventions in actual practice settings, and 4) the establishment of a number of nursing organizations committed to advancing the profession. These developments were followed in the 90s by the popular discovery of holism—holistic, alternative, and complementary care. Each of these issues is addressed in the following sections.

Holistically Oriented Nursing Theories

Throughout the 70s and 80s, academic nurses published theoretical perspectives on the discipline, and students in graduate nursing programs studied and developed various aspects of these theories. Most prominent in the 70s were Rogers' *Nursing: the Science of Unitary Man* and Watson's *Nursing: the Philosophy and Science of Caring.* Other theorists followed with books, such as Newman's, *Health as Expanding Consciousness;* Parse's *Human Becoming;* and Erickson and colleagues' *Modeling and Role-Modeling.* While these theories are distinct from one another, each incorporates aspects of the *holistic* view defined above. Each presented a distinct definition of nursing and a distinct view of the person: Watson emphasized "humancare," the caring-healing relationships between nurse and client; Rogers defined the person, not as merely more than and greater than the sum of the parts but as an irreducible whole—a human energy field; Parse also emphasized the notion of the person as irreducible, i.e., that which cannot be reduced to parts and is inseparable from and in mutual process with the environment and nursing as both a science and an art; Newman emphasized health as expanding consciousness that includes an individual's total energy field pattern and nursing as a caring support for people experiencing disruptive processes that can resolve in new patterns; and Erickson and colleagues emphasized *modeling the client's world,* meaning understanding the world from the client's perspective and modeling health behaviors from within the client's worldview. As nursing theory continues to develop today, it provides clear direction for *holistic* care and considerations about care that are grounded in holistic philosophy, nursing science and research, and thoughtful reflections. Table 12.1 presents a summary of these theoretical perspectives on the person and on nursing as presented in the early work of these theorists.

Nursing Language and Classification Systems

In 1972 a different group of nurses came together to define nursing's phenomenon of concern. These nurse leaders were attempting to define that which is nursing and that which a nurse is licensed to do independently, recognizing that much of nursing had been undocumented and undefined. They sought to describe aspects of care that could assist in understanding the discipline as a whole. While some of the nurse theorists were initially involved in this work, the nurse theorists did not continue with this effort and individuals such as Marjorie Gordon and Linda Carpenito became prominent in this field. They sought to establish a nursing language and classification system that would give voice to nursing's work and they certainly believed that nurses' work encompassed care of the whole person. Those involved ultimately established the North American Nursing Diagnosis Association (NANDA), which has become NANDA-International (NANDA-I) today. The NANDA taxonomy became a list of nursing's concerns and, from the beginning, included a call for nurses to document practice areas of physical, cognitive, emotional, spiritual, and family and community care. Criticisms emerged that this taxonomy and its related developments (such as the Nursing Interventions Classification [NIC] and the Nursing Outcomes Classification [NOC], which came later) were following a *wholistic* model that merely listed comprehensive aspects of care without addressing the true *holistic* nature of nursing's work (Mitchell, 1991). Others argued that the classification systems were atheoretical and could be used with any nursing theory to provide *holistic* care. They believed that the nursing language provided a means to describe and document the holistic components of care in a "shorthand" language system as necessary for charting and payment for nursing services (Kelley, Frisch, & and Avant, 1995; Frisch & Kelley, 2002; Potter & Guzzetta, 2005). These writers also noted that a majority of nursing diagnostic categories described and defined in the taxonomy were of a psychosocial and spiritual nature, requiring the nurse to address the client as a whole person. These debates about the use of standardized language systems in the delivery of holistic care are unresolved today and remain the critical challenge in the 21st century, particularly for holistic nurses entering the world of the computerized patient care record.

Table 12.1	Theoretical Perspectives on Holism in the 1970s and 1980s		
THEORIST (YEAR)	**THEORY**	**HOLISTIC VIEW: PERSON**	**HOLISTIC VIEW: NURSING**
Rogers (1970)	Science of Unitary Man	Irreducible whole; human energy field	The scientific study of human and environmental energy fields
Watson (1979)	Theory of Human Care	A holistic being that is greater than and different from the sum of its parts; each person is valued to be cared for and cared about	Mediated by human care transactions that are professional, personal, scientific, aesthetic, and ethical
Parse (1981)	Man-Living-Health (later renamed as the Theory of Human Becoming)	Human energy field that is open, indivisible, unpredictable, and ever-changing; in mutual process with the universe and co-constituting rhythmical patterns of relating	A basic science, the practice of which is an art
Erickson & Colleagues (1983)	Modeling and Role-Modeling	Greater than the sum of the parts; having biophysical, cognitive, psychological and social components with a genetic base and a spiritual drive	A process that involves interpersonal and interactive relationships and includes facilitation, nurturance, and acceptance
Newman (1986)	Health as Expanding Consciousness	Dynamic energy field; humans are identified by their field patterns	A profession moving toward an integrated role; nursing is caring

Writings of Nurses Who Applied Holistic Care and Modalities in Practice Settings

Practicing nurses who were discovering holism began to write about their experiences with nursing practice that truly touched themselves and their patients alike. In 1981, Kenner, Dossey, and Guzzetta wrote the first nursing text describing applications of holistic principles and interventions in critical and intensive care nursing settings. They described use of touch, sound, music, and relaxation techniques as part of nursing care and gave nurses guidelines for use of these modalities. At the time, the ideas expressed in this work were revolutionary in critical care settings. Within two years, Keegan, Dossey, and Guzzetta published the first edition of their now popular text, *Holistic Nursing: Handbook for Practice*. This book emphasized not only the holistic nursing interventions (touch, massage, imagery, and movement), it also addressed the role of "nurse self-care" in one's personal development and professional readiness for holistic practices. In these writings, for the first time nurses were able to see how others used interventions and strategies to provide comfort and support to treat the whole person in context of nursing's work. This work was followed by the establishment of newsletters (*Beginnings*) and professional journals (*Journal of Holistic Nursing, Australian Journal of Holistic Nursing,* and *Holistic Nursing Practice*) that continued to provide information, research findings, advice, and opportunities for dialogue for nurses embracing holistic care.

Nursing Organizations

The period of the 70s and 80s may well be described as the pinnacle of nursing organizations. Before that time, a few national organizations had prominence in the profession. In the 70s and 80s, nurses established and joined a number of specialty organizations. It was a time of excitement and hope as nurses participated in these organizations to move the profession to new heights. This period marks the establishment of several nursing organizations devoted to development of theory (e.g., the Society of Rogerian Scholars), organizations devoted to the use of modalities (e.g., Nurse Healers Professional Associates), and nursing organizations to support the nurse desiring to enter holistic practice (e.g., the American Holistic Nursing Association). These organizations each had a unique perspective on holism, and *holistic nursing* took on different connotations as the work of these organizations continued and newer organizations emerged in the decades that followed.

Popular Culture and Interest in Holism

To further complicate the meaning of holistic nursing, the popularization of complementary modalities in the 1990s drew public attention to alternative and holistic practices. In a United States study, Eisenberg's initial survey reported an astounding two thirds of people surveyed used complementary and unconventional remedies and did not report the use of these remedies to their care providers (Eisenberg et al., 1993). Eisenberg's work pointed out that a significant number of well-educated people were searching for something not included in conventional medical practices, and at least some of their search outside conventional practices was related to their desire for humanistic care that involved relational practices. Holistic nurses were in a position to provide some of the care demanded by the public, but so were other care providers, such as chiropractors, herbalists, acupuncturists, and massage therapists. For many consumers, the search for holism became the search for modality-based providers. Nurses who were developing holistic practices were also gaining knowledge and skills in alternative and complementary modalities and many carried modality-based certification. Thus, nurses who were certified in modalities such as aromatherapy, guided imagery, hypnosis, reflexology, or healing touch were developing what they called *holistic nursing practices*, whether or not these practices were based on holistically oriented nursing theory and whether or not these practices documented care in a nursing model. By 1998, in a survey of over 700 holistic nurses, researchers found that interventions such as acupressure, aromatherapy, biofeedback, guided imagery, presence, healing touch modalities and therapeutic touch, massage, music and sound therapy, and relaxation were commonly used in practice (Dossey, Frisch, & Forker et al.). Some of these nurses stepped into a market with "skills" and developed themselves as holistic nurse entrepreneurs in nurse-owned businesses providing consultation, healthcare assessments and treatment recommendations, life coaching, nurse professional development activities, and direct provision of specialized modalities to clients.

Thus, in the 21st century, nursing is left with a rich tradition of thought that developed nursing's art and continues to expand the theory of nursing in an abstract and conceptual manner. This tradition is steeped in academic nursing, theory development, and critique and is being carried forward by organizations devoted to the use of nursing theory. Nursing is also enriched by a language and classification system that has evolved worldwide through NANDA –I and other taxonomies, such as the International Classification of Nursing Practice that defines nursing, and through the NIC and NOC provides a means of recording and tracking nursing activities and outcomes. Many of these diagnoses, interventions, and outcomes describe care that is relational, humanistic, and meets the psychosocial and spiritual aspects of care typically associated with holistic interventions. Lastly, many nurses have become experts in alternative modalities that support care of the whole person and have sought modality-based certification. So it is not readily apparent what holistic nursing really is today and what it means to nurses. Nonetheless, the official voice for nurses is spoken through national professional associations, so it makes sense to review their documents and publications for an understanding of how holistic nursing is understood by national-level nursing organizations. For purposes of this chapter, the views of the nursing organizations in Canada, the United States, and Australia will be presented because their work is most prominent in the literature on holistic nursing.

MODERN HOLISTIC NURSING: A THREE-COUNTRY COMPARISON

The Canadian Holistic Nurses Association

Nurses in Canada who were committed to holism joined to form an organization to further the development of holistic nursing practice. In 1986 they formed the Canadian Holistic Nurses Association (CHNA) to ensure that professional health maintenance and promotion services are made available to the people of Canada. The philosophical statement of the association begins with a quotation from Leddy (2003) and states, "we believe that each person is a whole, unitary human being, and a unitary human essence field in continuous mutual process with the environmental essence field" (Canadian Holistic Nurses Association [CHNA], 2006). The association quotes the work of nurse theorist Martha Rogers in describing nursing as an art that is the creative use of science for human betterment and well-being and having values that include compassion and unconditional love. The goals of nursing listed by the association include: to "strengthen the coherence and integrity of the human-environment essence field . . . stimulate mind-body-spirit healing . . . [and] facilitate empowerment through the health patterning process" (CHNA, 2006). According to CHNA, holistic nursing practice is grounded in health patterning as described by Barrett's pattern manifestation knowing and mutual patterning process (1990, 1998) and Cowling's pattern manifestation knowing process (1990). The CHNA has taken an exclusively Rogerian view and the representative of the association's specialization committee (Dobbie) writes, "we believe that a nursing conceptual framework based on unitary human science, human environmental essence field theory and energy based nursing practice is the foundation of holistic nursing practice" (retrieved January 18, 2008 from http//:chna.ca/specialization.htm).

CHNA provides specialty determination for holistic nursing and provides a framework to guide practice based on unitary human universal essence field theory and unitary energy-based nursing practice. Without question, this approach to holistic nursing has taken the work of Rogers' theory and its expansion and development over the years and built a credible specialty practice and specialization program grounded in this theoretical point of view. The educational program for the specialty begins with coursework on Rogers' theory, field theory, and energy-based and other modalities. Progression requires completion of Level 1 Healing Touch (an introduction to the practice of energy work) or Reiki and further develops theories derived from and consistent with Rogers' work. Lastly, the final phase of the educational program expands to the study of nurse-theorists presenting unitary human wholeness and human-universe mutual process perspectives. A nurse completing the educational program and meeting requirements of the association carries specialization from the CHNA. Clearly, if one were to consider the CHNA's definition or description of holistic nursing, it would have to be theory-based practice grounded in Rogers' theory.

The American Holistic Nurses Association

The AHNA was founded in 1980 under the leadership of Charlotte McGuire and had as its mission "to unite nurses in healing with a focus on holistic principles of health, preventive education, and the integrations of allopathic and complementary caring-healing modalities to facilitate care for the whole client . . ." (Dossey, 2000, p. xv). AHNA's description of holistic nursing includes the basic statement that "holistic nursing embraces all nursing that has enhancement of healing the whole person from birth to death as its goal" (Dossey, 2000, p. xxvi). Further, the AHNA statement includes the ideas that holistic nursing can be practiced using more than one theoretical perspective; that the holistic nurse is an instrument of healing; and that practicing holistic nursing requires self-care and personal self-responsibility, reflection, and spirituality. Thus, the organization has had two simultaneous foci: the development of holistic nursing practices through research and education and assistance to its members in their own personal and professional development through networking groups, conferences, supports, and opportunities to "nurture the nurse."

AHNA has established Standards of Holistic Nursing Practice (Frisch, 2000; Mariano, 2007) grounded in core values of holistic nursing. The Standards of Holistic Nursing Practice provided a foundation for certification in holistic nursing as a specialty. The association members had many discussions on whether or not holistic nursing was truly a specialty area of practice or represented what all professional nurses do. The issue was simply that all registered nurses (RNs) have the obligation to carry out professional nursing care in keeping with their scope of practice and, in doing so, any professional nurse can (and should) have as a goal to address the needs of the whole person. However, it is also clear that there is a body of knowledge that is necessary to expand one's professional, legal practice in areas that demonstrate consistency with AHNA's core values that go beyond the practices legally required for RNs and tested for safe practice on the initial licensing exam. Therefore, the specialty certification is a means to document that individual nurses have knowledge, competencies, and skills beyond what is required for entry into practice as an RN. The certification is provided through the American Holistic Nursing Certification Corporation on the basis of academic credentials, portfolio submission and review, and examination and is offered at the basic (baccalaureate degree) and advanced (master's degree) levels. The certification is based on values encompassing holistic philosophy, self-care, cultural congruence, theory, ethics and research, and application of the holistic caring process. In 2006, the AHNA and the American Nurses Association joined in a mutual effort to recognize holistic nursing as a specialty in the United States.

The definition of holistic nursing presented by AHNA is broad and designed to encompass much of nursing practice. The emphasis on nurse self-care underpins the view that holistic nursing is a way of life. The certification that begins with knowledge of holistic philosophy emphasizes values that holistic nurses must hold.

The Australian College of Holistic Nurses, Inc. and Holistic Nurses Association of New South Wales

Nurses in Australia have had a longstanding interest in and commitment to holistic nursing. They established two organizations: Australian College of Holistic Nurses, Inc and the Holistic Nurses Association of New South Wales. These organizations are no longer active but did attract, support, and launch holistic nurses in their work and their quest for knowledge about holism and complementary modalities. The Australian College of Holistic Nurses, Inc. was devoted to education and support of nurses performing holistic practices. A former president of the organization, Rosalie Van Aken, reports that the 1990s were the most active period for membership (2008). The college sponsored annual conferences that included speakers on theory, complementary modalities, and self-care practices. In collaboration with Southern Cross University, the organization supported the Australian Journal of Holistic Nursing, a biennial, peer-reviewed publication that was printed from 1994 through 2005. The mission of the journal reflected the mission of the organization: to document the trends and issues that emerged from contemporary nursing practice.

Inspired by a national conference in natural therapies, the Holistic Nurses Association (HNA) of New South Wales was founded in 1995 (Redmond, 2000). The organization grew out of a "disenchantment with the mechanistic and reductionistic methods of modern healthcare" (Redmond, p. 95) and was founded with an intent to support nurses wishing to undertake holistic practices. The organization had a focus on assisting nurses to develop competence in complementary and alternative modalities. The HNA met its goals of supporting nurses by teaching complementary modalities and working with the regulatory bodies to gain legal support for use of these modalities in nursing practice. Thus, the HNA represented the point of view that holistic nursing is the use of alternative interventions in the practice of nursing for the purpose of meeting client needs.

The fact that these two organizations are no longer active does not necessarily mean that their interests are no longer relevant or valued in Australia. According to Dr. Van Aken, there are probably multiple factors that contributed to the closure of these organizations. Among these were two significant developments: the fact that many holistic nurses became active members of organizations related to complementary modalities (such as Healing Touch or Aromatherapy) and no longer maintained membership in the nursing organizations and the fact that the nurses in Australia (including the Royal College of Nursing) adopted the broader view that all nursing is holistic. In Australia, nurses have not sought to make holistic nursing a specialization as their counterparts in Canada and the United States have done. Many holistic nurses in Australia carry certification in various complementary modalities and continue to build nursing practice on holistic theory. Interest in holism certainly exists (as Dr. Van Aken reports that over one third of nursing students at her university take elective courses in holistic and integrated care), though it may be less visible than in the comparison countries where the holistic nursing organizations are still active.

International Comparison

The holistic nursing movements in these three countries represent differing perspectives and differing views about holistic nursing. Table 12.2 provides a comparison. Understanding the divergent views may bring nurses to a better understanding of the complexities of determining "what is holistic" and may, in turn, stimulate nurses to consider their personal and professional need to confront the differences. Nurses may ask themselves to what degree holistic nursing is 1) a specialty rather than an expectation of all nurses, 2) defined narrowly through adopting one theoretical perspective or more broadly based on the goal of care, and 3) related more to a philosophy of care or the performance of complementary modalities. All of the perspectives are legitimate and each brings value in nursing practice.

Table 12.2	Comparison of Holistic Nursing Organizations		
ORGANIZATION	**COUNTRY**	**FOCUS OF ORGANIZATION**	**DEFINITION OF HOLISTIC NURSING**
Canadian Holistic Nurses Association	Canada	To support the development of holistic nursing practice	Science of unitary human beings
American Holistic Nurses Association	United States	To unite nurses in healing	All nursing practice that has healing the whole person as its goal
College of Holistic Nursing, Inc.	Australia	To explore diverse trends emerging in contemporary holistic practice	Diverse definitions, focused on healing
Holistic Nurses Association of New South Wales	Australia	To support qualifications and training in complementary modalities	The practice of complementary modalities (inferred)

Given that the CHNA defines holistic nursing according to one theory, Canadian nurses certainly may question if that perspective represents the totality of holistic nursing or if one could practice holistic nursing without being an adherent of Rogerian science.

 ## PRACTICING HOLISTIC NURSING TODAY: ISSUES AND CHALLENGES

Modern nursing work is complex and challenging. The shortage of nurses in Canada (Maddalena & Crupi, 2008) and worldwide has attracted attention to what nurses actually do and plays into the discussions of what nurses will do in the future. Nursing theories have advanced in their development and contribute to nursing reflection and practice. However, nurses in practice see the results of mechanistic and reductionistic care. Nurses' work has been described as a series of tasks to complete, with little time to devote to client education, surveillance, and compassion (Tucker & Spear, 2006; Tucker, 2003). Writers have addressed the silencing of nurses (Gordon, 2005) and the emotional exhaustion felt by many nurses (Aiken et al., 2001). If nurses are to continue to serve as the "front-line" patient contact, holistic nurses must be in a position to provide care true to the "art" of nursing practice—those aspects of care described by Erickson (cited above) as the work of early holistic nurses who refused to accept nursing as a science of disease and illness. There are three important developments in current practice that should be addressed as one considers the role of holistic nursing today. These are the use of holistic principles in the evidence-based practice environment, the use of holistic principles with the computerized patient-care record, and the need for nurse self-care to sustain professionalism throughout a 21st-century nursing career.

Challenge 1: Evidence-Based Practice

Modern healthcare is steeped in a continuous search for quality through clinical practice guidelines and standardization based on sound research and an evaluation of the evidence. These are very good developments and have certainly helped to raise care standards so that people in one city or locality have the same access to quality care as people on other areas. There is, as it is described, the "national standard" of care that requires all providers to accept the prevailing view of "best practice" and provide such care to all. In healthcare, the 21st century arrived with a call for "evidence-based practice" (EBP) and a mandate to perform based solely on that evidence.

The challenge with this development for holistic nurses is that the EBP movement neither defines what evidence is nor does it readily examine the limits of the evidence one has. In modern medicine, evidence is usually determined by the "gold standard" of the randomized controlled clinical trial (RCT [Frisch, 2007]). The RCT certainly provides clear data on the average response to clinical or experimental interventions and can set parameters for the use of those interventions. Few, however, question if the RCT is the best research method to provide data, not for experimental purposes but for application to actual clinical situations in which clients do not meet the standard of homogeneity required of experimental subjects in clinical trials. Holmes and colleagues pointed out that the operationalization of EBP gives an unquestioned privilege to research designs that prioritize frequentist methods over qualitative ones (Holmes et al, 2006).

The challenge is for holistic nurses to learn and understand the research methods being used and to be in a position to articulate the use and the limits of application of those methods. All too commonly, holistic nurses embrace qualitative methods and develop an incomplete knowledge of the quantitative methods used by others. It will be impossible to negotiate holism in practice if nursing leaders do not have a level of sophistication in traditional quantitative research and statistics, a basic level of knowledge about newer approaches to quantitative analysis (such as Bayesian reasoning), and an understanding of qualitative methodologies as well. In an era where practice priorities and practice guidelines may be dictated by "evidence," holistic nurses need to be able to question and critique what evidence is used, based on what assumptions, and in what settings. This knowledge will be essential for holistic nursing leaders of the future.

Challenge 2: Computerized Patient-Care Records

The second challenge for holistic nurses is the inevitable move from paper to computerized patient-care records. This move will be forthcoming as health systems across the country seek to document all aspects of client care through various electronic systems. There is no question that these electronic systems provide an efficient means to record client data and client progress. In addition, they provide a means to track outcomes across client populations. The computerized record is seen as an interdisciplinary record so that each health professional can enter data into the system and that data can be retrieved by other professionals.

A challenge for nurses, particularly holistic nurses, is the decision of how nursing will be documented electronically. Current nursing language and classification systems provide a very shorthand means of describing nursing's phenomenon of concern. These phenomena may include (among many others): spiritual distress or spiritual well-being, anxiety, fear, states of grieving, states of coping, and issues related to health promotion. A review of the current NANDA-I taxonomy indicates that over half of the diagnoses are psychosocial and/or spiritual in nature (NANDA-I, 2007). Further, the nursing diagnoses also incorporate a multi-axial structure that permits documentation of the health–illness continuum of each nursing concern. Thus, the nurse may distinguish between a condition of actual health problem or need, risk of that problem or need, and a wellness condition of opportunity to enhance the client's level of functioning to move toward a condition of enhanced wellness (Potter & Frisch, 2007). The current nursing interventions classification includes numerous complementary modalities as reasonably practiced within the context of nursing, such as acupressure, simple massage, therapeutic touch, relaxation techniques, and imagery (Dochterman & Bulechek, 2003). Thus, it is possible to document the scope of holistic nursing assessment, interventions, and outcome electronically in the current structure (Potter & Frisch, 2007).

As stated previously, there has been dissension regarding the use of standardized nursing languages, and many holistic nurses have rejected the process of documentation through nursing diagnoses and related terms. At the same time, many have strived to make the standardized languages inclusive so that every area of nursing could be recorded. Today, holistic nurses who may have preferred narrative documentation are faced with the challenge of either using the standardized languages to give voice to nursing's work or to become silent in a system that will include only electronic entries based on coded terms. The challenge for holistic nurses may become to learn to use the standardized languages to their fullest extent and to engage as leaders in activities that promote recording of holistic practices in systems that could easily omit nursing and result in computerized medical records rather than a computerized healthcare record.

Challenge 3: Sustaining Self Over the Course of a Nursing Career

One of the definitions of holistic nursing discussed previously is that holistic nursing is a way of life. This perspective means that holistic nursing entails adopting a philosophy of holism, that is, a "philosophy based on a perspective that acknowledges and values the connectedness of the body-mind-spirit, the inherent goodness of human beings, and the ability of each person to find meaning and purpose in his or her own life, and the nurse's role of support to each client so that the client may find comfort, peace, and harmony" (Frisch, 2000, p.1). Having adopted such a philosophy of nursing, the

BOX 12.1 Examples of Nurse Self-Care Activities

- Engaging in health-promoting behaviors and health protecting behaviors
- Empowering self to modify attitudes and develop healthy life patterns
- Creating satisfying interpersonal relationships
- Using wellness programs
- Creating social networks
- Engaging in activities to awaken the inner spirit
- Developing a healthy self-outlook
- Ongoing reflection on one's own professional practice

nurse recognizes in herself or himself that person who is whole and who has capacity for growth, development, and healing. The holistic nurse becomes an instrument of healing when using unconditional presence and intention to support the healing process of another (Quinn, 2000). To do so, however, the nurse must attend to his or her own personal awareness and self-care. Self-care practices that assist the nurse to sustain health begin with an honest assessment of one's life demands and personal needs, one's risks for health problems, and forming a life pattern aimed at supporting one's own health. Secondly, holistic nurses must cultivate awareness and understanding of the deeper meaning and purpose of life and the connectedness with self and others, perhaps aided through ongoing reflections on their own nursing practice.

Self-care practices are highly individualized, such that practices that support one nurse may not be those that support another. However, all self-care practices give the nurse a strength and a balance or harmony that helps one to deal with the stressors, uncertainties, and demands of nursing's work-life. Considering the fact that nurses are at significant risk for vocational "burnout" and emotional exhaustion (Aiken et al., 2001), self-care practices may be the distinguishing difference between those who thrive in nursing and those who are unable to sustain the work-life demands. Box 12.1 lists examples of nurse self-care activities.

SUMMARY

This chapter has presented multiple views and definitions of holism and the meaning of holistic nursing. The 20th century was a time of considerable change and advancement in nursing and health science. That period was associated with advances in medical science and a concurrent need to articulate that which is nursing as distinct from the reductionistic view of a medical science of illness and disease. Holistic nursing theorists wrote prolifically and presented views about nursing's philosophy and outlook, successfully challenging the accepted world view of other healthcare professionals. Similarly, nurses sought to establish nursing standardized languages to give voice to that which had been silent. Nurses experimented with the application of holistic principles and modalities in acute- and chronic-care settings and began to share their practice experiences with one another. By the end of the century, nurses had established professional organizations to provide support, networking, scholarly exchange, and a collective voice of the discipline.

There have been a number of holistic nursing organizations, one in Canada. Each is committed to the general ideals of holism and each carries or carried out its work in a manner unique to the organization and its location. Nurses should consider each of the perspectives presented to gain a full understanding of the complexities of holism and its meaning for nursing.

Nursing as a discipline has many challenges entering the 21st century. How holistic nurses negotiate those challenges will dictate, in many ways, the future of the entire profession. The challenges discussed include: 1) the need to articulate holistic principles in a system devoted to evidence-based practice, 2) the requirement of documenting nursing in an electronic patient-care record, and 3) the nurse's need for self-care practices to sustain one's work over the course of a career.

The overriding issue for readers of this chapter may be deciding how holism fits with one's individual worldview and perspective on nursing. In many ways, all nursing care that is professional and compassionate is holistic care. Yet, there are certifications and specialty designations in holistic nursing. Each individual must consider the philosophy of holism and the work of nursing theorists who serve as guides to holistic practices. The questions at the end of the chapter are suggested for further exploration of the issues.

Add to your knowledge of this issue:	
Canadian Holistic Nurses Association	**info@chna.ca**
American Holistic Nurses Association	**info@ahna.org**
Nursing Theory Homepage	**http://sandiego.edu/academics/nursihng/**
Nanda International	**http://www.nanda.org/**

Online

REFLECTIONS on the Chapter...

1 Write you own definition or description of *holistic nursing*. What is the essence of holistic nursing? What perspective do you take regarding your own practice?

2 In what ways is your nursing practice holistic? In what ways is it not?

3 Do you subscribe to a theory of practice? If so, which one? Why is theory thought to be holistic?

4 Do you have experience with any modality or nursing intervention that may be considered alternative or complementary? Which one(s)?

5 Have you looked at the NANDA-I taxonomy of nursing and the NIC and NOC? Try to document the humanistic aspects of your care in this language. Does it work for you?

6 Do you practice self-care techniques and modalities? What do you believe is the single most important factor in sustaining yourself in a nursing career?

7 In what ways are you currently connected to other nurses in supportive ways? How will you continue those connections over time?

References

Aiken, L.H., Clarke, S.P., & Sloane, et al. (2001). Nurses' reports on hospital care in five countries. *Health Affairs, 20*(3), 43–53.

Barrett, E. (1998). Theoretical concerns: A Rogerian practice methodology for health patterning. *Nursing Science Quarterly, 11(4)*, 136–138.

_____. (1990). *Visions of Roger' science-based nursing*. New York: National League for Nursing.

Berman, A., Synder, S.J., & Kozier, B., et al. (2008). *Fundamentals of nursing: Concepts, process and practices* (8th ed.). Upper Saddle River, NJ: Prentice Hall.

Canadian Holistic Nurses Association. (2006). *Canadian holistic nursing practice standards*. Author.

Cowling, W.R. (1990). A template for unitary pattern-based nursing practice. In E.A.M. Barrett (Ed.), *Visions of Roger's science-based nursing* (pp. 45–65). New York: National League for Nursing.

Daniels, R. (2004). *Nursing fundamentals: Caring and clinical decision making*. Clifton Park, NY: Delmar Thomson Learning.

Dochterman, J. & Bulechek, G. (2003). *Nursing interventions classification (NIC)* (4th ed.). Philadelphia: Elsevier-Health Sciences Division.

Dossey, B. (2000). Introduction. In N. Frisch, B. Dossey, & C. Guzzetta, et al. (Eds.). *AHNA Standards of Holistic Nursing Practice* (pp. xv–xlii). Gaithersburg, MD: Aspen.

Dossey, B., Keegan, L., & Guzzetta, D. (2005). *Holistic nursing: Handbook for practice* (4th ed.). Sudbury, MA: Jones and Bartlett.

Dossey, B., Frisch, N., & Forker, J., et al. (1998). Evolving a blueprint for certification: Inventory of professional activities and knowledge of a holistic nurse. *Journal of Holistic Nursing, 16(1)*, 33–56.

Eisenberg, D.M., Kessler, R., & Foster, C., et al. (1993). Unconventional medicine in the United States: Prevalence, costs and patterns of use. *New England Journal of Medicine, 328(4)*, 246–252.

Erickson, H. (2007). Philosophy and theory of holism. *Nursing Clinics of North America, 42(2)*, 139–163.

Erickson, H., Tomlin, E., & Swain, M.A. (1983). *Modeling and role-modeling: A theory and paradigm for nursing*. Englewood Cliffs, NJ: Prentice-Hall.

Frisch, N. (2000) Holistic philosophy and education. In N. Frisch, B. Dossey, & C. Guzzetta, et al. (Eds.). *AHNA standards of holistic nursing practice* (pp. 1–22). Gaithersburg, MD: Aspen.

_____. (2007). Preface, EBP. *Nursing Clinics of North America, 42(2)*, xi–xiv.

Frisch, N., Dossey, B., & Guzzetta, C., et al. (2000). *AHNA standards of holistic nursing practice*. Gaithersburg, MD: Aspen.

Frisch, N. & Kelley, J. (2002). Nursing diagnosis and nursing theory: An exploration of factors inhibiting and supporting simultaneous use. *Nursing Diagnosis, 13(2)*, 53–56.

Gordon, S. (2005). *Nursing against the odds*. Ithaca, NY: Cornell University Press.

Holmes, D., Perron, A., & O'Bryne, P. (2006). Evidence, virulence, and the disappearance of nursing knowledge: A critique of the evidence-based dogma.*Worldviews, Evidence Based Nursing, 3(3)*, 95–101.

Kelley, J., Frisch, N., & Avant, K. (1995). A trifocal model of nursing diagnosis: Wellness reinforced. *Nursing Diagnosis, 6(3)*, 123–128.

Kenner, C., Dossey, B., & Guzzetta, C. (1981). *Critical care nursing: Body-mind-spirit*. Boston: Little Brown.

Levine, M. (1969). The pursuit of wholeness. *American Journal of Nursing, 69(1)*, 93–99.

_____. (1971). Holistic nursing. *Nursing Clinics of North America, 6(2)*, 253–264.

Maddalena, V. & Crupi, A. (2008) *A Renewed call for action: A synthesis report on the nursing shortage in Canada*. Ottawa: Canadian Federation of Nurses Unions.

Mariano, C. (2007). Holistic nursing as a specialty: Holistic nursing—scope and standards of practice. *Nursing Clinics of North America, 42(2)*, 165–188.

Mitchell, G.J. (1991). Diagnosis: Clarifying or obscuring the nature of nursing. *Nursing Science Quarterly, 4(2)*, 52.

Newman, M. (1986). *Health as expanding consciousness*. St. Louis: Mosby.

NANDA-I. (2005). *Nursing diagnosis: Definitions, and classification 2005–2006*. Philadelphia: Author.

Potter, P. & Frisch, N. (2007). Holistic assessment and care: Presence in the process. *Nursing Clinics of North America, 42(2)*, 213–228.

Potter, P. & Guzzetta, C. (2005). The holistic caring process. In B. Dossey, L. Keegan, and C. Guzzetta (Eds.). *Holistic nursing: Handbook for practice* (4th ed., pp. 341–372). Sudbury, MA: Jones and Bartlett.

Quinn, J. (1992). On healing, wholeness and the haelan effect. *Nursing Outlook, 10(10)*, 552–556.

_____. (2000). Holistic nurse self-care. In N. Frisch, B. Dossey, & C. Guzzetta (Eds.). *AHNA Standards of holistic nursing practice* (pp. 55–74). Gaithersburg, MD: Aspen.

Redmond, C. (2000). The Holistic Nurses Association of New South Wales: Our history, our present and our future. *Contemporary Therapies in Nursing and Midwifery, 6(2), 95–97.*

Rogers, M. (1970). *An introduction to the theoretical basis of nursing.* Philadelphia: F.A. Davis.

Tucker, A. (2003). Organization learning from operational failures. Doctoral dissertation, Graduate School of Business, Harvard University.

Tucker, A. & Spear, S. (2006). Operational failures and interruptions in hospital nursing. *Health Services Research, 41(3),* 643–662.

Van Aken, R. (2008). *Personal communication.* June 12, 2008.

Watson, J. (1988). *Human science and human care.* New York: National League for Nursing.

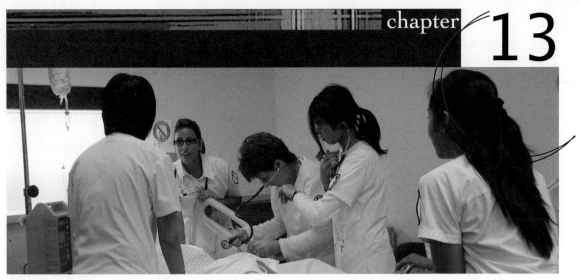

chapter 13

Students participate in a simulated learning experience. (Used with permission, University of Manitoba, Faculty of Nursing.)

Nursing, Technology, and Informatics: Understanding the Past and Embracing the Future

W. Dean Care, David Michael Gregory, and Wanda M. Chernomas

Critical Questions

As a way of engaging with the ideas in this chapter, consider the following:

1 What is your comfort level with the use of technology?

2 What are your assumptions about the usefulness of technology in nursing education and professional nursing practice?

3 Can you identify what your learning needs are with respect to technology and how they can be addressed?

4 How do you think that nursing compares with other professional practice disciplines in regard to the use of technology in practice and in education?

Chapter Objectives

After completing this chapter, you will be able to:

1 Discuss the relationship between nursing and technology.

2 Discern the technology and informatic foundations, theoretical and practical, expected in a baccalaureate nursing program.

3 Describe the role of technology and informatics in nursing.

4 Explore the possibilities of the use of technology and informatics in nursing.

5 Discuss the issues related to applying technology and informatics in education and practice.

Chapter Objectives (continued)

6 Identify the barriers to technology in education and practice contexts.

7 Formulate strategies for resolving these
barriers in practice settings.

It is the year 2010. You are a public health nurse with the regional health authority. Your primary responsibilities include following up on clients who have been discharged from the cardiac surgery program at the local tertiary care hospital. Clients are now being discharged 2 to 3 days after surgery. The care you provide includes teaching, wound care, symptom management, assessing and monitoring health status, and coordinating the interdisciplinary team. Most (90%) of the clients you serve have access to the Internet and personal computers (PCs) in their homes.

A typical day for you looks something like this: You arrive at work and log on to your desktop PC. You receive notice of the cardiac clients who were discharged yesterday. You call or e-mail five of these clients and set up appointments for the day. Having down-loaded their electronic medical records onto your desktop computer, you review the files in preparation for the home visits. You then transmit these files onto a wireless, handheld personal digital assistant (PDA), which accompanies you on all home visits. It provides access to your e-mail messages and Internet databases and it has an intranet feature that allows instant access to the other members of the team. This tool is also a cell phone, and it contains your appointment schedule, word processing documents, and address book; it is your personal organizer. It has 2 GB of memory and contains a voice recognition system that allows you to verbally record and store your "Nurse's Notes," which will be digital-ized and downloaded to a permanent record when you get back to your office.

Most of your clients wear electrocardiogram (ECG) leads. You are able to monitor their cardiac rhythms and vital signs from both your desktop and PDA. Each client has an e-mail account from which they can send you messages and ask you questions. Before you leave the office, you receive a call from a 5-day post-op client who is experiencing chest discomfort. You ask him to turn on his video web cam, a piece of equipment provid-ed to each client upon discharge. It is mounted on top of his desktop PC and allows you to view his appearance, assess his medical and emotional condition, and speak with him "face to face." He attaches a Dynamap to his arm, and you receive instant blood pressure and pulse readings; an oxygen saturation reading is transmitted from the finger probe he is wearing. Using your desktop computer, you upload his ECG to get a "real-time" image of the client's cardiac rhythm. Next, you upload a visual image of his normal cardiac rhythm and compare it to his current ECG. You decide to make a home visit to assess this client's situation more thoroughly.

This brief vignette sets the stage for a discussion of the issues and trends arising from technology and informatics as they apply to nursing. Like the vignette, this chapter focuses on common uses and applications of technology in nursing practice and education. It also identifies issues arising from this technology and broaches the future of technology in nursing and healthcare. Relevant historical events are introduced, particularly as they relate to the significant shift in Western society from an industrial focus to an information ethos. Both rely heavily on technology but in vastly different ways.

The Industrial Age (late 19th and early 20th centuries) was characterized by an emphasis on produc-tivity, efficiency, division of labor, and hierarchical organizations. In contrast, the Information Age (pres-ent era) is distinguished by a heavy dependence on telecommunications, knowledge and information explosion, global operations, decentralized organizations, and networked employees. The Information Age provides society with rapid access to and manipulation of information. In the area of healthcare, the Information Age fosters advances in health and telecommunications technology, which has had, and will continue to have, a profound effect on nurses and the organizations for which they work.

Historically, the relationship between technology and nursing has been marked by tension and unrest. Until recently, nursing and technology were framed as a dichotomy—nursing at one end and technology at the other—polar opposites, in a sense. Technology has been viewed as masculine, scientific, mechanistic, and reductionistic. In contrast, nursing in this dichotomous thinking has been conceptualized as feminine, nurturing, a soft science, humanistic, and holistic. Thus, technology has been identified as innately negative and dehumanizing to nursing—potentially obstructing or impeding nursing care (Gadow, 1988). The long-term utility of framing nursing and technology in this manner (i.e., masculine versus feminine, hard versus soft science, and reductionistic versus holistic caring) is questionable. Of course, the advent of new biomedical technologies can have ethical, moral, and philosophical implications for nursing and Canadian healthcare (e.g., genetic marker assessments, techno-treatments, diagnostic technology, etc.). Nurses are concerned with the resultant impact of technologies on the lives of patients and nursing practice.

In this regard, nurses do serve as "cultural brokers" between technology and patients. In this role, nurses translate technology for patients and provide explanations about the technology. On another plane of discussion, however, the development and adoption of information and communication technology (ICT) has the potential to optimize client and patient outcomes. ICT can permit nurses to readily access the knowledge they need to support their care (Mathieu, 2007). The Canadian Nurses Association ([CNA], 2006) recognizes the importance of nursing information and knowledge management.

> *Competencies in information management and the use of communication technology are integral to nursing practice. Competencies in information management and the use of communication technology are no longer add-ons to traditional methods of health-care delivery. Rather, these competencies are an integral part of health care and nursing practice. CNA supports the Health Council of Canada's statements that health-care providers "need reliable and accurate patient health information at the point of care and the best evidence available to determine treatment options" and that electronic tools to manage this information are a necessity (p. 1).*

 ## RELATIONSHIP BETWEEN NURSING AND TECHNOLOGY

What exactly is the relationship between nursing and technology? To date, nurses have rarely been "at the table" in regard to developing much of the biomedical technology that affects their practice. As a profession, nursing most often inherits or receives technology developed by other disciplines. Medical technology is not nursing technology, and yet this technology is most often imposed on nursing (Purnell, 1998). In contrast to the importation of biomedical technology, there is the promising presence of nurses in the development and application of ICT. For example, nurses were involved in the development of an electronic information gathering and dissemination system to support both nursing-sensitive outcomes data collection and evidence-based decision making at the point of patient care (Doran et al., 2007). At the point of patient care, nurses can use technology to improve the quality of patient and client care and generate data about nursing outcomes. This and other related technologies are thus poised to provide freedom to nurses, the freedom to engage in holistic and humanistic care for patients and clients and their families.

Despite such recent developments, there are several factors that may be contributing to a *technology lag* within the profession itself. A closer look at these factors may help us to better understand why this technology lag exists.

- As Booth (2006) observes, nursing education programs "have yet to conquer the larger issues surrounding the necessary knowledge, skills, and practice competencies required for nurses to function in the future" (p. 3). There has been little movement in Canadian nursing curricula to address such shortcomings in undergraduate nursing education Furthermore, there is a need for faculty development in the areas of e-Health (electronic health), including informatics, technology, and ICT. (See next section regarding e-Health.)

- Although new graduates from baccalaureate nursing programs may be lacking in literacy skills with respect to e-Health, the need for ongoing literacy education becomes clear when looking at the demographic profile of the profession. In 2006, more than 50% of practicing nurses graduated 20 years ago and just over 30% of all registered nurses (RNs) in Canada were aged 55 or older. In 2006, Canada had more RNs employed in nursing at ages 50–54 than any other age group (Canadian Institute for Health Information [CIHI], 2006). This is not to suggest that older nurses lack the capacity or aptitude to embrace and master technology or informatics. Rather, they likely have had to become techno-literate through individualized continuing education and staff development efforts. And if we consider that formal and informal education and socialization processes may disadvantage women with respect to e-Health literacy, then there may also be a gender gap within the profession, i.e., 94.4% of RNs are women; 5.6% are men (CIHI, 2006). Further research regarding the possibility of the gender–generation technology gap within nursing is required.

Recently, sectors within the Canadian healthcare system are implementing a range of e-Health–related technologies to improve patient care. Although the progress to date can be considered slow and ad hoc, the widescale adoption of new technologies will likely occur at a very fast pace over the next few years. This trend has significant—perhaps even dramatic—implications for the education of future RNs. Similarly, nurses currently working within the healthcare system in Canada will require adequate supports and education. For example, the Association Québécoise des Infirmières et Infirmiers en Systèmes et Technologies de l'Information is authoring a position paper on the need for the systemic training of nurses in the area of informatics (Mathieu, 2007). The need for nursing informaticists is clear as is the need for nurses to embrace technology and care. Thus, the stage is being set for future developments in the relationship between nursing and technology.

NURSING INFORMATICS

According to Simpson (1998, p. 22), "Part of the reason nursing informatics is so hard to define is because it's a moving target." A decade later, there remains some confusion regarding the concepts of health information technology, health informatics, and e-Health (Loiselle & Cossette, 2007). Booth (2006) suggests that "e-Health" serves as the umbrella term for many of these concepts, including ICT. In its broadest sense, nursing informatics is understood as the integration of information technologies and communications into nursing practice (Mathieu, 2007). Staggers and Bagley Thompson's (2002) definition is helpful in understanding the breadth and depth of nursing informatics:

Nursing Informatics is a specialty that integrates nursing science, computer science and information science to manage and communicate data, information and knowledge in nursing practice. Nursing informatics facilitates the integration of data, information and knowledge to support patients, nurses and other providers in their decision making in all roles and settings. This support is accomplished through the use of information structures, information processes and information technology (p. 255).

Today's nurse is affected by an ever-changing healthcare system dominated by a focus on outcomes, evidence, performance measurement, and the use of technology to provide and support care delivery. Information is key to effective decision making and integral to quality nursing practice (CNA,

2001). In their evolving role as "knowledge workers," nurses are increasingly being called on to access information systems to facilitate evidence-based practice. In addition, as more patients become comfortable with information technology, expectations will be placed on nurses to have similar skills. "In fact, nurses may find that their patient education encounters will increasingly occur through distance technology" (Gassert, 1998, p. 266).

APPLICATIONS OF NURSING INFORMATICS AND TECHNOLOGY IN PRACTICE

The application of nursing informatics as an umbrella concept takes various forms in practice. More recently, the term "eHealth" is used to refer to "the application of information and communication technologies in the health sector" (Health Canada, 2007, p. 1) reflecting the integration of telehealth technologies with the Internet (Riva, 2000). The proliferation of terms relating to care practices using distance technology has created confusion and difficulty when exploring related issues. Terms such as *telemedicine, nursing telepractice,* and *tele-education* are used in the literature. Collectively, they refer to different components of healthcare delivery through technology and, in certain instances, as subsets of telehealth. This section will discuss telehealth, emphasizing nursing telepractice with the telephone, electronic mail, and Web-based information as the vehicles for knowledge dissemination, information exchange, communication, and electronic health records.

Telehealth and Nursing Telepractice

The term *telehealth* encompasses a broad range of healthcare and service delivery systems provided through distance or electronic technology (Gassert, 2000). "Nursing telepractice is a nursing-specific application of telehealth that includes all client-centered forms of nursing practice and the provision of information, conferences and courses for health care professionals occurring through, or facilitated by, the use of telecommunications or electronic means" (CNA, 2001, p. 1).

The geographically dispersed population of Canada provides an ideal opportunity for the application of telehealth to reduce barriers related to healthcare access. Telehealth has the potential to provide borderless, seamless, and accessible healthcare in all reaches of the country, delivering fast, accurate diagnoses and treatments in situations where face-to-face visits may not be possible. For example, Alberta's extensive telehealth network offers clinical services including specialist consults and follow-up care, rehabilitation services, and patient education sessions (Alberta Telehealth, 2007).

Nursing telepractice uses the nursing process, within the context of the nurse–client relationship, to assess, plan, and implement care through the provision of information, referral, education and support, evaluation, and documentation (CNA, 2001).

In real time, nurses can perform a wide variety of assessment, education, and intervention skills at varying frequencies. They can listen to heart and chest sounds, read and interpret ECG results, assess wound status, review downloaded blood glucose information, and observe and facilitate the patient's self-care (Russo, 2001). Mobile phones and PDA technology exist to communicate health information, such as ECG and blood pressure readings, to clinicians anywhere in the world from a mobile consumer (Rasid & Woodward, 2005). The opportunities for nursing within this area may be limited only by the technologic resources available and the knowledge and ability of nursing to advocate for our expanded role in implementation, care, and evaluation.

Within telehealth, the need remains for nurses to practice according to the established standards of practice, codes of ethics, legislation, and competencies of their regulatory bodies. Several related issues and challenges are apparent within the telehealth environment. There are guidelines for telephone practice in some jurisdictions but not all have such policies for their practitioners. (See, for example, "Practice Guideline: Telepractice," College of Nurses of Ontario, 2005.) These telepractice guidelines address many of the broad practice expectations within a telehealth environment. CNA's position is that nurses' accountability lies within the jurisdiction of their registration (CNA, 2001). However, policies on the provision of telehealth across provincial registering bodies have yet to be developed through coordinated efforts. In addition, educational standards or credentials have not been established for this area of practice. Issues related to maintaining privacy and confidentiality pose challenges that are still being understood. Without a comprehensive consideration of the aforementioned issues, liability issues and employer responsibilities become unclear. The following question remains relevant: How do professional nursing organizations and regulatory bodies promote safe and competent practice, prevent substandard nursing practice, and intervene or investigate complaints as necessary when the RN and patient may be thousands of miles apart and their interactions are electronic (CNA, 2000)?

Care Delivery by Telephone

The earliest use of the telephone as a tool for providing public health or private duty nursing occurred in the early 1920s (Sandelowski, 2000). Nurses have long since been offering advice over the telephone, particularly from emergency rooms and public health areas. Today, eight provinces and one territory offer "24/7" access to nurses by telephone, thus ushering in a new era in nursing telephone practice (Goodwin, 2007).

In addition to the guidelines for telehealth practice noted above, a wide range of protocols also exists to support nurses' decision making and judgment. Questions and issues remain regarding the frequency of review of protocols, the qualifications and education required of the practitioner, and nurses' involvement in developing these standards.

Manitoba's Health Links is an example of telephone technology that provides 24-hour province-wide nursing access for health information and advice. Experienced RNs with a broad range of expertise and skills usually provide this service. Another example is British Columbia's HealthGuide NurseLine, which makes 24-hour, toll-free, province-wide nursing access available. Nurses use software to assist in guiding patients' healthcare decision making. NurseLine is part of an expanded program endorsed by the College of Registered Nurses of British Columbia. The program consists of a printed HealthGuide handbook and an online health database. Commercially available software can be customized, at a cost, to meet needs for evaluation and monitoring of calls, including the number and type of calls and users, automated evaluation of disposition or outcome, patient satisfaction, and patient knowledge of services.

Whether the protocols are available online or on paper, telephone nursing can be compared with more traditional triage. Telephone nursing uses nursing assessment to guide or coach the decision making of the patient concurrently with an empowerment approach rather than directed decisions. The inability for nurses to incorporate nonverbal patient behaviors can be viewed as a limitation, or as a challenge, to their assessment skills. However, the advent of visual images may address this limitation.

The Aboriginal Nurses Association of Canada supports the use of telehealth practices to improve the health of First Nations, Métis, and Inuit communities. According to a discussion paper, "inequities exist in the health and the health care services of Aboriginal people compared to the general population of Canada" (Aboriginal Nurses Association of Canada, 2001, p. 9). The Manitoba Telehealth First Nations Expansion Project links 10 northern, remote First Nations communities. Videoconferencing can now be used to improve access to specialist care, health-related education, and visits with family members located in healthcare facilities elsewhere in the province (Manitoba Telehealth, 2007). However, patients from these communities and others without phones, computers, or computer skills are at a disadvantage. The introduction of advanced technology in some communities may inadvertently create a "digital divide" that further marginalizes people in remote communities who do not have access to that technology. (Refer to the Digital Divide Web site for more information on this topic.)

Electronic Mail and the Internet

Electronic mail (e-mail) and the Internet are means of providing telehealth services in an e-Health world. As more patients become comfortable with and gain access to e-mail, this form of communication may be used increasingly as a means of contact and consultation with healthcare providers. Some patients may experience greater comfort using e-mail as a form of communicating, especially if their concerns are of a personal or sensitive nature. With e-mail, patients and nurses have some flexibility in regard to the timing of consultations, inquiries, and responses. However, the issues of privacy and confidentiality remain unresolved. Additionally, it may not be possible to verify that the individual initiating communication is indeed the patient and that the question and the nurse's response will not be read by others. The nurse's e-mail response could also be circulated to other care providers, with the potential for the nurse's response to be misinterpreted or taken out of context. The lack of live communication may belie the complexity of the patient's situation, leading to tendencies for both the patient and provider to inadvertently simplify or exaggerate their concerns, assessments, and responses. Liability for care practices and potential misdiagnoses or care provided through distance or electronic technology are issues warranting careful exploration.

Health-Seeking Behaviors

Similarly, the Internet has provided the opportunity for health-seeking behavior by patients, often before contact with a health professional. Potentially, the Internet offers privacy, immediacy, breadth of information, different perspectives, and infinite repetition of information (Bischoff & Kelley, 1999). The proliferation of Web-based resources provides individuals with access to health information not easily obtained prior to the advent of the Internet. Conversely, the amount of information, quality of presentation, and often-conflicting information can create confusion. Patients and care providers may be unaware of how to evaluate the accuracy and credibility of Web-based information. Provider resources for such evaluation are growing, as exemplified by the inclusion of guidelines and standards for Web-based publishing on many Web sites. The nurse may find her or his practice extending into patient education about how to evaluate Internet sites. Local public and academic libraries are beginning to provide information on how to evaluate the quality of Web-based information. The Canadian Health Network provides recommendations on locating trustworthy health information on the Internet. An example of an interactive Internet service that promotes health-seeking behaviors with palliative care patients is the Canadian Virtual Hospice. This service represents a network of information and support for people dealing with life-threatening illness and loss. After registration, people can access this Web site as a patient, friend or family member, healthcare provider, or volunteer. This is a credible and well-recognized health service offered by healthcare professionals. This site is in contrast to the myriad unregulated Internet sites that have been established and maintained by nonprofessional "experts" in various areas of healthcare. Consumers of health and those seeking healthcare information need to be aware of the potential for information that is not validated or credible being posted to authentic-looking Web sites.

Online Support Groups

In addition to its use for patient self-education, the Internet is used for support groups through online synchronous chat rooms (real-time discussion) and asynchronous interaction (anytime discussion), which provide patients with the opportunity to seek support and to consult with others independently. The content of online healthcare and related discussions may vary according to the nature of the disorder and the composition of the group (White & Dorman, 2000). Topics may revolve around general themes, such as personal experience and opinion, encouragement and support, treatment, symptoms, alternative therapies, caregiver concerns, and coping strategies. As with e-mail, using technology may ease communication for those who feel inhibited by face-to-face support groups, who seek the company of those who are similarly affected, or who are geographically isolated. Future research will need to explore the role that nurses play in such online support groups, how effective groups are conducted, and the role of such groups in health promotion. Active participation or "listening" to online support groups also helps the nurse to understand patients' concerns. Nurses need to be familiar with the opportunities that online support groups provide.

Despite the challenges of this technology, e-mail, the Internet, and telehealth practices have the potential to substantially decrease the indirect and social costs of healthcare. Costs associated with travel to healthcare facilities and absenteeism from family, school, or work may be reduced. This cost savings is particularly relevant to patients and families isolated by geography or care needs.

Electronic Health Records

Since 2001, Canada Health Infoway has been working with Canada's 14 federal, provincial, and territorial governments to improve the accessibility, safety, and efficiency of healthcare by developing private and secure *electronic health records* (EHRs). An EHR is the health record of a person that is accessible online from many separate, interoperable automated systems within an electronic network (Office of Health and the Information Highway [OHIH], 2001). This definition infers the complexity of the issues involving EHRs, such as the need for additional resources, infrastructure, and economic challenges related to accessing an integrated electronic network. Health Canada (2001 as cited in CNA, 2002) notes the following characteristics of EHRs:

- *Electronic*—voice, video, images, and data related to the client or patient are available electronically
- *Longitudinal*—data on the client or patient are collected and stored over time
- *Accessible*—authorized health professionals can access the record to support the delivery of care
- *Comprehensive*—the record includes service encounter data from various health professionals and across the continuum of health service delivery.

Thus, the EHR is a secure and private lifetime record of an individual's health and healthcare history, available to authorized healthcare providers. It is designed to tie together the output of a number of information systems. Some of these systems are in use today, while others are in development. Canada Health Infoway (2008), an independent and nonprofit organization, is involved in a number of projects to develop systems that form the essential building blocks of an EHR, such as digital imaging, summaries of drug prescriptions, immunizations, and lab test results. Provinces and territories across Canada are working together with Infoway to accelerate the development of these systems. The move to EHRs has been stimulated by technologic development, increased social mobility, public and government demand for accountability, and care by a wider range of healthcare professionals—all of whom will require information (OHIH, 2001). Healthcare decision makers and policy analysts increasingly require access to data for the evaluation and support of appropriate healthcare programming. The electronic availability of a patient's record promotes accessibility of the information by a variety of healthcare providers—linked to the network—who are involved in the patient's care. EHRs could eliminate duplication of services, improve efficiency of the system, and provide accurate documentation over time. With access to complete records, physicians and nurses will have far better information for decision-making. This information is especially critical when prescriptions and treatments are being provided by multiple care providers, or when a patient is in an emergency situation.

Limited patient access to health records also becomes a possibility with EHRs. Such access may support enhanced personal decision making in health behaviors. Potentially, patients can be more informed about their health status, which may facilitate discussions with healthcare providers. In this way, patients will be empowered to take a more active role in their health. Privacy and security are fundamental to EHRs. Health Canada Infoway (2008) is working with jurisdictions and privacy commissioners to implement an EHR information governance structure. The agency is also completing a conceptual EHR privacy impact assessment. In addition, it is planning to conduct (with the Office of the Privacy Commissioner of Canada and Health Canada) a comprehensive survey of public attitudes and concerns about privacy and electronic health. Ideally, only authorized healthcare providers will have access to confidential patient information.

The value of EHRs in relation to renal nurse practitioner care has been noted (Allen, 2007). Information technology in the form of the EHR "can profoundly affect clinical workflow, enhance and expand the NP's [nurse practitioner] ability to work with client data and information. EHRs have the potential to greatly improve client safety by making it possible for clinicians to have information available to enable them to make informed decisions" (p. 44). Thus, EHRs can offer point-of-care information to clinicians.

 ## ISSUES IN THE APPLICATION OF BIOMEDICAL TECHNOLOGY AND NURSING PRACTICE

In terms of biomedical technology, a study by Cooper and Powell (1998) revealed how such technology created extreme uncertainty and profound physical, emotional, psychological, and spiritual vulnerability among patients undergoing bone marrow transplantation. It was, however, nurses who attended to these vulnerabilities. The researchers observed the following about how nurses incorporated technology as part of their nursing care:

> It is no exaggeration to suggest that these nurses created a sacred space in this highly technologic enterprise for patients to do the work of making meaning of the experience . . . One extraordinary feature of this [nursing] care resides in the fact that it occurred in the context of a highly technical endeavor. Capturing the essence of this feat, one patient insightfully asked, "How can the nurses be at the end of technology [in a spectrum of technology and care] and thank goodness they are because I'm here today because of it—and then how can they be at this touch-feel end at the same time?" (p. 65)

Ethical Dilemmas

The nurse experiences firsthand the ethical dilemmas associated with new biomedical technology. Ethical and moral knowledge moves nurses to action in relation to technology. Reproductive technologies, for example, are a special concern of women, their families, and practitioners, and, within nursing, there is a substantial body of work related to the ethics of reproductive technology. Availability of genetic testing requires women to examine their personal situations and beliefs to determine whether they wish to access the technology. Nurses may need to provide counselling as a woman decides what is best for herself. Additionally, society at large varies in its perception of the right or the need of government, resource availability, funding, and community values to influence the utilization and distribution of technologies.

Decision Making

Decision making regarding access to available biomedical technology has further ethical implications when technology is costly or in limited supply. Who should have access? What criteria should be used? Who should develop the criteria for access? These are some issues that emerge in the face of new technology. For example, at this time, not all people who need dialysis have locally available access to this technology. One mechanism to address determination of access under high-demand, limited-availability situations is to refer decision making to review boards. Such boards establish criteria in reviewing candidates for access to the technology. Nurses may be members of such boards or they may be called on to assess a patient's suitability for access to the technology. Then, too, nurses are in positions to provide information, advocacy, and emotional support to patients and families denied access to these services.

Decision-making criteria to purchase technology or make it accessible to units are also limited (Purnell, 1998). In most instances, incorporation of technology onto nursing units occurs as a consequence of criteria established by medical and, increasingly, non-nursing administrators. As nurses are left out of technology development, they are similarly distanced from decision making related to technology application in their workplaces.

 ## ISSUES IN THE ALLOCATION OF TECHNOLOGY IN EDUCATION

> Timothy, a nursing student, is about to graduate and thinks he is well prepared to face a workplace filled with technology. Computers are commonplace in his life as a student. Nursing Informatics is a required course that he took at the beginning of his program. He uses a word processing program to construct and format papers. He finds that electronic mail and Internet access are helpful to search Web sites, stay in touch with classmates, keep informed about university and faculty information, and take courses offered by WebCT. He is adept at locating electronic information and is skilled at critiquing the quality and credibility of the information.
>
> Timothy is enjoying the high-fidelity simulation experiences that are part of the learning laboratory course. Because of the limited access to clinical practice sites, Timothy and his fellow students are now substituting a clinical day a week for a simulated learning experience. He is concerned that this reduced exposure to "real" patients in the clinical setting will reduce his ability to critically think and develop his competency as a practicing nurse.

Computer technology is a significant tool for nursing education and practice. However, according to Ehnfors and Grobe (2004), the largest dilemma facing nursing and health professional education is accurate identification of the future competencies that will be required to function in a technology-infused workplace. If nurse educators expect students to use technology in their practice as graduates, students must become proficient and comfortable with healthcare-related technology in their basic programs. The new generation of university students has been raised with an appreciation for and a working knowledge of technology. They bring with them thousands of hours of playing video games, text messaging, blogging, and social interaction on MySpace, YouTube, and Facebook. The challenge for educators involves taking these previously learned skills and adapting them to the world of healthcare informatics.

Extent of Computer Literacy

Computers are available in most schools of nursing but their use is neither systematically nor routinely included in programming, unlike the situation described in the previous vignette. Until recently, few programs in Canada had a required nursing informatics course. Postsecondary institutions may believe that incoming students possess the necessary computer skills because of their experience with computers in primary and secondary schools. However, empirical evidence shows that although nursing students had access to computers in primary and secondary schools, they had limited opportunity to use them for tasks other than word processing (Gassert, 1998) and social interaction.

The life experiences of today's students are vastly different from that of previous generations'. The new generation of postsecondary student, often called Generation X (comprising young adults in their late 20s to early 30s) and Generation Y (in their early to mid-20s), exhibits unique learning characteristics and needs (Hessler & Ritchie, 2006). These young learners function better in learning activities that are structured, involve teamwork and experiential activities, and include the use of technology (Collins & Tilson, 2001). This generation wants quick access to information; has little tolerance for delays; and prefers interactive, collaborative learning styles. Members of this generation represent a challenge for traditional instructors who rely on a teacher-centered lecture style of course delivery. Part of the tension that exists in higher education today is related to the disconnect between the needs and abilities of students versus the capacity of our educational institutions and faculty to adapt to these changes.

Many institutions of higher learning are increasing their use of teaching innovations. In some cases, technology is being used to address the issue of increasing student numbers, multiple-site campuses, declining numbers of faculty, and limited financial resources. The potential then exists for technology to become a means to address these complex administrative problems without due consideration for maintaining educational standards and quality programming. Educational facilities need to guard against the temptation of substituting quality of instruction for increased student access and financial gain.

Simulated Learning

Technology has always played an integral part in the learning laboratory experience. The era of using stationary models and filmstrips has evolved into the use of more high-fidelity simulated learning experiences. Nursing has followed high-risk professions like airline pilots and adopted simulated learning because of the concern for patient safety and quality care. Recently, increased enrollments in nursing programs, reduction in faculty numbers, and reduced access to clinical sites has caused a heightened interest in the use of simulated learning in nursing education. Early studies have shown that critical thinking, clinical judgment, and confidence levels can increase when nursing students are exposed to computer-based simulations in their programs of study (Lasater, 2007; Schoening, Sittner, & Todd, 2006). The recent movement toward substituting simulated learning experiences for clinical practice time requires further debate at the faculty level.

Options for Distance Learning

Nursing education is experiencing unprecedented changes in student characteristics. Students of the 21st century are more likely to be of diverse backgrounds and nontraditional in their learning styles. These characteristics are fueling the need for educational facilities to consider alternative approaches to teaching, such as distance-learning options. The same can be said for providing opportunities for practicing nurses who require enhanced job skills, such as physical assessment or leadership abilities.

Technology-based pedagogy enables us to conceive of education without the restrictions of the classroom; hence, the usual mechanisms and parameters around course delivery need to be rethought. For example, traditional lectures, which commonly are the foundation of knowledge delivery in higher education, become nonexistent in a learner-centered, Web-based environment. In this scenario, a faculty member and student may never see each other, despite having lengthy "discussions" that have the potential to shape a student's thinking for life. At the same time, nursing education values strategies that facilitate the learning of a wide range of skills. Nursing education also values knowledge that includes assessment skills, promotion of health in families, adoption of the ethical values of the profession, and communications skills. Jukes (2005) has suggested that engaging students in e-learning can make learning fun and relevant, can deliver learning faster, can encourage "just-in-time" learning, and can provide opportunities for multitasking, networking, and interactivity. However, two questions remain: how does e-learning address the affective domain; and how does e-learning influence socialization into the professional nursing role? Until these questions are answered, educators will remain skeptical of the merits of e-learning.

Learning Distribution Systems

There are four general categories of distributed learning systems that support instructional delivery and communication. These include (1) print, (2) audio conferencing, (3) videoconferencing, and (4) Web-based and blended delivery.

PRINT-BASED DELIVERY

Print-based and correspondence courses employ prepackaged courses and self-contained learning modules. Faculty–student interaction is limited to occasional telephone contact and written feedback on submitted assignments. In recent years, distance education providers have incorporated technology, such as facsimile machines, e-mail, and assignment submissions through the Internet, to supplement print-based courses. This mode of course delivery requires maintaining an expensive and extensive infrastructure and is not a popular method of choice today.

AUDIOCONFERENCE DELIVERY

Instructional delivery has been enhanced by advancements in digitalized audio capabilities. This medium includes two-way telephone interaction between the faculty member and groups of students gathered at remote sites. Courses can be offered anywhere in the world that has telephone lines. Audioconferencing provides for real-time delivery at a fairly reasonable cost. It is ideally suited to students who cannot attend courses offered on campus or who do not have easy access to computer technology. One drawback of this method is the lack of visual stimuli to enhance the teaching–learning experience. This drawback is especially evident for students who have been exposed to video games, television, virtual learning experiences, and other hi-tech classes with slide presentations and graphic illustrations of course materials.

VIDEOCONFERENCE DELIVERY

Interactive video networks use compressed digital video technology to deliver two-way audio signals and visual images to distant sites. Although the initial investment in videoconferencing requires an expensive technologic infrastructure, ongoing costs are usually limited to long-distance telephone charges and technical support. Student participation is encouraged through the use of multimedia presentations and interactive capabilities. Recent innovations in technology include the development of desktop video applications and simulations.

This form of delivery best approximates a face-to-face learning experience. It also permits students in remote locations to have access to faculty expertise that they may not have available in their locale. However, the expectations of this technology are often exceeded by the realities of the technical difficulties that can occur. The more complex the technology, the more complex the problems; this is one reason that more technical support is needed before and during course delivery. Preparing for a videoconference course requires considerable preliminary planning, knowledge of the technology, and the ability to solve problems and use the available technology to its fullest. Another drawback is that students on the receiving end tend to feel isolated from the faculty member, which may result in a perception of substandard and unequal treatment. Extensive faculty development is needed to assist educators to use this method of teaching.

A study by Care and colleagues (2006) showed that Aboriginal nursing students were often intimidated by the videoconference experience. They often positioned themselves off camera so they could remain anonymous and invisible to the remotely located instructor and students. Aboriginal students were often uncomfortable speaking out in class when videoconferencing with their more verbal southern counterparts. The study found that faculty who made the extra effort to personalize the video technology were more effective in fostering a positive teacher–student relationship.

WEB-BASED AND BLENDED DELIVERY

To participate fully in a Web-based course, students must have regular access to a computer with Internet capacity. Web-based delivery allows students to engage in online interaction with the teacher and other students in a virtual learning environment. The instructional medium is through such software programs as WebCT and Blackboard. Interaction occurs through bulletin boards, chat rooms, and e-mail. New hybrid learning technologies combine the use of audio, video, and computer applications, creating multidimensional course delivery options. Courses can be structured as synchronous (real time) and asynchronous (anytime) offerings. This delivery method virtually eliminates geographic and access barriers to education. Blended delivery, "the thoughtful fusion of face-to-face and online learning experiences" (Garrison & Vaughn, 2008, p. 5) is increasing in popularity. In this method, a portion of traditional classroom hours are restructured and replaced with appropriate online learning experiences.

The natural evolution of instructional technologies has created a need for a transformation in higher education. This transformation has resulted in the need to address a myriad of issues in nursing education.

 ## ISSUES IN ADOPTING TECHNOLOGY IN NURSING EDUCATION

The adoption of advanced instructional technology, like Web-based and blended delivery, has become commonplace in continuing and higher education. It has been viewed as both an educational boon and a technologic "money pit." Using advanced instructional technology in higher education also challenges educators to rethink the teaching and learning enterprise.

Changing Models and Roles

In the traditional paradigm of education, the educator was the "sage on the stage," with lectures being the dominant teaching practice. Students were expected to listen passively and absorb large quantities of content in a single serving. This "tell 'em and test 'em" approach saw the teacher as the expert and provider of information. In a learner-centered paradigm, the principles of constructivism, that is, "learning is a process of meaning making or knowledge building in which learners integrate new knowledge into a pre-existing network of understanding (Young & Maxwell, 2007, p. 9), can be applied in a Web-based course. In this constructivist paradigm, teachers facilitate the learning process and, as such, become "guides on the side" for students.

The adoption of technology in education requires a paradigm shift that has a dramatic impact on the roles of faculty and students. With online courses, faculty and students have limited or non-existent face-to-face interactions. The instructor is less likely to be the primary source of content expertise or information for the student. The role of facilitator has been commonly used to characterize how an educator functions in the technology-based pedagogy (Care et al., 2007). Specific aspects of the faculty role have been defined as assisting with access and navigation, explaining expectations for students, clarifying the faculty role, stimulating critical thinking, sharing professional expertise, and providing encouragement to online students (VandeVusse & Hanson, 2000). These changing responsibilities and relationships can affect the receptivity of students and faculty to embark on Web-based teaching and learning.

Carryover to Curricula

Rapid advances in the use of technology in practice have put pressure on faculty to integrate the types of technology used in healthcare and nursing into already "packed" undergraduate curricula. Educational programs need to make decisions about the extent of use of technology in the delivery of curricula. For example, the adoption of PDAs is becoming popular in nursing education. According to Martin (2007), PDAs help to reduce student anxiety in clinical practice by making readily available a large volume of information and evidence. In a rapidly changing healthcare system, current information about medications, policies and procedures, and laboratory tests and values are readily available on a PDA at the point of care. Access to empirical evidence and medical and nursing information has been shown to have a positive effect on reducing medication errors, delivery of more comprehensive care, improving the continuity of care, and reducing stress levels in healthcare practitioners (Martin, 2007).

Demands on Time and Career Activities

A troublesome area for faculty in regard to adopting technology into their teaching is time. The use of technology may actually increase the amount of time needed for teaching. This increased amount takes faculty away from other aspects of their academic roles and responsibilities such as scholarly and research activities. Bates and Poole (2003) suggest that online courses increase faculty workload in all aspects of course design and implementation. Halstead and Billings (2005) believe that "time management frequently becomes an issue for faculty teaching online courses because of the amount of student communication typically generated within the course through threaded discussion postings, e-mail, and phone calls" (p. 429). This additional time commitment can be offset by establishing policies about "capping" enrollment in online courses as well as allocating preparation time and reducing the teaching load for faculty engaged in online teaching. One of the greatest barriers to implementing Web-based instruction in higher education is the lack of recognition it affords faculty. University environments, in particular, place a high value on research and scholarly achievements in the criteria for tenure and promotion. Faculty members who persist in incorporating advanced instructional technologies in their courses serve the curriculum in significant ways, but the time spent on this activity may be perceived as detracting from their other academic roles. If so, faculty may be reluctant to take on this type of instruction. Faculties and schools of nursing need to make important decisions about the value placed on using advanced technologies in their programs. Sufficient resources and faculty development activities will help to reduce this significant barrier.

Gains and Losses

One of the benefits of Web-based, online instruction is increased access by students who live in remote locations. For example, education becomes a reality for underrepresented populations like the Aboriginal community. A concern with this instructional medium is the loss of face-to-face contact between teachers and students and among students themselves. What becomes of the high value placed on socialization, role modeling, and development of the student–teacher relationship? Can a chat session replace the level of dialogue and discourse that exists in a traditional classroom? It is only after these issues are resolved that faculty will feel comfortable adopting this approach on a large scale.

Isolation

The inherent nature of distance education includes the geographic separation of students from faculty and from other learners. This separation can often contribute to feelings of social and psychological isolation. Moore and Kearsley (1996) coined the phrase "transactional distance" to describe the psychological distance that occurs in learners. This transactional distance is often caused by miscommunication and psychological gaps occurring between learners and instructors. In a traditional classroom, students are in touch with the nuances of nonverbal communication. Their presence in class contributes to a sense of community with other students and the instructor. In a virtual classroom, the instructor must make a conscious effort to bridge the psychological distance experienced by learners. This bridge can be achieved by promoting the establishment of a community of learners among students.

Effect of Advanced Instructional Technology on Career Choices

There is a call for a critical examination of the use of and growing reliance on technology in education. Mallow and Gilje (1999) caution faculty about the rapidity of adopting technology in nursing education without careful thought about its impact. They note that research to date supports the effectiveness of technology in conveying factual information, and they report student satisfaction. However, little evidence exists regarding "student progress in affective domain criteria such as outcomes related to humanism, moral knowledge development, ethical development, interdisciplinary communication, or caring attributes." Mallow and Gilje recommend that educators consider the core values and social processes of the profession before using technology in the curriculum. Faculty often struggle to balance the use of technology with the need to develop valuable working relationships with students.

In Canada, it is becoming clear that certain clinical areas within nursing practice are "passed over" by students in favor of more technologically challenging environments. Nursing students are drawn to the "power and prestige" of technology. This theory was substantiated in a longitudinal study by Australian researchers (Stevens & Crouch, 1998). Of note was how nurse educators and nurses in clinical settings championed high-technology areas of nursing practice (e.g., emergency room and intensive care nursing) and created favorable technologic bias in students. The 156 students who were studied responded accordingly and, after graduation, gravitated toward these high-technology nursing practice domains. Because of this socialization by educators and clinicians, students valued specialized training experiences (e.g., intensive care, spinal trauma, and pediatric and neonatal intensive care) over basic nursing. Students and graduate nurses in the Australian study perceived that high-technology activities attracted power, prestige, and the nod from the elite of the profession, whereas basic nursing had low status and no power and was marginalized from the profession (Stevens & Crouch, 1998, p. 14). At issue then, is how the new generation of computer-literate, technologically savvy nurses will be attracted to and retained in low-technology practice areas, such as long-term care, or in practice agencies that do not have the financial means to support the newest technologies.

Information and instructional technologies can enhance the quality of the educational experience if used for the right purpose. The adoption of advanced technology in education does not in and of itself guarantee a positive outcome. How can this technology contribute to the overall effectiveness of the educational process in a way that maximizes student learning? Until this question is adequately addressed, educators must be cautious of wading into the technologic sea.

 # FUTURE OF TECHNOLOGY IN EDUCATION AND PRACTICE

Although the future is unclear, one thing is certain: Technology will continue to evolve and advance. The computer has become to the Information Age what the automobile was to the Industrial Age. The Internet is accessed by millions of people daily. The explosion of a digital society has brought about significant transformations in the way people interact, access and process information, and solve problems. Healthcare professionals are only beginning to appreciate the impact this revolution will have on the ability to deliver comprehensive and safe care. These challenging times call for healthcare professionals who can think critically and adapt to change quickly.

Impact of Nursing Science on Practice Technology

The development of nursing science, that is, knowledge relevant for nursing practice, will have an impact on the development and use of technology in nursing practice. Clinical nursing information systems for data categorization and storage depend on the taxonomic structures developed to reflect the phenomena of the discipline (Graves & Corcoran-Perry, 1996). If nursing science continues to be reflected in numerous classification systems, those that are selected to frame data management programs will have their presence more strongly embedded in the discipline.

Extent of Informatics in Curricula

At this point in nursing's history, it is not surprising that there is a need for more education, support, and research for optimal utilization of computer technology and information systems for practicing nurses, educators, and undergraduate and graduate students (Link & Scholtz, 2000; Smith et al., 1998). As the next decades unfold, improved understanding and skills among all these groups are likely, as is concurrent acceptance of advanced information technology as part of nursing.

The Canadian Nursing Informatics Association completed a national research study of undergraduate nursing education informatics in Canada (Clarke & Nagle, 2003). Among its recommendations, the study suggested a holistic approach to nursing informatics and that the use of information and communication technology be required in education, healthcare, research, and policy development. Schools of nursing should also plan and implement a strategy for faculty development in the area of nursing informatics. Progress to date has been limited, and there is the risk that Canadian nursing students will graduate without the requisite knowledge and skill related to informatics (Nagle, 2007).

As a result, the extent of inclusion of nursing informatics within nursing undergraduate curricula is now being discussed in faculties across the country. Fostering this discussion is the position statement on baccalaureate education and baccalaureate programs offered by the Canadian Association of Schools of Nursing (CASN). CASN notes that baccalaureate programs are "characterized by the presence of information technologies and infrastructures" (2006, p. 1). Existing and new curricula must demonstrate not only their commitment to ICT, but also the manner in which students are provided with the education and hands-on experience to make them e-Health literate. Research into the effectiveness of advanced technology in nursing education will provide valuable information in refining how we incorporate technology into delivering nursing knowledge in undergraduate programs.

Potential for Greater Learning Access

Technology has the potential to improve the availability of basic and continuing nursing education for those for whom geography or other barriers have prevented access, which is a particularly significant issue in Canada for nurses and students who live great distances from major cities where higher education or facility-based continuing education is more likely to be located. Today's public demands education that is convenient and flexible. Moreover, in the face of busy lives, the ability to access education from home is appealing. Developments in the kind of available distance education modalities have expanded the options and increased the quality of communication that is now possible with students who prefer to obtain degrees from their living rooms.

Faculty and student roles will change as the means of communication between faculty and students takes different forms. This can also be said about nursing practice as technology is further incorporated into the healthcare system. Although computer skills and knowledge will be important in the 21st century, interpersonal relations that rely on basic language and communication skills will remain significant in the provision of nursing care. Relationships with patients and their families can be facilitated through technologic advances, because it is the way nurses enact their knowing with patients that defines the practice. Technology facilitates and alters this but does not replace nursing knowledge about the work with patients.

Whatever technologic innovations emerge in the future, nursing must remember that technology offers the profession tools to use in its mandate to provide care to individuals and their families in illness and in health promotion. Technology is a means toward the goal of health and quality patient care. Thoughtful development and use can serve nursing and recipients of care well.

SUMMARY

Nursing informatics—the integration of information technologies and communications into nursing practice—has a profound effect on nurses and the organizations where they work. The relationship between technology and nursing is evolving and, literally, at a crossroads. The advent of nursing informatics presents challenges and opportunities. CNA recognizes that technology can improve healthcare, but technology without education and support may also negatively affect clients, families, healthcare professionals, and the health system in untoward ways.

Some applications of nursing informatics are telehealth (the use of advanced telecommunications technologies to exchange health information and provide healthcare from vast distances), videoconferencing, remote monitoring, and electronic health records.

Challenges associated with technology include "short-shifting," as real-time demands replace patient care with a litany of technical tasks and a focus on outcomes (evidence), performance measurement, and technical expertise that calls for acquiring related knowledge and competence in information technology.

Applied informatics will require nurses to adhere to standards of practice, codes of ethics, provincial legislation, and competencies established by regulatory bodies. To this end, nurses will need to develop or follow telephone standards of practice, policies on providing telehealth across provinces, educational standards and credentials, provisions for maintaining privacy and confidentiality, protocols to guide decision making and judgment, and advice on professional liability issues and employer responsibilities.

Additional challenges to nursing practice are the geographic invisibility of the client and liability for care practices—potential malpractice or misdiagnoses—delivered by distance or electronic technology. On the other hand, changes influenced by informatics will be incorporated into the healthcare system, offering nurses tools to use in promoting health and caring for the sick.

Benefits to practice include greater client involvement in health-seeking behaviors and health choices, possibly because electronic communication is perceived to offer privacy, immediacy, breadth of information, and different perspectives.

Additional benefits apply particularly to education. One of the benefits of Web-based, online instruction is increased access by students who live in remote locations. Information previously disseminated in classrooms and in textbooks and other print media is now available to students and faculty in remote locations at nontraditional times. The benefits are obvious, as are the challenges prompted by change. Faculty must clearly articulate the need for information technology in nursing curricula to ensure that all nurses have the skills needed to practise effectively. Faculty must acquire technical skills and adjust to altered roles as collaborators, facilitators, and guides of learning.

Technology is fundamental to ensuring that nursing remains at the forefront of healthcare and continues to contribute to its natural evolution. According to Simpson (2006), "nursing can either embrace technology and bend it to the profession's purpose or continue to wait in the wings, watching other industries and constituencies prosper and grow. Or, even worse, nursing can find itself replaced by the very technology it avoids in the name of patient care" (p. 249).

Add to your knowledge of this issue:	Online
Aboriginal Nurses Association of Canada: Technology Information	www.anac.on.ca/web/techinfo.html
Breakthru Counseling Care	www.therapyexpress.com
British Columbia Health Guide, B.C. Ministry of Health	www.bchealthguide.org/kbaltindex.asp
Canadian Network for Innovation in Education	www.cade-aced.ca
Canadian Agency for Drugs and Technology in Health	www.cadth.ca
Canadian Health Network	www.canadian-health-network.ca/
Canadian Nursing Informatics Association	www.cnia.ca
Canadian Society of Telehealth	www.cst-sct.org
Canada's Health Information Informatics Association	www.coachorg.com
Canadian Virtual Hospice	www.virtualhospice.ca/
Digital Divide	www.digitaldivide.org
Manitoba Telehealth	www.mbtelehealth.ca/
Office of Health and the Information Highway	www.hc-sc.gc.ca/ohih-bsi/menu_e.html
Telehealth Association of Ontario	www.rohcg.on.ca
Telemedicine Research Center	trc.telemed.org/telemedicine/education.asp

REFLECTIONS on the Chapter...

1 From your experience, consider the application of technology and informatics in your practice.

2 How would you describe the relationships among technology, informatics, and nursing practice in these examples?

3 Identify issues related to the use of technology in your practice or in practice situations you have observed.

4 What strategies have you used or observed being used to overcome barriers to the use of technology and informatics in practice?

5 What barriers have you experienced in using technology in your nursing studies?

6 What strategies have you used or could you use to overcome these barriers?

References

Aboriginal Nurses Association of Canada. (2001). *Impact of technology on Aboriginal nursing: A discussion paper.* Ottawa: Author. Retrieved January 29, 2008 from http://www.anac.on.ca/web/techinfo.html.

Alberta Telehealth (2007). *Telehealth services: Clinical telehealth services.* Retrieved January 28, 2008 from http://albertatelehealth.com/content.asp?category_id=5&root_id=2.

Allen, S. (2007). Benefits of electronic health records to renal nurse practitioner care. *The CANNT Journal, 17(3),* 44.

Bates, A.W. & Poole, G. (2003). *Effective teaching with technology in higher education: Foundations for success.* San Francisco: Jossey-Bass.

Bischoff, W.R. & Kelley, S.J. (1999). 21st century house call: The Internet and the World Wide Web. *Holistic Nursing Practice, 13*(4), 42–50.

Booth, R.G. (2006). Educating the future e-health professional nurse. *International Journal of Nursing Education Scholarship, 3*(1). Retrieved January 29, 2008 from http://www. bepress.com/ijnes/vol3/iss1/art13/.

Canadian Association of Schools of Nursing. (2006). CASN position statement on baccalaureate education and baccalaureate programs. Author. Retrieved January 29, 2008 from http://www. casn.ca/content.php?doc=33.

Canadian Nurses Association. (2000). Telehealth: Great potential or risky terrain? *Nursing Now: Issues and Trends in Canadian Nursing.* Ottawa: Author. Retrieved January 29, 2008 from http://www.can-Nurses.ca/CNA/ documents/pdf/publications/Telehealth_November2000_e.pdf.

_____(2001). *Position statement: The role of the nurse in telepractice.* Ottawa: Author. Retrieved January 29, 2008 from http:// www.cna-nurses.ca/CNA/documents/pdf/publications/PS52_Role_Nurse_Telepractice_Nov_ 2001_e.pdf.

_____(2001). What is nursing informatics and why is it so important? *Nursing now: Issues and trends in Canadian nursing,11,* 1–4.

_____(2002). Demystifying the electronic health record. *Nursing now: Issues and trends in Canadian nursing,13,* 1–4.

_____(2006). *Nursing information and knowledge management.* Ottawa: Author. Retrieved January 29, 2008 from http://www.cna-nurses.ca/CNA/documents/pdf/publications/PS87-Nursing-info-knowledge-e.pdf.

Canadian Institute for Health Information. (CIHI, 2006). *Workforce trends of registered nurses in Canada, 2006.* Author. Retrieved January 29, 2008 from http://secure.cihi.ca/cihiweb/dispPage. jsp?cw_page=AR_20_E.

Care, W.D., Gregory, D.M., & Russell, C., et al. (2006). Aboriginal students and faculty experiences with distance education. In R. Riewe and J. Oakes (Eds.), *Aboriginal connections to race, environment, and traditions* (pp. 101–109). University of Manitoba: Aboriginal Issues Press.

Care, W.D., Russell, C.K., & Hartig, M.T., et al. (2007). Challenges, issues, and barriers to student-centered approaches in distance education. In L.E. Young & B.L. Paterson (Eds.), *Teaching nursing: Developing a student-centered learning environment* (pp. 484–502). Philadelphia: Lippincott Williams & Wilkins.

Clarke, H. & Nagle, L. (2003). *OHIH research project: 2002–2003—Final report.* Retrieved January 29, 2008 from http://www.cnia.ca/OHIHfinaltoc.htm.

College of Nurses of Ontario. (2005). *Practice guideline: Telepractice.* Toronto: Author. Retrieved January 28, 2008 from http://www.cno.org/docs/prac/41041_telephone.pdf.

Collins, D.E. & Tilson, E.R. (2001). A new generation on the horizon. *Radiological Technology, 73,* 172–177.

Cooper, M.C. & Powell, E. (1998). Technology and care in a bone marrow transplant unit: Creating and assuaging vulnerability. *Holistic Nursing Practice, 12*(4), 57–68.

Doran, D.M., Mylopoulos, J., Kushniruk, A., Nagle, N., Laurie-Shaw, B., Sidani, S., Tourangeau, A.E., Lefebre, N. & Reid-Haughian, C., et al. (2007). Evidence in the palm of your hand: Development of an outcomes-focused knowledge translation intervention. *Worldviews on Evidence-Based Nursing,* Second Quarter, 69–77.

Ehnfors, M. & Grobe, S.J. (2004). Nursing curriculum and continuing education: Future directions. *International Journal of Medical Informatics, 73,* 591–598.

Gadow, S. (1988). Covenant without cure: Letting go and holding on in chronic illness. In J. Watson & M. Ray (Eds.), *The ethics of care and the ethics of cure.* New York: National League for Nursing.

Garrison, D.R. & Vaughn, N.D. (2008). *Blended learning in higher education. Framework, principles, and guidelines.* San Francisco, CA: Jossey-Bass.

Gassert, C.A. (1998). The challenge of meeting patients' needs with a national nursing informatics agenda. *Journal of American Medical Informatics Association, 5*(3), 263–268.

_____. (2000). Telehealth and nursing. In B. Carty (Ed.), *Nursing informatics: Education for practice.* New York: Springer.

Goodwin, S. (2007). Telephone nursing: An emerging practice area. *Nursing Leadership, 20*(4), 37–45.

Graves, J.R. & Corcoran-Perry, S. (1996). The study of nursing informatics. *Holistic Nursing Practice, 11*(1), 15–24.

Halstead, J.A. & Billings, D.M. (2005). Teaching and learning in online learning communities. In D.M. Billings and J.A. Halstead (Eds). *Teaching in nursing: A guide for faculty* (pp. 423–439). St. Louis: Elsevier Sanders.

Canada Health (2007). *eHealth.* Retrieved January 28, 2008 from http://www.hc-sc.gc.ca/hcs-sss/ehealth-esante/index_e.html.

Canada Health Infoway (2008). *Infoway: Electronic health record.* Author. Retrieved January 29, 2008 from http://www.infoway-inforoute.ca/en/ValueToCanadians/EHR.aspx.

Hessler, K. & Ritchie, H. (2006). Recruitment and retention of novice faculty. *Journal of Nursing Education, 45*(5), 150–154.

Jukes, I. (2005). *Understanding digital kids (DKs): Teaching & learning in the new digital landscape.* Retrieved January 28, 2008 from http://www.ldcsb.on.ca/schools/cfe/ internet_safety/documents/understanding%20digital%20kids.pdf.

Lasater, K. (2007). High-fidelity simulation and clinical judgment: Students' experiences. *Journal of Nursing Education, 46*(6), 269–276.

Link, D.G. & Scholtz, S.M. (2000). Educational technology and the faculty role: What you don't know can hurt you. *Nurse Educator, 25*(6), 274–276.

Loiselle, C. & Cossette, S. (2007). Health information technology and nursing care. Guest Editorial. *Canadian Journal of Nursing Research, 39*(1), 11–14.

Mallow, G.E. & Gilje, F. (1999). Technology-based nursing education: Overview and call for further dialogue. *Journal of Nursing Education, 38*(6), 248–251.

Manitoba Telehealth. (2007). *MBTelehealth Innovation: Current project highlights.* Retrieved January 28, 2008 from http://www.mbtelehealth.ca/innovation_research.php.

Martin, R. (2007). Making a case for personal digital assistant use in baccalaureate nursing education. Online Journal of Nursing Informatics (OJNI), *11*(2) [Online]. Retrieved January 29, 2008 from http://eaa-knowledge.com/ojni/ni/11_2/martin.htm.

Mathieu, L. (2007). Discourse. Nursing informatics: Developing knowledge for nursing practice. *Canadian Journal of Nursing Research, 39*(1), 15–19.

Moore, M.G. & Kearsley, G. (1996). *Distance education: A systems view.* Belmont, CA: Wadsworth.

Nagle, L. (2007). Everything I know about informatics, I didn't learn in nursing school. *Canadian Journal of Nursing Leadership, 20*(3), 22–25.

Office of Health and the Information Highway, Health Canada. (2001). *Toward electronic health records* [Online]. Retrieved January 29, 2008 from http://www.hc-sc.gc.ca/ohih-bsi/ehr/ehr_dse/ehr_dse_e.html#Overview.

Purnell, M. (1998). Who really makes the bed? Uncovering technologic dissonance in nursing. *Holistic Nursing Practice, 12*(4), 12–22.

Rasid, M.F.A. & Woodward, B. (2005) Bluetooth telemedicine processor for multichannel biomedical signal transmission via mobile cellular networks. *IEEE Transactions on Information Technology in Biomedicine, 9*(1), 35–43.

Riva, G. (2000). From telehealth to e-health: Internet and distributed virtual reality in health care [Electronic version]. *Cyberpsychology & Behavior, 3*(6), 989–998.

Russo, H. (2001). Window of opportunity for home care nurses: Telehealth technologies. *Online Journal of Issues in Nursing, 6*(3). Retrieved January 29, 2008 from http://www.nursingworld.org/ojin/topic16/tpc16_4.htm

_____. (2000). Thermometers and telephones: A century of nursing and technology. *American Journal of Nursing, 100*(10), 82–85.

Schoening, A.M., Sittner, B.J., & Todd, M.J. (2006). Simulated learning experience: Nursing students' perceptions and the educators' role. *Nurse Educator, 31*(6), 253–258.

Simpson, R.L. (1998). A few points about point-of-care technology. *Nursing Management, 29*(11), 19–22.

_____. (2006). Advancing with technology. In P.S. Yoder-Wise & K.E. Kowalski (Eds.), *Beyond leading and managing: Nursing administration for the future* (pp. 231–256). St. Louis: Mosby Elsevier.

Smith, C.E., & Young-Cureton, V., & Hooper, C., et al. (1998). A survey of computer technology utilization in school nursing. *Journal of School Nursing, 14*(2), 27–34.

Staggers, N. & Bagley Thompson, C. (2002). The evoluation of definitions for nursing informatics: A critical analysis and revised definition. *Journal of the American Medical Informatics Association, 9(3)*, 255–262.

Stevens, J. & Crouch, M. (1998). Frankenstein's nurse! What are schools of nursing creating? *Collegian, 5(1)*, 10–15.

VandeVusse, L. & Hanson, L. (2000). Evaluation of online course discussions: Faculty facilitation of active student learning. *Computers in Nursing, 18(4)*, 181–188.

White, M.H. & Dorman, S.M. (2000). Online support for caregivers: Analysis of an Internet Alzheimer mailgroup. *Computers in Nursing, 18(4)*, 168–179.

Young, L.E. & Maxwell, B. (2007). Student-centered teaching in nursing: from rote to active learning. In L.E. Young & B.L. Paterson (Eds.), *Teaching nursing: Developing a student-centered learning environment* (pp. 3–25). Philadelphia: Lippincott Williams & Wilkins.

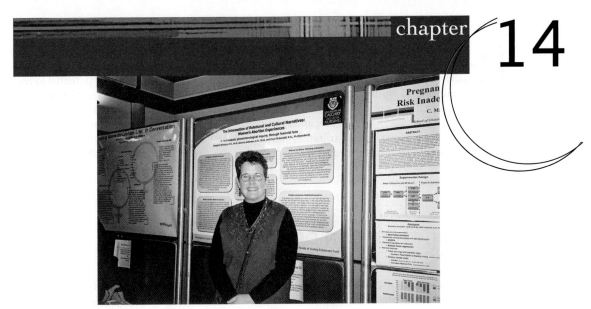

Publications, professional conferences, poster sessions, and scholarship exchanges are key ways to disseminate the nursing research findings that are central to determining what constitutes "best practice." (Photography by Beverly Anderson. Used with permission.)

The Realities of Canadian Nursing Research

Dorothy Pringle

Critical Questions

As a way of engaging with the ideas in this chapter, consider the following:

1. How do you understand the claim that research conducted by nurses is not necessarily "nursing research"?

2. What areas of research, apart from nursing research, do you imagine that nurses draw on in practice?

3. In your practice so far, what questions have come up for you that might benefit from research or inquiry?

Chapter Objectives

After completing this chapter, you will be able to:

1. Appreciate the history of nursing research in Canada.

2. Identify significant milestones in the evolution of nursing research in Canada.

3. Describe obstacles nurses and nursing have had to overcome to develop research.

4. Describe how nurses can use research in their practice.

5. Identify challenges confronting the continued development of nursing research.

6. Discuss ways in which these challenges can be overcome.

R esearch has become an important force in Canadian nursing. This evolution has not happened quickly, and, whereas the ultimate impact of research is still not clear, it has the potential to revolutionize nursing. To illuminate the impact of research in nursing, this chapter traces the evolution of nursing research in Canada, examines the influence it currently has on nursing practice and education and how it exercises that influence, and speculates on the potential influence of nursing research. This chapter also explores the contribution nursing research has made to the health of Canadians. Finally, this chapter discusses issues regarding getting nurses to become involved in the utilization of research and the future of nursing research in Canadian healthcare.

 ## THE EVOLUTION OF NURSING RESEARCH IN CANADA

This section could easily have been called "The Revolution in Nursing Research in Canada" because the last four decades of the 20th century represent no less than a revolution. Revolutions are not one-battle affairs. They are fought over time and include many skirmishes as well as a few large-scale battles. Usually, only the battles make their way into the history books. Although there were no declarations of war and no lives lost, nurse researchers in Canada struggled to establish nursing research firmly during the second half of the century and finally achieved that status in the 1990s.

Before tracing this development, it is important to discuss what the term "nursing research" refers to and where it fits into the spectrum of human sciences research. The boundaries around nursing research are quite fuzzy; in some quarters, nursing research is understood to refer only to research undertaken to develop the scientific basis of nursing practice. However, others include research on nursing education and nursing administration under the rubric of nursing research, and still others would argue that nursing research is any research undertaken by nurse scientists. In this chapter, the term "nursing research" will be used to refer to research that informs clinical practice, education, and nursing administration and the focus will be on what nurse scientists have contributed.

Bloch (1981) developed a model of nursing research and nursing science that nicely locates these within the larger landscape of science. She describes a communal pool of what she calls "fundamental research" to which researchers of all disciplines contribute. This pool includes knowledge about life, health, and disease. Before this knowledge can be applied directly in practice, it first must be translated into a series of interventions. Nursing develops its interventions based on this fundamental knowledge, as do all other applied disciplines, such as psychology and medicine. An important message in Bloch's perspective is that nursing must draw on knowledge developed by many other disciplines to develop interventions that are unique to its practice. These interventions are tested, and their results, taken together, form nursing science or the science of nursing practice and the sciences of nursing education and nursing administration. Nurse researchers have a responsibility to contribute to the pool of fundamental knowledge as well as to address the questions that affect all aspects of nursing. This perspective does not preclude researchers from other disciplines undertaking research on nursing practice, education, and administration and quite a number have; however, most frequently it is nurse scientists' direct knowledge of practice, education, and administration and their work with nurses involved in these arenas that reveal the issues from which questions and, in turn, research develops.

The evolution of Canadian nursing research can best be appreciated against the landscape of its counterpart in the United States. Canada followed the American model of nursing education rather than the British model in that it identified nursing education as appropriately located in universities. This does not mean that all or even most nursing education occurred there, but in Canada from 1919 onward when the University of British Columbia commenced a degree program to prepare nurses for public health, nursing was associated with universities. This association was very important in the evolution of nursing research because universities and their affiliated teaching hospitals are where the vast majority of health-related research occurs. Furthermore, the usual academic progression of baccalaureate to master's to doctoral education was adopted in Canadian nursing (as it was in the United States), and this set the pattern for the preparation of nurse researchers in the same mold as other academic disciplines.

In Britain, the voyage has been more difficult than in North America because of early decisions that nursing education should occur in hospitals and that specialization should be through hospital-based certification programs rather than through the pursuit of master's degrees. Nursing education essentially did not move to universities until the 1990s. There were exceptions, such as the University of Edinburgh, which established the first university nursing program in the United Kingdom in 1956, but few British nurses pursued their initial nursing education through university programs.

Publishing Nursing Research

Nursing research began in Canada in the 1920s with a focus on nursing education. However, over the next half century, only occasional studies were conducted by the few people prepared to undertake research (Ritchie, 1992). This trend contrasts with that of the United States, where nursing research began developing momentum in the 1940s and 1950s. *Nursing Research*, the first research journal in nursing, was initially published in the United States in 1952. The first nursing research text, *Better Patient Care Through Nursing Research* (Abdellah & Levine), appeared in 1965. The impetus for much early nursing research came from McGill University and the leadership of Dr. Moyra Allen. Dr. Allen completed her Ph.D. at Stanford University and returned to Canada and to McGill. She saw the need for a nursing research journal to serve Canadian researchers, and *Nursing Papers* was launched in 1969 with just two editions per year. In 1975, *Nursing Papers* became bilingual, publishing both French and English articles and providing abstracts of the articles in the other language. The French language name, *Perspectives en Nursing*, was added (Gottlieb, 1999) at that time. It was renamed the *Canadian Journal of Nursing Research/Revue Canadienne de Recherche en Sciences Infirmiéres* in 1988. Gottlieb traced the history of this journal in the editorial that introduced the 30-year anniversary edition published in 1999. Maintaining this journal represents one of the struggles in the development of nursing research in Canada. There was never enough money, manuscripts—particularly in the early days— were hard to come by, and circulation was low. However, it was crucial and remains so for Canadian nurse researchers to have a vehicle in which to publish their works, some of which address topics of particular interest to the Canadian scene. For example, in 2002, Butler and colleagues produced a report on a workshop that was held to develop a national strategy for integrating supportive care in research, practice, and policy. In addition, the editorials reflected issues in Canadian healthcare and nursing education and what research had to bring to these issues (Gagnon, 1999). The journal remains at McGill, and four issues a year are published.

Many other journals have been established in Canada since 1969, including journals that support specialty fields, for example, the *Canadian Journal of Cardiovascular Nursing,* the *Canadian Journal of Nursing Leadership,* and the *Canadian Gerontological Nurse,* the journal of the Canadian Gerontological Nurses Association. Several of these journals began by publishing articles about clinical practice with very little research reflected in them. This lack of research has changed over the years. They all now publish reports of research on topics relevant to practitioners in their specialty areas. Most have introduced peer review, which means that the reports submitted by the researchers are reviewed by people with research expertise in that field to determine whether the research is sufficiently sound to warrant publication. The reviewers are not informed who the authors are; hence, the peer review is called a "blind" review. This prevents the reviewers from bringing positive or negative biases colored by any relationships they might have with the authors of the research.

Canadian researchers publish well beyond journals based in Canada and well beyond nursing journals. Many excellent nursing research journals are now available, including *Nursing Research,*

Research in Nursing & Health, the *Journal of Nursing Scholarship* (formerly *Image*), *Qualitative Nursing Research,* and the *Western Journal of Nursing Research.* Despite the excellence of many journals and the filter of the peer-review process, the caveat "reader beware" still holds true. Consumers of research must bring a critical perspective to reading all published research to determine whether the findings of the study can or should be applied to their own practice.

Funding of Nursing Research

Until the mid-1990s, being a nurse researcher in Canada was challenging because of the lack of resources available. Conducting research takes funds, and funds were scarce to support the kinds of research that nurses undertook. The Medical Research Council (MRC) of Canada was launched in 1960 with a mandate to "promote, assist and undertake basic, applied and clinical research in Canada in the health sciences" (MRC Act), but because of the meager funding available, MRC decided to limit its support to biomedical research. This limitation did not change in any fundamental way until the mid-1990s and, as such, did not support research by nurses.

The alternative major national source of funding available to nurses (and other nonbiomedical researchers) was the National Health Research and Development Program (NHRDP) of Health Canada (previously Health and Welfare Canada). Unlike MRC, which operated in an arm's-length relationship with the government and could develop its own research priorities, NHRDP was a department of the government and was expected to support research that assisted the government to meet its objectives. The size of their budgets differed enormously: When MRC and NHRDP merged into the Canadian Institutes of Health Research (CIHR) in 2000, MRC's budget was $350 million and NHRDP's was about one tenth of that. Furthermore, NHRDP's budget fluctuated every year depending on the government's largesse. Because NHRDP was the major general research fund (i.e., not limited to a specialty area) available at the national level to nurses and several other nonbiomedical disciplines like epidemiology, occupational therapy, and family medicine, the competition was fierce and the size of the available grants was limited. Grants could be as large as $300,000 for a 2-year project but most were less than $100,000 annually.

Despite the constraints of both a limited budget and government-directed focus, NHRDP proved to be a great benefactor of nurses. Many nurses who pursued doctoral education from 1975 until 2000 received fellowships from NHRDP that supported them during their studies. Nurses won these fellowships in national interdisciplinary competitions that demonstrated their ability to compete head-on with the best candidates from other health disciplines. The scientists who gained this training went on to become some of the best researchers in the country. Academically able, they were admitted to excellent research training programs in nursing and other disciplines in Canada and elsewhere and worked with some of the best supervisors available.

NHRDP was also a source of project grants required by nurses for research. Charitable organizations with special interests in particular diseases, for example, the Heart and Stroke Foundation, the Diabetes Association, the Alzheimer Society, and the Cancer Society, raise money to support research in those diseases. Most began their funding programs favoring biomedical research because of an orientation to seek cures rather than to focus research on caring for individuals with the disease. Even under these circumstances, some nurses were successful in receiving grants from competitions held by these organizations and built important research programs based on this funding. Fortunately, the policies of these foundations have evolved over the years, and nursing research is now part of the range of studies they fund.

Because of the very limited funding available at the national level, the Canadian Nurses Foundation (CNF) was established by the Canadian Nurses Association (CNA) in 1962 initially to provide support for nurses studying at the master's and doctoral levels. (See Ritchie [1992] for a description of the development of the CNF.) In 1984, small grants for research were added. As with many nursing-based endeavors, the CNF has struggled since its inception to secure sufficient funds to keep itself in business. Much of its support has come from donations from nurse researchers themselves. In the days before NHRDP and MRC funding, CNF was frequently the sole resource nurses could turn to. Even today, CNF will fund studies that address topics unique to nursing that would not likely be successful in interdisciplinary competitions. The investigation of nursing-specific themes, such as the nature of the nurse–patient relationship, is appreciated as vital to understanding nursing as a discipline in peer-review committees dominated by nurses. This is not necessarily true of interdisciplinary committees unless a strong nursing research advocate is a member of the committee. In 2002, CNF entered into a partnership with the Canadian Health Services Research Foundation (described later) to increase their resources substantially.

The Social Sciences and Humanities Research Council of Canada (SSHRC) has been and continues to be an important source of funding for many nurse researchers. SSHRC is a national foundation established in 1977 on the same basis as MRC, that is, funded by but at arm's length from the federal government. (The third national body in Canada that makes up the research funding triumvirate is the Natural Sciences and Engineering Research Council.) SSHRC has always had a substantially smaller budget than MRC and its successor, CIHR. In 2007–2008, its budget was $312,700 million while CIHR had a budget of $700 million. As its name suggests, the SSHRC funds research that examines questions relevant to the social, cultural, economic, technological, environmental, and wellness dimensions of life. For many qualitative nurse researchers and those interested in the ethical, historical, and psychosocial dimensions of nursing, SSHRC is a major source of funding. The peer-review committees understand and value qualitative methods to address questions and have expertise in content areas relevant to nursing. Nurses also have received doctoral fellowship support from SSHRC. However, the size of the overall budget dictates that most SSHRC grants are relatively modest in comparison to those available from CIHR.

Some provincial granting bodies have had a tradition of providing funds to nursing research, for example, the Fonds de Researche Scientifique du Québec, the Michael Smith Foundation for Health Research in British Columbia, and the Alberta Heritage Foundation for Medical Research (AHFMR). These three foundations have developed a variety of innovative ways to support research studies and researchers in their provinces, and nurses have successfully capitalized on these opportunities.

The history of research funding in Alberta, however, helps to illustrate the challenges that have faced nurses as they have developed research as a critical dimension of the discipline. In 1980, Alberta was enjoying a booming economy, and the government decided to invest some of the money not needed for current provincial needs into AHFMR. A $300 million endowment was created to fund basic biomedical and medical research. New research positions were created, and new competitions for doctoral and postdoctoral training were initiated. Nurses in the province objected because they were not eligible to apply, and, after a major initiative led by Dr. Shirley Stinson of the University of Alberta, the Alberta Nursing Research Foundation (ANRF) was established in 1982 and provided with an expendable $1 million yearly budget. This amount contrasted with the large endowment provided for biomedical research but, nevertheless, was a breakthrough for nursing research in Canada.

ANRF was certainly welcomed by nurse researchers in the province, but the fund was too limited to award large grants, for example, more than $100,000 per year for several years. Furthermore, it separated nursing from the more intense interdisciplinary competitions at AHFMR. Provincial competitions are good training grounds for learning to write strong, coherent grant applications that will survive and be successful when researchers compete at the national level. ANRF was terminated in 1994, but Alberta nurses once again successfully mounted a campaign, and AHFMR expanded its mandate to include nursing research and nurse researchers among those eligible to compete for their funds. Since then, nurses have successfully competed for grants, doctoral and postdoctoral training awards, and research scholar awards to support young investigators. In fact, AHFMR has become a major source of support for nurse researchers in Alberta and is a model of an innovative granting body for the rest of the country.

At the national level, a lot happened in the 1990s.

The Canadian Health Services Research Foundation (CHSRF) was established in 1997 with an initial endowment of $66.5 million that was increased by an additional $60 million in 1999. Its mandate is to fund research on health services management and policy. In 1999, as a result of successful lobbying of Health Canada led by Dr. Mary Ellen Jeans, who at that time was the executive director of CNA, $25 million was allocated to CHSRF for the funding of nursing research over a 10-year period. CHSRF was the recipient of the funds because CNA argued that workplace difficulties and workforce shortages were at crisis levels in Canada and required serious research attention. The agreement between Health Canada and CHSRF specified that $500,000 per year was to be spent on clinical research; the rest was to go to health services and policy research relevant to nursing. CHSRF and CNF have developed the Nursing Care Partnership Fund for the administration of the clinical research dollars.

Almost simultaneously with the CHSRF developments, MRC—led by Dr. Henry Friesen—undertook a national study that resulted in a reinterpretation of its mandate to embrace all types of research. New peer-review committees were developed, and nurses and researchers from other disciplines, such as occupational and physical therapy, epidemiology, and family medicine, were able to compete. This reinterpretation was followed quickly by a redevelopment of the entire health research enterprise. CIHR was approved by the government of Canada in June 2000. MRC and NHRDP ceased to exist, and CIHR became the major source of health research funding for the nation.

Thirteen "virtual" interdisciplinary institutes were created to represent such diverse areas of science as genetics, aging, cancer, Aboriginal health, and gender and health. Each institute reflects four areas of research: basic biomedical, clinical, health services, and population health. A scientific director heads each institute and is assisted by an advisory board. CIHR started with a budget of $339 million, which had increased to slightly more than $730 million by 2008–2009. A target had been set to try to achieve $1 billion in funding annually by 2006 but clearly this target was not met. This shortfall is a problem for all health researchers and speaks to the limited commitment of the federal government to research relative to other countries, such as the United States, where the National Institutes of Health, the American equivalent of CIHR, had a budget of $28 billion dollars in 2008.

Nurses are an integral part of CIHR. Dr. Nancy Edwards, an outstanding nurse researcher who holds a CHSRF nursing research chair in the School of Nursing at the University of Ottawa, was a member and, for a time, chaired the Governing Council, which is the policymaking body of the CIHR. Nurses have been the scientific directors of the Institute of Gender and Health since the beginning; Dr. Miriam Stewart of the University of Alberta was the first and she was followed by Dr. Joy Johnson at the University of British Columbia. There are nurses on most institute advisory boards, and nurses sit on all the appropriate peer-review committees. They chair some committees and serve as scientific officers on others. Nurse researchers now compete for the much larger grants available through the CIHR and take their place alongside scientists from all other disciplines.

The structure of CIHR was not what nursing had hoped for. Given the frustration created by MRC's exclusion of nursing research for so many years and the tentative steps to include an applied research agenda in the 1990s, nursing had hoped that the new approach to research funding would include an institute for nursing research. However, very early in its development, the CIHR embraced a strictly interdisciplinary agenda and declared that no institute would be disciplinary based. Despite this assertion, the Canadian Association of Schools of Nursing and the Canadian Association of Nurse Researchers mounted a campaign for a nursing-specific institute. The two organizations successfully competed for funds from SSHRC and CHSRF to undertake a planning exercise for a new institute. Representatives met and debated the relative advantages of advocating for a nursing research institute versus a nursing and caregiving research institute. The latter was seen to accommodate an interdisciplinary thrust while acknowledging nursing as the lead discipline. The decision was made to go with the latter, and a proposal for such an institute was developed and submitted to the CIHR interim council, which acted as a planning committee. The application was not successful. In hindsight this may have been a good decision because it has led to nurse researchers being embedded in virtually all the CIHR institutes.

In the United States, nursing research has had a different history. After many years of concerted and well-coordinated lobbying by nurses, a National Center for Nursing Research was created in 1985 as part of the National Institutes of Health. The center was elevated to the status of a National Institute of Nursing Research (NINR) in 1992. The American National Institutes of Health are organized very differently from their Canadian counterparts in that they have dedicated buildings, they conduct research within the institutes (intramural research), and they mount competitions for researchers to apply for funds (extramural research). The NINR's autonomy and resources (a budget of $137,800 million USD in 2008) mean that American nurses are able to identify areas of particular interest to nursing or areas that require special attention and establish directed competitions (in addition to their regular competitions) to drive research into them. For example, they have identified seven core areas that require specific nursing research attention: cardiopulmonary and critical care science, chronic conditions and infectious diseases, end-of-life and long-term care, health behavior and minority health, HIV/AIDS and oncology, neuroscience and reproductive, and child and family health.

Canadian nursing cannot do this under the CIHR structure and must seek other routes to gain attention for special needs areas. This battle for the recognition of nursing research is not over. Nurses are well positioned within the CIHR, and there is no reason to believe that individual nurse researchers will not continue to do well in competitions for grant support, but nursing has yet to develop strategies within the unique funding opportunities in Canada that will allow it to focus on areas of unique or special interest to nurses.

Preparation of Nurse Researchers

Conducting nursing research depends on having well-prepared researchers. This requires programs of study and funds for students while they study. Preparation at the doctoral level is seen as necessary for most people to undertake the role of principal investigator, the person who takes major responsibility for designing and managing research studies. Canada was late to develop doctoral programs in nursing relative to other countries. Our first programs occurred in the early 1990s, whereas the United States already had four doctoral programs by 1975. By 1990, the United States had 45 programs, and Finland, Japan, Korea, and Thailand all had doctoral programs in nursing.

In the mid-1980s, McGill University, followed closely by the University of Alberta, began to plan in earnest for doctoral programs in nursing. In the case of McGill, the governing body of the Faculty of Medicine—in which the School of Nursing is located—challenged the plan. The Faculty of Medicine did not think that nursing had demonstrated sufficient resources or a sufficient body of knowledge to justify a Ph.D. degree in the discipline. The Faculty of Nursing at the University of Alberta saw their program approved at the university level, but the government was not prepared to provide funding for it. The faculty decided that it should not try to mount the program in the absence of funds; essentially, they determined that if the doctoral program could be mounted without additional government funding, even if it was difficult, the government would never provide the funds.

Both programs went on hold while these internal and external political situations were resolved. However, both McGill and the University of Alberta had provisions within the universities that made it possible to admit individual students to studies in areas in which doctoral programs were planned. Both nursing schools used these provisions to admit nurses to ad hoc studies, and several nurses were able to complete the requirements for a Ph.D. in nursing before formal programs were established. One of these nurses was Dr. Francine Ducharme, the first person to complete a Ph.D. in nursing in Canada. Dr. Ducharme completed her doctoral program at McGill University.

Although it took a long time to initiate doctoral education in Canada, once started, five programs began within a 3-year period. After intensely lobbying the government, the University of Alberta received funding to begin a formal doctoral program in nursing in January 1991, and the University of British Columbia followed with a program later that same year. The University of Toronto opened a program in 1993, and a joint bilingual program between McGill University and the University of

Montreal also opened in 1993. McMaster University completed this quintet with a program in 1994. In 2008 there are 15 Ph.D. programs in nursing in universities across the country, so it is now possible for nurses who wish to pursue a Ph.D. in nursing to choose from many excellent programs. Importantly, nurses who find that they are not able to relocate in order to undertake a Ph.D. in nursing are much more likely to find a program within commuting distance than was true a decade ago. It is important to point out, however, that ease of access to a program should not be the primary, or even among the top two or three, criteria for choosing a program. Much more important are the reputation of the program for graduating excellent researchers, access to a supervisor who has a strong reputation both as a researcher in the field of interest and as a supervisor, and financial support so the majority of time can be spent studying rather than working. In 1995 when the first five Ph.D. programs were up and running, a total of 53 students were enrolled in them and five students had graduated with Ph.D.s in nursing. Compare that with 2006, when a total of 390 students were enrolled across all the nursing Ph.D. programs and an additional 327 had graduated (Canadian Nurses Association/Canadian Association of Schools of Nursing 2004).

The graduates of these early programs are among the major Canadian nurse researchers of the early 21st century. Several hold research chairs: Dr. Ducharme at the University of Montreal, Dr. Bonnie Stevens at the Hospital for Sick Children in Toronto, Dr. Carole Estabrooks at the University of Alberta, and Dr. Cindy-Lee Dennis at the University of Toronto.

Like everything else in the establishment of the nursing research enterprise in Canada, the mounting of doctoral programs did not come easily. Nursing had to prove itself once again as a legitimate academic field of study in several of the universities. Only a few faculties and schools actually received additional funding to support these programs, and the rest stretched their budgets to include this new resource-intensive activity. This most important battle can now be declared won.

These programs provide the infrastructure for the continued production of researchers without which all the other elements of the conduct of research could not proceed. Furthermore, after 15 years of experience, a clearly Canadian model of the Ph.D. degree in nursing has emerged. Canadian programs require only a few courses, four to five on average, including a course on the philosophic underpinning of science (in general) and nursing science (in particular), one or two research design and statistics courses, and one or two courses on theories and content specific to the students' research. The dissertations are a very large component of the programs and are begun immediately upon entering the program. These dissertations are substantial in scope, and the supervisory committee is usually interdisciplinary in composition.

This model contrasts markedly with the design of doctoral programs in the United States, which include a large number of courses, usually around 20, a smaller dissertation that the doctoral candidate does not begin until completing much of the course work, and a supervisory committee composed largely of nurse scientists. In Britain, there is usually no required course work, and the entire focus of the Ph.D. degree program is on conducting research, which is supervised by one individual.

All of these models are consistent with the approach to doctoral work in general in their host countries. One design is not superior to another, but they do tend to produce researchers with somewhat different strengths. Graduates of Canadian programs have strong research design skills and an appreciation of what other disciplines bring to research even when that research is focused on answering questions relevant to nursing. This is an important orientation given the strong interdisciplinary bent of the national funding agencies.

Funding to support nursing doctoral students has not proved as buoyant as the programs themselves. The absence of a specific source of funds for nurses is felt every time the CIHR releases the list of successful candidates for doctoral fellowships. There is an enormous demand for doctoral support, and the CIHR funds fewer than 20% of the applications it receives. The limited access to funds means that many doctoral students work full-time or part-time throughout their programs. This necessity tends to slow their progress and creates a great burden on the individual, who may be raising a family at the same time. This is a continuing struggle and one that requires creative solutions by nursing agencies.

Although completion of a doctoral program used to be sufficient to commence a research career, now it is common for graduates to undertake 2 to 3 years of postdoctoral studies before accepting an academic or research position. The graduates of Canadian nursing Ph.D. programs have achieved a high level of success in national and provincial competitions for funding to support their post-doctoral work. Most Canadian funding sources require candidates to change their locations and their supervisors to get the maximum benefit from further studies. Postdoctoral work is intended to turn young researchers into independent researchers and position them to be competitive for grants, which Ph.D. studies alone sometimes cannot or do not do.

Research takes time: time to undertake the review of the current state of knowledge in the area of interest; time to assemble a research team and to meet with them; time to determine the most appropriate design, data gathering approach, and measurement instruments; time to figure out the data analysis strategies; and time to write the grant and get ethics approval. Because it is so time intensive, research commonly is relegated to second or third place behind other responsibilities. Nurses in academic settings find themselves with heavy teaching loads, a situation that requires them to fit research into weekends and evenings. Similar dilemmas are faced by administrators and clinical nurse specialists, who have heavy demands on their time but are expected and encouraged to do research. One way of managing this load is for the researcher to apply for a "personnel award." These awards have a number of different titles depending on the granting agency and the stage of the individual's career: research scholar, career scientist, scientist, national scientist, and research chair, among others. Personnel awards provide a researcher's employer with at least half of the researcher's salary, with an expectation that 75% of the person's time can be spent on research.

These awards are very important, particularly to young scientists who are just launching their independent research careers. As noted earlier, because MRC and most disease-related funding charities did not support nurses, young scientists depended on NHRDP and a few provincial funding agencies for personnel awards. In the 1970s, Dr. Moyra Allen at McGill won an NHRDP National Health Scientist award to study the health-promoting activities nurses undertook at the nursing-run health station in Montreal. A few other nurses were awarded the NHRDP research scholar funding. In the 1970s, awards were granted to Dr. Shirley Stinson of the University of Alberta and Dr. Jacqueline Chapman at the University of Toronto; in the 1980s, awards went to Dr. Sharon Ogden Burke at Queen's University, Dr. Gina Browne at McMaster University, Dr. Joan Anderson at the University of British Columbia, and Dr. Janice Morse at the University of Alberta. These were important breakthroughs for nursing as a discipline, but they were too few to move the development of nursing science ahead at a pace that reflected the size of the profession. Much more was needed, particularly to assist young investigators to launch their research careers.

Dr. Ginette Rodger was executive director of the CNA in the 1980s, and, in 1986, she was appointed to the MRC council. Only one nurse before her, Dr. Dorothy Kergin, then the director of the McMaster University School of Nursing, had ever sat on the decision-making body of MRC. Dr. Rodger used this opportunity to encourage MRC to work with NHRDP to create a new set of research scholar awards for nurses only. After huge initial resistance, the agencies capitulated, and the Joint MRC/NHRDP Research Scholar awards were launched in 1988. Schools of nursing had to compete for these awards on behalf of their best young researchers. The program got off to a rather slow start, but, over the subsequent seven years of its existence, 17 nurse researchers from eight universities received 5-year awards.[1] Building on their earlier successes, some went on to compete for and receive NHRDP research scholar awards for another five years. Many of these awardees went on to become leaders in nursing research in Canada.

---

[1]The 17 were Drs. Hilary Llewellyn-Thomas and Diane Irvine (now Doran), University of Toronto; Annette O'Connor, University of Ottawa; Celeste Johnston, McGill University; Louise Levesque, Francine Ducharme, Lise Talbot, and Sylvie Robichaud, University of Montreal; Lesley Degner and Linda Kristjanson, University of Manitoba; Sharon Ogden Burke and Carol Roberts, Queen's University; Marilyn Ford-Gilboe and Helene Berman, University of Western Ontario; and Janice Morse, Jane Drummond, and Beverley O'Brien, University of Alberta.

Nurse researchers now compete for CIHR personnel awards along with all the best scientists from other health disciplines. Is this another battle won on the road to research respectability and achievement or one that is still in progress? After seven years of experience competing within the interdisciplinary programs of CIHR, it is possible to say that nurse researchers are doing well because they are in several provincial funding programs (Ontario, Alberta, British Columbia, and Quebec) that offer these types of competitions. Another battle won.

Research chairs are now a major resource on the national scene. There have been research chairs for many years, but the 1990s saw an avalanche of new chairs become available. The creation of named chairs became a popular fundraising target for universities and hospitals. Dr. Ellen Hodnett assumed the first endowed research chair in nursing in Canada, the Heather M. Reisman Chair in Perinatal Nursing Research, a joint chair between Mt. Sinai Hospital and the University of Toronto. CHSRF added five more nursing chairs in 2000. These chairs are not endowed but will support the incumbents for 10 years. Research chairs are filled by researchers who have international reputations for their work and who have made outstanding contributions to specific fields of knowledge. We are now at the point where the number of endowed chairs is outstripping the number of senior nurse researchers available to fill them. This is a new phenomenon for nursing (i.e., to have more resources than it is able to absorb), and it puts pressure on the discipline to continue to support young investigators, protect their time, and assist them to develop the reputations that will make them eligible to assume chairs in the future.

A final indicator of the maturation of nursing research in Canada is reflected in the amount of funding nurses are receiving to conduct their research. The statistics from CIHR demonstrate that nurses who served as principal investigators, i.e., took the leadership role in designing the research study, received increased amounts of funding from 2000/2001 through 2006/2007 (Fig.14.1) Funding rose from just slightly more than $2 million to more than $10 million over this time. When funds for fellowships and personnel awards are added to the amounts received for research project grants, the amount peaked in 2006/2007 at just over $16 million (Fig. 14.1).

Much of this increase in success can be attributed to the first graduates of the Canadian doctoral programs in nursing. The beginning productivity of this new stream of researchers bodes well for the future of research. Nurses are now successfully competing for funds provincially, nationally, and internationally.

INFLUENCE OF RESEARCH ON NURSING PRACTICE AND EDUCATION

Influence on Practice

Throughout the 1970s and part of the 1980s, much was made of nurses delivering theory-based practice. This term commonly referred most frequently to the grand theories that a number of nurses had developed to understand and explain patient behaviors and the relationships between what nurses did and patients' responses to these interventions. Among these were King's Interacting Systems Framework, Rogers' Science of Unitary Human Beings, and Neuman's Systems Model (Fawcett, 1989). The term *theory-based practice* is rarely heard now because the era of evidence-based practice has replaced it.

Evidence-based practice, which is sometimes referred to as *best practice,* means that the type of care delivered (or in health promotion arenas, the health promotion strategy used) is based on the best research evidence about that practice integrated with knowledge about the patient's preferences, culture, emotional status, information needs, and unique physiologic responses, among other things.

**CIHR: Total annual funding of all grants & awards
2000-2007**

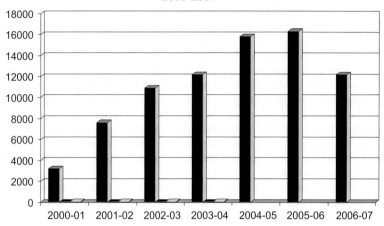

CIHR: Annual funding of nursing operating grants 2000-2007

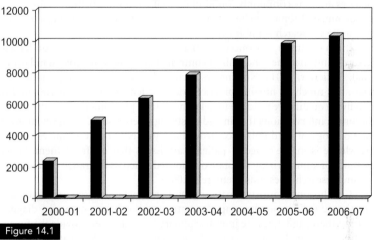

Figure 14.1

Funding for nursing research. Amounts shown in millions. (Source: Dr. Mary Ellen Jones with data provided by the Canadian Association of Schools of Nursing, 2008.)

Research is now regarded as central to the determination of what constitutes best practice. Basing care on research evidence was not possible until recently because there was simply not enough research available in most areas of nursing practice to influence the decision. This is still the case in some areas of nursing practice, such as the care of patients with dementia or chronic psychiatric disorders. Nevertheless, the evidence is mounting, and increasingly nurses can turn to research studies to help them determine what is best for individual patients or classes of patients, for example, patients being supported by mechanical ventilation or recovering from coronary artery bypass surgery. This ability represents a significant change in how nurses approach patient care and will change the view that nurses turn to each other rather than to research literature to answer questions about what is the most current thinking on the care of patients with specific problems.

One research study in an area tells us something about that area but is rarely sufficient in scope or size to support a change in practice. An exception might be a large, multisite, randomized controlled trial with thousands of patients enrolled such as the study on breech births referred to earlier. Clinicians seek out a series of studies that focus on a specific type of practice but this requires a method for integrating the findings from across the studies so a determination can be made of what the true conclusion is. Two approaches are used: systematic reviews and meta-analysis. In systematic reviews (sometimes called *integrated reviews*), all the studies that relate to a topic are retrieved from published and unpublished sources, the individual studies are assessed for their methodologic quality, and then the findings from all the studies, taking into account the quality of the research, are examined to reach a decision on what is the state of knowledge on that topic (Mulrow & Cook, 1998). If possible, a recommendation is made to change practice. However, if the evidence is conflicted or the quality of the studies is poor, then a recommendation for further research is made specifying the questions it must address and the designs needed before a conclusion can be reached.

A meta-analysis takes the systematic review a step further and integrates the actual data from all the studies to reach a statistical decision about whether a particular intervention improves outcomes. These data are reported in the form of an odds ratio or an effect size, depending on whether the data are continuous or dichotomous (Lau, Ioannidis, & Schmid, 1998). This latter technique is applied mainly to analysis of findings from randomized controlled trials. Systematic reviews and meta-analyses are now commonly found in journals, and the Cochrane Library provides meta-analyses on a wide range of topics, including many that are relevant to nursing. These analyses are updated regularly as new research is published.

It is a common misconception that systematic reviews can be undertaken only on experimental research and that the randomized controlled analysis is the gold standard for all research (Jennings, 2000; Petticrew, 2001). Nursing research includes an increasing number of randomized controlled trials, but much of nursing practice does not lend itself to experimental treatment. Nursing relies heavily on qualitative research to help understand phenomena from the perspective of the patient; furthermore, interventions that include a strong interpersonal component are difficult to subject to the methodology of randomized controlled analysis. Nevertheless, nurses need to know what the state of knowledge is in the range of patient care issues that confront them. Systematic reviews provide a method for summarizing the state of knowledge across the range of research methods used to address nursing research questions (Petticrew, 2001).

Conclusions from systematic reviews and meta-analyses frequently are integrated into clinical practice guidelines or care maps for patients who share a common diagnosis or clinical condition. Most of these guidelines are interdisciplinary in nature and provide the type and timing of tests, interventions, and medications across all the disciplines providing patient care.

The development of electronic databases has made the search for and location of research studies and systematic reviews immensely easier. Access to these databases in all hospital libraries and commonly through computers located on hospital patient care units or public health units has provided nurses with findings from research never before possible. Additionally, there are Internet web sites that house clinical practice guidelines that teams of practitioners can access rather than having to start from scratch every time to develop their own. In practice, however, most teams find it difficult to incorporate other teams' guidelines without studying the issues, reading the original research or at least the systematic reviews, and finally adapting the guidelines to their own environments and patient populations.

As difficult as it is to believe, doing the research and accessing the research reports, the systematic reviews, the meta-analyses, and the clinical practice guidelines on patient care units are the easy parts of evidence-based practice. The difficult part is getting the individual practitioner—whether that person is a nurse, physician, or physical therapist—actually to change her or his practice to conform to the evidence. There is a huge gap between what is known as a result of research and its application in patient care. Research utilization, also called knowledge translation, is a developing area of science, and a Canadian nurse scientist, Dr. Carole Estabrooks and her colleagues at the Knowledge Utilization Studies Program at the University of Alberta Faculty of Nursing, have taken the lead in explicating the factors that influence health professionals to use research findings in their practice (Estabrooks et al., 2007; Cummings et al., 2007). It seems that simply knowing what works best does not usually lead to practising on the basis of that knowledge. The reasons are complex and involve issues at the level of the individual nurse and the context in which the nurse practices. Estabrooks et al. (2007) have identified factors that contribute significantly to research utilization, which include nurses who use the Internet more and feel less emotionally exhausted at work; higher levels of nurse-to-nurse collaboration; someone available to facilitate the uptake of research; high levels of nursing autonomy; organizations that are innovative, responsive, employ adequate staff and are supportive of them; and, finally, the presence of nursing leadership.

Several theories (Rycroft-Malone, 2007) have been developed to try to guide research utilization. The difficulty with many of them is their linearity (Kitson, Harvey, & McCormack, 1998); that is, there are a series of steps that, if followed in a simple straightforward manner, will result in practice changes. The reality is quite different. Kitson and coworkers have proposed a conceptual framework labeled PARiHS, Promoting Action on Research Implementation in Health Services, that acknowledges how messy and complex the process is. Their framework for implementing research in practice is based on the formula: SI = f (E, C, F). That is, Successful Implementation is a function of Evidence, Context, and Facilitation. Rather than treating this as a linear formula, the elements of evidence, the environment, and the presence of a facilitator whose role it is to make things easier for those being asked to change are considered simultaneously. Each of these components has several dimensions:

- Evidence includes research, clinical expertise, and patient choice.
- Environment incorporates an understanding of the culture and of human relationships as explicated in leadership roles and how the organization measures its system and service performance.
- Facilitation involves determining how the facilitator uses interpersonal and group skills to influence change.

In this framework, context and evidence are assessed along a continuum (high to low). Depending on what this assessment reveals, the facilitation approach changes (Kitson et al., 1998). An analysis of 10 years of experience using PARiHS by Kitson et al. (2008) has led to the conclusion that the framework should be used as a two-stage process: first, as a diagnostic and evaluative measure of the components of evidence and context, and second, using what has been learned to determine what type of facilitation is required.

None of the research utilization theories guarantees successful change to best practice; however, the theories represent the state of the art of our understanding about how to bring about practice changes early in our experience. Clearly, this is an area of great potential for future development, but the patients and the practitioners cannot wait until the "right" theory comes along that will guide change with more predictable results. The facilitators, nurse educators, and clinical leaders must use the theories and frameworks available now to approach research utilization in as systematic a way as the theories allow.

A second force for research on the horizon is an increasingly better-educated nursing workforce. Research will increasingly influence the way nurses practice as more nurses are educated to read research with understanding, to conduct systematic reviews, and to seek out research as their first resource when trying to answer practice questions.

So far, this discussion on evidence-based practice has skirted the question of how much research actually influences current practice because the question cannot be answered definitively. In some settings, typically the highly specialized areas of practice like intensive care units, coronary care units, and transplantation units, clinical practice guidelines that incorporate best practices are widely used.

Nurses in these units are challenging long-standing practices such as the routine introduction of saline solution into artificial airways to facilitate suctioning of mucus. A number of well-designed studies demonstrate that saline solution does not necessarily improve suctioning and may harm the patient (Druding, 1997). In other units, the concept of best practice has not yet been discovered, let alone incorporated into daily life. This lag will not continue for long. Nursing in Canada is in the very early days of research production and utilization. Nursing practice will be influenced and changed as more nurses are educated to use research and as more nurses attend conferences in their specialty areas and hear presentations on research on common practices. Nursing practice will be influenced and changed as more nurses read their specialty journals and encounter not "let-me-tell-you-how-we-do-it-on-our-unit" articles but articles describing why questions were raised about a nursing practice and how research was conducted to answer those questions. Nursing practice will be influenced and changed as nurses change employment and move from units or organizations that operate on best-practice principles to ones that do not. It is possible to predict that, by the end of the first decade of the 21st century, nursing practice will be greatly influenced by research. The term *best practice* may not be heard very commonly then because it will be so embedded in the daily lives of nurses as not to require comment or attention.

Influence on Education

Nursing education has been profoundly affected by the development of research in terms of what is taught and who teaches it. Forty years ago, faculty members in university programs were educated at the baccalaureate or master's levels, and teachers in diploma programs themselves had only diplomas or baccalaureate degrees. Research had little presence in the programs by virtue of the fact that little existed. Textbooks were the cornerstone of course work. In the 21st century, that trend has changed dramatically. Most university professors of nursing now hold a Ph.D., and the minimum preparation found throughout nursing education programs is the master's degree. These are not just paper qualifications. They mean that the faculty in nursing programs are both educators and researchers, thus profoundly changing teaching.

The journal replaces the textbook as the source of knowledge. Students are guided to use the journal collection as their major resource. Increasingly, the assigned readings for courses are collections of research articles assembled and printed, in accord with Canadian copyright laws, and sold to students. Course content focuses on findings from research on the topic. Faculty members bring their own research into the classrooms to teach the content students are to acquire. If courses in the 21st century are taught the same way as they were even 10 years earlier, they are not reflecting the changes in knowledge or the source of knowledge.

In larger research-intensive university programs, opportunities are available to undergraduate students to work as research assistants on research projects throughout their education. These opportunities commonly serve as incentives for students to pursue graduate education immediately to acquire the research skills that will allow them to become principal investigators. They get bitten by the research bug, and they want to do it all.

Nursing is still struggling with how to make research an attractive and attainable career goal for an increasing number of students entering the profession. Most students enter nursing to realize their desire to care for people who are ill. In the course of their studies, they find that many different career paths are available to them. If they are exposed to research and have the opportunity to participate actively in it, they might come to see research as a possible future.

In schools of nursing with master's and doctoral programs, undergraduate nursing students are exposed to graduate-level students in those programs. The students interact in their roles as teaching assistants or in social encounters. This interaction makes graduate education very real and attainable. If undergraduate students are not in a research-intensive environment, then faculty members have to use imaginative ways of making research live for the students. It may mean attending research days at other universities; having days when faculty and graduate student research is presented; or having researchers or doctoral students come and meet with students, present their work in interactive seminars, and discuss the realities of research careers. Students need encouragement to see graduate school as a logical step in their career plans. They also need tangible financial support to be able to pursue their education. Students who are excited by the possibilities of research, who in the course of their studies raise questions that have been investigated or can be investigated using research methods, and who challenge current practice are excellent candidates for future research careers in nursing.

CONTRIBUTION OF NURSING RESEARCH TO THE HEALTH AND HEALTHCARE OF CANADIANS

It would be very nice if the contributions of nursing research to Canadians' health could be numbered and neatly listed. It is not that simple. Nursing research has contributed in many different ways to Canadians' health and healthcare, but the nature of the research undertaken by nurses does not usually result in products like the identification of the gene for muscular dystrophy, the discovery of insulin, or the development of pablum—all the outcomes of medical research by Canadian scientists. Instead, nursing research has helped us to understand how parents manage multiple encounters with the healthcare system when they have a chronically ill child (Burke et al., 1991), how pain is experienced by premature infants in pediatric intensive care units (Stevens & Johnston, 1994; Stevens, Johnston, & Horton, 1994), how chronic illness is experienced and how people change their lives to cope with it (Paterson, 2001; Thorne & Paterson, 2001), how patients are comforted during painful treatments in emergency rooms (Morse & Proctor, 1998), and how patients with cancer want to have control over the type and amount of their treatments (Degner, 1992). Much of what nursing research has done to date is inform clinicians (nurses and all healthcare professionals) of what patients are experiencing and what they prefer in the way of treatment, information, and approach. This knowledge positions the clinicians to work in more sensitive, helpful, and therapeutic ways with patients. Nurses increasingly are undertaking experimental research, whether it be randomized controlled trials or theory-based experimental studies advocated by Sidani as more appropriate for many of nursing's questions (Sidani & Braden, 1998). Randomized controlled trials have demonstrated how to control pain in babies undergoing such procedures as heel sticks (Stevens et al., 1999), how to help family caregivers of older people with dementia adjust to the institutionalization of their relatives (Ducharme et al., 2001), and how to use exercise to manage fatigue in patients with cancer (Graydon et al., 1998). These few examples all focus on what research by Canadian nurse researchers has contributed to our understanding of how to care for people having a variety of illnesses or undergoing medical treatments. Clearly there is much more; the journals are replete with reports of studies.

Nurses have also contributed research that has improved the health of Canadians. They have explored how to assist pregnant women and new mothers to stop smoking or to extend periods of nonsmoking (Johnson et al., 2000), and they have studied how to help mothers protect their infants from environmental smoke (Ratner, Johnson, & Bottoroff, 2001). Much work has been done on how to reduce falls among individuals living in the community and in institutions because falls are a major contributor to morbidity, reduced quality of life, and premature death (Edwards, Cere, & Leblond, 1993; Gallagher & Scott, 1997; Morse, 2001). An inventory has been compiled of interventions carried out by public health nurses and other community health workers that are effective in improving health and preventing morbidity and mortality (Ciliska et al., 1996; Ploeg et al., 1996).

An area to which nurse researchers, and Canadian nurse researchers in particular, are making impressive contributions is in our understanding of how to staff and manage the healthcare system. Doran and McGillis Hall at the University of Toronto have undertaken a series of studies on the impact of staffing ratios and nursing-skill mix (the proportion of registered nurses [RNs], licensed practical nurses, and nonprofessional workers) on a variety of patient outcomes and several aspects of nurses' work (Doran et al., 2002; McGillis Hall et al., 2001). Tourangeau and colleagues (2002) at the University of Alberta have demonstrated that better nurse–patient ratios reduce the death rate among patients with cardiovascular disease and shorten their hospital stays. An interdisciplinary team of researchers with nursing leadership (O'Brien-Pallas et al., 2002) found that nurses with baccalaureate degrees working in home care reduced the number of visits patients required to achieve the desired outcomes. O'Brien-Pallas (2002) has launched a program of research to develop a model for explicating the complex phenomenon of determining the size and nature of the nursing workforce required to meet Canadians' healthcare needs in the future.

This type of research, which relies heavily on databases that house information about patient case mix, lengths of stay, and mortality rather than on the collection of primary data, is increasingly important to our understanding of how to staff the healthcare system to achieve maximum efficiency and maximum patient outcomes. It is relatively new to nursing and requires that nurse researchers have the expertise to use, link, and extract data from these types of databases, which are a national resource. The Canadian healthcare system makes it possible to establish national databases drawn from the systems in each of the provinces that house information about patients, their diagnoses, treatments, lengths of stay, use of medications, and outcomes in terms of morbidity. Ontario has funded the development of a clinical database called Health Outcomes for Better Information and Care. It consists of patient outcomes that research has shown are influenced by nursing care or how nurses are deployed, such as whether care is deliverd by an RN, practical nurse, or healthcare aide. Nurses assess patients on their functional status, level of symptom control (pain, nausea, dyspnea, fatigue, etc.), falls, and pressure ulcers and determine their ability to care for themselves (therapeutic self-care) on admission to and discharge from whatever sector of the healthcare system they enter. This information remains available to them in a form that allows them to compare any one patient with all others on the unit and it also populates a database that can be linked to other provincial and national databases. These databases will allow questions to be answered regarding the relationship between nursing inputs, such as skill mix, the number of nursing hours per patient days, and the educational level and experience of nurses as well as a range of nursing care interventions and patient outcomes. This database should be fully established in Ontario by 2010 as well as in some other provinces (Nagle et al., 2007; White & Pringle, 2005).

 ## ISSUES FACING NURSING RESEARCH

A number of issues have been identified throughout this chapter, but the following three, in particular, deserve special attention:

- the need to produce sufficient researchers for the future
- the need to use the CIHR's structure and resources to serve nursing research and the role of interdisciplinary research in nursing's future
- the need to increase research utilization in practice.

Shortage of Nurse Researchers

Canada entered the 21st century in the throes of a nursing shortage and with the probability that this shortage would intensify over the next decade. The shortage is distributed across all dimensions of the profession. There are insufficient staff nurses, too few nurse educators, not enough senior researchers to fill the chairs available, and not enough junior researchers to replace the cohort of researchers who will retire during the next 10 to 15 years.

Canada needs more nurse researchers, not fewer. Medical science is making enormous progress in addressing the treatment of disease. For every development in medical care, nursing must respond by determining patients' responses and needs and by developing interventions that complement the medical treatment. For every advance in our understanding of what promotes health or prevents disease, nursing must develop programs at the individual and population levels that build on this new knowledge. Furthermore, there is much catching up to do. Because the undertaking of nursing research is so recent, most of what nurses do and most of what patients experience and need to understand about their health situations has not been studied.

In an overall nursing shortage, every dimension of nursing competes with every other to attract nurses. When there are lots of well-paying clinical positions, it can be very difficult to convince undergraduate students to forego immediate employment and stay in school to pursue research training or to leave well-remunerated positions and return to school. This difficulty is compounded in situations of insufficient funding to allow students to remain in school. The increasing cost of nursing education has resulted in more students graduating with debt. Many find it untenable to take on more debt in the course of acquiring graduate degrees.

Because nurse researchers compose the majority of nurse educators, unless incentives are put in place to make it possible for nurses to undertake graduate work, there will be not only insufficient researchers but also insufficient educators to prepare the nurses to staff the health system. In the United States in the 1960s, the federal government put in place "nurse traineeships" so all students undertaking graduate degrees in accredited nursing programs received a tuition waiver and a monthly stipend. Over the years, this program allowed the federal government to manage shortages in selective areas, such as psychiatric nursing, by offering more traineeships in these areas and fewer in areas where numbers were greater.

There are alternative strategies that serve as incentives for nurses to seek advanced preparation:

- academic debt forgiveness programs if students pursue research training
- tuition reimbursement programs
- special graduate scholarships
- awards available to schools with graduate programs.

With the exception of the small MRC/NHRDP research scholar program of the early 1990s, Canadian nursing has not been the beneficiary of incentive programs designed specifically to support nurses to achieve or accelerate research careers. And they are needed now more than ever before. However, they will not be successful unless young nurses see research or academic careers as attractive, achievable, and rewarding. Interested students need to be exposed to successful nurse researchers who are enthusiastic about their career choice and can serve as role models and mentors to less experienced nurses. Developing opportunities for young nurses or nursing students to work as research assistants to successful and positive researchers is an important recruitment device.

Creating incentive programs to support nurses while they pursue graduate education and developing creative and stimulating opportunities to help undergraduate and graduate students see research as a viable and desirable career choice are desperately needed to ensure the future of nursing research.

Canadian Institutes of Health Research Structure

As noted earlier, Canadian nursing does not have its own institute within the CIHR structure and must seek other routes to attract attention for special needs areas. Furthermore, the CIHR emphasizes interdisciplinary research. Nurses are well positioned within the CIHR institutes, but the discipline has yet to develop strategies for working with the various institutes so nursing is heard when new initiatives are required to better understand issues that are either unique to nursing or in which nurses play a major role.

The peer-review committees that review applications and make recommendations for grants to support research projects and personnel awards are separate from the CIHR institutes. Many of these peer-review committees include nurses but usually not more than one or two in a total membership of 12 to 15. When applications from nurses reach these committees, the nurse members may find themselves having to interpret the relevance of the project and argue for its worth. Nursing must find a way to ensure that there are nurses on all peer-review committees to which nursing proposals might be assigned so proposals are reviewed by knowledgeable researchers who respect the nature of the work.

Additionally, nursing needs to continue to develop ways of connecting with all the CIHR institutes. These connections might be made through nursing's specialty organizations, such as the cancer' nurses association, the cardiovascular nurses group, and the gerontologic nursing societies. These specialty organizations could develop special relationships with their institute counterparts to design special initiatives that would serve nursing. Keeping in mind that the institutes must be interdisciplinary in their orientations, the initiatives would have to be of interest to other disciplines and incur their support. *Interdisciplinarity* in research has become the watchword of CIHR. As an organization, CIHR is convinced that better research results from investigators from a variety of relevant disciplines working together and merging their expertise. This theory may be true. However, interdisciplinarity results from individuals well prepared in their own disciplines coming together. Interdisciplinarity depends first on disciplinarity. Preparing experts in their own disciplines in an environment that rewards interdisciplinary teams who write grants and conduct research is a real challenge and, in Canada, one that nursing needs to continue to address.

Nurses will have to be creative to work with CIHR to ensure that nursing's unique needs and orientation are addressed. It will take imagination and relationship building different than the routes available to American nurses, who have their own NINR; however, it is not impossible, and nurses' presence in important positions throughout the institutes and on the CIHR council is a good starting place.

Research Utilization

A third critical issue facing nursing research is the need to accelerate the translation of research into practice. As discussed earlier, the uptake of research into best practice is at an early stage of development in nursing and in all the health disciplines. The rate of research production in nursing, however, means that if the transfer process does not accelerate, research knowledge will languish in journals years before it is used in patient care. This sluggishness is wasteful and unfair to the public who has funded the research in the first place. Nursing needs an understanding by and commitment from all practicing nurses to attend to research findings and to seek opportunities to use the results of research in their practice, which means that nurses must be prepared in their initial education or through continuing education opportunities to read, comprehend, and critique research. It puts a special demand on nursing practice leaders, such as nurse managers, clinical nurse specialists, and nurse educators, to assist nurses to appreciate the value of research and to find creative ways of bringing research into practice. Organizations that employ nurses have a special responsibility to provide the resources and the infrastructure supports that make it possible for nurses to access research, to have time to read it, and to have individuals available to them to assist them in using it.

 # THE FUTURE OF NURSING RESEARCH

Notwithstanding the challenges confronting nursing and nurses in the creation of nursing research, the future has never been more encouraging, more robust, or more exciting. Nursing internationally, and particularly in Canada, has never before in its history had so many well-prepared and productive researchers. They are increasingly successful in funding competitions; they see their research published in the best nursing journals and highly regarded interdisciplinary and medical journals; they are sought out to participate in research studies examining a wide range of health issues; and they are well placed in the new structures that support Canadian health research. The doctoral programs that were created in the 1990s and more recently have proved to be solid and sustainable. Their graduates are credible and successful. The research conducted by the students is sound and relevant.

Canadians have every reason to be confident that the money they are investing in nursing research is paying off in better understanding of what matters to them about their health, how they can sustain their health, how their healthcare and nursing care can be better designed and delivered, and how they can achieve their objectives through the healthcare system. It is a good time to be a nurse researcher.

SUMMARY

Nursing research has been developing since the 1960s in Canada, and enormous strides were made in the 1990s. Doctoral programs in nursing were launched, and more nurses than ever before achieved doctoral preparation. The funding environment changed, new sources of funds became available to support nursing research, and a number of opportunities developed to allow nurses to devote more of their time to conducting research. Nursing research achieved an increasing share of the research dollars that are distributed annually. These changes did not come easily. Opposition both inside and outside universities had to be overcome before the Ph.D. programs became established, but nurses worked strategically to ensure that they gained access to the new sources of funding.

Research is now regarded as central to determining what constitutes best practice, that is, care delivered based on the best research evidence available combined with knowledge about the patient's unique circumstances. An understanding of how to bring about best practice and research utilization more broadly is in its infancy, but new theories and robust programs of research are slowly contributing to knowledge in this area.

Nursing education has been profoundly influenced by research. Nurse educators are better prepared and bring knowledge about research into their teaching. Increasingly, students are assigned journal articles and critical appraisals of sets of articles on specific topics rather than textbooks as their first source of information about patient care.

Despite its relative youth, nursing research has made major contributions to our understanding of what patients are experiencing and what they prefer in the way of treatment, information, or approach to their care; how to better care for patients experiencing a variety of health conditions; how to run the healthcare system more effectively and efficiently; and how to help people to live healthier lives. The potential for even more substantive contributions is immense, particularly because more research funding is available and more nurse researchers are in positions to design, develop, and conduct programs of studies.

Of the many issues facing nurses, three stand out: the challenge to prepare sufficient researchers to replace those who will retire over the next 10 to 15 years and to meet future demand,; the challenge of using the structure and resources of the new CIHR to meet the needs of nursing research, and the challenge of dramatically increasing research utilization in practice.

Future nursing research will help Canadians better understand how to sustain their health and how healthcare and nursing care can be better designed and delivered. Nurses have never before been as well prepared or had the amount of support available to them to meet these expectations.

Online

Add to your knowledge of this issue:	
Alberta Heritage Foundation for Medical Research	www.ahfmr.ab.ca
Canada Association for Nursing Research (CANR)	www.canr.ca
Canadian Association of Schools of Nursing (CASN)	www.casn.ca
Canadian Health Services Research Foundation (CHSRF)	www.chsrf.ca
Canadian Institutes of Health Research (CIHR)	www.cihr-irsc.gc.ca
Canadian Nurses Association (CNA)	www.cna-nurses.ca
Canadian Nurses Foundation (CNF)	www.canadiannursesfoundation.com
Fonds de Researche Scientifique du Québec (FRSQ)	www.frsq.gouv.qc.ca
Michael Smith Foundation for Health Research (MSFHR)	www.msfhr.org
Natural Sciences and Engineering Research Council of Canada (NSERC)	www.nserc-crsng.gc.ca
Social Sciences and Humanities Research Council of Canada (SSHRC)	www.sshrc.ca

REFLECTIONS on the Chapter...

❶ Identify one or two nurse researchers whose work interests you. Trace their publications through electronic databases such as the Cumulative Index to Nursing and Allied Health Literature and MEDLINE. What journals are they publishing in? Are they working alone or with a consistent team of collaborators? How would you summarize their contributions?

❷ Think about an area of practice that interests you, for example, managing the symptoms of children being treated for cancer or helping mothers maintain a sense of control during labor, and then develop a nursing practice question. Go to the electronic databases and search for research that addresses that question. Has research been done on it? If there is research, who has done it, and how much of it has been done by nurses? If there is no research, are there opinion pieces, editorials, or descriptions of how various places manage? Describe the state of knowledge at this time on the practice. Would you recommend research or more research on the question?

❸ Think of one practice setting you have been in. What strategies are in place to apply research findings to practice? How successful are they? If there are no obvious strategies, describe what could be done to bring research to practice.

❹ Go to the CIHR Web site, http://www.cihr-irsc.gc.ca/. Visit the Web pages of the 13 institutes. Review their mission statements and the types of research they are interested in. How many are focused on research that is relevant to nursing? Look at their staffing and the members of their advisory boards. How many have nurses on their boards? Is there a relationship between mission and research focus and the membership of their boards?

References

Abdellah, F.G. & Levine, E. (1965). *Better patient care through nursing research.* New York: Macmillan.

Bloch, D.A. (1981). Conceptualization of nursing research and nursing science. In J. McCloskey & H. Grace (Eds.), *Current issues in nursing* (pp. 81–93). Oxford, UK: Blackwell.

Burke, S.O., Kauffmann, E., Costello, E., et al. (1991). Hazardous secrets and reluctantly taking charge: Parenting a child with repeated hospitalizations. *Image: The Journal of Nursing Scholarship, 23,* 39–45.

Canadian Association of Schools of Nursing (CASN). (2002). *Nursing research funding database.* Retrieved from http://www.causn.org/Databases/nursing_research_database.htm.

Canadian Nurses Association/Canadian Association of Schools of Nursing (CNA/CASN). (2004). The *national student and faculty survey of Canadian schools of nursing 2002–2003.* Retrieved from www.cna-nurses.ca/_frames/resources/statsframe.htm.

Ciliska, D., Hayward, S., & Thomas, H., et al. (1996). A systematic overview of the effectiveness of home visiting as a delivery strategy for public health nursing interventions. *Canadian Journal of Public Health, 87*(3), 193–198.

Cummings, G.G., Estabrooks, C.A., & Midodzi, W.K., et al. (2007). Influence of organizational characteristics on research utilization. *Nursing Research, 56*(4S), S24-S39.

Degner, L. (1992). Patient participation in treatment decision making. *AXON, 14,* 13–14.

Doran, D.I., Sidani, S., & Keatings, M., et al. (2002). An empirical test of the nursing role effectiveness model. *Journal of Advanced Nursing, 38*(1), 29–39.

Druding, M.C. (1997). Re-examining the practice of normal saline instillation prior to suctioning. *MEDSURG Nursing, 6,* 209–212.

Ducharme, F., Levesque, L., & Gendron, M., et al. (2001). Development process and qualitative evaluation of a program to promote the mental health of family caregivers. *Clinical Nursing Research, 10*(2), 182–201.

Edwards, N., Cere, M., & Leblond, D. (1993). A community-based intervention to prevent falls among seniors. *Family & Community Health, 15*(4), 57–65.

Estabrooks, C.A., Midodzi, W.K., & Cummings, G.G., et al. (2007). Predicing research use in nursing organizations. *Nursing Research, 5*(4S), S7–S23.

Fawcett, J. (1989). *Analysis and evaluation of conceptual models of nursing* (2nd ed.). Philadelphia: F.A. Davis.

Gagnon, A.J. (1999). Do editors have anything to teach us? A review of 30 years of journal editorials. *Canadian Journal of Nursing Research, 30*(4), 23–26.

Gallagher, E.M. & Scott, V.J. (1997). The STEPS project: Participatory action research to reduce falls in public places among seniors and persons with disabilities. *Canadian Journal of Public Health, 88*(2), 129–133.

Gottlieb, L.N. (1999). From nursing papers to research journal: A 30-year odyssey [Editorial]. *Canadian Journal of Nursing Research, 30*(4), 9–14.

Graydon, J., Sidani, S., & Irvine, D., et al. (1998). Literature review of cancer-related fatigue. *Canadian Oncology Nursing Journal, 8*(Suppl 1), S5.

Hannah, M.E., Hannah, W.J., & Hewson, S.A., et al. for the Breech Trial Collaborative Group. (2000). Planned caesarian section versus planned vaginal birth for breech presentation at term: A randomized multicentre trial. *Lancet, 356,* 1375–1383.

Jennings, B.M. (2000). Evidence-based practice: The road best traveled? [Editorial]. *Research in Nursing & Health, 23,* 343–345.

Johnson, J.L., Ratner, P.A., & Bottoroff, J.L., et al. (2000). Preventing smoking relapse in postpartum women. *Nursing Research, 49,* 44–52.

Kitson, A., Harvey, G., & McCormack, B. (1998). Enabling the implementation of evidence-based practice: A conceptual framework. *Quality in Health Care, 7,* 149–158.

Kitson, A.L., Rycroft-Malone, J., & Harvey, G., et al. (2008). Evaluating the successful implementation of evidence into practice using the PARiHS framework: Theoretical and practical challenges. *Implementation Science, 1,* 3. (http://www.implementationscience.com/content/1/1/3).

Lau, J., Ioannidis, J.P., & Schmid, C.H. (1998). Quantitative synthesis in systematic reviews. In C. Mulrow & D. Cook (Eds.), *Systematic reviews.* Philadelphia: American College of Physicians.

McGillis Hall, L., Doran, D.I., Baker, G.R., et al. (2001). *The impact of nursing staff mix models and organizational strategies on patient, system and nurse outcomes. Final report.* Toronto: University of Toronto.

Medical Research Council of Canada. [Online]. Retrieved April 2, 2005, from http://strategis.ic.gc.ca/epic/internet/inrti-rti.nsf/en/te01458e.html.

Morse, J.M. (2001). Preventing falls in the elderly. *Reflections on Nursing Leadership, 27*(1), 26–27.

Morse, J.M. & Proctor, A. (1998). Maintaining patient endurance . . . the comfort work of trauma nurses. *Clinical Nursing Research, 7*(3), 250–274.

Mulrow, C. & Cook, D. (1998). *Systematic reviews.* Philadelphia: American College of Physicians.

Nagle, L.M., White, P., & Pringle, D. (2007). Collecting outcomes in spite of our systems. *Canadian Journal of Nursing Informatics, 2*(3), 4–8.

O'Brien-Pallas, L. (2002). Where to from here? *Canadian Journal of Nursing Research, 33*(4), 3–14.

O'Brien-Pallas, L.L., Doran, D.I., Murray, M., et al. (2002). Evaluation of a client care delivery model, Part 2: Variability in client outcomes in community home nursing. *Nursing Economics, 20*(1), 13–21.

O'Connor, A.M. & Bouchard, J.L. (1991). Research activities in Canadian university schools and faculties of nursing for 1988–1989. *Canadian Journal of Nursing Research, 23*(1), 57–65.

Paterson, B. (2001). The shifting perspective model of chronic illness. *Journal of Nursing Scholarship, 33*(1), 21–26.

Petticrew, M. (2001). Systematic reviews from astronomy to zoology. *British Medical Journal, 322,* 98–101.

Ploeg, J., Ciliska, D., & Dobbins, M., et al. (1996). A systematic review of adolescent suicide prevention programs. *Canadian Journal of Public Health, 87*(5), 319–324.

Ratner, P.A., Johnson, J.L., & Bottoroff, J.L. (2001). Mothers' efforts to protect their infants from environmental tobacco smoke. *Canadian Journal of Public Health, 92,* 46–47.

Ritchie, J.A. (1992). Research issues. In A.J. Baumgart & J. Larsen (Eds.), *Canadian nursing faces the future.* St. Louis: Mosby.

Rycroft-Malone, J. (2007). Theory and knowledge translation. *Nursing Research, 56*(4S), S78–S85.

Sidani, S. & Braden, C.J. (1998). *Evaluating nursing interventions: A theory-driven approach.* Thousand Oaks, CA: Sage.

Stevens, B.J. & Johnston, C.C. (1994). Physiologic responses of premature infants to a painful stimulus. *Nursing Research, 43,* 226–231.

Stevens, B., Johnston, C., & Franck, L., et al. (1999). The efficacy of developmentally sensitive interventions and sucrose for relieving procedural pain in very low birth weight neonates. *Nursing Research, 48,* 35–43.

Stevens, B.J., Johnston, C.C., & Horton, L. (1994). Factors that influence the behavioural pain responses of premature infants. *Pain, 59,* 101–109.

Thorne, S. & Paterson, B. (2001). Health care professional support for self care in chronic illness: Insights from diabetes research. *Patient Education and Counseling, 42,* 81–90.

White, P. & Pringle, D. (2005). Collecting patient outcomes for real: The nursing and health outcomes project. *Canadian Journal of Nursing Leadership, 18*(1), 26–33.

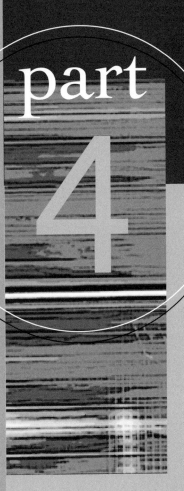

WORKPLACE REALITIES

part

4

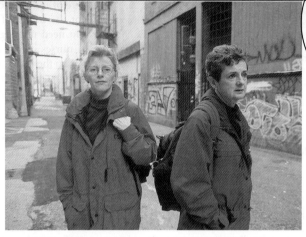

Nurses work in many environments and adapt to many conditions. The setting for these nurses is the inner city. (Photography by Chuck Russell. Used with permission from *Canadian Nurse*.)

Issues Arising From the Nature of Nurses' Work and Workplaces

Carol McDonald
Marjorie McIntyre

Critical Questions

As a way of engaging with the ideas in this chapter, consider the following:

1. Before beginning your nursing education, where did you imagine that nurses worked? How has that changed for you?

2. Before your first practicum experience, what work did you imagine nurses would do? How does this fit with the realities of your nursing experience?

3. What do you think nurses would identify as their major concerns around their work and their workplaces?

4. As a student, what, if any, concerns do you have about your future work and workplaces?

Chapter Objectives

After completing this chapter, you will be able to:

1. Articulate issues arising from the nature of nurses' work and their workplaces.

2. Frame and analyze issues arising from the nature of nurses' work and the places in which that work is carried out.

3. Identify barriers to resolving issues arising in nurses' work and workplaces.

4. Formulate strategies for resolving issues arising in nurses' work and workplaces.

5 Trace the links between nurses' work, nurses' health, and the health of Canadians.

6 Recognize the conflicting loyalties between the goals of organizations and nurses' professional goals.

This chapter highlights relevant issues arising from the nature of nurses' work and the significance of these issues for the health of nurses and the health of Canadians who need nursing care. Issues arising from the nature of nurses' work are closely related to and sometimes overlap the issues arising within the environments in which nurses' work takes place. However, there is increasing Canadian and international research substantiating the importance of understanding the nature of nurses' work as distinct from nurses' work environments. Thus, this chapter highlights some of the distinctions between the issues arising from the work that nurses do and the places in which this work takes place.

THE NATURE OF NURSES' WORK

Themes throughout the literature on the changing nature of nurses' work include confusion about what constitutes nurses' work, the increasing demands of nurses' work, the lack of control that nurses have over the work they do, and the incongruity between what nurses are prepared as professionals to do and what they are expected to do in practice.

The lack of clarity in defining nurses' work is due in part to the lack of clear boundaries between nurses' work and non-nurses' work and the increasing expectation that nurses perform work other than nursing care. Changes in administrative structures and in the way auxiliary workers are utilized means nurses take on work that has been traditionally performed by others. In other situations, nursing practices have been relinquished to auxiliary workers. In addition to the increasing demand to do more work, nurses are also faced with the increasing demands of the work itself. Patients in care are more acutely ill, and the care nurses provide is increasingly complex. There are demands on nurses for increasing technical competence.

In practice, nurses are often faced with a lack of control over the work they do. Decisions about what care will be provided, who will provide that care, and in what setting the care will be provided are made by someone other than the nurses expected to provide the care. Nurses' work often occurs in a climate of diminished resources without support to meet the demands of their work with competence and confidence. The increased demands of nurses' work and the lack of support provided to sustain the work may contribute to the disturbing reality that nurses are unable to nurse in the ways that they have come to expect they should. Nurses increasingly experience incongruities between the work that they are prepared to do, both educationally and philosophically, and the expectations that they encounter in practice.

THE NATURE OF NURSES' WORKPLACES

The nature of nurses' work and the workplaces themselves are interrelated; both contribute to nurses' experiences of job satisfaction, recruitment and retention, and well-being. For example, many writers and researchers have linked Canada's current nursing shortage to inadequate and inferior work environments (Ceci & McIntyre, 2001). Baumann and others (2001) claim, "Canada's nursing shortage is at least in part due to a work environment that burns out the experienced and discourages new recruits. But that environment can be changed" (p. iii). Despite the seriousness of the real and potential shortcomings of nurses' work environments, there is evidence that governments, employers, and nurses are taking action to improve the situation. Further, there is an acknowledgment on the part of these groups that they must work together to create and maintain healthy nurse workplaces. Research suggests that recruitment and retention strategies will be successful only if this action is implemented on a large scale (Sochalski, 2001). More recently, Laschinger (2001) suggests that despite our knowledge of what constitutes healthy workplaces for nurses, we have yet to act on this evidence.

Understanding what constitutes a healthy work environment and selecting those environments in which to work will positively affect not only the individual's work-life experience but also the quality of care that individual is able to deliver. As more desirable work environments are created, nurses already in practice will undoubtedly be attracted to those employment situations, promoting the continued production of healthy work environments. Some employers offer nurses and other employees onsite services that have been identified as indicative of a quality work environment, such as fitness centers, hot food services 24 hours a day, wellness programs, and provision of onsite childcare (Baumann et al., 2001).

THE SIGNIFICANCE OF NURSES' WORK ISSUES

Issues arising from the nature of nurses' work relate directly to the recruitment and retention of nurses, the health of the nursing workforce, and the quality of care that nurses are able to deliver. The belief that all we need to do to address the recurrent shortages of nurses is to produce more nurses overlooks the point that it is the issues arising from the nature of nurses' work that sustain and perpetuate nursing shortages. Unless these issues are addressed, it is unlikely that existing vacancies will be filled, that student enrollments will increase, or that nurses, given other opportunities, will stay in nursing. This chapter challenges the inevitability of healthcare systems doing more with less in the short term when downsizing and restructuring occur at the expense of nurses' health and well-being (Table 15.1).

For the most part, nurses' work environments are and always have been complex, and barriers to providing quality professional practice environments are considerable. However, given the authority, adequate resources, and support of colleagues, it is assumed at the outset of writing this chapter that nurses can provide such quality practice environments as those envisioned by the Canadian Nurses Association (CNA).

Table 15.1	Employment Predictions for Nurses in 2011		
BETWEEN 1993 AND 2011 NUMBER OF NURSES MUST INCREASE	LOW GROWTH: 23%	MEDIUM GROWTH: 34.5%	HIGH GROWTH: 46%
Number of RNs employed, 1993	235,630	235,630	235,630
Number of RNs employed, 1996	227,830	227,830	227,830
Projected number of RNs required, 2011	290,000	317,000	344,000
Additional RNs required, 2011	62,000	89,000	116,000
Projected number of RNs available, 2011	231,000	231,000	231,000
Projected shortage of RNs	**59,000**	**86,000**	**113,000**

Source: Compiled from data collected by the Canadian Nurses Association. Used with permission.

According to the CNA position statement (2001, p. 1) on nurses' work environments, nurses have an obligation to their patients to "demand practice environments that have the organizational and human support allocations necessary for safe, competent and ethical nursing care." The CNA position states that a quality nursing practice environment for professional nurses is one in which "the needs and goals of the individual nurse are met at the same time the patient or client is assisted to reach his or her individual health goals, within the costs and quality framework mandated by the organization where the care is provided" (p. 1). The CNA holds that the development and support of quality practice environments for professional nurses are responsibilities shared by practitioners, employers, regulatory bodies, professional associations, educational institutions, unions, and the public.

In November 2006 the CNA Board of Directors approved a joint position statement titled "Practice Environments: Maximizing Client, Nurse and System Outcomes," jointly developed by the CNA and the Canadian Federation of Nursing Unions (CFNU). This document extends the earlier CNA position statement by identifying seven characteristics of quality practice environments (Box 15.1).

 ## ISSUES ARISING IN NURSES' WORK AND WORKPLACES

In the face of indisputable evidence that there are too few nurses to fill current positions and predictions that the shortage will worsen, recognition that issues related to the nature of nurses' work can and must change is only beginning. In any discussion of nurses' work, one cannot overlook the nature of the work itself and the availability of nurses to do this work.

Despite the positive initiatives of select groups of employers, for many Canadian nurses the realities of the workplace continue to be reflected in themes of professional and social isolation; disrupted workplaces, resulting in alienation from nurse leaders, peers, and other professionals; inadequate educational, mentorship, and orientation programs; decreased levels of support for professional development; and the failure of governments and the public to recognize and support the need for change in nurses' workplaces. Despite the well-documented lack of control over their work and work environments, nurses continue to be held accountable for and, in some cases, hold themselves accountable for providing quality practice environments and safe, competent, and ethical care. The following sections contain an expanded discussion of each of these issues.

Increasing Demands of Nurses' Work

Although one can cite many examples of the increasing volume of nurses' work, it is important not to overlook the demands of increasing acuity and complexity of patient care. Baumann and coauthors (2001) conclude that the discrepancy between the work demanded of nurses and what nurses can reasonably give because of increased patient acuity and complexity of care creates an imbalance that threatens the health of nurses and "puts patients throughout Canada at risk" (p. 4).

The care provided by nurses is thought to be more complex than ever before. O'Brien-Pallas and associates (2001) reported that the acuity of patients has increased steadily since 1994. Nurses have the added responsibility of providing care not only to individual patients but also to families and communities; this suggests that nurses' work is increasingly physically, intellectually, and emotionally demanding (Baumann et al., 2001). Studies also show that, in addition to the increased demands brought on by patient acuity and complexity of care, the effects of hospital downsizing and restructuring have intensified nurses' work.

BOX 15.1 Characteristics of Quality Practice Environments

Quality practice environments identified in the "Canadian Nurses Association & Canadian Federation of Nurses Unions Joint Position Statement" demonstrate the following characteristics:

1. *Communication and collaboration*—Quality practice environments promote effective communication and collaboration throughout the system: among nurses, between nurses and clients, between nurses and other health and non-health professionals, between nurses and unregulated workers, and between nurses and system managers and employers.

2. *Responsibility and accountability*—Nurses are professionals; they are responsible and accountable for their practice. Therefore, nurses must be supported in their practice environments to participate in decision making that affects their work, including developing policies, allocating resources, and providing client care.

3. *Realistic workload*—Quality practice environments support continuity of care and enable nurses to maintain competence, develop holistic therapeutic relationships, and create work-life balance. There must be sufficient nurses to provide safe, competent, and ethical care. Together with supportive employer policies and effective relationships with team members, sufficient time will allow nurses to practise at their full level of competence, to meet the "Code of Ethics for Registered Nurses" and to meet jurisdictional standards of practice.

4. *Leadership*—Effective leadership is important in all nursing roles and is an essential element for quality practice environments. Nurses who are employers have a direct impact on nurses' work environments, but nurses who act as collaborators, communicators, mentors, role models, visionaries, and advocates for quality care also play a leadership role.

5. *Support for information and knowledge management*—Quality practice environments include enabling technologies to support optimal information and knowledge management as well as critical thinking (e.g., electronic health records and decision support tools). Adequate time for nurses to access these technologies is important.

6. *Professional development*—Quality practice environments must be adequately funded to allow nurses to access professional development opportunities to develop and maintain competence. These opportunities include continuing education, formal education, online learning, and mentoring.

7. *Workplace culture*—A quality practice environment creates a workplace culture that values the well-being of clients and employees. The culture must be continually assessed and evaluated with an interest in improving client, nursing, and system outcomes. Contributions to a positive workplace culture include, but are not limited to, policies that address ethical issues, support safety, promote employee recognition, and ensure adequate resources.

Source: Canadian Nurses Association (CNA) & Canadian Federation of Nurses Unions (CFNU) Joint Position Statement. *Practice environments: Maximizing client, nurse and system outcomes* (2006).

Other research highlights the "load" that nurses' work puts on nurses (Gaudine, 2000). In a descriptive study in which 31 nurses were interviewed, Gaudine offers compelling narration of the experiences of workload—and work overload—from the accounts of these nurses. Although nurses' descriptions of what constituted work overload varied significantly, a brief glimpse of the richness of these accounts is offered in the following examples.

Simultaneous demands were apparent in situations in which study subjects talked about being expected to do more than one thing at a time and to be in more that one place at a time:

A doctor is asking me questions. . . . Meanwhile a patient's relative is standing beside me and wants something, and the phone is ringing. I have to get a patient ready to go to X-ray. Then the doctor wants a dressing changed and I know the vitals need taking on my patient receiving blood (Gaudine, 2000, p. 24).

In a second example of work overload, Gaudine (2000) describes "qualitative work overload," in which the nurses' experiences of work overload are attributed by the nurses to the unfamiliar nature of the work. The following example richly illuminates one nurse's experience with this:

It was the night shift, and I had never done [total parenteral nutrition (TPN)] before. I had eight charts to look over. The TPN lines hadn't been changed on days and had to be done for around 8 PM. I spent a half hour with the procedure manual, which for me is useless. I want to see it, not just read it. The dressing set didn't have what the procedure book said it would. It was 9:30 PM by the time I finished it, and I hadn't even looked at the other patients' charts (p. 25).

"Heavy load" is another dimension of the work that Gaudine (2000) describes. Heavy load involves situations in which there is just too much work to do and is exemplified by this nurse's response:

I can't believe we have to be here for twelve hours and often have to miss our breaks. And I just get the expectations of nurses is really, like super nurse, to do an incredible amount, and I think it is just too much. To work twelve hours, and I can't even go out to lunch, like at any other job (p. 25).

The final example of work overload is illustrated by a situation in which nurses are, by virtue of their competence and experience, responsible directly for the care of the patients assigned to them and also responsible indirectly for the patients assigned to other nurses on their unit. One of the nurses in Gaudine's (2000) study talks about this dilemma in a way that resonates with other accounts throughout the literature: "Most [nurses] are more junior than me and may have trouble doing new things . . . Just to be cautious, I stayed on the unit at break today, because there was a very sick child and so many new nurses" (p. 25).

Many researchers and practicing nurses identify workload as the most significant issue for nurses directly and indirectly because of links between nurses' work, nurses' health, and the health of patients in their care (Baumann et al., 2001; Burke & Greenglass, 2000; Cockerill & O'Brien-Pallas, 1990; Laschinger & Leiter, 2006; O'Brien-Pallas et al., 1997; Shullanberger, 2000; White, 1997).

Incongruities Between Nurses' Work as Taught and Practised

The lack of clarity about what constitutes nurses' work and the increasing demands of nurses' work life have hindered the development of a professional role for nurses. The professional role of nurses is further hindered by incongruities that exist between "nursing as taught and nursing as practiced, between nursing as experienced by nurses and nursing as perceived by others" (Ceci & McIntyre, 2001, p. 123). The incongruities that are raised "when nurses find themselves unable to nurse as they had envisioned, as they can or believe they should" (p. 123), undermine the meaning that nurses find in their work. Researchers who interviewed practicing nurses claim "nurses find meaning in their work when they are able to care for patients performing in a way that conforms to the philosophy of care held by the nursing profession" (Baumann et al., 2001, p. 8).

In considering the meaning that nurses find in their work, it is important to recognize that nurses have a different experience than other members of the healthcare system. And this difference, rather than being trivial or blatantly obvious, "holds ethical and political meanings and implications for nurses and for our practices" (Ceci & McIntyre, 2001, p. 127). The professional role for nurses (i.e., their understanding of their scope of practice) develops through both education and practice experiences. For many nurses, this scope of practice makes central a holistic approach to the care of patients and their families. However, in contemporary practice, a "treatment-oriented medical model" often overrides the nurse's scope of practice (Baumann et al., 2001, p. 9). When faced with demanding workloads and the dissonance of conflicting approaches to care, nurses' work becomes reconfigured as tasks. In addition, when nurses' interpretations of what is occurring in practice are excluded from policy discussions, "a sense of being incorrect, in some essential sense, in their understanding of themselves and their work comes into play" (Ceci & McIntyre, 2001, p. 123).

Lack of Control Over Nurses' Work

Commitment and Care: The Benefits of Healthy Workplaces for Nurses, Their Patients and the System, by Baumann and others (2001), makes an important contribution to our understanding of issues arising from the nature of nurses' work in Canada. Drawing on the earlier work of Kristensen (1999), Baumann identified six principles that constitute an optimal work environment for nurses' social and psychological well-being. Baumann's work incorporates a review of current literature, including relevant policy documents on the topic as well as the findings of focus group discussions with nurses in practice across Canada.

This chapter draws on the findings of Baumann's work to support discussions of issues of control and support in nurses' work. The term *control* as it is used here can be understood as both control over the work that nurses do and control over the ways in which that work is organized in practice. Baumann and colleagues introduce the finding that "establishing a professional role is a prerequisite for establishing control over practice" (2001, p. 9). They further link control over practice to job satisfaction and greater latitude in decision making to decreased turnover of nurses in practice.

Baumann and others reported that focus group participants strongly supported the need for nurses to have input into the "patient-care decisions related to their practice" (2001, p. 9). Nurses stressed the importance of having their say in "all aspects of care within their scope of practice, including serving as patient advocates" (p. 9). Nurses in this study experienced difficulty in playing "significant roles in policy-making" or in communicating "effectively with decision makers" because of being "under-represented in institutional hierarchies" (p. 10).

For nurses to experience control over their work, they must be central in the policy decisions that direct work-life issues, such as scheduling, full-time to part-time staff ratios, casual nurses, and auxiliary workers. Although nurses are often left with the responsibility of calling in relief staff and implementing mandatory overtime, there are still too few instances in which nurses have meaningful input into the policies that determine these arrangements. The failure to gain control over and have meaningful input into one's practice, generated by the demands of mandatory overtime and the high rates of relief staff, influences nurses' commitment to their practice and the decisions they make about remaining in practice. Nurses who are satisfied with their work and the organization of their work schedules show a higher commitment to their practice. Research shows that the job satisfaction level of the nursing staff strongly determines the satisfaction level of the patients in their care (Baumann et al., 2001).

Lack of Support for Nurses' Work

Central to the discussion of nurses' work is the decline of emotional and cognitive support available to nurses in their workplaces (Baumann et al., 2001). In place of full-time positions, in which nurses knew the people they worked with and were familiar with their places of work, many working nurses have "moved away from the traditional workplace to a world where employers may offer part-time or casual work and employees have several jobs" (Baumann et al., 2001, p. 7). In full-time, long-term work situations, nurses' social support for dealing with professional and personal issues came from managers, supervisors, and colleagues. Cognitive support came from preceptors, mentors, and organizational policies that provided the needed in-service and continuing education for professional and career development.

In the absence of leaders to protect them from overwork, some nurses have turned to absenteeism as a way to deal with feelings of diminished competence, work overload, and mandatory overtime (White, 1997). Research shows a relationship between nurses' satisfaction with support in their work and absenteeism (Blythe, Baumann, & Giovannetti, 2001). It is significant that nurses have lower rates of absenteeism in part-time than in full-time work, suggesting that absenteeism may be related to the strain of working longer hours (Burke & Greenglass, 2000).

Table 15.2	Levels of Education Among Canadian Nurses The highest levels of education in nursing reported by registered nurses (employed in nursing) in Canada are as follows:	
EDUCATION IN NURSING IN 2005	**EDUCATION IN NURSING IN 2000**	
66.0% (166,004) Diploma	75.6% (175,801) Diploma	
31.5% (79,306) Baccalaureate	22.7% (52,927) Baccalaureate	
2.4% (5,954) Master's	1.6% (3,652) Master's	
0.1% (394) Doctoral	0.1% (186) Doctoral	

Source: Canadian Nurses Association: Highlights of 2005 Nursing Statistics.

During the restructuring of healthcare services, as nurses face increasing demands in their workloads, the cognitive or educational support that could once be counted on has been withdrawn. In spite of the recognition of mentoring and educational support as a characteristic of quality work environments (CNA, 2006), financial and professional support for ongoing education and in-servicing has diminished at a time when there is an increasing pressure for nurses to account for their continued competency. Despite the profession's commitment to advanced education among its members, employers provide little support or remuneration for the pursuit and attainment of advanced degrees (Table 15.2).

Workplace Isolation

A review of literature on social support in the workplace and an examination of employer practices suggest that nurses' commitment to their employing organizations has decreased (Baumann et al., 2001). This diminished commitment is due, at least in part, to a belief that employers no longer support them. The dismissal of chief nursing officers, head nurses, and middle managers during restructuring has meant that nurses receive less professional support on the job. Unit nurses do not have the opportunity to build relationships with their managers, an important source of professional and social support in the past. The nurse working in the practice environment has no one to turn to for professional support such as for advice on patient- or unit-related problems.

Nursing teams that take time and commitment to build have been decimated by the redeployment of nurses from their usual practice environments. This redeployment of nursing teams has also reduced the collaboration in patient care and relationships with other healthcare professionals because of the uncertainty of professional practice environments.

One example of organizational initiatives to create healthy workplaces is the Victoria Order of Nurses in the Ottawa region. In this setting, nursing teams have been established to support nurses working with specialized groups of patients. On these teams, in whic nurses are able to develop and use their expertise, nurses not only nurse better but also derive more satisfaction from their work (Baumann et al., 2001).

Although many, if not all, nurses experience some degree of professional and social isolation in their workplaces, rural nurses, community health nurses, and new graduates are nurses whose sense of isolation can be linked clearly to the workplace. The following sections discuss these select groups of nurses (Table 15.3).

THE EXPERIENCES OF RURAL NURSES

Whereas nurses working in rural locations have more independence in their practice than other nurses have, they have other workplace issues to contend with. (See also Chaper 2.) Rural nursing

Table 15.3	Where Do Canadian Nurses Work?	
LOCATION	PERCENTAGE (%) OF REGISTERED NURSES	NUMBER OF REGISTERED NURSES
Hospital	62.5	157,489
Community health	13.3	33,419
Nursing home/Long-term care	11.5	28,965
Other	11.3	28,369
Not stated	1.4	3,433

Source: Canadian Nurses Association: Highlights of 2005 nursing statistics.

environments often include both inpatient and outpatient practice areas, and rural nurses attend to medical, surgical, obstetric, pediatric, and emergency room patients, possibly on the "same shift and frequently alone" (Winters & Mayer, 2002, p. 79). Scharff (1998, p. 20) describes experienced rural nurses as "expert generalists" because they must know a great deal about a "variety of practise areas," possess a "high level of flexibility, work independently, [and] transition smoothly from one task to another and one patient to another" in constantly changing environments. However, not all nurses working in rural settings have the experience and education needed to provide care in such varied situations. Nurses working in isolated communities seldom have the opportunities to update their knowledge and skills that nurses working in major centers have. Additionally, rural nurses face professional isolation in that there are not always other nurses to draw on.

These nurses may find themselves alone with professional care and decision making while being highly visible to the community. "Nurses working in sparsely populated areas lack anonymity, which means they are visible and identifiable within their communities and experience diminished personal and professional boundaries" (Winters & Mayer, 2002, p. 79). An example of the conflict that can arise from high visibility or lack of anonymity for nurses in small communities is demonstrated by nurses' privileged access to confidential information about community members. Unlike nurses in larger centers, rural nurses cannot avoid social interaction with patients and their families. In instances in which a patient's circumstance has social consequences, such as alcohol or substance abuse, the nurse can be placed in an uncomfortable or a situation that conflicts with her or his own values.

COMMUNITY AS WORKPLACE

Although much of the distance nurses experience from leaders, peers, and other professionals can be attributed to restructuring and the deployment of nurses, in some cases the particular workplace undermines the relationship of nurses and the leaders who work there. Home-care nurses practise in isolation and commonly provide nursing care that remains invisible to administrators of home-care services and to the decision makers who fund these programs. Nurses who work in home-care settings may be asked to exclude from their caseloads patients to whom they have been providing nursing care. These excluding practices are based on criteria set by administrators rather than on what the home-care nurses know from providing care (Ceci, 2006). Purkis (2001) describes how home-care nurses find themselves caught in the tension between what they know particular patients need and what administrators and government agencies expect nurses to provide.

Nurse administrators who supervise home-care nurses are also caught in a tension, but their conflicts are different. Nurse administrators are situated between the home-care nurses' desire to base their decisions for excluding patients from services on their professional assessments and the pressure they face as administrators "to reduce the deficits in the face of major cuts in federal health and social spending" (Purkis, 2001, p. 142).

MENTORSHIP AND ORIENTATION PROGRAMS FOR NEW GRADUATES

Another group of nurses for whom the professional practice environment is an issue is new graduates whose precarious job situations as occasional "on-call" nurses have become a way of life (Viens, 1996). To understand better what it means for new graduates to fit into current practice environments and to understand the rate at which new graduates leave the profession, Viens explored the experiences of 31 new graduates over 18 months from five different Quebec hospitals. In this study, new graduates discovered very early on that "they have entered a brave new world where the work situation proves to be very different from what they have been taught" (p. 44). In the absence of the stability that a consistent environment might bring, new graduates struggle for "professional survival." Adapting to a constantly changing environment produces what Viens (1996, p. 44) dubbed the "functional nurse"—the nurse who learns to be "available at all times, to provide care with no continuity and without any hope of ever belonging to a unit." Is it any wonder these new graduates question the quality of care they give or their future as nurses? How is it that new graduates are expected to take their places in this constantly changing practice environment?

Numerous innovative programs across the country support new graduates and their mentors through the provision of release time and reduced responsibilities for both participants. Examples of these programs are in St. Michael's Hospital in Toronto, in the Winnipeg Health Authority, and through British Columbia's Health Action Plan (Baumann et al., 2001).

Disrupted Workplaces

During restructuring, healthcare organizations decreased their level of support for professional development. The shift to program management meant that mentoring and evaluating junior nurses became less common and resources for continuing education were often eliminated. Today, staff shortages make attendance at educational courses difficult even when they are available. In 1988, the CNA developed a position statement on nurse administrators that emphasized the role of the nurse administrator in providing an environment conducive to quality patient care and nurses' well-being. In 1993, the CNA developed a position statement on the role of chief nursing officers, and, in 1996, it developed a position paper on nursing leadership. These statements have been repeatedly updated and offer clear direction for change (CNA, 1996a, 1996b).

However, hospital downsizing and restructuring have undermined existing leadership structures and the vision the CNA documents provide for nursing. Significantly, positions such as the chief nursing officer are being eroded. In some instances, they have disappeared altogether. Changes in the role of nurse managers have led to these roles becoming more diffuse with "a broader scope of services to administer and more managerial tasks to accomplish" (McGirr & Bakker, 2000, p. 7). These changes tend to distance managers from practice and give added professional practice and coordination responsibilities to staff nurses at a time when fewer nurses are available.

Framing and Analyzing Issues Arising From the Nature and Conditions of Nurses' Work

Issues arising from the nature of nurses' work and the conditions within and under which this work is performed are not new. Although the rationale for making nurses' work-related issues a priority has varied across time, overall, governments, employers, and even nurse leaders have failed to address these issues in a way that resulted in lasting effects.

Clearly, more than the temporary provision of resources or superficial changes in nurses' working conditions is at stake in this issue. Each of these elements—numbers, working conditions, and work satisfaction—incorporates underlying and unexamined assumptions about the nature of nurses' work, nursing knowledge, and the relationship of each to power structures in healthcare and society. What follows is a discussion of different frameworks for analysis and the possibilities they generate for understanding issues arising from the nature and conditions of nurses' work.

Historical Understandings of Nurses' Work

In reviewing historical literature, one gets a sense that the nature of nurses' work has always been idealized—and less than ideal (Gibbon & Mathewson, 1947). What we can learn from historical analysis is how the issues have been sustained over time and the implications this has for the current situation and for long-term planning of healthcare provision.

Despite the evidence of declining enrollments and an inadequate supply of nurses to fill current positions, many employers continue to assume that one can still "recruit women interested in self-denial, servitude and the expression of their natural qualities as women . . . the workplace still operates to some extent on that basis—expecting nurses to work harder than ever for less and less" (Stuart, 1993, p. 22). Although many nurses in the past expressed a deep dissatisfaction with nurses' work, what has changed is that, today, nurses are more likely to view themselves as professional and their work as a career rather than to understand nursing as a calling to servitude. With this view of professional work, nurses who stay in the profession do so knowing they have choices. Nurses now have many more opportunities to leave the profession and work elsewhere than they did in the past.

Social and Cultural Analysis

Priorities placed on nurses' work and the value attributed by society and by nurses to this work have often been linked to economic rather than social realities (Donner, Semogas, & Blythe, 1994). The issues arising from the nature of nurses' work would benefit from a social and cultural analysis that considers the social realities of nurses' lives, nurses' health, and the quality of patient care.

A social and cultural analysis reminds us that considering the realities of nurses' lives must include consideration of the realities of the lives of women in our society. Nurses facing issues of increasing demands and lack of support for their work simultaneously experience the demands of the multiple roles in their nonworking lives as women. Prevailing attitudes in society suggest that work and personal lives are separate domains. This attitude privileges particular members of society and fails to take into account the realities of the lives of women as mothers, care providers, community supporters, and volunteers juggled alongside their paid work as nurses. Issues that arise from mandatory callback, overtime, and the increased workload demands of nursing compromise the quality of nurses' lives, their well-being, and their energy to participate fully in both their personal and professional lives.

Professional organizations and individual nurses have lobbied, and continue to lobby, government representatives for changes that would empower nurses to control their workplaces and that would provide the resources needed for safe, competent, and ethical nursing care. Yet as our history unfolds, it is the values and priorities of the dominant culture rather than those that are representative of nursing or the recipients of nursing care that continue to influence this issue.

Despite a growing awareness of how professions whose members are predominantly women are disadvantaged, decisions about nurses' work and their workplaces continue to be made by non-nurses. Decisions about nurses' work and nurses' work environments are increasingly based on criteria derived from business, management, and economic models rather than on the needs of the populations nurses serve (Taft & Steward, 2000; White, 1997).

Nurses and their managers continue to hear explanations of budget cuts that have forced them to reconceptualize services without the opportunity for nurses or their leaders to provide input about what patients need in terms of care. Moreover, nurses have insufficiently understood and critiqued the

Table 15.4	Age of Registered Nurses Employed in Canada in 2005	
AGE	**NUMBER**	**PERCENTAGE (%)**
<25	6,238	2.5
25–29	19,100	7.6
30–34	24,944	9.9
35–39	30,164	12.0
40–44	37,723	15.0
45–49	40,209	16.0
50–54	43,778	17.4
55–59	31,043	12.3
60–64	14,243	5.7
65–69	3,441	1.3
70+	781	.3
Not stated	11	<0.0

The average age of a registered nurse employed in nursing in 2005 was 44.7; the average age in 2003 was 44.5; and the average age in 2000 was 43.3.
Source: Canadian Nurses Association: highlights of 2005 nursing statistics.

ways in which these values and priorities put the needs of the dominant culture over other members of society (Davies, 1995).

The aging of the nursing workforce is well documented in the literature (Table 15.4). Dominant views of society regarding the devaluing and dispensability of older workers threaten to undermine the contribution that nurses continue to make to the profession as they age. Operating on a framework that views all nurses as the same, with expectations that each nurse will perform the same work in a given setting, erases the realities of the differences among nurses, including the differences that may be associated with aging. A British Columbia setting provides a useful model that recognizes both the realities of nurses' lives and the contribution that is fluid throughout nurses' careers. This program enables senior nurses to be relieved of up to 30% of their patient assignment in return for mentoring new nurses (Baumann et al., 2001).

Political Analysis

Typically, issues arising from the nature of nurses' work come to the foreground when recruitment and retention issues arise, but these issues tend to fade from public awareness and concern once the numbers (shortages) problem is averted. Significantly, once vacant positions are filled, concern about nurses' work tends to be put aside as a topic for serious debate. The failure of governments, employers, professional organizations, and nurses to address adequately the issues arising from the nature of nurses' work is linked to the failure to understand the implications of such conditions and their significance for the health of Canadians.

A political analysis asks who benefits from this issue being resolved and who benefits from things staying the same. Nurses and the patients they care for stand to benefit from the resolution of issues arising from the nature of nurses' work. Employers, however, may benefit from some of these issues remaining as they are. For example, the lack of clarity between nursing and non-nursing work allows employers to exploit nurses in assigning multiple roles to them. This exploitation serves managers well as nurses take on the work of other professionals and clerical staff when needed but it undermines the control that nurses have over what constitutes nurses' work. When nurses are engaged in non-nursing work in addition to their patient care, it is the patient care, the real work of nurses, that is compromised.

Critical Feminist Analysis

A critical feminist analysis directs us toward the consideration of power structures and ideologies and to the question of what it means to be a subject of one's own life. This analysis highlights how realities, such as other people defining and controlling nurses' work, influence how nurses see themselves. As the subject of their own work life, nurses would retain control of their work and work arrangements rather than be objects that are manipulated and controlled by structures of power.

Nurses are complicit in the maintenance of power structures when they fail to make central their own beliefs and ideas or the ideas of nurse leaders. *Complicity* as it is used here refers to nurses perpetuating power structures and unexamined ideologies that work against them.

Although the nursing literature and other human-care literature highlight the importance of relationships accompanied by an ethic of care in the work of nursing, there is still an unquestioned assumption that implicitly or explicitly nursing is an expression of women's natural capacities, a view that effectively erases the knowledge required by nurses to comprehend and respond to the needs of another (Ceci & McIntyre, 2001, p. 128). Still "other discourses obscure or slide over the emotional labor and stress involved in nurses' work and instead emphasize the instrumentality [of nurses' work], the tasks that need to be done and [the] pairs of hands" (p. 128) needed to perform them. It is not difficult to see how "these ideas about women, about women's work and how it does or does not require significant knowledge, responsibility and skill are embedded in nursing and become part of nursing's taken for granted reality" (p. 128).

Ethical Analysis

Professional codes, such as the CNA "Code of Ethics" and the provincial and territorial scope of practice guidelines, direct nurses to advocate for patients in the provision of healthcare. Legislative acts, such as the Canada Health Act and the Health Professions Act, mandate nurses as professionals to provide competent, ethical care. Collective bargaining and labor laws are in place to protect nurses from the demands of overwork, to control the hours of work, and to ensure safe practice standards. Despite these multiple levels of regulation of nurses' work, governmental agencies and employers continue, uninterrupted, to demand work of nurses that erodes these guidelines.

Ethical questions are raised about the health of nurses and the subsequent healthcare provided to patients. These quandaries include the risks to patients when a nurse who has worked many shifts without leave or entire shifts without a break becomes vulnerable to fatigue and a consequent increased risk for making errors. Ethical questions may also evolve from the added responsibility felt by nurses when they are working with other nurses whose competence is compromised by unfamiliarity with the work demanded of them or with the fatigue of overwork.

Economic Analysis

An economic analysis highlights how the forces of supply and demand work in a particular issue. For issues related to nurses' workplaces, one may explore the influence nurse leaders have in challenging purely cost-containment strategies when the health of Canadians is thought to be at risk. A purely economic analysis of these issues could lead, and has led, to nurses being asked to do more with less. Sochalski (2001, p. 15) reminds us that "economics provides the framework for the allocation of resources," and the economics question facing nursing is not what the value of nursing care is but rather "how to allocate this valuable resource to best meet the health care needs of our patients and our population."

The difficulty with talking about healthcare and nursing care in purely economic terms is that it overlooks other costs. What needs to be made more transparent to the public is the high cost and incredible waste of resources resulting from the short-term slashing of funds, the closure of needed health facilities, and the withdrawal of life-sustaining services. A point to consider here is that the position statement obligating nurses to demand quality practice environments includes a phrase suggesting that this be done "within the costs and quality framework mandated by the organization where the care is provided" (CNA, 2001, p. 1). The concern is that such wording supports the claim that governments would provide differently if they could, a point that, in many cases, has been accepted without question.

 ## BARRIERS TO RESOLVING WORK AND WORKPLACE ISSUES

One of the largest barriers to making decisions about the amount and nature of work one nurse can be expected to do is that there is little, if any, consensus on what nurses' work is and what it is not. For example, many systems designed to measure nurses' workload measure only a portion of the work done (O'Brien-Pallas et al., 1997). Typically, the focus of such systems is tasks performed without taking into account the complexity of the patient assignment, the nurses' knowledge and skill to provide the required care, and the context in which the care is to be provided. Incomplete assessment of what nurses know and do in their practice results in nursing effort and expertise being inadequately recognized or compensated (Baumann et al., 2001, p. 5).

"Nurses' views of the world are both overshadowed and undermined" by the views of others who "define what nurses are and what nurses are for" (Ceci & McIntyre, 2001, p. 126). This places nurses in the "uncomfortable position of trying to render their perspectives believable or credible using terms of reference which are not necessarily their own" (p. 126). Many employers think of nurses as versatile. In addition to the care their education and experience have prepared them to give, they are known to be able to provide "services for which the hospital sometimes employ nurses' aides, secretarial and clerical personnel, lab technicians, pharmacists, physical therapists, and social workers. They commonly assume hospital management roles after hours and (under certain circumstances) substitute for physicians in the community" (Stuart, 1993, p. 22).

A second major barrier to changing the issues arising from the nature of nurses' work is the failure of Canadians generally and governments and employers specifically to acknowledge the impact of the nature of nurses' work on nurses' health and on the health of patients. Nurses' work, in particular adequate staffing levels, has been linked through research to improved patient outcomes (Aiken, Sloane, & Sochalski, 1998) and to the health of nurses (O'Brien-Pallas et al., 2001).

The reality that staffing decisions are based on funding rather than on the level of nurse preparation or the number of nurses needed to achieve the desired outcomes is the third barrier to resolving these issues. Despite the tools and systems available to help with making staffing decisions, the literature reviewed expresses skepticism about these tools and the need for senior nursing positions, whereby those with the expertise would make these decisions. The staffing of patient care units must be based on the needs of the patients and the corresponding "staffing required to achieve desired outcomes" (Blegen, Goode, & Reed, 1998, p. 49).

A fourth barrier that undermines the control that nurses have over their work and that interfaces with the lack of clarity about what constitutes nurses' work is the balancing of the ratio of registered nurses to auxiliary workers. It is not always easy or even possible to assess accurately how many registered nurses are needed to achieve desired outcomes of care. As discussed earlier, difficulty in assessing nurses' work is compounded by difficulties distinguishing nurses' work from other work that nurses do. Although existing tools for determining a good skill mix have been judged inadequate, there is support among nurses for refining these tools. In addition to the limitations of existing tools, however, the literature is very clear that much more important than the tools are the relationships among nurse managers, nurses, and other team members involved in and influenced by the staffing decisions made (Gaudine, 2000).

A fifth barrier to resolving issues of nurses' work conditions is a failure to see the link between job security and nurses' absenteeism from work, nurses' organizational commitment, and nurses' satisfaction or dissatisfaction with work. Similar to other workers involved in research studies, nurses reported that job security (i.e., being able to count on full-time work despite changes and restructuring) was associated with less absenteeism from work, more commitment to employers, and better physical and emotional health (Blythe et al., 2001).

STRATEGIES FOR RESOLVING WORK AND WORKPLACE ISSUES

Recent research studies provide compelling evidence that the issues arising from the nature of nurses' work can and must change (Baumann et al., 2001). They challenge the notion that these issues are a problem for nurses to address; instead, the studies assign responsibility for the current situation of nurses' work and the threat of a system-wide shortage of nurses to governments, employers, and professional organizations.

Strategies to overcome the existing barriers to resolving issues that arise from the nature of nurses' work are those that "enable nurses to practice in a way that optimises the use of their knowledge and expert judgment" in their practice (Laschinger et al., 2001, p. 240). "Work environments that provide opportunities to learn and grow" and "support creative strategies" in nurses' work are those that will be considered health promoting for nurses and those to whom they provide care (p. 240). Strategies increasing "decision-making latitude" (the extent to which a worker has control over the job and how it is done) will "moderate the effects of high levels of psychological demands" (p. 239) and enhance the quality of nurses' work lives.

In her research on work overload, Gaudine (2000) stressed the importance of administrators listening carefully to the accounts of nurses' experiences of workload as part of verifying what a particular workload might be. Although one can make use of the tools available to get some indication of workload, one should not interpret the findings of such tools without considering the particularities of the nurse or nurses involved. An additional insight gained from Gaudine's study was that even in situations in which it is not possible to alter the workload or change the conditions at that particular time, taking the time to understand a particular nurse's experience of workload or work overload can make a contribution to the quality of a nurse's work life through validation and support.

In the United States and elsewhere, research on magnet hospitals (i.e., hospitals that embody a set of organizational attributes that nurses find desirable and that are conducive to better patient care [Aiken, Smith, & Lake, 1994]) may provide valuable direction for strategies to mediate some of the issues arising from the nature of nurses' work. Kramer and Schmalenberg (1988, p. 13) suggest that "magnet hospitals may be dealing effectively with the nursing shortage by creating organizational conditions conducive to eliminating the shortage." They identified the following attributes of magnet hospitals:

- innovative policies and practices
- intelligent use of staff (nurses are not treated as replaceable parts in the bureaucratic machinery; rather, they are moved in teams)
- informal communication lines and open-door policies
- pervasive and deliberately promoted and promulgated quality care values, including (1) advocacy of education, (2) drive for quality, and (3) the importance of autonomy (including the freedom to act and the freedom to act and fail).

Aiken and colleagues (1994) extend the work on magnet hospitals, which they identify as "like other hospitals except in the organization of nursing" (p. 784). They produced evidence to show that the magnet hospitals in their study had lower mortality rates, suggesting that factors such as the organization of nursing care can be linked to better patient outcomes. Research is one of the most convincing strategies to support the link between nurses' work and positive patient outcomes.

In their work on "moral climate," understood as "the implicit and explicit values that drive healthcare delivery and shape the workplaces in which healthcare is delivered" (2006, p. 24), Rodney et al. offer valuable insights for addressing many of the workplace issues discussed earlier in this chapter. Drawing on their studies with nurses on the enactment of moral agency and ethical policy and practice, these researchers have made a significant contribution to the knowledge needed for change to occur. This group of authors note that nurses in pratice already know what is needed to create a moral climate, what is required is "the opportunity for self-reflection and for true collaboration with their colleagues in management, administration and other health-care disciplines to make it happen" (p. 27) (Box 15.2).

In making reference to the many challenges and limited benefits that nursing offers today, the report of Baumann and associates (2001) on the benefits of a healthy work experience for nurses predicts that if nursing is to "remain a viable profession, its status must be enhanced and the welfare of nurses promoted" (p. 13). In their policy synthesis on the benefits of a healthy work experience for nurses and the patients they care for, Baumann and associates (2001) stressed that governments, professional organizations, employers, educators, and researchers must act together to promote patient welfare by facilitating healthy work experiences for nurses. What follows are a selection of the key points identified by this research team (Baumann et al., 2001).

 ## BOX 15.2 Creating a Safer Moral Climate in the Workplace

- An explicit ethical and moral (value-based) dimension must be included in research on nursing practice and nurses' workplaces.
- The moral climate of healthcare workplaces shapes the safety of patients and the safety of healthcare providers.
- Nurses in all facets of the profession need to be supported in using the language of ethics to name problems in nursing practice and in the quality of care they deliver, including matters of patient safety.
- To improve ethical practice, nurses must work proactively with other disciplines to identify problems in the moral climate in which they practice and to come up with solutions.
- Nurses in advanced practice and in other leadership positions are well situated to identify problems in the moral climate of nursing and interdisciplinary practice.
- In the current moral climate, nurses in direct-care delivery roles often feel powerless when confronting problems with the structural and interpersonal resources available to them. These nurses must be actively and systematically involved in planning, implementing, and evaluating changes in their practice environments.
- Nurses in all facets of the profession (practice, research, management, and education) need more opportunity to reflect on their practice, on the quality of their interactions with others, and on the resources they need to maintain their own well-being.
- While personal reflection and individual action are important, collective action is necessary if meaningful changes are to be made to work environments. This collective action must involve nurses in direct care and in leadership roles.

Source: Rodney, Doane, Storch, Varcoe. (2006). Toward a safer moral climate. *Canadian Nurse, 102*(8), 27.

Key points for governments include the following:

- Revise funding formulas to better support the many dimensions of nursing practice.
- Set rules for using the funds, and monitor how they are spent.
- Support the welfare of nurses by providing funds to increase staff so managers can assign workloads that consider the acuity and complexity of patient care.
- Ensure the supply of nurses in the future by investing in continuing education, including baccalaureate and postgraduate education.

Key points for professional associations and councils include the following:

- Continue to advocate for nurses and advise governments and employers to allow nurses to practise to their full scope.
- Share recruitment and retention strategies, and promote nursing through advertising and marketing strategies.

Key points for employers include the following:

- Address staffing issues by hiring sufficient nurses to ensure a reasonable workload.
- Address issues of staff mix and full-time and part-time statuses.
- Work with unions to develop flexible scheduling that suits both nurses and employers.
- Engage nurses on units in the recruitment and hiring processes.
- Adopt the most effective tools for measuring and allocating workload.
- Recognize effort and achievement with economic remuneration and other rewards.
- Support nursing leadership and professional development.
- Monitor nurses' health.
- Promote recruitment and retention of graduates into the workforce.

Key points for educators include the following:

- In partnership with employers, governments, and nursing associations, integrate new nurses into the workplace through such strategies as clinical internships and cooperative programs.
- Ensure a match between the curriculum and the skills required in the workplace.
- Teach leadership skills, healthcare policy, and work–life health issues for nurses.
- Work with nursing associations on scope-of-practice issues.

Key points for researchers include the following:

- Develop databases, workload-measurement instruments, and human resources forecasting tools.
- Conduct studies to evaluate the effectiveness of strategies to improve nurses' well-being.

The strategies suggested in this chapter are directed toward individuals and groups with the power to sustain or to revise the structures and ideologies that underlie the issues arising from the nature of nurses' work. Societal and cultural analysis, in particular, helps us to recognize that the burden for the resolution of these issues does not rest with individual nurses but with governments, professional groups, employers, and labor groups.

What, then, is the role of the individual nurse in coping with and contributing to the establishment of a healthier work experience for nurses and, subsequently, to improved patient care? Perhaps the most powerful action that individual nurses can take is to disrupt or to interrupt the dominant discourse in healthcare and in society regarding the versatility and subservience of nurses. When given the opportunity, nurses can make their voices heard with governments, professional associations, and labor groups by broadcasting the issues of justice and health arising from the nature of nurses' work as it is currently experienced.

SUMMARY

Although historically the nature of nurses' work has been less than ideal, the changes in nurses' work and the issues that have arisen from this work in the past decade have seriously compromised nurses' ability to provide quality care in some circumstances and even adequate care in others. Nurses' work has undergone dramatic changes without corresponding support to moderate the effect of these changes. Increased workloads and work overload, higher patient acuity and care complexity, and increased job insecurity in the workplace have had an overwhelming effect on how nurses experience their work. The impact of the issues that arise from the nature of nurses' work can be seen in the way nurses care for their patients and ultimately contributes to both the quality of nurses' work and the quality of care they are able to provide.

There is significant research evidence presented in this chapter to support the links between nurses' work, nurses' health, quality of nursing care, and patient outcomes. Studies support the link between the practice of nursing and hospital mortality and nurses' work satisfaction with better patient care (Aiken et al., 1994; Laschinger et al., 2001).

Barriers to resolving the issues arising from the nature of nurses' work are many, but the need to overcome these barriers and begin to address these issues has never been more urgent. Strategies for resolution involve the cooperation of governments, professional organizations, employers, educators, and researchers. The time to act is now.

Add to your knowledge of this issue:	
Canadian Federation of Nurses Unions	www.nursesunions.ca
Canadian Nurses Association	www.cna-nurses.ca
International Council of Nurses	www.icn.ch
Provincial and Territorial Organizations	
Alberta Association of Registered Nurses	www.nurses.ab.ca
Association of Nurses of Prince Edward Island	www.anpei.ca
Association of Registered Nurses of Newfoundland and Labrador	www.arnn.nf.ca
College of Nurses of Ontario	www.cno.org
College of Registered Nurses of Manitoba	www.crnm.mb.ca
College of Registered Nurses of Nova Scotia	www.crnns.ca
Nurses Association of New Brunswick	www.nanb.nb.ca
Ordre des Infirmières et Infirmiers du Québec	www.oiiq.org
Registered Nurses Association of British Columbia	www.rnabc.bc.ca
Registered Nurses Association of the Northwest Territories and Nunavut	www.nwtrna.com
Registered Nurses Association of Ontario	www.rnao.org
Saskatchewan Registered Nurses Association	www.srna.org
Yukon Registered Nurses Association	www.yrna.ca

Online

REFLECTIONS on the Chapter...

1 From your own experiences in practice, describe situations that support or challenge what you have read about the nature of nurses' work.

2 How do you account for the current issues arising from the nature of nurses' work in your practice or practicum areas? Who might you ask or where might you look to gain an understanding of these current issues?

3 Researchers have located the responsibility for the issues arising from the nature of nurses' work with governments, employers, and professional organizations. Support or challenge this view.

4 The idea of strengthening the moral climate has emerged from recent studies with nurses in practice. Reflect on your practice experiences in which there might have been evidence of moral distress.

5 What other strategies might you suggest for resolving issues related to the nature of nurses' work?

References

Aiken, L., Sloane, D., & Sochalski, J. (1998). Hospital organization and outcomes. *Quality of Health Care, 7*(4), 222–226.

Aiken, L.H., Smith, H.L., & Lake, E.T. (1994). Lower Medicare mortality among a set of hospitals known for good nursing care. *Medical Care, 32*(8), 771–787.

Baumann, A., O'Brien-Pallas, L., & Armstrong-Strassen, M., et al. (2001). *Commitment and care: The benefits of health workplaces for nurses, their patients and the system. A policy synthesis.* Canadian Health Research Foundation. Ottawa: Government of Canada.

Blegen, M.A., Goode, C.J., & Reed, L. (1998). Nurse staffing and patient outcomes. *Nursing Research, 47*(1), 43–50.

Blythe, J., Baumann, A., & Giovannetti, P. (2001). Nurses' experiences of restructuring in three Ontario hospitals. *Journal of Nursing Scholarship, 33*(1), 61–68.

Burke, R.J. & Greenglass, E.R. (2000). Effects of hospital restructuring on full time and part time nursing staff in Ontario. *International Journal of Nursing Studies, 37*(2), 163–171.

Canadian Nurses Association. (1996a). *Chief executive officer.* Ottawa: Author.

_____. (1996b). *Nursing leadership.* Ottawa: Author.

_____. (2001). *Position statement: Quality professional practice environments for registered nurses.* Ottawa: Author. Retrieved April 19, 2005, from http://www.cna-nurses.ca/CNA/documents/pdf/publications/PS53_Quality_Prof_Practice_Env_RNS_ NOV_2001_e.pdf.

_____. (2002). *Code of ethics for registered nurses.* Ottawa: Author.

_____. (2006). *Joint position statement: Practice environments: Maximizing client, nurse and system outcomes.* Joint CNA and CFNU Position Statement. Ottawa: Author. Retrieved July 10, 2008, from www.cna-aiic.ca.

Ceci, C. (2006). Impoverishment of practice: Analysis of effects of the economic discourse in home care case management practice. *Canadian Journal of Nursing Leadership, 19*(1), 56–68.

Ceci, C. & McIntyre, M. (2001). A "quiet" crisis in health care: Developing our capacity to hear. *Nursing Philosophy, 2*(2), 122–130.

Cockerill, L. & O'Brien-Pallas, L. (1990). Satisfaction with nursing workload systems: Report of a survey of Canadian hospitals. Part A. *Canadian Journal of Nursing Administration, 3*(2), 17–22.

Davies, C. (1995). *Gender and the professional predicament in nursing.* Philadelphia: Open University Press.

Donner, G., Semogas, D., & Blythe, J. (1994). *Towards an understanding of nurses' lives: Gender, power and control.* Toronto: Quality of Nursing Worklife Research Unit.

Gaudine, A.P. (2000). What do nurses mean by workload and work overload? *Canadian Journal of Nursing Leadership, 13*(2), 22–27.

Gibbon, M. & Mathewson, M. (1947). *Three centuries of Canadian nursing.* Toronto: MacMillan.

Kramer, M. & Schmalenberg, C. (1988). Magnet hospitals: Part 1, Institutions of excellence. *Journal of Nursing Administration, 18*(1), 13–24.

Kristensen, T.S. (1999). Challenges for research and prevention in relation to work and cardiovascular diseases. *Scandinavian Journal of Work, Environment and Health, 25*(6), 550–557.

Laschinger, H. & Leiter, M. (2006). The impact of nursing work environments on patient safety outcomes: The mediating role of burnout and engagement. *Journal of Nursing Administration, 36*(5), 259–267.

Laschinger, H.K.S., Finegan, J., & Shamian, J., et al. (2001). Testing Karasek's demands-control model in restructured health care settings: Effects of job strain on staff nurses' quality of worklife. *Journal of Nursing Administration, 31*(5), 233–243.

McGirr, M. & Bakker, D. (2000). Shaping positive work environments for nurses. *Canadian Journal of Nursing Research, 13*(1), 7–14.

O'Brien-Pallas, L., Irvine, D., & Peereboom, E., et al. (1997). Measuring nursing workload: Understanding the variability. *Nursing Economics, 15*(4), 171–182.

O'Brien-Pallas, L., Thomson, D., & Alksinis, C., et al. (2001, May). The economic impact of nurse staffing decisions: Time to turn down another road? *Hospital Quarterly, 4*(3), 42–50.

Purkis, M.E. (2001). Managing home nursing care: Visibility, accountability and exclusion. *Nursing Inquiry, 8*(3), 141–150.

Rodney, P., Doane, G., & Storch, J., et al. (2006). Toward a safer moral climate. *Canadian Nurse, 102*(8), 24–27.

Scharff, J. (1998). The distinctive nature and scope of rural practice: Philosophical bases. In H.J. Lee (Ed.), *Conceptual basis for rural nursing* (pp. 19–38). New York: Springer.

Shullanberger, G. (2000). Nurse staffing decisions: An integrative review of the literature. *Nursing Economics, 18*(3), 124–132, 146–148.

Sochalski, J. (2001). Nursing's valued resources: Critical issues in economics and nursing care. *Canadian Journal of Nursing Research, 33*(1), 11–18.

Stuart, M. (1993). Nursing: The endangered profession. *Canadian Nurse, 89*(4), 19–22.

Taft, K. & Steward, G. (2000). *Clear answers: The economics and politics of for-profit medicine.* Edmonton: Duval House.

Viens, C. (1996). The future shock of nursing graduates. *Canadian Nurse, 92*(2), 40–44.

White, J.P. (1997). Health care, hospitals, and reengineering: The nightingales sing the blues. In A. Duffy, D. Glenday, & N. Pupo (Eds.), *Good jobs, bad jobs, no jobs: The transformation of work in the 21st century.* Toronto: Harcourt & Brace.

Winters, C. & Mayer, D. (2002). Special feature: An approach to cardiac care in rural settings. *Critical Care Nursing Quarterly, 24*(4), 75–82.

Zeytinoglu, I., Denton, M., & Davies, S., et al. (2006). Retaining nurses in their employing hospitals and in the profession: Effects of job preference, unpaid overtime, importance of earnings and stress. *Health Policy, 79*(1), 57–72.

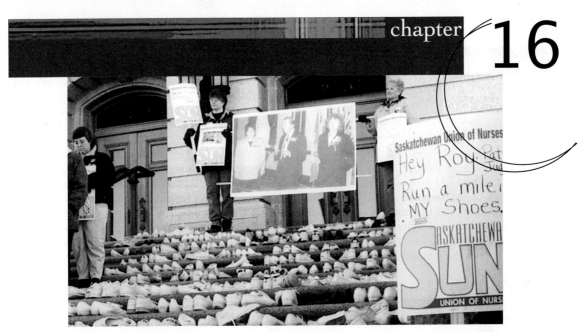

Nurses in Saskatchewan took very public steps to communicate their response to nursing cutbacks and other work environment issues that "invalidate their concerns, fragment their practices, and disallow their understandings." They marched and left their shoes as a calling card, inviting officials and others to "run a mile in [a nurse's] shoes." (Photo by larry lemoal, Saskatchewan union of nurses. Used with permission of *Canadian Nurse*.)

The Nursing Shortage: Assumptions and Realities

Marjorie McIntyre
Carol McDonald

The authors wish to acknowledge the contribution of Christine Ceci to an earlier version of this chapter.

Critical Questions

As a way of engaging with ideas in the chapter, consider the following:

1 What are your views about whether or not there is a shortage of nurses in Canada?

2 What, if anything, have you read in the media about the nursing shortage?

3 Is there evidence from your practice experience of a shortage of nurses currently?

Chapter Objectives

At the completion of this chapter, you will be able to:

1 Identify relevant issues in relation to the nursing shortage.

2 Articulate selected frameworks for analyzing issues arising from the nursing shortage.

3 Analyze selected strategies to address these issues.

4 Identify past and current barriers to resolution of the nursing shortage.

5 Discuss strategies for resolution of the nursing shortage.

This chapter challenges existing assumptions about the nursing shortage in order to generate new ways of understanding it and new possibilities for resolving it. At the outset, it is assumed that the recurrence of nursing shortages relates directly to an inability to see beyond the immediate problem of not enough nurses to the larger issues that have sustained and perpetuated shortages. The chapter then challenges the acceptance of the inevitability of recurrent shortages and the ethos of nurses as expendable, interchangeable, and easily replaced. Finally, questions are raised about the relationship between recurrent shortages and the conceptualization of nurses' work, women's work, and nursing knowledge. The arguments proposed on these pages resist the notion that the predicted scarcity of nurses is a problem that can be solved by simply increasing the numbers of graduating nurses. Instead, different perspectives on the issue are presented in an effort to generate new possibilities for its resolution.

NATURE OF THE NURSING SHORTAGE

The Canadian Nurses Association (CNA) has highlighted an impending shortage of nurses who have the skills and knowledge to meet the healthcare needs of the Canadian population, a shortage, according to the CNA, that has been unequaled in past decades (2002). Historically, nursing shortages have alternated with periods when too many nurses were available for the positions offered by employers. The question that arises, then, is what, if anything, is different now? Before answering the question, we must consider how the complexity of the issue precludes finding quick solutions, such as hiring more nurses, recruiting more students, or paying higher wages.

Hospital administrators, board members, leaders in professional nursing organizations, collective bargaining groups, and all people involved in staffing nursing positions have been and continue to be concerned with the numbers of nurses available for work. When the inability to fill vacant positions is conceptualized simply in terms of shortage, as a temporary and easily corrected mismatch of supply and demand, mainly instrumental or quick-fix solutions suggest themselves. The concern with these quick-fix solutions is that there is an element of distress that remains unaccounted for, suggesting perhaps that nurses suffering and exodus from the workforce "may arise not only from the conditions of their work but also more existentially, from having one's way of understanding the world unacknowledged" (Ceci & McIntyre, 2001, p. 123).

Oulton (2006), the Canadian chief executive officer of the International Council of Nurses, notes that there is "both a real shortage and a pseudo-shortage, in which there are enough nurses but not enough willing to work under available conditions" (p. 35S). This view suggests that if we increase the number of new graduate nurses without addressing the working conditions for nurses, the situation will remain the same. It is important here to view the working conditions not only as the physical environment in which the work is carried out but also as including the factors that sustain the professional and personal well-being of the nurses themselves.

The issue of nursing shortages will ultimately be discussed many times in this book in relation to many other topics. This chapter, for example, provides a critical analysis of the way in which the nursing shortage has been conceptualized and of the strategies aimed at its resolution.

FRAMING AND ANALYZING THE ISSUE

Like other complex issues, the nursing shortage can be best understood as multiple problems—all raising issues for nurses, healthcare providers, and Canadians seeking healthcare. Viewed simply as a problem of numbers, the nursing shortage could be resolved by producing more nurses. Viewed as a problem of working conditions, the issue could be resolved by mobilizing resources to improve working conditions. Viewed as problem of work satisfaction, the issue could be resolved by addressing nurses' concerns about salaries and other contractual issues. Studies on work satisfaction for nurses have identified alleviating work pressures, security and workplace safety, support of managers and colleagues, opportunities for education, professional identity, control over practice, scheduling, and leadership as elements that are as important to nurses as remuneration (Baumann et al., 2001).

Clearly, more than the provision of resources or changes in nurses' working conditions is at stake in this issue. Each of these elements—numbers, working conditions, and work satisfaction—incorporates underlying and unexamined assumptions about the nature of nurses' work, nursing knowledge, and the relationship of each to power structures in healthcare and society. What follows is a discussion of different frameworks for analysis and the possibilities they generate for understanding the nursing shortage, its recurrence, and its resolution.

HISTORICAL ANALYSIS OF THE NURSING SHORTAGE

The point is to write about and render historical what has hitherto been hidden from history

Joan Scott, 1992

The purpose of an historical analysis is to show how a particular issue has evolved and how it has been, and continues to be, analyzed in relation to different points of view. If we draw on the work of feminist historians, such as Joan Scott (1992), we quickly realize that histories are written from different perspectives. Historical analysis helps us to understand the views we currently hold or could hold about an issue. It may also provide insights into how we have come to hold them.

What Constitutes a Shortage of Nurses?

Some questions to answer through historical analysis include the following: What exactly constitutes a shortage? Who decides that a shortage is a shortage? To begin these discussions, consider the following comments that appeared in a 1943 issue of the *Canadian Nurse:*

How would you answer the age-old imponderable—Is there a shortage of nurses? A study made not long ago showed that on November 20, 1942, there were 986 vacancies for nurses reported in Canada. A statement from all registries revealed the fact that 1133 nurses were on call that same day. We do not know what a statistician would make of these figures . . . but, so long as these conditions persist, we must say there is a shortage of nurses in certain vital services (Kathleen Ellis, p. 269).

Sound familiar? What makes these words written more than 60 years ago so relevant today is that there is still no consensus about what constitutes a shortage and the relationship between persistent vacancies and the apparent availability of nurses to fill them. Despite the confusion about whether or not there is a shortage, Ellis feels bound to say there is a shortage as long as there are vacancies in particular areas.

What has continued since, and likely preceded, Ellis' clear conceptualization of the confusion about what constitutes a shortage is this: Until we know better what is going on when faced with vacancies in nursing positions, we will continue to talk about the situation as a shortage. To support what Ellis brings into question, it is not just that the shortage is expressed in numbers that must be challenged but that the number often reflects vacant positions as opposed to nurses available.

Who Is the Authority on What Counts as a Shortage?

The literature contains ample evidence that shortages are recurrent in nursing history. What is less clear and never really made explicit is whose and what authority defines a shortage? Does what we mean by a shortage depend to some extent on the authority of the speaker? That is, does what actually counts as a shortage in nursing rely less on what is happening at a particular moment in history and depend more on *who* claims that a shortage exists? You may ask, for example, if one nurse is doing the work that to be done competently should be done by two, is there a shortage? Or, if nurses are mandated to work past their 12-hour shift, on days off or holidays, is there a shortage? Or, if nurses on a particular unit are overworked, but there are no vacant positions for nurses, is there a shortage? Whether these situations represent a problem of numbers or a problem of management is unclear.

In many instances, nurses are excluded from important decisions about the number of nurses needed, how nursing positions are best managed to provide care, and even what constitutes adequate care. In situations in which well-qualified nurse managers are present, the best-planned staffing can be undermined by so-called cost-containment strategies. Thus, it is not always clear to others or even to nurses what it is that we are short of when we talk of shortages (Ceci & McIntyre, 2001).

How Are Nursing Shortages Created?

In considering how shortages come about in the first place, we need to take into account how strategies for dealing with shortages, such as unfilled registered nurse (RN) positions, are commonly based on the assumption that not enough nurses are being produced or maintained in the system. In some ways, this assumption is true. In other ways, it is a limited understanding of how shortages are created. In many ways, shortages are linked to an increased demand for what it is that professional nurses are thought to provide—nursing care. These questions confound the issue: What creates an identified need, and is this need linked to a clearly articulated need for nursing care? Nurse positions are created for many reasons—which are not always clearly linked to the need for nursing service.

Aiken and Mullix (1987) reported that the versatility of RNs in performing a wide range of other functions "including those assigned at other times to secretarial and clerical personnel, laboratory technicians, pharmacists, physical therapists and social workers" and the ability of RNs to "substitute for physicians" and "assume management roles after regular hours" made it advantageous for hospitals to create nurse positions rather than other positions, because RNs "require little supervision and can assume responsibility for a wide range of duties" (p. 646). Aiken and Mullinex link the increased demand for nurses who for "relatively low wages" (1987, p. 646) can do much more than provide nursing care to a created demand for and, therefore, a shortage of, nurses.

This and other studies do not mention the effects of hospitals taking advantage of nurses' presumed versatility on nursing practice. That it is unimaginable that a pharmacist, physiotherapist, or physician would be asked to take on a role usually assigned to others suggests that nurses are viewed differently than their contemporaries in practice are. Other professionals clearly have the same ability to assume responsibility with minimal supervision for a wide range of duties outside their own practice fields, and yet no one would consider this possibility, making it clear that nurses' work is viewed differently from the work of other professionals (Fawcett, 2007).

Another way to illuminate the picture of how shortages come about is to consider the relationship between shortages and surpluses. For example, the nursing shortages of the 1980s can be linked to the development of new technologies leading to increasing demand for medical services. The expansion of services and increased use of medical technologies increased the demand for nurses, who were now needed to administer and monitor the new technologies. Given that nurses could also take on the care provided by other nursing personnel, the numbers of licensed practical nurses and orderlies decreased. These shortages, created by demand for more nurses to incorporate the advances in technology into patient care, became, in the context of healthcare restructuring and government cost-containment strategies, the nursing surplus of the 1990s (Donner et al.,1994).

What is important to grasp here is that there was no significant change in the number of nurses available. More often, what changed was the demand for nurses, not a decline in the supply of nurses. Increased medical services increased the number of RN positions needed. Later, the reduced funding available for structures that provided nursing positions, such as hospitals and health units, created the impression that a surplus of nurses existed where once there was a shortage. In reality, the number of nurses available for work had scarcely changed.

What is even more important to understand from the past, and what remains important today, is that structural changes seldom mean improved healthcare services. Many would argue and produce substantial evidence to support the claim that these changes have decreased the quality and availability of healthcare services (Taft & Steward, 2000).

Across Canada, the previous decades of restructuring and downsizing have had profound effects. Without a plan of how care would be provided and concern for the welfare of nurses whose positions were cut or those nurses who remained in a system decimated by the cuts, extensive layoffs of nursing positions took place. Nurses struggled and continue to struggle to provide care in environments characterized by heightened patient acuity, intensified workloads, and limited resources. Experienced RNs and new graduates were abandoned by the system they had prepared themselves to serve through advanced education and years of clinical service. Recurrent shortages and surpluses continue to be viewed in relation to numbers of nursing positions left vacant. What remains unacknowledged are the underlying conditions that created the surplus and the conditions—now about a decade later—that have led to a predicted nurse shortage of crisis proportions. What also remains unacknowledged are the effects of all this on nurses. The problem for nurses who make these claims and who continue to gather data to support these claims is that the predictions, however compelling, were not and are not accompanied by authority to act. The concerns of nurses have not been heard (Ceci & McIntyre, 2001).

Another issue that remains unacknowledged and unaccounted for is the weak link between the creating and cutting of nursing positions and the health of Canadians. United States studies of magnet hospitals have shown lower mortality rates, suggesting that the "organization of nursing care" can be linked to improved care outcomes (Aitken et al., 1994). Although a shortage of nurses to provide care undoubtedly puts the health of all Canadians at risk, the biggest and most commonly overlooked risk is to the health of Canadian nurses. Canadian studies show that the nature and conditions of nurses' work (increased workloads, work overload, patient acuity, and the complexity of care) increasingly affect the health and well-being of nurses themselves (Baumann et al., 2001).

SOCIAL AND CULTURAL ANALYSIS OF THE NURSING SHORTAGE

The purpose of social and cultural analysis is to provide the background to how particular issues develop in particular contexts that influence both the way the issue is understood by others and its possibilities for resolution. Important questions to guide social and cultural analysis include, but are not limited to, the following:

- What are the prevailing attitudes in society about this issue?
- What values and priorities of the dominant culture influence this issue?
- In what ways, if any, do these values and priorities privilege the dominant culture over other members of society?

The topic of the nursing shortage is prevalent in the literature and media discussions both within and beyond the discipline of nursing. Since 2002, the global nursing shortage has, in fact, been termed a "global crisis"; "in developing countries the situation is dramatic—a chronic nursing shortage is worsened by the migration of nurses in search of better working conditions and quality of life" (Oulton, 2006, p. 35S). In her paper on the global nursing shortage, Oulton (2006) identifies factors contributing to the increasing demand and decreasing supply of nurses. Demands include shortened hospital stays and increased acuity of care, a shift to ambulatory and community care, and

Percentage Distribution
Age of RNs Employed in Nursing, Canada, 1966 – 2001

Year	Employed RNs by Age					Total
	<25	25–34	35–44	44–54	55+	
1966	19.2 %	35.2%	19.2 %	15.8 %	10.5%	100.0 %
1967	18.7	37.3	19.3	14.9	9.8	100.0
1968	17.6	38.6	19.6	14.6	9.6	100.0
1969	16.8	39.0	19.8	14.3	10.1	100.0
1970	15.9	40.0	20.2	13.9	10.1	100.0
1971	18.0	40.7	19.9	12.7	8.7	100.0
1972	15.9	41.7	20.5	13.1	8.9	100.0
1973	16.3	41.2	20.8	13.1	8.5	100.0
1974	16.2	40.8	21.4	13.1	8.4	100.0
1975	15.5	39.6	21.7	13.8	9.4	100.0
1976	11.5	40.4	23.4	14.9	9.7	100.0
1977	13.3	40.4	23.2	14.4	8.7	100.0
1978	12.7	40.9	23.9	14.3	8.2	100.0
1979[1]	6.2	43.2	26.5	15.5	8.6	100.0
1980	4.7	42.4	28.0	16.0	8.9	100.0
1981	8.2	40.8	27.7	15.6	7.8	100.0
1982	7.5	40.4	28.9	15.6	7.6	100.0
1983	6.5	39.4	30.1	16.2	7.8	100.0
1984	6.1	37.3	31.9	16.8	7.9	100.0
1985	5.9	36.5	32.8	16.5	8.3	100.0
1986	5.7	34.4	33.4	18.2	8.4	100.0
1987	5.3	32.6	34.3	19.1	8.7	100.0
1988	4.8	31.3	35.0	20.2	8.7	100.0
1989	4.2	29.9	35.3	21.3	9.3	100.0
1990	3.9	29.2	35.9	21.9	9.1	100.0
1991[2]	3.5	28.2	35.8	23.1	9.4	100.0
1992	3.2	27.1	35.6	24.4	9.7	100.0
1993	2,7	26.1	35.4	25.8	9.9	100.0
1994	2.2	25.1	35.1	27.2	10.4	100.0
1995	1.9	24.4	34.8	28.4	10.5	100.0
1996	1.9	23.5	34.5	29.5	10.7	100.0
1997	1.9	22.0	33.7	31.2	11.3	100.0
1998	1.9	21.0	33.3	32.2	11.5	100.0
1999	2.0	20.0	32.5	33.3	12.2	100.0
2000	1.8	19.2	31.3	34.3	13.4	100.0
2001	1.7	18.4	30.5	35.0	14.4	100.0

Source: CNA, Statistics Canada & CIHI; Calculations by E. Ryten

Figure 16.1

Percentage distribution age of registered nurses employed in nursing, Canada, 1966–2001. (Source: Canadian Nurses Association, Statistics Canada, and Canadian Institutes of Health Information; Calculations by E. Ryten.)

publicizing the aging of the population. The decreased supply of nurses is influenced by the aging and retiring workforce, fewer applicants and new graduates, and nurses leaving the profession citing unfavorable work environments (Figure 16.1).

The disparity between what society believes it means to be a nurse—a belief that draws many students into nursing—and the reality of the nature and conditions of nurses' work continues to grow. Although the nature and conditions of nurses' work have not changed significantly over time, the attitudes toward the nature of work, the conditions of nurses' work, and the availability of other possibilities for work have changed. In fact, the reasons given for leaving the profession by nursing students in the 1940s, such as mandatory overtime, the valuing of non-nursing tasks over the delivery of nursing care, and reproach for sick time taken (Cohen, 1948 in West, Griffith, & Iphofen, 2007), are not dissimilar from current day workplace realities.

The attitudes discussed above are those commonly held by societal members, including nurses, as the "reasons for the shortage." What is less understood are the assumptions and discourses that underlie these conditions, the values that are attached to nurses' work that perpetuate unsatisfactory or, in many cases, intolerable working conditions. Oulton (2006) reports that "nurses are changing jobs, leaving the country, and leaving nursing" (p. 37S), as she gives voice to nurses' parting comments: "I'm leaving because of understaffing, because we don't have the human resources, because the skill mix is not right, because I go home at night and I am frustrated and unhappy and dissatisfied with myself that I cannot give the kind of care that I want to give" (p. 36S). Other voices say, "I am frustrated and tired because of the lack of support, because I do not have professional parity, because there is not the team work I wanted to see, because my salary and benefits are not what I want. There is not the opportunity for autonomy and for control of workload" (p. 37S). This international work by Oulton raises many issues that are relevant for Canadian nurses; the remaining question is, why, for over 50 years, have unsatisfactory working conditions for nurses prevailed?

ECONOMIC ANALYSIS OF THE NURSING SHORTAGE

An economic analysis can highlight how the forces of supply and demand work in a particular issue. What some call a nursing "shortage" may manifest itself principally as a "problem of numbers," which, in turn, can be most effectively addressed by managing or rebalancing supply and demand. Put another way, nurses are viewed as "an application of technology, as objects to be controlled, managed and understood primarily in practical instrumental ways" (Ceci & McIntyre, 2001, p. 123).

For example, the view of the current situation in nursing as principally an imbalance of supply and demand is considered to be so self-evident by some healthcare planners that it is seldom discussed as merely a point of view. The numbers currently quoted suggest that there will be an expected shortfall of 113,000 RNs in Canada by 2016 (Canadian Nurses Association, 2002). It should be noted that this same number (113,000) was once predicted as the shortfall for the earlier date of 2011. Nonetheless, for some people, particularly those who have either lived or read the history of the shortage, this focus on numbers—on supply and demand—inadequately accounts for what is happening. This inadequacy suggests that more convincing interpretations are now necessary. For some, though, it is difficult to move past the idea that, the nursing "shortage," be it current or forecasted, is a problem with obvious solutions: "We need more nurses and we need them faster," is a view that has shown itself to be short-sighted, failing to address the concerns of actual nurses in its preoccupation with providing sufficient "cover" or pairs of hands (Davies, 1995).

Although understanding the economic elements of any issue is important, this point of view has limitations. Its effects have created problems for nursing—particularly in relation to nursing shortages. What makes an economic analysis so useful is not just what the numbers are telling us but what they do not tell us. For example, vacancy rates are frequently cited as evidence of a shortage of nurses. However, vacancies only indicate "the inability to recruit people or retain them in a particular position" (Ross, 1996, p. 201). There is no analysis of how the numbers of needed nursing positions are determined or of who determines this. New RN positions can be created for many reasons. Ideally, positions are created or added in response to an identified need for the knowledge and skills an RN provides. What is notable is that numbers tell us very little about the different knowledge, skills, and experience that the new positions require. In addition, what an analysis of numbers of nurses or numbers of positions may overlook is the hidden and non-nursing work incorporated in what many positions involve.

In an interesting forum, speaking of the United States nursing shortage, Fawcett (2007) suggests that efforts to rapidly increase seats for nursing students in the "shortest and least professionally focused programs" (p. 98) will flood the market and contribute to the undervaluing of professional nurses in the market place. Fawcett underscores a point made earlier by Sandelowski that a "deliberately controlled shortage of physicians . . . preserves their market value" (2007, p. 97).

These examples are raised to point to alternative understandings that, in the case of Fawcett, raise disciplinary knowledge and practice as critical to analyzing the shortage. In addition, these voices raise questions that ask, for example, how are the decisions to create new nursing positions or to cut back on the number of nurses made? Who makes these decisions? It is not so much that a good economic analysis is not useful in making these decisions, but rather, how are other perspectives taken into account? How much influence do nurse leaders have in challenging purely cost-containment strategies when the health of Canadians is thought to be at risk? Influence is discussed further in the following section on political analysis.

POLITICAL ANALYSIS OF THE NURSING SHORTAGE

Politics is often talked about as the art of influencing another person. When individuals and groups with disparate values enter into decision-making processes, politics shapes the content of what is discussed and the decision-making process itself. Although some nurses claim they are not political, others insist there is no escaping politics. A political analysis can be useful in highlighting the relationship between knowledge and power. To be able to persuade others that nurses working to their full capacity will produce different outcomes, that practice could be restructured to maximize nurses' skills and knowledge, and that nurses are a scarce resource that cannot be spared to do non-nursing tasks is to have power. Put another way, knowledge is power and may be nurses' greatest source of power. Although many nurses have recognized the importance of developing political skills, using their knowledge to influence health and nursing policy has not been that easy. What structures keep nurses from using what they know to influence others?

Ideologies are the voices of power and of authority within a culture. Ideologies are how we come to know who we are, what we are to think, and how we are to behave. Ideologies are ways through which we come to understand ourselves. The power of ideologies lies in the authority they have to define many of our social arrangements as obvious or natural (Althusser, 1971). How do dominant ideologies keep a nurse from accepting one's own ideas or the ideas of one's leader over those imposed by other authorities? The concept of power is not generally associated with nursing. The concept usually refers to the power of major corporations, politicians, trade unions, medical associations, and male-dominated organizations. Despite nurses' numbers and roles in healthcare, it is not that common for the nursing profession and nurses to be considered powerful.

A political analysis points to the conditions that influence us to act or not on that which we know. What follows are examples of changing conditions that have enabled nurses to use knowledge to pursue or influence decision making and policy development. In many provinces, nurses have, through changing legislation, acquired legal powers that legitimize various nurse roles. In several provinces, roles such as the nurse practitioner and clinical nurse specialist have been created, accepted by the public, and integrated into the healthcare system. In addition to the clinical expertise nurses in these roles provide, these advanced practitioners also contribute to the larger system. Through serving on advisory boards and acting as preceptors, these nurses are able to monitor and influence course content in schools of nursing. Through their involvement in research, evidence-based practice, and quality assurance, these nurses have opportunities to monitor activities and facilitate change in service settings. Most importantly, through these changing conditions, nurses' power base is expanded. Nurses have begun to encourage and support nurse candidates for political office and are increasingly involved in professional organizations' lobbying efforts.

 ## CRITICAL FEMINIST ANALYSIS OF THE NURSING SHORTAGE

A feminist analysis looks beyond the experiences of a particular nurse—man or woman—to the structures and ideologies that influence these experiences. Although one could use many different approaches to guide feminist analysis, the questions selected for this chapter are the following:

- What are the structures and ideologies in our world that contribute to errors or myths about a nurse's abilities or realities?
- Is this issue influenced by the power inequities or the hierarchic or patriarchal structures of institutions over patients?
- In this situation, is expert power given authority over the right to be the subject of one's life?

STATUS OF NURSING KNOWLEDGE

Despite our significance in healthcare settings, nurses are thought by many to be "marginal players, and this marginality affects our sense of ourselves and our possibilities for practice" (Ceci & McIntyre, 2001, p. 128). Although the marginal position of nurses can be linked to the "subordinate status of women" and the value of what is commonly thought of as "women's work, nursing marginality is also specifically related to the subordinate status of nursing knowledge" (p. 128). Despite the significant contributions of nurses to health and healthcare, the question of whether or not nursing is "a practice that requires a substantive knowledge base" is still asked, particularly by those outside of nursing (p. 128). As Rafferty (1996) has suggested, this anti-intellectual prejudice attaches to women's work in general. For nurses this becomes a prejudice that contributes to their social and intellectual subordination.

Nowhere is this more apparent than in discussions of how to address the current so-called nursing shortage. Discussions of shortage are all too easily transformed into arguments concerning what constitutes an adequate nursing education. Shortages are and have always been accompanied by discussions of how to shorten the time needed for nursing education, assuming that "skilled and intelligent nursing care may be accomplished in the absence of a broad and substantive knowledge base. Not only does it seem that anyone can be a nurse but that any nurse is better than no nurse—again a claim hard to argue with but one that merely reinforces the intellectual subordination of nurses" (Ceci & McIntyre, 2001, p. 128).

STATUS OF NURSES' WORK

Although the nursing literature and other human care literature highlight the importance of relationship accompanied by an ethic of care in the work of nursing, there is still an unquestioned assumption that implicitly or explicitly nursing is an expression of women's natural capacities, a view that effectively erases the knowledge required by nurses to comprehend and respond to the needs of another (Ceci & McIntyre, 2001). Still "other discourses obscure or slide over the emotional labor and stress involved in nurses' work and instead emphasize the instrumentality [of nurses' work], the tasks that need to be done and [the] pairs of hands" (p. 128) needed to perform them. It is not that difficult to see how "these ideas about women, about women's work and how it does or does not require significant knowledge, responsibility and skill are embedded in nursing and become part of nursing's taken for granted reality" (p. 128).

IDENTIFYING BARRIERS TO RESOLUTION OF THE NURSING SHORTAGE

That nurses are considered expendable as evidenced by cost cutting in the 1990s (1993–1996) was, in no sense, inevitable but rather the result of values, beliefs, and choices among possibilities. An outcome of these choices that seems not yet to be appreciated by the public or by policymakers, at least not in any deep sense, is the way in which these actions and policies have precipitated a certain suffering among nurses, a suffering which needs to be understood as now contributing to both a scarcity of nurses and a deficiency of nursing care (Ceci & McIntyre, 2001). One of the most important strategies for moving an issue toward resolution is identifying barriers that may impede the resolution process. Once the barriers are identified, chances for resolution through mediation, collaboration, and negotiation increase. What makes identifying barriers so useful in issue resolution is that we may lack awareness of the taken-for-granted assumptions that sustain an issue and obstruct its resolution. Nowhere is this truer than in the nursing shortage issue.

The biggest barrier to resolving what has been called a nursing shortage is the way this issue has been conceptualized and understood. Typically, shortages have been viewed as short-term problems solved temporarily either by educating more nurses or by recruiting nurses internationally. Although it can be argued that a focus on the recruitment and retention of student and graduate nurses would go a long way in addressing the current shortage, history has shown that it does not effectively address many of the underlying issues that sustain and perpetuate the ongoing cycle of surplus and shortage.

A second barrier that follows from the first is viewing nurses as temporary workers created to fill a gap in services. In this view, the gap is thought to be easily addressed by accelerating training, increasing head counts, and adding full-time equivalent positions, actions that undermine attempts at long-term recruitment and retention (Brush, 1992).

A third barrier to resolving the nursing shortage is the incongruity between the complex nature of nursing practice and the status of nurses' work and nurses' knowledge. In nursing history and today in practice, it is disturbing how "significant knowledge, insight, and experience that nurses require in their practices can be so effortlessly rendered invisible. How does this trivialization of the knowledge of nursing work itself contribute to what is called a nursing shortage?" (Ceci & McIntyre, 2001, p. 124).

We would like to suggest that it is the persistent undervaluing of nurses' knowledge and the status of nurses' work that accounts for a declining applicant pool for nursing education, increased attrition of students and new graduates, and continuing difficulties with retention. This failure to acknowledge the disciplinary knowledge required for professional nursing practice keeps the focus on numbers of nurses needed to fill vacant positions, assuming any nurse will fill any position.

A fourth barrier is government's failure to consider the long-term ramifications of cost cutting on healthcare and of the nurses who are central to its provision. One cannot overlook the possibility that the negative impacts on the health and well-being of nurses contribute to nurses leaving the profession, nurses not being available for work, and nurses not being able to contribute effectively at work. We should consider the possibility that nurses are refusing to tolerate work environments that "invalidate their concerns, which fragment their practices, and disallow their understandings" (Ceci & McIntyre, 2001, p. 126). Perhaps a large part of the current situation in nursing has to do with how these conditions of practice conflict with "nurses' beliefs about what is necessary in terms of care. Nurses, it seems, are refusing to accept such unreasonableness as part of what it means to be a nurse" (p. 126).

DEVISING STRATEGIES TO RESOLVE SELECTED ISSUES

Nurses, when they have a choice, will go where they are respected, rewarded for their competencies and problem-solving skills, challenged appropriately, and given opportunities for personal and professional development. Creating those conditions need not be costly and will go a long way to resolving the nursing shortage.

Oulton, 2006

Following the articulation, analysis, and discussion of barriers to resolution of a nursing issue, strategies for resolution must be generated. Although there are a wide variety of effective strategies to choose from, complex issues such as the nursing shortage call for particular strategies for resolution. As the analysis of the nursing shortage in this chapter clearly shows, long-term strategies are most important in moving this issue toward resolution. Also, given that the focus on numbers and instrumental solutions has been conceptualized as part of the problem, the strategies section deliberately highlights other possibilities for resolution. Finally, given the concern that nurses have been left out of many of the discussions involving the nursing shortage, emphasis is placed on the contributions that nurses have to make in its resolution. Strategies that nurses can carry out are central, beginning with what nurses must change to move the nursing shortage issue to resolution.

A first and, likely, a pivotal strategy is to acknowledge that nurses' concerns have been largely ignored in the past decades. There is no point in continuing strategies that history clearly shows have not worked. Concerns about the knowledge and skills needed for entry to practice, predicted shortages due to an aging workforce and declining enrollments, and the restructuring of the healthcare system in the 1990s have been articulated clearly by nurses and supported with research. Professional organizations have lobbied all levels of government on behalf of nurses, the health of Canadians, and the healthcare system. History tells us that nurses have not been heard.

Specifically, the strategy proposed here is this: Rather than discounting nurses' experiences or interpreting nurses' differing viewpoints as simply wrong, we might profitably ask why it is that we, as nurses, interpret our experience of the healthcare system and its workings differently from others. In taking up this point, Ceci and McIntyre (2001) suggest, "difference may be most productively interpreted not as mere diversity but as difference in experience and perspective which both reflects and establishes differences of power" (p. 127). The point these authors stress is that "nurses have a different experience of health care systems ... this difference holds ethical and political meanings and implications for nurses and for our practices," and this "difference always plays itself out in a material world" (p. 127).

The specific action that would follow from this strategy would be to challenge ourselves and others to hear what nurses have to say as significant. Put another way, we need to insist that concerns, which are sometimes dismissed as groundless complaints, be seen as the "beginnings of a critique . . . of the dominant modes of thinking that organize the work of health care" (Ceci & McIntyre, 2001,

p. 126). The term *critique*, as used here, is not to suggest that nurses are right and that dominant modes of thinking are somehow misinformed. Rather, the point is to suggest that there is room in the discussion of healthcare concerns for the different perspective that nurses can bring. To sum up this first strategy then, nurses are well positioned by their knowledge and experience of the healthcare system to critique dominant ways of thinking that inform healthcare decisions. The point is not that dominant ways of thinking are wrong, but that they are simply insufficient to handle important issues in the Canadian healthcare system, of which the nursing shortage is one example.

Emanating from this first strategy of listening to what nurses have to say and hearing their views as significant among others' views is the second strategy of developing issues to put forward for consideration. First, nurses, nurse educators, and nurse researchers can draw on a feminist analysis to raise questions about assumptions and beliefs about the nature and value of women that obscure or distort the realities of nursing from those outside of nursing. Second, we must become critically aware of how nurses and women may be implicated in self-invalidation. It is essential that we explore our own complicity in ways of thinking that diminish nursing.

A third strategy is to look to understanding nursing contexts as involving and expressing questions that provide the foreground to the relations of power inherent in the hierarchies of gender, the ideologies of knowledge, and the dominant institutional realities that constitute our practice. By addressing these three dimensions, our understanding, including self-understanding, can change how we understand what we, as nurses, are meant to do and be in our practice.

SUMMARY

Those who understand nurses as something more than a pair of hands or more than technical support for the real work of medicine will recognize the need to question the current situation that has been named the nursing shortage. As we have discussed in numerous ways throughout this chapter, nurses' views of the world are both overshadowed and undermined by more dominant views that define who nurses are; the work they do; and, in many cases, the knowledge and skill needed to do this work. Until we can move beyond thinking of recurrent nursing shortages as inevitable; of the ethos of nurses as expendable, interchangeable, and easily replaced; and of the immediate problem of not enough nurses to the larger issues that have sustained and perpetuated shortages, the current situation is unlikely to change. Questions raised about the relationship between recurrent shortages and the conceptualizations of nurses' work, women's work, and nursing knowledge must be addressed.

Add to your knowledge of this issue:		Online
Canadian Nurses Association	**www.cna-nurse.ca**	
International Council of Nurses	**www.icn.ch**	
National League for Nurses	**www.nln.org**	
Canadian Association of Schools of Nursing	**www.casn.ca**	

REFLECTIONS on the Chapter...

1 What do you think of Fawcett's comment that the "continual quest for additional students in our programs as a response to the periodic shortages has resulted in undervaluing nursing in the market place" (2007, p. 98)?

2 How do you understand the ethics of internationally recruiting nurses, who are greatly needed in their own countries?

3 In this chapter there are several examples of working conditions that nurses have found intolerable. Which of these in your opinion is the most important for nurses and the profession?

4 Identify an additional barrier to the resolution of the nursing shortage that has not been discussed in the chapter.

5 Suggest a strategy for the barrier you have named above.

References

Aiken, L., Smith, H., & Lake, E. (1994). Lower Medicare mortality among a set of hospitals known for good nursing care. *Medical Care, 32*(8), 771–787.

Aiken, L. & Mullix, C. (1987). Special report: The nursing shortage—myth or reality. *New England Journal of Medicine, 317*(10), 641–646.

Althusser, L. (1971). Ideology and ideological state apparatuses. In L. Althusser (Ed.), B. Brewster (Trans). *Lenin and philosophy and other essays* (pp. 123–173). London: New Left Books.

Baumann, A., O'Brien-Pallas, L., & Armstrong-Strassen, M., et al. (2001). *Commitment and care—the benefits of a healthy workplace for nurses, their patients and the system: A policy synthesis.* Ottawa: Canadian Health Services Research Foundation.

Brush, B. (1992). Shortage as shorthand for the crisis in caring. *Nursing & Health Care, 13*(9), 480–486.

Canadian Nurses Association. (2002). *Planning for the future: Nursing human resource projections.* Retrieved July 28, 2008 from www.cna-nurses.ca/cna/documents.

_____. *The quiet crisis in health care: A submission to the House of Commons Standing Committee on Finance and the Minister of Finance.* Ottawa: Author.

Ceci, C. & McIntyre, M. (2001). A quiet crisis in health care: Developing our capacity to hear. *Nursing Journal of Nursing Philosophy, 2*(2), 122–130.

Davies, C. (1995). *Gender and the professional predicament in nursing.* Philadelphia: Open University Press.

Donner, G., Semogas, D., & Blythe, J. (1994). *Towards an understanding of nurses' lives: Gender, power and control.* Toronto: Quality of Nursing Work Life Research Unit Monograph Series.

Ellis, K. (1943). Some pertinent questions. *Canadian Nurse, 39*(4), 268–271.

Fawcett, J. (2007). Nursing qua nursing: The connection between nursing knowledges and nursing shortages. *Journal of Advanced Nursing, 59*(1), 97–99.

Oulton, J. (2006). The global nursing shortage: An overview of issues and actions. *Policy, Politics and Nursing Practice, 7*(3), 34S–39S.

Rafferty, A. (1996). *The politics of nursing knowledge.* New York: Routledge.

Ross, E. (1996). From shortage to oversupply: The nursing workforce pendulum. In J. Kerr & J. McPhail (Eds.), *Canadian nursing: Issues and perspectives* (pp. 196–207). St. Louis: Mosby.

Scott, J. (1992). Experience. In J. Butler & J. Scott (Eds.), *Feminists theorize the political.* London: Routledge.

Taft, K. & Steward, G. (2000). *Clear answers: The economics and politics of for-profit medicine.* Edmonton: Duval House Publishing.

West, E., Griffith, W., & Iphofen, R. (2007). A historical perspective on the nursing shortage. *MEDSURG Nursing, 16*(2), 124–130.

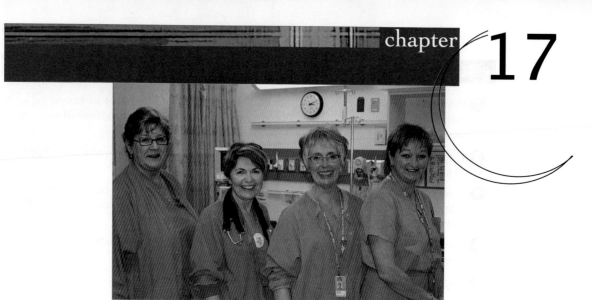

These nurses provide over 144 years of nursing experience on one unit in an Alberta hospital; we can't afford to lose them. (Used with permission of the Canadian Federation of Nurse's Unions. Photographer Keith Wiley.)

Taking Power: Making Change and Nurses' Unions in Canada

Pat Armstrong
Linda Silas

Critical Questions

As a way of engaging with the ideas in this chapter, consider the following:

❶ How do you understand the difference between the mandate for collective bargaining organizations and professional associations and colleges?

❷ What assumptions do you hold about the relationships between nursing as a profession and nurses as members of collective bargaining units?

❸ Attitudes toward collective bargaining vary significantly from province to province and territory to territory in Canada. What do you already know about the nature of your province or territory that might influence these attitudes?

❹ Consider what changes within society and in the nursing profession, as you understand it, might contribute to the changing face of unions and collective bargaining.

Chapter Objectives

After completing this chapter, you will be able to:

❶ Understand the historical background of nurses and nurses' unions in Canada.

❷ Understand the role of collective bargaining.

❸ Articulate and analyze issues that arise in nurses' workplaces.

❹ State past and current barriers to workplace representation.

❺ Formulate strategies to resolve nurses' workplace issues.

For well over a century, nurses in Canada have worked together to improve conditions not only for themselves but also for those in their care. It has not been a smooth or uncontentious ride. Today, the overwhelming majority of nurses belong to a union and many also participate in other collective organizations. New issues are continually emerging and old ones linger. This chapter is about why nurses are highly unionized and what unionization means in nursing today.

The chapter begins by tracing the historical developments that have shaped collective organizing among nurses. The direction and content of this chapter are based on the assumption that in order to fully understand nursing and its organizations today, we have to understand forces that operate at global, national, and local levels. Additionally, it is important to understand forces within medicine that have influenced the demographics of nursing, how nursing is done, and why nurses formed unions. Politics and economics have played a role in shaping this understanding. So have physicians and ideas about both gender and healthcare. It is no accident that the overwhelming majority of nurses are women; nor is it accidental that nurses have turned to unions to protect themselves and their conditions for providing care.

After setting the stage, this chapter then moves on to look at nursing today. Given that over 80% of nurses belong to unions, it is important to understand the structure and organization of these unions. It is equally important to understand the current context for healthcare services, because this context influences not only how unions operate but also the issues they need to address on behalf of nurses and those in their care. While there are some new political and economic forces at work, there are also many old ideas and pressures that continue to structure healthcare, nursing, and nursing unions today.

HISTORICAL INFLUENCES

The nursing schools established in late 19th century Canada can themselves be understood as a form of collective action and resistance from women. Florence Nightingale was undoubtedly the single most important woman in that struggle, although she was certainly not alone. In mid-1900's England, a woman of her class was expected to seek marriage and, in that marriage, to be obedient and passive. Nightingale's early rebellion took the form of writing a novel that was a thinly veiled description of her own life. In *Cassandra*, she attacks the conditions that limit women's minds as well as their bodies. "The accumulation of nervous energy, which has had nothing to do during the day, makes them feel every night, when they go to bed, as if they were going mad" (Showalter, 2007, p. 64). She, like other women of her class, was at risk of being defined as mentally ill, and she saw their best hope in being exposed to "the practical reality of life—sickness, crime and poverty in masses" (Showalter, 2007, p. 65). The industrial revolution had helped create this class of protected women, many of whom started to rebel.

Nightingale used her class position to initiate the first nursing schools, after she had refused marriage, opposed her family, and exposed herself to the conditions of the Crimean War. From such a woman it is hard to see the early motto of nursing schools, "I See and Am Silent," as primarily a call for obedience and passivity or as based exclusively on assumptions about women's innate caring skills.

Of course, women were nursing in Canada long before nursing schools in the Nightingale tradition were established. Aboriginal women practiced midwifery and provided most of the care, commonly saving the lives of the white men who came from abroad to exploit the natural resources (Van Kirk, 1980). Jeanne Mance is recognized as being the first lay nurse to practice in North America. She is also known as the founder of Montreal and its first hospital, the Hôtel-Dieu de Montréal, built in 1645 (Library and Archives Canada, 2005). She served as hospital administrator until her death in 1673. There were also nuns who worked in hospitals from the time the French settled in Canada. Indeed, the training systems they developed became models for care before Nightingale (Nelson,

2001). Many other women did what could be defined as paid nursing work. Hospitals tended to be either military ones that employed mainly male nurses or religious ones that employed nuns, with some charitable hospitals and private homes employing other women. "By the mid-nineteenth century in English Canada, it can be said that nursing had become a 'trade' carried out by working class women (and a few men) of varying skills and respectability" (Young & Rousseau, 2005, p. 16). There is evidence that even before formal nursing programs were introduced in Canada, physicians relied on skilled nurses. As industrialization contributed to the development of both cities and prosperity for some classes, the demand for nurses to work in private homes grew.

The St. Catherines, Ontario nursing school established in 1874 by a physician and two Nightingale nurses marked a significant change (Coburn, 1987, p. 447). They sought to meet "the desperate need of nursing services in Canada as well as of establishing nursing as a respectable profession for women," based on formal education in nursing skills (Coburn, 1987, p. 448). This successful school coincided with rapid industrialization and new developments in healthcare that contributed both to the expansion of hospital care and its effectiveness. "The emergence of the 'trained' nurse followed dramatic changes such as surgery, new diagnostic tools, and other medical techniques successfully undertaken in the hospital setting" (Keddy & Dodd, 2005, p. 440). The development of nursing schools also coincided with increasing activism among women in the prosperous classes who had lots of time to do good work, including the promotion of skilled care by women. At the same time, governments became more active in delivering care; thus, public hospitals became increasing involved in educating nurses who provided labour in return for education.

One of the most notable examples of developments in nursing was the founding of the Victorian Order of Nurses (VON) by Lady Ishbel Aberdeen, wife of Canada's then governor-general, Lord Aberdeen. At a meeting for the National Council for Women in Halifax, Nova Scotia, Lady Aberdeen was asked to create an order of visiting nurses in Canada to respond to the desperate need for medical care for families in rural areas and rapidly developing cities and towns (Victoria Order of Nurses [VON], 2004). In February 1897, VON's inauguration was hosted at Rideau Hall by then Prime Minister Sir Wilfred Laurier as a memorial for the 60th anniversary of Queen Victoria's ascent to the throne. The services provided by the VON have helped Canada through many historical events, including both World Wars and the Halifax Explosion. One of their first major projects was a desperate call to women to join their Klondike contingent to care for the many victims of the typhoid epidemic in Dawson, Yukon Territory (VON, 2004). The VON continues to be well known for their dedication to community building and homecare. Due to their charitable status, their work relies on a large number of volunteers in addition to staff, and they remain dedicated to providing universal, not-for-profit healthcare.

Although the work of activists improved the skills and reputations of nurses, and even some of their working conditions, most nurses were working up to 14 hours a day in return for room, board, a small allowance, and education (Keddy & Dodd, 2005). In Montreal in 1889, the few graduate nurses employed were paid less than the hospital's rat catcher (Coburn, 1987). Some graduate nurses worked as supervisors if they were single or widowed, typically living in the hospital where their life was their work and their pay suggested religious devotion rather than reward for a day's work. Other graduate nurses were employed in private homes, although these women were single or widowed as well. Married women were not likely to be hired, and there was nothing preventing employers from refusing to hire them.

Hospitals were organized along hierarchical lines, not surprising given the tradition established by military and religious organizations. The male physicians were in charge. Indeed, they significantly outnumbered the nurses. In 1901, the census recorded 208 student and graduate nurses, compared to 5,000 physicians (Coburn, 1987). The training emphasis was on establishing nurses' respectability as well as their skills, reflecting both the influence of the upper class women reformers and women's subordinate status in the larger society. With students who were pushed out after three years training as the primary hospital nursing labour force, with graduate nurses working in private homes, with male physicians in charge and with dominant ideas about female respectability, it is not surprising that these nurses did not join together to rebel.

ORGANIZING PRACTICES OF PROFESSIONAL NURSES

As their numbers and jobs grew, however, nurses started to work together for more than recognized training schools. The first recorded collective opposition was in 1878, when a group of Nightingale nurses threatened to return to England unless the Montreal General Hospital improved their working conditions (Canadian Federation of Nurses Unions [CNFU], n.d.). Such action was rare, however. Not surprisingly, their primary model for organizing was the physicians. Long before most of their techniques were effective, physicians had started organizing to defend their interests and to establish standards for education (Naylor, 1986). By the beginning of the 20th century, the allopathic physicians had been largely successful in controlling who became a physician, by establishing their power within health services and by requiring university education. They were also successful in convincing others that their organizations were about public interests rather than personal ones. Abraham Flexner, writing a report on North American medical schools that was profoundly influential in 20th century health services, claimed that professions are intellectual disciplines, taught in educational institutions, based on a body of knowledge that is practical rather than theoretical, organized internationally, and perhaps most importantly, motivated by altruism. However, Flexner made it clear that nurses did not meet the criteria (Kerr, 1988); they were less esteemed than physicians.

Equally unsurprising is the leadership of a Toronto nursing superintendent, Mary Agnes Snively (Mansell & Dodd, 2005), a nurse with a full-time job, who worked regularly with the physicians and who was most concerned about achieving legitimacy, power, and autonomy along physician lines. Snively held the position of Lady Superintendent of Nurses at the Toronto General Hospital's School of Nursing from 1884 to 1910. She began by working with others of her rank to organize alumnae associations, providing the basis for later formation of the Graduate Nurses Association of Ontario. Each province but Prince Edward Island had formed provincial associations by 1914 (Mansell & Dodd, 2005). The 1907 Canadian Society of Training Schools for Nurses became the Canadian Association of Nursing Education, which, in turn, created the Canadian National Association of Trained Nurses ([CNATN] in 1908) and, in 1924, the Canadian Nurses Association (CNA). The CNA, then, was organized primarily by nursing managers and teachers, although the structure allowed for representation of nurses in private duty, in public health, and in hospitals (Mansell & Dodd, 2005). While the CNATN sought "mutual understanding and unity among nurses in Canada" (Mussallem, 1988, p. 401), it also wanted to create a high standard of education and professional honor (Jensen, 1992). Like the physicians before them, the CNA worked to control who could practice and what they would learn. They also wanted schools devoted to "the education of the nurse, and not as under the present system, to lessening the cost of nursing in the hospitals" (Mussallem, 1988, p. 403)

Just as the Crimean War had helped legitimate Nightingale and the other nurses who provided care there, so too did Canadian nurses gain leverage based on their work in World War I (WWI) and II (WWII). Wars made the contributions of nursing visible, contributed to shortages at home, and enhanced women's sense of their own power. In WWI, military nurses "received the rank of lieutenant, along with all the advantages of rank: salary, leaves, retirement plan" (Allard, 2005, p. 157), and the recognition of their work was a factor in the success of nursing organizations in the period immediately after the war. Similar patterns are evident during and after WWII.

This is not to argue for war as a strategy for improving the reputation of and conditions for nursing. Rather, it is to stress the importance of taking context into account in understanding strategies for change. In spite of their enhanced reputations, nurses found it very hard to find employment after the 1929 stock market crash that marked the beginning the Great Depression. One report estimated that "40 percent of the private duty nurses in Canada were almost continuously unemployed and another 20 per cent were only employed intermittently" (Toman, 2005, p. 176). Until the end of WWII, 60% of nurses were in private duty, usually working in private homes, making collective organization difficult (Richardson, 2005, p. 213).

It is important to note that these nurses associations were not nearly as successful as the physicians in their search for control over admission to their profession. Although their lobbying was successful in getting registration and the recognition of the title "registered nurse" (RN) in all provinces by 1922, the first mandatory registration was not introduced until the 1950s (Kerr, 1988). After years of effort, they only had a small degree of self-regulation and did not have the power to police their own (Mansell & Dodd, 2005, p. 202). It took just as long to end the dependence on student labour and develop schools that did not involve free labour. Even when employing strategies similar to those used by physicians, efforts did not bring the power and prestige nurses sought. This was likely because physicians' power did not result primarily from their skills, their education, or the nature of their work. Rather, it mainly followed their effective organization, their class, their position in the health hierarchy, and their gender. Even though nurses managed to meet all Flexner's criteria for professionalization when they officially adopted the International Council of Nurses' Code of Ethics in 1955, they still did not have nearly the pay, prestige, autonomy, or power as physicians had (Mansell & Dodd, 2005). Nursing was still a low paid, insecure profession, commonly with long or split shifts without benefits, few vacations, no job security, and little protection from the whims of employers and supervisors.

In short, nurses were busy doing more than caring for patients in the century from the 1850s to the 1950s. They worked together to establish nursing schools and the regulation of nursing, which in turn helped ensure standards of care and enhance the reputation of nursing. They were supported in their efforts by the growing demand for skilled nursing in the wake of industrial expansion, urbanization, and new techniques in medical care. However, they were limited by physicians' power, the organization of hospitals, and the extensive use of private care as well as by ideas about women and the lack of legal or other protections for their paid work. It was mainly the women superintending the nursing students and those teaching them, along with those working in public health, who organized in professional associations that followed the model set by physicians. These associations were eventually successful in reaching most of the criteria said to define a profession, but they were much less successful in achieving the power, prestige, pay, and autonomy that other professions enjoyed. Clearly, these criteria were not the only critical factors. Indeed, war was almost as important as the nursing schools and associations in enhancing nurses' power and pay.

EMERGENCE OF UNION PRACTICES

WWII, in particular, marked a major turning point for Canada, for women, for our healthcare system, and for the nurses who worked in it. The war ended the Great Depression and Canadians emerged from it to jobs, with a new faith in government and demands for more public services and more human rights. One of those demands was for public health services. They sought access to the medical advances developed during the war that made hospitals safer places that could provide effective care (Armstrong & Armstrong, 2003). Women joined the labour force and the military in large numbers during the war, earning significantly better wages than they had before and gaining experiences that made many unwilling to return to prewar inequities (Armstrong & Armstrong, 2001). Nurses, too, wanted better conditions and more equitable treatment. A number of factors contributed to both their increasing demands and their move to unionization to achieve them.

TRANSFORMATIONS IN HEALTHCARE

First, hospitals expanded and the demand for nurses grew. When the federal government failed right after the war to get provinces to agree on a national healthcare plan, they instead invested in hospital construction and training for physicians and nurses. In 1941, the census recorded 26,626 graduate nurses. By 1961, when public hospital insurance was in place, there were 61,553 of them. The number of nurses-in-training also doubled during this 20-year period (Dominion Bureau of Statistics, 1961). Most of these graduate nurses were employed in hospitals rather than in private homes, and they now outnumbered the supervisors and teachers significantly. Working together allowed them to share their concerns, and working as general duty nurses gave them experiences that were different from most of the nurses who had formed the associations.

Finally, in 1984 the Canada Health Act was passed unanimously in Parliament, and Medicare, Canada's universal public health insurance system, was firmly established (Silversides, 2007). Funded through transfer payments to provinces and supported by public taxation, Medicare was created to provide all Canadians with access to medical care regardless of ability to pay. Five principles were created to govern the administration of Medicare: (1) public administration (on a non-profit basis accountable to the provincial or territorial government), (2) comprehensiveness (all medically necessary services covered), (3) universality (coverage for all on uniform terms and conditions), (4) portability (coverage provided in all provinces) and (5) accessibility (access must be reasonable, uniform, and free of barriers, including user fees).

TRANSFORMATIONS IN UNIONS

Unions were growing rapidly and achieving considerable success. "Between 1939 and 1945, the number of organized workers doubled" (White, 1993, p. 49). Although unions had been organized in Canada in the 19th century, it was not until the war that unions won legal recognition and formal procedures for the certification that was the indication of legal recognition. Labour shortages added to their strength. Employers were required to recognize a union that represented a majority of its employees and were required to bargain in good faith with the recognized union. Collective bargaining, the process of negotiating terms and conditions of work between an employer and a union, became entrenched in industrial relations. In 1944, the year that emergency Order-in-Council P.C. 1003 legislation was passed, the CNA approved collective bargaining in principle (McIntyre and McDonald, 2006) and recommended that the provincial associations be certified as bargaining agents.

Unions not only grew, but their composition changed significantly. Government employees, many of whom defined themselves as professionals and many of whom were women, started to demand real collective bargaining rights. Prohibited from negotiating contracts on the grounds that their work was essential, public sector employees became increasingly restless as they saw gains made by private sector unions for people in similar jobs. Quebec led the way by striking illegally in the 1960s, winning the right to bargain and even strike. By 1975, those in other provinces gained the right to bargain collectively, too, although the right to strike was not granted in all provinces (White, 1993). This meant that half of unionized workers were in the public sector and the majority of those were women. Perhaps surprisingly to those who think of unions as defending private interests, the union movement in Canada has long supported programs such as public education that would promote the general good. In the period after WWII, unions became particularly active in supporting public healthcare services.

Lay nurses in Quebec had formed a union as early as 1939. Following the 1946 Quebec Nurses' Act that provided for collective bargaining, they organized a union with assistance from the Quebec Federation of Labour (Richardson, 2005). They, like nurses who were part of government bargaining units, saw their wages rise and conditions improve as a result. But they did not win these improvements without a struggle. Although the threat of a strike was enough to gain concessions from one Montreal Hospital in 1962, a year later, nurses in the same city went on strike for 30 days before winning not only better salaries and working conditions but also the right to negotiate workloads and to require all nurses to pay union dues (Canadian Federation of Nurses Unions [CFNU], 2003). This requirement, known as the Rand formula—whereby all employees are required to pay union dues even when they do not belong to a union—is now widely accepted. The principle is based on the argument that, although people may not be required to join the union, they still benefit from collective bargaining and should therefore contribute to the costs. Such funding also strengthens the union by providing economic stability.

CNA INFLUENCES ON THE MOVE TO UNIONIZATION

The CNA did not support unionization, and in 1946 passed a resolution against "any nurse going on strike at any time for any cause" (Richardson, 2005, p. 215). The organization did recognize that the poor conditions of work and pay required some action. In jurisdictions that prohibited provincial associations from acting as legal bargaining agents when they included managers in their membership, the CNA suggested associations establish a group to serve as their certifiable bargaining committee and a labour relations committee. The CNA offered advice through its own committee and through a labour consultant. There were several reasons why this was not a very satisfactory solution.

Perhaps most importantly, these collective bargaining agents had nothing to back up their requests. As Joan Harte, former provincial vice president of the Newfoundland and Labrador Nurses Union explained in an interview about her experiences before unionization, "We had no power because we were not organized to bargain . . . nurses were getting whatever government wanted to give us because we had no power; we weren't a union" (Andrews, 1993, p. 1). "When we became a staff association we negotiated and got some things on paper, but we had no power to enforce provisions" (Andrews, 1993, p. 3). The things they won on paper disappeared in practice. With voluntary dues and membership, the association also lacked a firm financial base and evidence of commitment to bargaining agent negotiations. In addition, there were disagreements within the associations between those who did managerial work and those who did general duty nursing. Such disagreements weakened their overall position. The fact that other bargaining units were getting more benefits was something else under scrutiny. As Christine Kavanaugh, former Employment Relations Officer in the Prince Edward Island Nurses Union put it, "the real catalysts [sic] was that nurses who were unionized in the civil service a year or two earlier had gotten significant increases, better working conditions, and pensions" (Andrews, 1993, p. 13). In some case, as Madelaine Steeves, former President of the New Brunswick Nurses Union explained, RNs "actually found themselves behind in salary compared to co-workers they were responsible for . . . I was an operating nurse and I would be in a theatre with an OR [operating room] technician who make [sic] more per hour than I did and I was responsible for her, the patient, and the theatre" (Andrews, 1993, p. 20). The issues nurses faced, and had difficulty addressing in associations that represented both management and workers and that opposed action against employers, went beyond pay and pensions. In hospitals, lack of protection for patients and reporting mechanisms for nurses who tried to stand up for patients were of significant concern. "Nurses were caught in some really difficult employment situations—threats, intimidation," and "there was no onus on the employer to follow standards" (Steeves in Andrews, 1993, p. 22)

The CNA support for collective bargaining actually helped move nurses into unionlike activities, and their opposition to action (e.g., strike or other methods) also helped drive the momentum towards unionization. Nurses' lack of success in trying to improve working conditions and wages with the help of CNA pushed nurses further towards unionization. Then the law relating to unions changed. In 1973, the Supreme Court ruled that the Saskatchewan Registered Nurses Association could not represent nurses in collective bargaining because nurse managers were members of the governing body of the association, creating an inherent conflict of interest (Richardson, 2005). Nurses in Ontario already had separate bodies, and nurses in others provinces had begun to act more like unions by taking various kinds of actions against their employers when the CNA personnel policy approach failed (Andrews, 1993). Thus, the Supreme Court decision reinforced a trend that had already begun.

After the decision, many associations helped establish independent nurses' unions and within a decade (by 1978) all provinces except Prince Edward Island and Quebec had one. In that same year, CNA drafted a code of ethics that would imply nursing strikes were unethical because they placed self-interest, high wages, and improved working conditions before the needs of patients (CFNU, n.d.). Nurses' unions across the country won the right to strike after many long and arduous struggles. Led by Saskatchewan Union of Nurses, Newfoundland and Labrador Nurses' Association, and Prince Edward Island Nurses' Union, a committee was formed to discuss the potential organizational structure, funding, and constitutional provisions that would be needed to create a national organization to represent the voice of unionized nurses. Discussions, which began in 1978, led to the founding convention of the Canadian Federation of Nurses Unions (CFNU) in April 1981. The CFNU allows nurses to share their skills and experiences and to develop national strategies related to their work. For example, the CFNU has taken a leadership role in the Canadian Health Coalition, an organization that works to defend and expand public health services, and has worked internationally with unions in other countries to collaborate on strategies for healthcare change.

Beginning with a mission statement (Box 17.1), CFNU's constitution outlines the structure of the organization, its members, and its officials. The constitution explains that CFNU shall be governed by a National Executive Board when the convention is not in session and that the board shall comprise a president and secretary treasurer who are elected by membership at convention and national officers who are the presidents and or vice presidents of provincial nurses' unions. Currently, the following provincial unions and their members hold membership with CFNU: Prince Edward Island Nurses' Union, the Newfoundland Labrador Nurses Union, the Nova Scotia Nurses Union, the New Brunswick Nurses Union, the Ontario Nurses' Association, the Manitoba Nurses' Union, the Saskatchewan Union of Nurses, the United Nurses of Alberta, and the British Columbia Nurses' Union. A recent addition to the National Executive Board is the President of the Canadian Nursing Students' Association. Provincial unions and the CFNU are entirely funded by dues-paying members. While CFNU has a broad mandate to protect the health of patients and the national health system and to promote nurses and the nursing profession at the national level, provincial unions focus more on workplace administration of collective agreements, grievances and occupational health and safety, and, of course, collective bargaining.

 BOX 17.1 Canadian Federation of Nurses Unions Mission Statement

The birth of the Canadian Federation of Nurses Unions (CFNU) in 1981 marked a new era for interaction among nursing unions in Canada and provided a united front for action on problems that directly or indirectly affect the unionized nurses and the quality of healthcare.

The rebirth of CFNU in 1999 as the national affiliating body for nurses to the Canadian Labour Congress marks another era for nursing unions in Canada. Through this formalized relationship we have deepened and expanded our involvement and influence on the national labour scene.

The core purpose of CFNU is to be a proactive, unifying national voice for quality healthcare and the socioeconomic welfare of nurses and others.

CFNU is driven by the core values of democracy, collectivity, action, social justice, inclusion, and advocacy.

CFNU's vision of the future is to become both a truly strong national organization for unionized nurses, representing all nursing unions in Canada, and part of a world voice for unionized nurses. We will have both the capacity and the influence as the experts on quality healthcare and healthcare policy.

The strategic focus of CFNU will be on building a strong, clear, unified, national voice for the role of nurses, the protection and preservation of public healthcare, the advocacy of social justice and equity, and the development of an international network and international solidarity.

CHANGES IN NURSES' THINKING ABOUT COLLECTIVE BARGAINING

Unionization of nurses both reflected and reinforced a major shift in ideas about the public sector, professions, nursing, and women's work. Until the 1960s, those employed in the public sector were called civil servants, in part because it was widely assumed that they were dedicated to the public good and guided by that commitment as well as protected by a benevolent government. Professionals maintained they were governed by ethical considerations that would preclude forming organizations to defend their interests and unions were often seen as simply defending their own interests. For nurses, the notion of commitment to patients was combined with ideas about women's submission to others and about the value linked to professions. These perceptions undermined progress in the profession as nurses were constantly associated as akin to mothers, saints, and servants.

THE GENDERED NATURE OF ISSUES SURROUNDING COLLECTIVE BARGAINING

As Christine Kavanaugh explained (Andrews, 1993, p. 12), "the idea of nurses unionizing was considered demeaning" and those who unionized were seen as "less compassionate." This idea partly reflected an association in their minds with violence, with ideas that unions "are nasty, they damage homes, they threaten people in their homes," as Joan Harte put it (in Andrews, 1993, p. 4). It also reflects women's place. She also recalls that there is "a lot of interference from husbands and boyfriends telling their wives and girlfriends what was good for them and what wasn't . . . There was a lot of patronizing attitudes from hospitals, employers, treasury boards, husbands—everybody" (Andrews, 1993, p. 12). Until the mid-1970s, nurses were discouraged from questioning their working conditions or salaries. There were neither laws prohibiting employers from firing women when they got married or pregnant nor laws requiring women to be paid on the same basis as men, in part because it was assumed women would be supported financially by men.

All of this had started to change right after WWII, but the big transitions took place in the 1960s and 1970s—especially during the height of the women's movement. The relationship between the women's movement and nursing is complex, and, from a historical perspective, it has often been characterized by contradiction and conflict (Bunting and Campbell, 1990). Although this chapter will not explore this relationship in depth, it is valuable to note that the two—nursing and the feminist movement—have impacted each other in significant ways, though not always positively. Despite the fact that some believe the relationship should have been mutually enhancing, thanks to so many shared understandings between the two groups, particularly their common belief in a holistic approach to women's healthcare (McBride, 1984), feminists have often criticized nursing for a lack of commitment to women's movements (Bunting and Campbell, 1990) and nurses have criticized the feminist movement for ignoring and devaluing their work. Hunt's (1998) review of nursing and feminism's "turbulent history" offers a possible explanation that "a fear of feminism related to negative stereotyping and discrimination against feminist nurses, and the fear of losing nursing's 'caring' aspects, are some reasons why nurses did not want to be labeled as feminists. Ironically, this 'caring' aspect is thought to be the reason feminists have often excluded nurses." This, along with differing experiences and reactions to patriarchy in medicine and society in general, provide us with a sense of where tensions lay during these formative years.

Meanwhile, in the workplaces, public sector employees began recognizing that they would have to become more assertive if they were to match conditions and pay with their private sector counterparts. Commitment did not pay the rent, and governments were not necessarily good employers. The character of unions changed as many more professionals became union members. During this period, women moved into the labour force in large numbers, primarily because they needed the pay but also because many wanted the other rewards of paid jobs (Armstrong & Armstrong, 2001). Women also began entering universities in large numbers, having won battles to gain more equity in access and in financial support. Nursing education was moved from hospitals, where nurses provided much of the free labour and where they were closely supervised in residences, to colleges and universities where they enjoyed more freedom and saw more challenges to old ideas. Experiences with discrimination in both education and paid work in turn contributed to their dissatisfaction with the old inequities in the workforce and in unions. Feminists in and out of unions successfully fought not only for the right to their jobs after marriage and pregnancy and for access to birth control but also for paid maternity leave. Within unions they fought for equality as well as for women's issues to be placed high on the agenda (White, 1993). As a result, nurses stayed much longer in their jobs. Employed in large hospitals, they could share their grievances and work together over time for real change. Meanwhile, the experience of involvement in union actions (such as mass resignations in New Brunswick in 1969) made nurses more militant and promoted their negotiating skills.

Just as they saw that it was possible to be mothers and employees, so, too, did nurses start to see that they could unionize to fight for better working conditions, job security, and pay while maintaining their commitment to care and their code of ethics. Strikes still seemed to go against what all nurses were committed to as nurses, even though some physicians had resorted to such action. What was often thought of as "professional conduct" had not won them many of these traditional union benefits. Asking nicely did not work for nurses or their patients. Indeed, it became increasingly clear that good conditions for work and job security were necessary for good care. Job security gave nurses the right to say no to practices that would harm patients without fear of reprisal, allowing them to fulfill their professional role as patient advocates. It gave them the right to say no to sexual harassment and other forms of discrimination that could undermine their capacity to fulfill their professional responsibilities. Contracts also helped equalize conditions among nurses by addressing favouritism. With job security, decent conditions, and appropriate pay, nurses can provide better care. A 2002 United States study demonstrates this idea by showing a positive relationship between outcomes and unionization. Patients were significantly less likely to die after a heart attack if they were treated at a unionized hospital (Seago & Ash, 2002). Although strike action is the last resort, an action taken when all other avenues fail, nurses also learned that the public continued to support them even when they went on strike.

Joyce Gleason, former Executive Director of the Manitoba Nurses Union (MNU), recalls that in their 1975 strike, the physicians supported the nurses and even helped look after the patients (Andrews, 1993, p. 31). The dramatically improved pay and conditions that followed union negotiations and actions helped many nurses change their ideas about unions. However, outside perceptions of what it means to be a unionized nurse often leaves a lot to be desired. In the media, unionization is often associated with negativity, anger, and aggression. This type of imagery when linked with nursing paints a picture of an oppressed profession, despite innumerable testimonies from nurses who report feeling a great sense of personal and professional satisfaction from their work.

Nurses' unions have had to take dramatic steps to achieve benefits and to protect rights. The most significant example of such steps was probably the United Nurses of Alberta (UNA) hospital strike of 1988. In the fall of 1987, UNA began hospital negotiations with two employers who tabled major regressions, takeaways, and rollbacks. UNA was not willing to be forced into concessions at the bargaining table, and when no Memorandum of Settlement could be ratified, all hospital nurses were called out on strike. Since the strike was deemed to be illegal, the employers went to the Labour Relations Board and charged UNA with causing a strike (United Nurses of Alberta [UNA], n.d.). A timeline highlighting important events during the strike is contained in Box 17.2.

At the end of the strike, UNA was charged almost $427,000 in fines, but cash donations of support helped with their payment. It was not until negotiations in 1990 that most of the benefits of the 1988 strike were realized. In this round of bargaining, hospital nurses received many additional benefits, including an additional day of rest every 4 weeks (8-hour shifts) or every 6 weeks (12-hour

BOX 17.2 United Nurses of Alberta Hospital Strike 1988

- January 25th: The Labor Relations Board granted some employers the right to cease the collection of union dues for 6 months. In displays of support and solidarity with the United Nurses of Alberta (UNA), unions from across Canada began sending telegrams and letters with funds to prevent the financial destruction of UNA.
- January 26th: A permanent court injunction was granted to prevent picketing at three Crown hospitals, but over 1,000 nurses responded by picketing those hospitals nevertheless.
- January 27th: Individual nurses began being served with civil contempt of court charges. Over 75 charges were laid and heard by the end of the strike. This same day, UNA was also charged with criminal contempt of court.
- January 29th: UNA was served with a notice to appear at a hearing to be held February 1st. The government of Alberta requested a $1,000,000 fine and sequestrations of the union's funds and assets.
- February 3rd: Civil contempt hearings for individual nurses proceeded in courthouses in Calgary and Edmonton.
- February 4th: UNA was found guilty and fined $250,000.
- February 9th: UNA paid the $250,000 fine at the courthouse and was served a notice of motion of a second criminal contempt charge.
- February 10th: Termination notices were given to individual nurses as "punishment."
- February 11th: Fines up to $1,000 each for criminal contempt started being imposed on individual nurses. This same day, employers tabled an improved offer.
- February 12th: Hearings on the second criminal contempt charge began and UNA was fined $150,000. UNA members voted to accept the employers' latest improved offer and a settlement was reached.
- February 13th: Striking nurses returned to work.

shifts); a 19% wage increase over 2 years; an additional 8th increment worth 3%; a guarantee of two weekends off in four; language expressly prohibiting employers from making individual agreements that contravene the Collective Agreement; and many others as well (UNA, n.d.).

A number of strategies undertaken by nurses' unions had an impact on how nurses view nursing and how nursing is viewed. Perhaps the clearest example is the case of pay equity in Ontario. The Ontario Nurses Association (ONA) was active in the Equal Pay Coalition, an organization that brought together unions and community groups to work for equal pay for work of equal value. Once their efforts were successful in achieving legislation, ONA then focused on making sure it worked for nurses. In two ground-breaking cases heard by the Ontario Pay Equity Tribunal (Haldimand-Norfolk, 1989; Women's College, 1990), ONA was successful not only in making sure the skills, effort, responsibility, and working conditions involved in nursing were made visible and valued but also in establishing criteria for job evaluation that are used throughout the world. The result was more than higher pay, it was public and legal recognition of the valued work nurses do every day in their jobs.

NURSES' WORKPLACES

The most recent data on the distribution of RNs in Canada according to their place of work shows that more than half of RNs work in hospitals. Table 17.1 highlights findings from the Canadian Institute for Health Information's report "Workforce Trends of Registered Nurses in Canada" (2007).

The vast array of settings and conditions under which nurses work makes it difficult to describe the nature and quality of their practice environments. What can be said, however, is that when work

Table 17.1	Canadian Registered Nurse Workforce Distribution from 2003–2006			
	NUMBER OF NURSES		PERCENTAGE (%) OF NURSES	
PLACE OF WORK	2003	2006	2003	2006
Hospital	150,513	157,699	62.4%	62.3%
Community health agency	31,251	34,477	13.0%	13.6%
Nursing home/long-term care facility	25,292	27,754	10.5%	11.0%
Other	30,927	29,751	12.8%	11.8%
Not stated	3,359	3,267	1.4%	1.3%

Source: Canadian Institute for Health Information (2007). Registered Nurses Database, http://secure.cihi.ca/cihiweb/en/downloads/nursing_registered_profile_can_2006_e.pdf.

satisfaction is low, patient care may be compromised (McDonald & McIntyre, 2006). Job satisfaction cannot be measured using a simple set of indicators or formulae; issues both resulting from and contributing to the nature of nurses' work are interconnected to their unique experiences of satisfaction. This chapter has provided some insight into conditions that both contribute to and detract from a positive work environment. Research shows that the quality of the work environment, retention and recruitment of nurses, and the nursing shortage can all be interrelated and, consequently, play a role in shaping our nursing workforce.

Workplace challenges including excessive workload, high rates of overtime, injury, and stress are all detrimental to the health and safety of nurses. The Canadian Labour Code requires a number of measures be taken to protect the health and safety of workers in all workplaces. One mechanism by which this is accomplished is through the creation of a joint health and safety committee. The role of this committee is to ensure that workplace and legislative health and safety policies are applied in practice. Members of the committee generally include occupational health and safety (OH&S) experts as well as representatives from labour and management so that in-depth, practical knowledge of the work is brought together with company policies and procedures to enhance cooperation and the resolution of health and safety problems (Canadian Centre for Occupational Health and Safety, 2007).

Two major examples of OH&S issues that are of concern to nurses in the current work environment are workplace violence and control of infectious disease. Research has demonstrated that among healthcare personnel, nurses are most at risk of workplace violence (Kingman, 2001). This includes physical, verbal, and psychological violence that is perpetrated by patients as well as by other staff members. In 2005, one in six nurses reported having been bullied at work in the past 12 months (MacDonald, 2006), while 3 out of 10 nurses said they had been attacked by a patient in the previous year (Canadian Institute for Health Information, 2007). Emergency preparedness and infectious disease outbreak have been of particular concern as OH&S issues since 9/11, the severe acute respiratory syndrome (SARS) outbreak in 2003, and as the threat of pandemic influenza looms. Perhaps the single most valuable result of the SARS Commission is its advocacy for the precautionary principle (Campbell, 2006). The precautionary principle states that when an activity raises threats of harm to human health or the environment, precautionary measures should be taken even in the absence of full scientific certainty. (See Box 17.3 for CFNU's position on how this principle should be applied to pandemic planning.) Following this principle, in the event of a health emergency such as a pandemic, healthcare workers must be assured that all reasonable health and safety precautions are being taken to protect them from exposure to the threat. Applying the precautionary principle, many nurses' unions and OH&S experts agree that nurses and all allied healthcare providers should have regular fit-testing for N95 respirators, access to antiviral medication for prophylactic administration, and be trained in emergency procedures in the case of a public health emergency.

Despite the many challenges that nurses face in the workplace, they continue to provide safe, competent care to patients—and are highly trusted and respected as healthcare professionals. Furthermore, it should be noted that unions have taken many steps to improve the conditions of the work environment for nurses. There are many examples across Canada, but the British Columbia Nurses' Union (BCNU) is often a leader in advocating for improvements to workplace health and safety and patient care. BCNU encourages nurses across the province to use a professional responsibility reporting process—detailed in their collective agreement—to inform managers about workplace situations needing change (McPherson, 2004). This initiative has resulted in documentation by emergency room (ER) nurses who have identified the need to increase the number of full-time RNs on ER staff to reduce waiting times for patients and improve the workload and safety of both nurses and patients. "RNs on regular medical and post-surgical wards have been using their professional responsibility report forms to ask for more electric beds and overhead lifts to reduce injuries. Younger nurses are documenting the need to keep older nurses in the workplace to serve as mentors and use their experience to provide support" (McPherson, 2004). These are just a few examples of how unions work to improve the workplace environments for nurses and also patient safety. Another method is to bring solutions—proven by research—into action in the workplace; CFNU is working to promote balance and satisfaction in the workplace through the development of pilot projects that promote continuing education, mentorship, and professional development. These will be explored in more detail later in the chapter.

BOX 17.3 Safety Is Not Negotiable: A Position on Personal Protective Equipment when Planning for a Pandemic

- The precautionary principle be applied and N95 respirators (or greater) be used as the minimum standard for the protection of healthcare workers. We must not wait and monitor unknown viruses; rather we need to use the precautionary principle to ensure the health of workers, patients, and the public.
- This standard should apply for all viruses that are known or suspected to be airborne and any virus with an unknown transmission route.
- Develop policies and programs to ensure N95 respirators are fit-tested annually and health workers receive training, including information about the health risks present in an emergency pandemic situation so that protective equipment is used properly at all times.
- Require all healthcare workers to carry identification indicating the size of the fit-tested N95 respirator needed.
- Insist that employers develop institutional pandemic plans in consultation with nurses and other healthcare workers and provide education to all staff immediately.
- Insist that all provinces and the federal government demand the same standard for personal protective equipment and pandemic planning.

Conclusion

We must ensure the safety of the population, including that of healthcare workers, by requiring a proper standard of safety and training of healthcare workers in the event of a pandemic. We cannot take the risks associated with not providing adequate equipment in terms of the proper safety devices or in the quantity of stockpiled equipment.

COLLECTIVE BARGAINING

"Collective bargaining is a very broad concept that has the potential to involve and strengthen all nurses" (New Brunswick Nurses Union, n.d.). As nurses work to provide safe and effective care to the public, it is the job of unions to support them in achieving this important task by protecting their health, safety, and well-being. The collective bargaining process now addresses issues that range far beyond wages and benefits, including workplace health and safety issues and workload. These are addressed by articles on flexible staffing and scheduling measures, mentoring, professional training and development, and measures to reduce violence in the workplace. Nurses' unions in at least five provinces have brought workload issues into contract negotiations (CFNU, 2007a).

It has been said that collective bargaining is more of an art than a science; it's a process in which creativity is more valuable than analysis, in order to come to an agreement that is mutually acceptable to both the employer and the employee (Teplitsky, 1992). Unions vary in their procedures and techniques to negotiate collective agreements, but this section highlights a series of processes that generally take place throughout the course of the bargaining process. Negotiation teams often examine research, explore contract language, and develop goals and priorities to be reviewed at bargaining conferences where local presidents are in attendance. Following preparations, prenegotiations begin whereby proposals are exchanged between the union and the employer's negotiating committee. At this time, procedures and processes are established for future meetings. After both parties commence discussion and explore options for settlement, each negotiating team attempts to persuade the other side to their position. As both sides move toward reaching a tentative agreement, each offers a "final" or "minimum position" on the issues at hand. When an impasse is reached—the two parties cannot come close enough together to form an agreement—a Conciliation Officer or Commissioner (title and process may change for each province because these are based on provincial labour relations legislation) may be engaged to meet with both groups separately in an attempt to facilitate negotiations. Sometimes, as a last resort, a strike vote is taken by members of the union to put pressure on the employer to meet the collective bargaining demands. A strike vote does not automatically mean that a strike will occur, but it sends a strong message to the bargaining table that members support the demands brought forth by the negotiating committee. Finally, when the union's negotiation team receives a final position from the employer that they feel is the best possible settlement, it is considered to be a tentative agreement. Ratification occurs after the majority of voting union members vote in favour of the settlement. Despite the structure and tradition of the collective bargaining process, it is important to recognize that (1) collective bargaining processes may vary from union to union and (2) a number of external factors influence the nature and context for negotiations as well. Public opinion and the current political environment are two major factors. The public's high regard for nurses is something that strengthens their position, while government policies, such as legislated wage freezes, negatively affect bargaining power. It should also be noted here that although not all provinces have the right to strike, all have the right and power to influence decision making by placing political pressure on employers and government by raising public awareness of issues that are important to the healthcare work environment.

Bargaining power is further strengthened by numbers, cohesion and commonality of objectives within membership. Although provincial nurses' unions negotiate individually, their collective membership with CFNU allows them to receive information that will strengthen their individual bargaining power. By sharing information like the comparative contract shown in Table 17.2, provincial unions can use the successes of other provinces as a model for their own negotiations. However, it is important to note that the focus of collective bargaining is not solely monetary. As the example with BCNU highlighted above, making strides towards achieving improved working conditions and patient safety are also fundamental objectives.

Table 17.2	Canadian Federation of Nurses Unions Contract Comparison Document: Salary at Contract Expiry (2008)

| UNION | DOLLARS PER HOUR | | ANNUAL INCOME | | STEPS | CONTRACT EXPIRY | ANNUAL HOURS |
	MINIMUM	MAXIMUM	MINIMUM	MAXIMUM			
UNA	32.340	42.450	62,117.06	81,535.84	8	3/31/2010	1920.75
ONA	29.360	41.802	57,252.00	81,513.90	8	3/31/2011	1950.00
BCNU	29.020	38.100	54,534.38	71,597.52	8	3/31/2010	1879.20
MNU	29.544	34.830	59,531.16	70,182.45	6	9/30/2009	2015.00
NSNU	29.235	34.169	57,008.25	66,629.55	6	10/31/2009	1950.00
SUN	26.900	32.960	52,422.72	64,232.45	5	3/31/2008	1948.80
FIQ	21.410	31.890	40,497.02	60,319.94	12	3/31/2010	1891.50
NBNU	26.380	31.490	51,638.85	61,641.68	6	12/31/2007	1957.50
PEINU	25.130	30.620	49,003.50	59,709.00	6	3/31/2008	1950.00
NLNU	23.478	30.002	45,782.21	58,503.90	7	6/30/2008	1950.00

Note that not all contract expiry dates are updated because at the time this chapter was written, some member organizations were in the process of bargaining. It should also be noted that some organizations offer long-term recognition steps beyond the standard salary scales and signing bonuses. The Canadian Federation of Nurses Unions provides this and other wage comparison documents through their Web site: www.nursesunions.ca.

 MOVING AHEAD

By the 1980s, Canada had public hospitals, physician care, and a highly unionized public sector as well as more egalitarian ideas, laws, and practices in relation to women. More than 9 out of 10 nurses were women and three quarters of the nurses were unionized. This suggests that women who are nurses no longer see commitment to care and professional conduct as incompatible with being a woman and being in a union. This is not to suggest that all issues have been resolved or the tensions have disappeared, but it is often the unions—who have great strength in numbers— that are fighting to protect workers from external influences that damage their working conditions. A recent example of this is the case of Bill 29, the Health and Social Services Delivery Improvement Act, passed by the government of British Columbia in 2002. A number of health-care unions (led by the British Columbia Government and Service Employees' Union, BCNU, and the Hospital Employees' Union representing over 100,000 healthcare workers in British Columbia) appealed the legislation that would have eliminated key long-standing contract provisions like protections against contracting out, seniority rights, and labour adjustment programs. Unions argued that Bill 29 violated rights guaranteed under the Canadian Charter of Rights and Freedoms and, in particular, those sections relating to liberty and security of the person, freedom of association and equality rights (National Union of Public and General Employees, 2003). On June 8, 2007, the unions won their case, as the Supreme Court of Canada struck down key provisions of the 2002 law, ruling them to be in violation of the Charter of Rights and Freedoms. The Supreme Court of Canada has required that within one year the British Columbia government must bring the legislation into compliance with the Charter (British Columbia Government and Service Employees' Union, 2007).

UNIONS TODAY AND TOMORROW

Beginning in the 1980s, global pressure developed to turn back the clock on the development of public services. International organizations such as the World Bank and the International Monetary Fund promoted dramatic reductions in both public services and government regulation of private services. In Canada, growing government debts and deficits were used as a justification for "devolving responsibilities to other levels of government and to the private and voluntary sectors; reducing transfer payments to provinces, individuals and businesses; applying private sector management techniques to those federal activities that remain" (Swimmer, 1996, p. 2). Provincial governments had little choice but to follow this lead, although several did so enthusiastically.

Healthcare was one of the hardest hit, because it was one of the largest government expenses and because the private sector wanted to expand in health services, not only in providing services but also in managing care. Healthcare is primarily based on labour, and nurses are the largest single occupational group in health services. It is perhaps not surprising, then, that nurses were among the primary targets for cost cutting and new managerial techniques taken from the for-profit sector. It should be noted, however, that it has been widely recognized that the most rapidly rising costs in health services are technologies and pharmaceuticals, not labour—and certainly not nurses labour.

Nurses' unions found it difficult to resist this rising tide of cutbacks. They did manage to ensure orderly, fair layoffs and to maintain wages for the jobs that remained. They also maintained the right to say no for the nurses with jobs and the right to expose discrimination. But many nurses no longer had full-time jobs and some lost work altogether. To counter the trend, nurses' unions worked with health coalitions and other unions throughout the country to convince Canadians that public healthcare is the most effective and efficient way to deliver health services and that nurses are critical to care provision. When deficits, and even debt, could no longer be used as a justification for cutbacks in nursing, the strategy of working with others to support public care started to bear fruit. Governments began to put money back into health services and into nursing. Indeed, nurses' unions have been working with governments to address the growing nursing shortage that reflects not only the fact that the bulk of the nursing labour force is approaching retirement age but also that working conditions have deteriorated.

According to a Statistics Canada (2006) report on the work and health of nurses, the average age of a nurse is 44.7 years old, and 17% of the nursing workforce is between the ages of 50 and 54. For every nurse under the age of 35, there are two over the age of 50. Canada is expected to have a shortfall of 78,000 nurses by 2011, which will grow to 113,000 by 2016. A symptom of this shortage results in over one half of nurses regularly working unpaid overtime—estimated at approximately 4 hours per week. Also troubling is the fact that in 2005, over 3 in 10 nurses had experienced pain serious enough to prevent them from carrying out their normal daily activities (Statistics Canada, 2006). Recent research provides us with an overview of the Canadian nursing workforce; see Box 17.4.

In addition to addressing conditions of work and relating these to conditions of care, nurses' unions have been struggling to promote fair treatment on a range of issues.

In their early forms of existence, most of the nurses' unions focused on negotiating contracts, handling grievances, and other labour relations issues. However, annual general meetings revealed that a number of issues relating to the healthcare system and social justice were also very important for nurses. For example, in 1982, MNU brought a resolution to the special convention that CFNU join the Canadian Health Coalition to champion Medicare and other social justice issues. They have

BOX 17.4 Employment Trends of the Registered Nurse Workforce in 2006

In 2006, the number of registered nurses (RNs) submitting a registration for practice increased by 0.9% from the previous year and by 4.8% from 2003. These registrations include both employed and unemployed RNs.

In 2006, 56.3% of RNs were employed full time, while the proportion employed part-time and on a casual basis was 32.8% and 10.9%, respectively.

Between 2005 and 2006, the number of registrations increased in most of Canada's provinces and territories. Prince Edward Island decreased slightly by 0.6%.

In 2006, 83.1% of the RN workforce (excluding Quebec) lived in urban areas of Canada.

In 2006, 4,814 RNs with Canadian registration lived and/or worked outside of Canada. Of these, 84.4% (4,063) were employed in the United States.

Source: Canadian Institute for Health Information (2007). Available from http://secure.cihi.ca/cihiweb/products/workforce_trends_of_rns_2006_e.pdf.

also developed contract language on both sexual harassment and discrimination against racialized groups at the same time as they have sought to educate their members and the public on these issues. They have successfully demanded changes on health and safety matters, such as needles and reporting medical errors—matters that are critical to safe and effective care. Unions have also increasingly been at the forefront of demands for healthcare reforms that both recognize nurses' skills and protect equitable access to high quality, public care.

Advocacy, lobbying, and campaigning efforts often land CFNU at annual Council of the Federation meetings on Parliament Hill and in the media. Since 1998 CFNU has been an active member of the Canadian Labour Congress (CLC), the largest democratic and popular organization in Canada. With over 3.5 million members, the CLC joins national and international unions, the provincial and territorial federations of labour, and 136 district labour councils (Canadian Labour Congress, 2007). Included in this group of affiliates is the International Trade Union Confederation, which is the world's largest trade union organization, representing over 166 million people in 156 countries around the world (International Trade Union Confederation, 2007). In Canada, the CLC works to adapt policy and influence political agendas on issues like health and safety, pensions, and employment insurance. More recently their campaigning has focused on childcare, education, pension protection, pay equity, and the development of a national pharmacare program. As members of the CLC Executive Council, the strong collaborative relationship that the CFNU shares with the CLC provides all member nurses' unions with support for collective bargaining in areas such as occupational health and safety, pensions, and benefits.

CFNU's elected officials and National Executive Board members have met with premiers, developed and released peer-reviewed papers and position statements, and hosted discussion panels and press conferences to address national nursing and healthcare system issues. However, nurses' unions do not simply wait for change; they create change by applying creative, positive solutions as revealed through research into workplace action. Examples range from the advocacy for increased in-house education opportunities, to enhancement of access to personal protective equipment, to promotion of strategies to prevent the practice of hallway nursing.

The CFNU has been working with its member organizations to address staffing shortages and stressful working conditions in the workplace. In Nova Scotia and Saskatchewan, two pilot projects have been implemented with funding from Human Resources and Social Development Canada's Workplace Skills Initiative to improve the recruitment and retention of nurses. These projects have allowed nurses in two health regions to participate in continuing education or mentorship programs. Plans to expand these and other models of pilot projects across Canada are currently underway. Additionally, a recent partnership developed between the government of Saskatchewan and the Saskatchewan Union of Nurses to stabilize and rebuild Saskatchewan's dwindling nursing workforce and ensure that their province can deliver high quality, timely, and accessible care to residents. In recognition of the need to retain a large number of experienced and skilled nurses, while also planning aggressive recruitment initiatives to increase the numbers of practicing nurses, several concrete strategies were put in place. Examples of strategies include the establishment of quarterly retention and recruitment targets, the recruitment of internationally educated nurses, and the provision of incentives for senior nurses to remain in the workforce longer by recognizing long-term service and providing opportunities to mentor new graduates and immigrant nurses (Saskatchewan Union of Nurses, 2008).

Another mechanism by which nurses' unions aim to address issues of retention and recruitment is by remaining current and informed about the changing needs of the workforce. By inviting the Canadian Nursing Students' Association (CNSA) to sit on the National Executive Board, CFNU now represents over 158,000 members and associate members, making it the largest nursing organization in Canada. By working with the CNSA it is hoped that the future of nursing is well represented in current union activities and priorities.

SUMMARY

In short, there are very good reasons why 3 out of 4 nurses in Canada today belong to a union, and why most of their unions have joined with other unions to promote their rights. Despite historical tensions between the notion of professionalism and unionization, nurses today experience support brought by union values and activities that bring continuous learning, challenges, and many rewards to their profession. Without unions, but with other forms of collective action, nurses were able to obtain registration and some control over the process of getting and retaining the right to be called an RN. However, until they formed unions, they were unable to significantly improve their conditions of work and, thus, the conditions for care. Today, these unions work not only to promote the prestige and power of nurses but also to maintain a safe, accessible healthcare system that offers high-quality care. CFNU is a member of the Quality Worklife Quality Health Care Collaborative (QWQHC) (2006), a national interprofessional coalition of healthcare leaders who are working together to develop an integrated action-oriented strategy to transform the quality of worklife for Canada's healthcare providers in order to improve patient care and system outcomes.

The QWQHC (2006) maintains that "a fundamental way to better healthcare is through healthier healthcare workplaces; and it is unacceptable to work in, receive care in, govern, manage and fund unhealthy health care workplaces." Although a primary focus of nurses' unions is to ensure that nurses receive the same attention and care that they give to their patients, when nursing unions work in collaboration with local employers, governments, and nursing stakeholders, the overall result can be seen in improvements not only in the quality worklife of nurses but also in increased quality healthcare and better patient safety.

Add to your knowledge of this issue:	
International Council of Nurses	http://www.icn.ch
Canadian Federation of Nurses Unions	http://www.nursesunions.ca
Canadian Nurses Association	http://www.cna-nurses.ca
Canadian Labour Congress	http://canadianlabour.ca
Canadian Health Coalition	http://www.healthcoalition.ca
British Columbia Nurses Union	http://www.bcnu.org
United Nurses of Alberta	http://www.una.ab.ca
Manitoba Nurses' Union	http://www.nursesunion.mb.ca
Saskatchewan Union of Nurses	http://www.sun-nurses.sk.ca
Ontario Nurses Association	http://www.ona.org
Nova Scotia Nurses Union	http://www.nsnu.ns.ca
New Brunswick Nurses Union	http://www.nbnu-siinb.nb.ca
Prince Edward Island Nurses' Union	http://www.peinu.com
Newfoundland and Labrador Nurses Union	http://www.nlnu.nf.ca

Online

REFLECTIONS on the Chapter...

1 How would you describe the transformation of nurses' unions in Canada?

2 Identify the appropriate documents that provide direction for nurses and their employers in the provision of professional practice environments.

3 What are the barriers in your practice environment to nurses providing safe and ethical care? How could you resolve these?

4 What are your views on the strengths and limitations of the strategies presented in the chapter or that you have seen utilized in the practice setting?

5 Identify at least one issue for nurses in the provision of a safe professional practice environment for their work.

6 What are the benefits and challenges associated with collective bargaining processes?

7 What other strategies can you suggest for the resolution of these issues?

8 How would you describe the stand of your provincial nurses' union on issues? How would you account for this stand?

References

Allard, G. (2005). Caregiving on the front: The experience of Canadian military nurses during World War I. In C. Bates, D. Dodd, & N. Rousseau (Eds.), *On all frontiers: Four centuries of Canadian nursing.* Toronto: University of Toronto Press.

Andrews, J. (1993). Notes on the history of collective bargaining in current members of the CFNU: Interviews with key informants. Ottawa: Canadian Federation of Nurses Unions, May 1993.

Armstrong, P. & Armstrong, H. (2001). *The double ghetto: Canadian women and their segregated work* (3rd ed.). Toronto: Oxford University Press.

_____. (2003). *Wasting away: The undermining of Canadian health care* (2nd ed.). Toronto: Oxford University Press.

British Columbia Government and Service Employees' Union. (2007). *Bill 29 victory for workers.* Retrieved November 15, 2007 from http://www.bcgeu.bc.ca/Bill_29_ victory_for_workers.

Bunting, S. & Campbell, J. (1990). Feminism and nursing: Historical perspectives. *Advances in Nursing Science, 12*(4), 11–24.

Campbell, A. (2006). *Final report of the SARS Commission.* The SARS Commission, p. 254.

Canadian Centre for Occupational Health and Safety. (2007). *What is a joint health and safety committee?* Retrieved December 15, 2007 from http://www.ccohs.ca/oshanswers/hsprograms/hscommittees/whatisa.html#_1_4.

Canadian Federation of Nurses Unions. (n.d.). *Defending nurses and health care.* Ottawa: CFNU.

_____. (2003). Nursing unionism in Quebec. A bit of history (n.d.). *The Story of Canadian Labour.* Workshop handouts. Ottawa: CFNU.

_____. (2007a). *Creating positive solutions at the workplace: Time to work together.* Presented in Geneva, Switzerland, March 23, 2007.

_____. (2008). *CFNU contract comparison document.*

Canadian Institute for Health Information. (2007). *Workforce trends of registered nurses in Canada, 2006.* Retrieved November 15, 2007 from http://secure.cihi.ca/.

Canadian Labour Congress. (2007). *Welcome.* Retrieved November 15, 2007 from http://candianlabour.ca.

Coburn, J. (1987). I see and am silent: A short history of nursing in Ontario, 1850–1930. In D. Coburn, et al. (Eds.), *Health and Canadian society* (2nd ed.). Toronto: Fitzhenry and Whiteside.

Dominion Bureau of Statistics. (1961). *Census of Canada labour force occupation and industry trends.* Ottawa: Minister of Trade and Commerce.

Hunt, J. (1998). *Feminism and nursing: A turbulent history.* Retrieved November 15, 2007 from http://www.ciap.health.nsw.gov.au/hospolic/stvincents/stvin98/a5.html.

International Trade Union Confederation. (2007). Report on the International Trade Union Confederation. Retrieved November 15, 2007 from http://www.ituc-csi.org/.

Jensen, P. (1992). The changing role of nurses' unions. In A. Baumgart & J. Larsen (Eds.), *Canadian Nursing Faces the Future.* St. Louis: Mosby.

Keddy, B. & Dodd, D. (2005). The trained nurse: Private duty and VON home nursing (late 1800s to 1940s). In C. Bates, D. Dodd., & N. Rousseau (Eds.), *On all frontiers: Four centuries of Canadian nursing,* pp. 43–56. Toronto: University of Toronto Press.

Kerr, J. (1988). Professionalization in Canadian nursing. In J. Kerr & J. McPhail (Eds.), *Canadian nursing issues and perspective,* pp. 23–30. Toronto: McGraw-Hill Ryerson.

Kingman, R. (2001). Workplace violence in the health sector: A problem of epidemic proportion. *International Nursing Review, 48*(3), 129–130.

Library and Archives Canada. (2005). *Celebrating women's achievements: Women in science: Jeanne Mance.* Retrieved November 15, 2007 from http://www.collectionscanada.gc.ca/women/002026-410-e.html.

MacDonald, P. (2006). Bullying in the workplace *Practice Nurse, 32*(10), 1–4.

Mansell, D. & Dodd, D. (2005). Professionalism and Canadian nursing. In C. Bates, D. Dodd, & N. Rousseau (Eds.), *On all frontiers: Four centuries of Canadian nursing,* pp. 197–212. Toronto: University of Toronto Press.

McBride, A. (1984). Nursing and the women's movement. *Journal of Nursing Scholarship, 16*(3), pp. 285–302.

McDonald, C. & McIntyre, M. (2006). Issues arising from the nature of nurses' work and workplaces. In M. McIntyre, E. Thomlinson, & C. McDonald (Eds.), *Realities of Canadian nursing: Professional, practice and power issues,* pp. 303–316. Philadelphia: Lippincott Williams & Wilkins.

McIntyre, M. & McDonald, C. (2006). Unionization: Collective bargaining in nursing. In M. McIntyre, E. Thomlinson, & C. McDonald (Eds.), *Realities of Canadian nursing: Professional, practice and power issues,* pp. 303–316. Philadelphia: Lippincott Williams & Wilkins.

McPherson, D. (2004). BC nurses seek solutions for better patient care. *British Columbia Nurses' Union*. Retrieved November 15, 2007 from http://www.bcnu.org/whats_new_media/news_releases/2004/May10_2004.htm.

Mussallem, H. (1988). The changing role of the Canadian nurses' association in the development of nursing in Canada. In J. Kerr & J. McPhail (Eds.), *Canadian Nursing Issues and Perspectives*, pp. 35–46. Toronto: McGraw-Hill Ryerson.

Nelson, S. (2001). *Say little. Do much: Nurses, nuns and hospitals in the nineteenth century*. Philadelphia: University of Pennsylvania Press.

New Brunswick Nurses' Union. (n.d.). *How the NBNU negotiates your contract*. Retrieved November 15, 2007 from http://www.nbnu-siinb.nb.ca/pdf/negotiates.pdf.

National Union of Public and General Employees. (2003). *Unions will appeal. Bill 29 B.C. Supreme Court ruling*. Retrieved November 15, 2007 from http://www.nupge.ca/news_2003/n15se03a.htm.

Naylor, D. (1986). *Private practice. Public payment*. Montreal: McGill-Queen's University Press.

Ontario Nurses' Association vs. Women's College Hospital, Ontario Pay Equity Tribunal, 1990.

Ontario Nurses' Association vs. Haldimand Norfolk, Ontario Pay Equity Tribunal, 1989.

Quality Worklife Quality Health Care Collaborative. (2006). *Overview*. Retrieved November 15, 2007 from http://www2.cchsa.ca/qwqhc/.

Saskatchewan Union of Nurses. (2008). *Partnership between the government of Saskatchewan and the Saskatchewan union of nurses*.

Seago, J.A. & Ash, M. (2002). Registered nurse union and patient outcomes. *Journal of Nursing Administration, 32*(3), 143–151.

Showalter, E. (2007). *The female malady: Women, madness and English culture 1830–1980*. London: Virago.

Silversides, A. (2007). Medicare timeline. In *Conversations with champions of Medicare*. Ottawa: Canadian Federation of Nurses Unions.

Statistics Canada. (2006). *2005 National Survey of the Work and Health of Nurses*. Catalogue no-83-003-XIE.

Swimmer, G. (1996). An introduction to life under the knife. In Gene Swimmer (Ed.), *How Ottawa spends: Life under the knife*. Ottawa: Carleton University Press.

Toman, C. (2005). Ready, aye ready: Canadian military nurses as an expandable and expendable workforce (1920–2000). In C. Bates, D. Dodd, & N. Rousseau (Eds.), *On all frontiers: Four centuries of Canadian nursing*. Toronto: University of Toronto Press.

United Nurses of Alberta. (n.d.). *1988 Hospital Strike*. Retrieved November 15, 2007 from http://www.una.ab.ca/conferences/F00014095/UNA%20History/UNA%20History%20-%201988.

Van Kirk, S. (1980). *Many tender ties: Women in fur trade society in Western Canada, 1670–1830*. Winnipeg: Watson and Dyer.

Victorian Order of Nurses. (2004). *A century of caring*. Retrieved November 15, 2007 from http://www.von.ca/about_history.html.

White, J. (1993). *Sisters & solidarity: Women and unions in Canada*. Toronto: Thompson Educational Publishing

Young, J. & Rousseau, N. (2005). Lay nursing from the New France era to the end of the nineteenth century (1608–1891). In C. Bates, D. Dodd, & N. Rousseau (Eds.), *On all frontiers: Four centuries of Canadian nursing*. Toronto: University of Toronto Press.

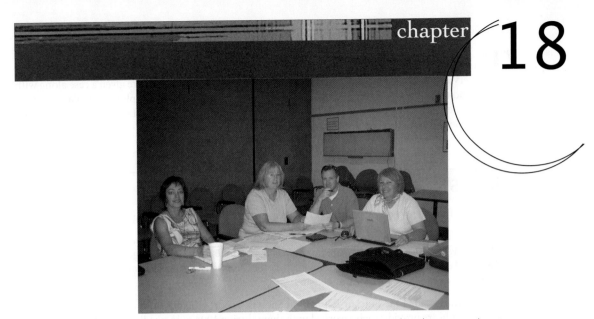

Left to right: Cathy Parsons, nurse and corporate facilitator; Tina Hurlock-Chorestecki, advance practice nurse; Kevin Coughlin, neonatologist; Laurie Hardingham, clinical ethicist.

Ethical and Legal Issues in Nursing

Laurie Hardingham

Critical Questions

As a way of engaging with the ideas in this chapter, consider the following:

1. What knowledge do you already have of ethics that will inform your reading of this chapter?

2. Reflecting on what you already know about the nurses' "Code of Ethics," what ethical issues do you imagine might arise for nurses in practice?

3. How might we account for the increasing interest in ethical dilemmas among nurses in practice?

Chapter Objectives

After completing this chapter, you will be able to:

1. Articulate relevant ethical and legal issues.

2. Understand the implications for individual nurses and for the nursing profession when ethical and legal issues are not resolved.

3. Identify some of the barriers to, and strategies for, resolving ethical and legal issues.

4. Identify some of the ethical and legal resources available to nurses.

This chapter introduces readers to some ethical and legal issues in nursing and provides an overview of their significance to nursing practice. Specifically, readers are given a case along with its legal and ethical issues. Examining the case will help readers to discern, explore, articulate, analyze, and generate resolutions to the issues. This chapter also focuses on bioethical issues, with a particular emphasis on those that arise for nurses and in the nursing profession.

 ## STORY: THE WINNIPEG NURSES

Chapter 1 of the *Report of the Manitoba Pediatric Cardiac Surgery Inquest* begins:

> *Pediatric cardiac surgery is one of the most professionally difficult and personally satisfying medical disciplines in which to work. It demands precision and accuracy from the surgeon, as well as a high degree of efficiency and teamwork from other doctors, nurses, and technicians who form its operating-room teams (Sinclair, 2000, p. 3).*

Sometimes called the Sinclair Report, the inquest report tells the story of 12 children who died and the healthcare providers who worked with them during 1994 in the pediatric cardiac surgery program at the Winnipeg Health Sciences Centre.

The program was suspended in February 1995, following an external review. When many parents of the children who died demanded a public inquiry into their children's deaths, the chief medical examiner for the province of Manitoba ordered an inquest, which commenced hearings in December 1995. The hearings lasted until the fall of 1998; the report was released in the fall of 2000.

The 900-plus page report found that the program had a mortality rate more than twice as high as similar programs. Two of the four central themes recorded at the inquest were the heartrending narratives of the children and their parents and the stories about the treatment of nurses.

History of the Program and Nursing Concerns

When the cardiac surgery program was restarted in 1994, after a break due to the previous surgeon leaving Winnipeg, the operating room and intensive care nurses began to have concerns about the lack of preparation, about the problems in surgery, and about the many complications the young patients were experiencing. As the deaths of infants began and continued, the nurses voiced their concerns to their supervisor, to physicians and surgeons, and to the director of nursing.

The nurses "were never treated as full and equal members of the surgical team" (Sinclair, 2000, p. viii). Their concerns were ignored, and the program continued. The nurses continued to keep notes and speak out to their supervisors. Finally, after the 12th child died, the program was suspended.

Inquest Findings

The report found that the nurses did nothing wrong; in fact, they did many things that were right. However, the nurses continue to wonder if events might have been different had they acted differently.

After several children had died, one of the nurses, Carol Youngson, decided to attempt to limit her contact with parents. She would no longer take the children from their parents' arms into the operating room. She told the officials at the inquest that she had considered telling parents to "take your baby and run" (Sinclair, 2000, p. 355). When asked why she did not warn the parents, she stated that had she done so, "all hell would have broken loose." She felt that she would have been perceived as overly emotional and that, although she could have perhaps saved one child, there would have been more children coming in, and nothing would have changed. She would have lost her job. Less experienced nurses would be hired, and the program would continue; it would not have been stopped (Sinclair, 2000, p. 355).

Using this story as a background for analysis, nurses can examine relevant ethical and legal issues and try to uncover what it means to practise ethically and legally in the difficult environment that is healthcare today. Although the story of the nurses in the Winnipeg Pediatric Cardiac Surgical Program is a particularly dramatic one, it raises many issues that concern nurses across the country on a daily basis.

WHAT IS ETHICS? WHAT IS BIOETHICS?

Ethics is the philosophical study of morality, the study of what is right and wrong behavior. Studying ethics enables us to examine the things that influence our moral decisions, our obligations and duties to others, our character, the nature of "good," and the underpinnings of what makes a good society.

A subset of ethics is applied ethics, in which ethical theory is applied to real-life situations. This can be divided into various categories, such as bioethics (the study of ethics in the life sciences), business ethics (the study of ethics in the business world), and environmental ethics (ethics related to the natural world and our relationship to it).

Bioethics can be broken into several subspecialties, for example, biomedical ethics (the study of ethics in the medical profession), healthcare ethics (ethics in the healthcare setting), nursing ethics (applied ethical theory in nursing), or clinical ethics. Clinical ethics concerns issues that are morally sensitive arising within the context of patient care and the relationships between the people involved. Doing clinical ethics involves a process of critical reflection on moral and ethical problems faced in healthcare settings that helps people to:

- Decide *what* we should do (what actions are ethically right or acceptable).
- Explain *why* we should do it (giving reasons or justifying our decision in ethical terms).
- Describe *how* we should do it (the method of our response).

This is a process we should all participate in, because ethical decisions are made by everyone on a daily basis. Note that in this definition, ethics is an activity, something we do, and that the plural is used, as ethics is best done in community with others.

RECOGNIZING ETHICAL ISSUES

Because ethics is the study of right and wrong behavior, it involves the analysis of what we "ought" to do, what our duties and obligations are to other people, and what kinds of behavior we should expect from others.

What guides this analysis? How do we determine what is the right (and the wrong) action in specific situations? When other people think differently about what actions are morally right, how do we defend our beliefs and question others about theirs? And should we do this?

Moral philosophers and ethicists are not moral experts claiming to have the answers to these questions. They can, however, be a resource to healthcare professionals, offering rational grounds or bases for our moral beliefs and helping us sort out difficult problems. They can help the decision makers in a situation to make the best decisions possible. Although they cannot be the "moral conscience" of society, ethicists have knowledge of moral theory, which is the systematic, critical study of the basic underlying principles, values, and concepts used in thinking about moral life (Boetzkes & Waluchow, 2000).

IDENTIFYING AND ARTICULATING ETHICAL ISSUES

The identification of an ethical issue is not always a straightforward activity. For example, when consent for surgery was obtained but the problems in the pediatric cardiology surgery program were not divulged, the surgeon might have justified the situation by claiming that he was maintaining public confidence in the program. And perhaps the administrators viewed the issue as one of risk management. The nurses, on the other hand, saw the problem as an ethical issue. They believed that the parents were not given all the information they needed to be able to give an informed consent that was consistent with their values and beliefs. This is, in fact, what made it an *ethical* issue—it concerned deeply held values and beliefs about how we treat other people and about the values and beliefs of the children's parents and of the healthcare professionals who were involved.

The issue of informed consent was identified both by the nurses and later by the Sinclair Report as an important ethical issue in the Winnipeg situation. This issue can be examined in greater detail to see how ethical analysis can help in identifying difficult problems.

Informed Consent: Example of an Ethical Issue

One of the major issues explored in the report was whether the families of the deceased children were fully informed of the risks and benefits of surgery before giving their consent to the surgical procedures involving their children. The following story is told in the report.

> Mary Jane Wasney's nephew was scheduled for cardiac surgery in June 1994 at the Health Sciences Centre (HSC). Mary Jane, a surgical nurse at HSC, had heard about the deaths of a number of children undergoing cardiac surgery, and she knew that operations were taking longer than expected. Concerned, she spoke with Carol Youngson, the senior nurse in charge in cardiac surgery. Carol advised her to speak with Joan Borton, a nurse clinician at HSC. Mary Jane went to Joan in tears, worried that her nephew was going to die. Joan suggested that Mary Jane could get her nephew "referred out of the province" and advised her to talk to the acting section head of pediatric cardiology. The cardiologist acknowledged that there was a "learning curve in any new program" but stated that he was confident that Dr. Odim could do the nephew's surgery.
>
> Still concerned, Mary Jane asked several of the anesthetists in the program for advice. In her testimony at the inquest, she recalled that all three anesthetists she spoke with recommended against having the operation done in Winnipeg. In the end, her nephew was operated on in Saskatoon (Sinclair, 2000).

Many people do not have access to the information that Mary Jane had. If you were the parents or a close relative of this child, would you have wanted to be informed about the problems in the surgical program? The inquest judge thought that you would and went on to make several recommendations regarding informed consent that, if adopted, would change our thinking about what is sufficient information needed by people to give truly informed consent.

THE RIGHT TO BE INFORMED

It is now widely recognized that a capable patient has the right to be informed about a proposed treatment and to decide whether to consent to that treatment. For consent to be valid, it must have the following attributes:

- It must be provided by a competent person.
- It must be informed (appropriate and sufficient information must be given in a way that the patient understands, and the informer must be satisfied that the patient understands).
- It must be voluntary (without undue coercion or pressure).

How much information must a physician provide? Until recently, the courts recognized a professional standard: Physicians must provide the amount of information that the average, prudent, reasonable physician would provide in a similar situation. Physicians would have fulfilled their legal obligations if they provided information to a patient in accordance with the practices among their colleagues. However, the law of medical consent has changed recently. The current standard appears to be patient centered. The information provided is sufficient if it meets the standard that a reasonable, average patient in that patient's situation would expect (Baylis et al., 2004).

The Sinclair Report (2000) reviews recent case law that suggests it is not only the patient or guardian (rather than the physician) who should decide whether medical treatment will be performed (and where and by whom it will be performed) but it is also a doctor's duty to inform the patient or guardian of all material risks. What is material is determined by asking the question "What would a reasonable patient or guardian want to know?" Material risks are also those risks that pose a real threat to the patient's life, health, or comfort.

Merely having a signed consent form in which it is acknowledged that the nature of the operation has been explained to the patient does not necessarily prove that the duty to inform has been observed. For example, in an Ontario case, a surgeon had failed to disclose to his patient that he had little experience with the technique being used. In this case, the trial judge held that the surgeon failed in his duty to his patient by not disclosing his inexperience and by failing to give his patient the opportunity to have the procedure performed by another, more experienced surgeon (Sinclair, 2000).

In light of such cases, the report states that when a person has been deprived of the opportunity to make a proper decision regarding treatment and when there is a significant risk that would affect the judgment of a reasonable patient, then in the normal course, it is the responsibility of the physician to inform the patient or guardian of that significant risk—if the information is needed by the patient to determine for himself or herself what course he or she should follow (Sinclair, 2000).

The report concludes that the evidence suggests that the parents of the children involved in the Winnipeg cases were not as fully informed as they were entitled to be. The report made several recommendations to both the Manitoba Department of Health and the hospital aimed at improving the process of consent and communication with families. These recommendations suggest that the information required is much more than is commonly given; it is the kind of information that the Winnipeg nurses wanted to give to the parents.

Increasing the standard for informed consent certainly involves not only physicians but also others in the healthcare environment. Those who recognize problems with consent in specific cases have a moral obligation, if not a legal obligation, to ensure that fully informed consent is obtained.

ETHICS INFORMS LAW

The last chapter in the *Report of the Manitoba Pediatric Cardiac Surgery Inquest* concludes:

> *The thrust of the recommendations in this chapter is not punitive. The need is to improve the health-care system so as to prevent the recurrence of events that occurred in 1994. It is necessary to accept that the health-care system will not improve if people act solely on the basis of a fear of consequences for themselves or their careers. Instead, the recommendations are intended to establish a structure within which highly skilled and talented people can establish a health-care team that continually works together to provide a high standard of care. All of the comments and recommendations in this chapter are intended to fulfill this objective (Sinclair, 2000, p. 466).*

The report also clearly points out that often nurses are the first people on the healthcare team to perceive a problem in the informed consent process. This is because nurses have access to information about healthcare professionals, programs, and institutional problems that most patients do not. Because they typically are more familiar with patient and family values, nurses can appreciate when these patients and families need to know more to make an informed and reasoned decision about medical care.

The law is ethics codified. It is shaped by what a society believes is ethical. Because it takes so long to enact laws, the legal system tends to lag behind society's ethical thinking. Typically what the law requires us to do is the minimum, while ethics obliges us over and above what is required by law. For example, the "Code of Ethics for Registered Nurses" (Canadian Nurses Association [CNA], 2002) is not a legal document, but spells out what behaviours, values, and ethical actions are expected of registered nurses.

The standards of informed consent imposed by recent court decisions and recommended by the Winnipeg inquest report have implications for nurses. Nurses need to be aware of the requirements for informed consent and the kinds of disclosure that are seen as relevant by the courts (Hardingham, 2001a, 2001b). The inquest report also recommended that laws be put in place to protect whistle-blowers in healthcare, an action that, although most citizens would agree is needed, has not yet been accomplished.

LEGAL RESPONSIBILITIES OF NURSES

What legal responsibilities do nurses have regarding informed consent? To answer this question, it is important, first of all, to distinguish between two kinds of situations:

- getting patient consent for what nurses do
- participating in the consent process for what other healthcare professionals do.

For the first kind of situation, the Canadian Nurses Protective Society (CNPS) cautions: "A nurse carrying out an invasive nursing procedure should provide an explanation and document that the explanation was given and consent obtained" (Canadian Nurses Protective Society, 1994, p. 13). Further, the CNPS states:

> Any touching of a client requires verbal, and in some cases, written consent. Legal experts suggest that the person carrying out the treatment should provide the relevant information to the client. So, nurses should be aware of disclosure and consent requirements, and they should be sure to chart that these requirements were met. Failure to obtain consent can result in professional sanctions, civil liability and/or criminal charges (p. 13).

For the second type of situation (e.g., when nurses witness the signing of a consent form for a surgical or medical procedure to be performed by a physician), nurses are not responsible for providing information. The physician, as the caregiver performing the treatment, must provide this. Nurses do, however, have an ethical responsibility to inform the physician when there is evidence that the patient does not have enough information to make an informed decision or that the decision is otherwise not fully informed. If the physician does not remedy the situation, nurses have a role to play as patient advocates. Under both the "Code of Ethics" and nursing practice standards, each nurse as an individual practitioner has responsibilities to the patients in his or her care. For example, under the value of "choice," the "Code of Ethics" (CNA, 2002) states:

> Nurses provide the information and support required so that clients, to the best of their ability, are able to act on their own behalf in meeting the health and health care needs. Information given is complete, accurate, truthful, and understandable. When they are unable to provide the required information, nurses assist clients in obtaining it from other appropriate sources.

These ethical responsibilities may become legal responsibilities if the provincial nursing practice standards or the "Code of Ethics" (CNA, 2002) are recognized by a court of law as guidelines for what a reasonable nurse would do in a specific situation.

For both types of situations, it is important to remember that informed consent is a process, not an event. Getting a patient's signature on a form is not the consent, but simply evidence that the patient agrees that he or she has been informed about the procedure and its consequences.

ETHICAL OR LEGAL ISSUE? ALIKE BUT DIFFERENT

As the preceding analysis points out, ethical and legal issues are closely linked. A legal action and an ethical action one might consider taking may be the same action—but not necessarily. For example, a nurse working in an emergency setting might be reluctant to report suspected child abuse to the authorities, which is required by law. The nurse may feel that by doing so she or he might lose the trust of the family and in turn discourage them from seeking needed medical help for their child or children in the future. The nurse's values suggest that the ethical thing to do would be to work with the family as long as possible to determine whether there is actual abuse or to refer the family to appropriate resources to help them resolve significant problems. The correct legal action would be to report any suspected abuse.

Like all professionals, however, nurses operate within a framework of legal as well as ethical rules and guidelines. (See Box 18.1 for a review of informative resources.) The legal rules that nurses must follow include those that apply to all members of society. In addition to these, nurses as professionals have legal and ethical duties that flow from their obligation to serve the public interest and the common good (Keatings & Smith, 2000). Having a unique body of knowledge, skills, and expertise, nurses have been granted certain rights and privileges by society, and, in return, society holds nurses to high standards of professional, moral, and ethical competence. To balance these responsibilities, nurses must be familiar with the legislation that governs nursing practice and the relevant policies, codes, and standards of practice.

The Need to Understand Legal Requirements

There are four reasons why nurses should be familiar with the law and have a basic understanding of Canada's legal system. First, the CNA "Code of Ethics" and each provincial regulatory body impose certain requirements with respect to nurses' levels of professional knowledge and skill. If nurses do not meet these requirements, they are open to disciplinary action from their professional governing bodies and, if the conduct is serious enough, the courts.

Second, nurses have access to drugs that are regulated both by legislation and hospital procedures governing their use, dispensation, and handling. They need to know the relevant laws and policies that apply to drugs.

Third, nurses need to be familiar with legal requirements because everyday actions and decisions made by nurses affect the basic rights of their patients. Nurses need to know what those rights are and how to respect and protect them.

Finally, nurses have access to confidential information about individual patients, and they are both legally and ethically obligated to keep such information confidential and not divulge it without patient consent. In some cases, however, nurses are required to divulge such information in court—in the form of testimony—or to report information, such as that related to child abuse (Keatings & Smith, 2000).

The legal system is founded on rules and regulations that guide society in a formal and binding manner. Although constructed by individuals and capable of being changed by the judiciary or legislative enactments, the legal system is a general foundation that gives continuing guidance to healthcare professionals regardless of their personal views and values systems. For example, the law recognizes the competent patient's right to refuse treatment. A patient has this right whether or not the healthcare providers agree with the patient's choice. This right, however, is not absolute. If there are overriding state interests, treatment may be mandated against a patient's or parent's wishes. Some examples of this are a court order to fluoridate the water supply or to perform a blood transfusion for a child whose parents refuse such treatment because of religious beliefs. One may have difficulty reconciling law and ethics in areas that transect both, such as issues of death and dying, abuse of others, or futility of healthcare; legal and ethical issues are often entwined.

BOX 18.1 Book Review

The following resources are suggested for increasing knowledge and skills for legal and ethical practice.

- Keatings, M. & Smith, O.B. (2000). *Ethical and legal issues in Canadian nursing* (2nd ed.). Toronto: W.B. Saunders Canada.

This book explores the ethical and legal challenges that nurses meet in everyday practice. It is a good resource for nurses on the Canadian legal system, how nursing is regulated in Canada, and professional conduct, misconduct, and malpractice.

- Yeo, M. & Moorhouse, A. (Eds.). (1996). *Concepts and cases in nursing ethics* (2nd ed.). Peterborough: Broadview Press.

Focusing on the ethical dilemmas faced by nurses who work in the "front lines" of the health care system, this book has many excellent case studies that illustrate how ethical theory can be applied in nursing practice.

- Boetzkes, E. & Waluchow, W. (2000). *Readings in health care ethics.* Peterborough: Broadview Press.

This anthology contains an excellent introductory chapter on ethical justification and theory, "Ethical Resources for Decision Making," as well as a well-chosen selection of readings, both well known and newly written, in the main areas of health care ethics.

- Thomas, J. & Waluchow, W. (1998). *Well and good: A case study approach to biomedical ethics* (3rd ed.). Peterborough: Broadview Press.

This text uses a case study approach to health care ethics, with a brief but good discussion on ethical theory. Included are some well-known Canadian cases, such as the "mercy killing" by Robert Latimer, the assisted suicide of Sue Rodriguez, and the pregnancy solvent-abuse case of Mrs. G., as well as little-known real-life cases.

- Canadian Nurses Association. (2002). *Ethical research guidelines for registered nurses.* Ottawa: Author.

This document links ethical guidance for nurses involved in research with humans to the ethical guidance offered by the Code of Ethics for Registered Nurses (CNA, 2002).

- Canadian Nurses Association. (2003). *Everyday ethics: Putting the code into practice* (2nd ed.). Ottawa: Author.

This updated study guide is intended to be used along with the *Code of Ethics for Registered Nurses* (2002). It is a practical tool that brings the code to life, with case studies and suggestions for using the *Code of Ethics.*

- Chambliss, D.F. (1996). *Beyond caring: Hospitals, nurses, and the social organization of ethics.* Chicago: University of Chicago Press.

This book, written by a sociologist, is based on more than 10 years of field research and shows how nurses, patients, and others become objects of the bureaucratic machinery of the healthcare system.

- Storch, J.L., Rodney, P., & Starzomski, R. (Eds.). (2004). *Toward a moral horizon: Nursing ethics for leadership and practice.* Toronto: Pearson Prentice Hall.

This book is written by current leaders in Canada who are researching nursing ethics and is for the study of ethics at an advanced level. It relates the application of moral knowledge to ethical problems in everyday nursing practice, education, research, and management of nursing care.

One way of differentiating between legal and ethical issues is that laws may be seen as external to oneself, being imposed from the outside. Ethics, on the other hand, can be viewed as something internal. Although this is often true, there are exceptions. Professional codes of ethics may be seen by some as imposed externally, although the aim might be to have nurses internalize their professional ethics during their education. If people agree with the laws of society, they may have internalized them. Someone might believe that it is always ethical to obey the laws of the society in which they live.

Another distinction might be that one should obey the law because it is prudent to do so, that actions that disobey the law might result in some harm. Ethical actions, on the other hand, are done not out of fear of punishment but because they are the right things to do.

The Need to Incorporate Law and Ethics Into Practice

In the story at the beginning of this chapter, the Winnipeg nurses advocated repeatedly for their patients but seemed to get nowhere. Here we might ask the following question: If nurses are unable to fulfill the requirements in the "Code of Ethics" and their nursing practice standards, are these requirements, then, empty ones? Empty requirements are those that cannot be fulfilled by nurses, for example, if there is a shortage of nurses to deliver the care laid out in the requirements. If they are not empty, then nurses must be able to incorporate them into their nursing practice.

However, a nurse who chooses to be a patient advocate by disclosing directly to a patient that there are problems with a specific healthcare professional or program may be legally open to a charge of defamation. If following the requirements means that nurses must perform heroic acts, such as putting their jobs at risk by repeatedly taking their concerns to upper management or by blowing the whistle (informing) on wrongdoers or on unsafe practices or conditions, then, for most nurses, the requirements may seem to be empty. Is this an unsolvable problem for nurses?

ISSUES OF MORAL INTEGRITY

A major issue that arises for nurses facing difficult situations is how they can maintain moral integrity, or a sense of moral wholeness between their values and their actions, when their values go unheeded and they see themselves as powerless to act or to influence change. As Redman and Fry (2000) point out:

> It is no surprise that nurses experience ethical conflicts while providing care. They are individuals with personal and professional values; they ply their skills in institutions in conjunction with other professionals—all of whom have different values. They provide nursing care to patients who may have religious, cultural, and moral values quite different from their own (p. 360).

These value conflicts often lead to problems within healthcare settings. In an analysis of five studies on ethical conflicts faced by nurses, Redman and Fry (2000) found two underlying themes:

1. Evidence of widespread conflict between professional, corporate, and societal definitions of adequacy of care
2. Evidence of differences in the philosophical orientations of the various health professions. For example, some nurses believe that they value patient autonomy more than physicians value patient autonomy.

Redman and Fry ask two questions: Will the differences and the concerns of nurses be seen as worthy of attention? In practice settings, what kind of moral agency of nurses will be supported? These are important questions because nurses make daily decisions in their work with patients. Some of these are moral decisions, and when nurses act deliberately on moral decisions, they are moral agents. As moral agents, nurses are required to examine, or reflect on, their actions.

Familiar to anyone who has taken a philosophy course, Socrates' assertion that "the unexamined life is not worth living" indicates how important thinking, self-analysis, and reflection are to understanding the world and our part in it. When feelings of distress arise, almost everyone examines the choices they have made and wonders if things would have turned out differently if they had made different decisions or pursued different actions.

Healthcare professionals do so frequently and, in fact, are encouraged to do so. For example, the College & Association of Registered Nurses of Alberta requires, in their Continuing Competence Program, that nurses conduct a "review of one's own nursing practice to determine learning needs and incorporate learning to improve one's own practice." The key to this process is the reflective practice approach (College & Association of Registered Nurses of Alberta, 2005, p. 2).

Reflection is serious thinking about something, thinking that "reflects" back to us what we believe or value, so that we can understand why we think that way. If we can find no good reasons for our beliefs, then we may need to think about whether we should change them.

Thomas and Waluchow (1998) use the notion of "reflecting" in their description of three levels of response to a moral question or problem:

1. the expressive level
2. the prereflective level
3. the reflective level

At the expressive level, responses are unanalyzed expressions or feelings, which, in themselves, do not constitute any kind of justification or reason for the response. The emotional response, "This is just not right!" is an example of the expressive level.

At the prereflective level of response, justification is given by reference to values, rules, and principles that are accepted uncritically. Most often, justification is made by reference to a "conventional" or commonly agreed-on standard or rule. We do not stop to think why we should act or base our judgments on these rules or whether they are good standards to adopt. For example, a nurse might say, "This is not right because it goes against hospital policy."

At the reflective level of response, moral judgments are based not entirely on blindly accepted conventional norms but rather on principles, rules, and values to which we ourselves consciously subscribe. A rational moral agent operating at the reflective level should be prepared to offer a reason for a moral judgment. Thus, moral reflection serves to concentrate one's thoughts back on a problem or an idea. This is not a new activity; it is something most of us have been doing all our lives. However, as moral agents, we need to continuously and consciously think in a reflective way about constructing and evaluating the reasons for our rules and beliefs and to set out standards we can use to judge these reasons as good or poor ones. We need to direct our attention explicitly toward things that we normally take for granted, to examine carefully our beliefs and opinions and the evidence we have for them.

Reflection and Integrity

May (1996) includes critical thinking as an important aspect of moral integrity. As people and professionals, when we refer to our moral integrity, we think about the relationship of our actions to our beliefs. This relationship is very important to our self-concepts.

According to May, the development of a critical point of view means that we need to view moral integrity not as holding steadfastly to a code of conduct or rules that others have provided—even if we approve of the code or rules—but rather "as a form of maturation in which reflection on a plurality of values provides a critical coherence to one's experiences" (1996, p. 16). Achieving integrity means developing a critical perspective, a standpoint from which one can examine and then endorse or reject new social influences.

Implicit in this view is the requirement that our choices must be our own. We mature not only by being socialized to accept certain values and beliefs but also by becoming committed to certain values and beliefs as a result of our own critical reflection. When our actions are in harmony with those values and beliefs, we have personal integrity. Acting at the prereflective level is a type of externally directed behavior, the blind following of standards or norms set by someone else. Although not necessarily bad (often conventional norms are capable of reasoned defense and can be fully justified morally), our conventional standards and rules must always be subject to scrutiny. Perhaps there are much better rules that we should try to persuade others to adopt, or perhaps existing conventions are morally objectionable. An example is the practice of slavery, which was believed to be acceptable by many people until the middle of the 19th century.

What happens when moral integrity is compromised? Webster and Baylis (2000) distinguish among three kinds of experiences:

Moral uncertainty occurs when one is unsure what moral principles or values apply, or even what the moral problem is. Sometimes all that is required is more information to resolve the uncertainty, but, at other times, the uncertainty can persist.

Moral dilemmas arise when there are obligations to pursue two or more conflicting courses of action and no obvious reason to prefer one course over the other. Moral dilemmas can also arise when some evidence suggests that a particular course of action is morally right, other evidence suggests that it is morally wrong, and in each case the evidence is inconclusive.

Moral distress is experienced when there is an inconsistency between one's beliefs and the actions that one takes. This inconsistency is usually because the person knows what the right thing to do is, but fails to do it for such reasons as an error of judgment, a personal failing, or other circumstances beyond one's control, such as when one lacks the authority to act or an honest mistake is made.

Redman and Fry (2000) found that studies of nurses and ethical conflicts show that moral uncertainty is rare. Most nurses believe that they understand the nature of the conflict; however, about one third of the nurses studied experienced moral distress. Nurses also perceived an organizational disinclination to deal with physicians when the ethical conflicts involved physicians. In such cases, nurses believed that these kinds of conflicts were unresolvable.

When situations that contribute to moral distress are not resolved, the result can lead to *moral residue*, "that which each of us carries with us from those times in our lives when in the face of moral distress we have seriously compromised ourselves or allowed ourselves to be compromised" (Webster & Baylis, 2000, p. 218). Moral residue results from the lingering distress that comes when a person compromises his or her basic values and principles. Moral residue can be profound and lasting, concentrated in our thoughts, and usually very painful because it threatens and sometimes betrays deeply held and cherished beliefs and values.

Carol Youngson, the Winnipeg nurse who could no longer take the children from their parents' arms into surgery, experienced profound moral distress, which remains with her as moral residue (Armstrong, 2001). Youngson and the other nurses involved in the pediatric cardiac surgery program found that their personal moral integrity was compromised because a combination of fear, uncertainty, and doubt led them to question their values and their actions. They set aside actions that they might have performed, such as warning the parents or going to the press, because these actions did not appear to be open to them at the time.

Unfortunately, in today's healthcare system, each professional may not have the time and the environment for the kind of critical reflection on values that might be required. It is also not clear that a distinction can be drawn between personal and professional integrity. In the same way, it is difficult to distinguish between errors caused by individual actions and errors resulting from systemic causes. However, in both situations, the individual is harmed when she or he experiences serious moral compromise. As May (1996) and Webster and Baylis (2000) point out, compromised integrity irreversibly alters the self. "One does not experience serious moral compromise and survive as the person once was" (Webster & Baylis, 2000, p. 224). When such change prompts the person to know with greater clarity what actions or situations he or she will or will not tolerate or cooperate with in the future, then it can be change for the better. The change can be harmful, however, if the person adapts by constantly shifting his or her values. As time passes, the person's values become so changeable that it is nearly impossible to articulate what she or he sincerely believes. The person then becomes desensitized to wrongdoing and willing to tolerate morally questionable or morally impermissible actions.

Webster and Baylis (2000) also suggest that moral residue may actually lead to error. Commonly, the error will take one of three forms:

1. denial of the incoherence between beliefs and actions,
2. trivialization of the incoherence between beliefs and actions, or
3. unreflective acceptance of the incoherence between beliefs and actions.

Commonly, the structure and culture of the clinical setting are factors that contribute to such errors. For example, ethical issues can be camouflaged in the ordinariness of things, when familiar nonmoral language and categories are used to describe normative issues. The culture can appear to be willing to dismiss or trivialize certain ethical concerns and overlook or sidestep others. Therefore, we need to ask not only about the quality and clarity of thinking in terms of knowledge and analytical skills but also about what place we hold in situations that arise and about the relationships we have, or expect to have, with colleagues and the wider healthcare community.

Moral Dilemmas

Bruce Jennings (1996) makes a useful distinction between two types of moral dilemmas. There are those moral dilemmas inherent in the human condition such as the fact that all people die sooner or later. And then there are those moral dilemmas created by institutional structures such as policies that prohibit us from doing what we think is the right thing. The first type of dilemma, Jennings says, is unavoidable. The second type can often be avoided by altering institutional structures. Jennings claims that an important part of professional ethics is to be open to the possibility of avoiding some moral dilemmas by modifying the institutions within which professionals work. In other words, we need to identify whether the moral dilemmas that we face are somehow inherent in our moral agency itself or whether the dilemmas are artifacts of specific institutional structures.

Those types of moral dilemmas that are artifacts of specific institutional structures require change in those structures. Both the "Code of Ethics" and the many nursing practice standards recognize this, calling attention to the value of practice environments conducive to safe, competent, and ethical care and to the organizational supports needed in the practice setting. What is implicit in both the "Code of Ethics" and standards of practice documents is that professional nurses working in institutional settings cannot practise ethically without the required support.

Does this let nurses off the hook? Not exactly. First of all, even if nurses recognize that without change in the institutional structure they cannot practise ethically, they are still in a difficult situation, often facing severe moral distress. The Winnipeg nurses agonized over the deaths of the children. They continued to press for change, despite sarcasm and criticism from other members of the healthcare team (Sibbald, 1997). Second, the "Code of Ethics" explicitly states that nurses must work both individually and in partnership with others to improve practice environments and to address unsafe practice issues (CNA, 2002).

Nurses and Professional Integrity

As we saw earlier, acting at the prereflective level is a type of "externally directed behaviour," whereby standards or norms set by someone else are followed blindly (Thomas & Waluchow, 1998). This blind acceptance is not necessarily bad, because conventional norms that are capable of reasoned defense and can be fully justified morally can be good standards to adopt. However, our conventional standards and rules must always be subject to scrutiny. Perhaps there are much better rules, and we should try to persuade others to adopt them, or perhaps existing rules are morally objectionable. For example, the convention—followed until fairly recently—whereby nurses always deferred to physicians and obediently complied with their orders, never questioning them, is now seen as unacceptable and archaic. Most nurses would agree now that if the nurse feels physician orders are not right for the patient, they should be questioned.

To have moral integrity, nurses need to assess the standards, codes, and rules that they are asked to follow in their practice. They must have good reasons for accepting them. This acceptance requires not only reflection on whether their practice follows codes of ethics and nursing practice standards but also reflection on the codes and standards themselves. Nurses ought to determine whether they are genuinely in accord with them and why. Reflective practice means thinking about standards, codes, and practices from a critical point of view and sharing this responsibility with other nurses

Reflective practice takes time! It takes time to become familiar with the standards and practices nurses are asked to follow in their professional lives as well as to subject these standards and practices to a critical point of view. Nurses do not always have time for reflective practice, but they need to find space for reflection because nurses are morally and legally required to do so. Reflective practice might be time consuming and frustrating, yet it offers the best hope for nurses' work to be responsive to the needs of their patients and society. Clinical ethicists and professional associations offer resources to nurses to do this work.

BARRIERS TO RESOLVING ETHICAL AND LEGAL ISSUES

Nurses are accountable to individual patients, their families, healthcare team members, employers, the profession, and society as a whole. They also have rights as professionals. These multiple obligations can present difficulties and complicate the identification of barriers to the resolution of problems.

Lack of Workplace Supports

Kelly (1998) carried out a study that describes, explains, and interprets how new graduate nurses perceived their adaptation to the "real world" of hospital nursing. This study examined the major influences on the new graduates' moral values and ethical roles in the 2 years after their graduation. Kelly found that the nurses went through a complex psychosocial process to preserve moral integrity and maintain a valued professional identity. This process resulted in a struggle that led to moral distress. Kelly concluded that the self-doubt and confusion from intense stress resulted in greater reliance on others as references for self-evaluation. She found also that individual ethical standards are influenced by group norms and that the environment in which nurses work and the practice and support of their more experienced colleagues are very important in the maintenance of professional values and a professional identity. With the results of Kelly's work in mind, it is very important to have a practice setting that some authors have described as a "moral community" (Storch, 1999, Webster and Baylis, 2000). A moral community is one in which "there is coherence between what healthcare institutions publicly profess to be—namely, helping, healing, caring environments that embrace the virtues intrinsic to the practice of healthcare and what employees, patients, and others both witness and participate in" (Webster & Baylis, 2000, p. 228).

When there is a gap between how professionals say they behave and the way they actually behave and practice, it is very difficult for individual practitioners to practice with *integrity.* The person with integrity can be relied on to act in a way that is responsive to a well-thought-out view of the relation between his or her beliefs and actions, but for people who practice in healthcare institutions, the ability to have integrity rests within the kind of organization they are a part of and can be said to be a relational concept. This is because when we work in a large institution, we rely on and have obligations to many other people, not just to our patients. Many bioethicists make a strong argument that such moral concepts as integrity and responsibility need to be understood as embedded in social structures (May, 1996; Sherwin, 2000; Webster & Baylis, 2000; MacDonald, 2002). These arguments suggest that approaches that emphasize the individual decision making of particular healthcare professionals (whether based on principles or cases or ideals of virtue) "will always be inadequate and that a more satisfying perspective on healthcare ethics must shift attention to the social relations and institutions that distribute power" (MacDonald, 2002, p. 288). For a professional, this means that professional ethics not only are embedded in an individual conscience but also result from interactions between persons. Thus, to have moral integrity as a professional, an individual must do more than simply adhere to what his or her conscience says. The person needs to evaluate critically the standards that he or she as a professional is required to follow both as an individual and collectively with others in the profession. If the standards are lacking or nurses are constrained from following them, then they must work as a group to develop new ones or to find ways of following them. Thus, maintaining our integrity is a relational process in which we need to reflect within ourselves and with others we work with (Hardingham, 2004a).

Conflict: Ambivalent Views and Approaches to Issues

Another barrier exists in the ways that society views healthcare hierarchies and concepts. For example, the notion of respect for patient autonomy, broadly recognized as the principle that patients have the authority to make their own decisions about their healthcare, occupies a prominent place in bioethics. However, Sherwin (2000) points out that feminists and others feel deeply ambivalent about the autonomy ideal. Although it is woven throughout many feminist approaches, Sherwin suggests that this ideal is something in need of a specifically feminist analysis.

Although there are many good reasons why respect for personal autonomy is important, there are also many problems with the autonomy ideal. For many feminists, the main problem is the focus on the individual that it usually takes, because life, especially for women, is not lived in a vacuum in which the decision maker acts in isolation. Decisions are made taking into consideration the relationships to other human beings, whether they are close relationships, such as those with parents, children, and partners, or less intimate relationships, such as those within communities or in professional–client relationships.

Sherwin proposes an alternative conception of autonomy, which she calls "relational autonomy." Although not denying that autonomy ultimately resides in individuals, Sherwin's concept takes into account the impact of social and political structures, especially sexism and other forms of oppression, on the lives and opportunities of individuals. "It realizes that the presence or absence of a degree of autonomy is not just a matter of being offered a choice. It also requires that the person have [sic] the opportunity to develop the skills necessary for making the type of choice in question, the experience of being respected in her decisions, and encouragement to reflect on her own values" (Sherwin, 2000, p. 79).

Applying the term *relational autonomy* to the full range of human relations, both personal and public, allows a political dimension to come in. It "makes visible the importance of considering how . . . social factors affect women's decision making" (Sherwin, 2000, p. 82) and how the place of nurses within the institutional context influences their ability to provide good nursing care.

Looking again at the Winnipeg nurses' story, the notion of relational autonomy is an excellent one. The nurses were concerned about their relationships with the children who were their patients, with the parents and families, with other members of the healthcare team, and with the wider community. In their decision making, they considered all of these groups, as well as the kinds of authority and influence that nurses had within the team, and decided that such actions as quitting or going public with their concerns would not be helpful and indeed, might cause more harm. They continued to press for change through the proper channels but remained distressed about taking the children into the operating room. Their worry that the parents didn't know enough about the program to make good decisions for their children's treatments was a constant source of pressure for them. On the other hand, the nurses realized the complexity of the relationships in healthcare and that the relationships depended on trust and cooperative action. Warning the parents or going to the press could do irreparable damage to trust and cooperation. The nurses felt that their own autonomy was diminished when their concerns went unheeded, leading some of the nurses to "silence themselves" (Sinclair, 2000, p. 478).

Limited Resources

Relational theory reminds us that material restrictions, including very restricted economic resources, "constitute real limitations on the options available to the agent. Moreover, it helps us to see how socially constructed stereotypes can reduce both society's and the agent's sense of that person's ability to act autonomously. Relational theory allows us to recognise how such diminished expectations readily become translated into diminished capacities" (Sherwin, 2000, p. 79).

The diminished capacities of the Winnipeg nurses resulted from, among other things, the lack of vehicles through which nurses could report incidents and concerns without risk of professional reprisal, the subservient position that nursing occupied within the organization, and the failure to involve nurses in the planning process of the pediatric cardiac surgery program (Sinclair, 2000).

 ## STRATEGIES FOR RESOLUTION OF ETHICAL AND LEGAL ISSUES

Once an ethical or legal issue for nurses is identified and analyzed, many strategies can be implemented to address and resolve it. Strategies include, but are not limited to, the following:

- Review the "Code of Ethics." The code is reviewed every 5 years, and nurses' input is invited for this process. If you identify an issue that does not seem to be addressed, you could volunteer to contribute to the code's review.
- Become familiar with the legislation, standards, codes, and policies that apply to nursing practice. When you cannot conform to them, document the problems. Incident report forms, professional responsibility forms, and other ways of reporting and discussing concerns should be utilized as often as possible to draw attention to unsafe and unethical practice.
- Ask for advice and support. Nurses' stories are of immediate interest in the political sphere, especially those that deal with ethical issues. Respect confidentiality, but try to find ways to broaden the approach to your issues. For example, contact your professional association or union for advice, support, and assistance to resolve concerns.
- Work to establish a moral community in your workplace. Participate actively on ethics committees, ethics rounds, and the like in hospitals and healthcare organizations. Most healthcare organizations have an ethics committee, an ethics consultation service, or other ways of dealing with ethical issues, and are becoming more concerned about ethics for accreditation purposes (Canadian Council on Health Service Accreditation, 2008). Bringing instances or concerns forward can often bring them to the attention of people who can take action to resolve them. Suggest a nursing ethics interest group or brown-bag lunch in your workplace to learn more about ethics and to discuss problems.
- Identify what you can do both as an individual and as part of a group to build a supportive moral community in your workplace. Research shows that the culture, the amount of support from

colleagues, and the kind of environment in which nurses work are important components to ethical practice (Kelly, 1998).

- Bring up ethical concerns with your colleagues and with the interdisciplinary team. Chances are that if you have a concern about something, other people in your workplace may as well. Remember, ethics is not just something you read about or study, but a practice, something you do. It requires dialogue and reflection on right action among members of a community; it also requires self-reflection. Organize a journal club or request educational sessions on ethical issues that arise. Use resources such as the "Code of Ethics for Registered Nurses" (CNA, 2002).

- Call the risk management committee (or coordinator) to bring their attention to a legal problem or a potential legal problem in a hospital or other healthcare facility where you work. This call alone may be enough to have action taken. Also, for legal issues, expertise and assistance are available from professional nursing organizations.

- Review ethically troubling cases retrospectively with colleagues. Take time to get together after a difficult case to discuss feelings, values, and beliefs about the case as well as what might be done differently the next time a similar case arises. Consider doing "preventive ethics" to put processes and procedures in place that might prevent ethically troubling situations (Hardingham, 2004b). If your organization has an ethicist or an ethics committee, ask for their assistance.

SUMMARY

Consider again the distress of the Winnipeg nurses in the pediatric cardiac surgery program. They were not facing moral uncertainty; they did not have a moral dilemma. They knew what the right thing to do was, and they did it. However, their concerns and attempts to use proper process did not help. They could have said, "We followed the policies, we took our concerns to the people we were supposed to report to, and so our responsibility is ended." But they did not: They continued to reflect on their concerns and continued to speak up for their patients. They decided that whistle-blowing or warning the parents might cause more problems. They thought it better for the children if they remained on the job and continued to try to work for institutional change. Carol Youngson and the other nurses suffered moral distress, and the resulting moral residue remains with them, possibly forever (Armstrong, 2001).

The issues around informed consent are not the only legal and ethical issues arising out of the Winnipeg story. Other issues include those of truth telling, whistle-blowing (going outside of the organization with information about harms or wrongdoing), nurse–patient relationships, conflicts between members of the healthcare team, and gender issues. However, the analysis presented around informed consent may act as a prototype that gives the reader a sense of what approaches to take to other issues.

Legal and ethical issues are significant to nurses, and they should be familiar with laws, codes, standards, and policies that apply to nursing practice.

Additionally, nurses should be able to identify, articulate, and understand ethical and legal issues and the problems that result when they are not able to do so. Identifying barriers to ethical and legal nursing practice is an important step for nurses to take.

The task of overcoming those barriers is one that cannot be undertaken only by individuals. Nurses as individuals are vulnerable when faced with legal and ethical issues. They require knowledge about the law and about ethics as well as the realization that they need to work individually and collectively to move identified issues toward resolution.

Add to your knowledge of this issue:	
Canadian Nurses Association (CNA)	www.cna-nurses.ca
Canadian Nurses Protective Society (CNPS)	www.cnps.ca
Bioethics for Clinicians	www.cmaj.ca/cgi/collection/bioethics_for_clinicians_series
NursingEthics.ca	www.nursingethics.ca
University of Toronto Joint Centre for Bioethics	www.utoronto.ca/jcb
The Canadian Bioethics Society (CBS)	www.bioethics.ca/english
Provincial Health Ethics Network (Alberta)	www.phen.ab.ca

Online

REFLECTIONS on the Chapter...

1 From your practice experience, identify examples of ethical and legal issues. How do you know that they were either ethical or legal issues? Were the two categories intertwined? If so, how, and how did you approach them?

2 Have you experienced moral uncertainty? A moral dilemma? Moral distress? What steps did you take? Looking back, what, if anything, would you do differently?

3 Think of the resources that are available to you to help you with ethical and legal issues. How would you go about accessing them?

4 Identify at least one ethical issue that seems to be prevalent in nursing practice. Is this issue one that is discussed publicly? What are the barriers to effective resolution of this issue? How are nurses approaching this issue and the problems it presents?

5 This chapter focuses on bioethical issues, with a particular emphasis on those that arise for nurses and in the nursing profession. What other approaches to ethics might inform nursing practice?

References

Armstrong, S. (2001). The crying shame. *Chatelaine,* pp. 86–94.

Baylis, F., Downie, J., & Hoffmaster, B., et al. (Eds.) (2004). *Health care ethics in Canada* (2nd ed.). Toronto: Nelson.

Boetzkes, E. & Waluchow, W. (2000). *Readings in health care ethics.* Peterborough: Broadview Press.

Canadian Council on Health Services Accreditation (2008). *CCHSA's Accreditation Program, 2008.* Ottawa: Author.

Canadian Nurses Association. (2002). *Code of ethics for registered nurses.* Ottawa: Author.

Canadian Nurses Protective Society. (1994). *Consent to treatment: The role of the nurse.* Ottawa: Author.

College & Association of Registered Nurses of Alberta. (2005). *Continuing Competence Program.* Edmonton: Author.

Hardingham, L.B. (2001a). Ethics in the workplace: Raising the standards of informed consent. The Winnipeg Inquest. *Alberta RN, 57*(1), 22–23.

_____. (2001b). Ethics in the workplace: Nurses and informed consent: Lessons from the Winnipeg Inquest. *Alberta RN, 57*(2), 22–23.

_____. (2004a). Integrity and moral residue: Nurses as participants in a moral community. *Nursing Philosophy, 5*(2), 127–134.

_____. (2004b). Managing ethically. In A. Crowther (Ed.), *Nurse managers: A guide to practice* (pp. 23–36). Melbourne, Australia: Ausmed Publications.

Jennings, B. (1996). The regulation of virtue: Cross-currents in professional ethics. In R.A. Larmer (Ed.), *Ethics in the workplace: Selected readings in business ethics* (pp. 397–404). Minneapolis/St.Paul: West Publishing.

Keatings, M. & Smith, O.B. (2000). *Ethical and legal issues in Canadian nursing* (2nd ed.). Toronto: W.B. Saunders Canada.

Kelly, B. (1998). Preserving moral integrity: A follow-up study with new graduate nurses. *Journal of Advanced Nursing, 28*(5), 1134–1145.

May, L. (1996). *The socially responsive self: Social theory and professional ethics.* Chicago: University of Chicago Press.

MacDonald, C. (2002) Nurse autonomy as relational. *Nursing Ethics, 9*(2), 194–201.

Redman, B.K. & Fry, S.T. (2000). Nurses' ethical conflicts: What is really known about them? *Nursing Ethics 2000, 7*(4), 360–366.

Sherwin, S. (2000). A relational approach to autonomy in health care. In E. Boetzkes & W. Waluchow (Eds.), *Readings in health care ethics.* Peterborough, ON: Broadview Press.

Sibbald, B. (1997). A right to be heard. *Canadian Nurse, 93*(10), 22–28, 30.

Sinclair, C.M. (2000). *Report of the Manitoba pediatric cardiac surgery inquest* [Online]. Winnipeg: Manitoba Provincial Court. Retrieved from http://www.pediatriccardiacinquest.mb.ca.

Storch, J. (1999). Ethical dimensions of leadership. In J.M. Hibberd & D.L. Smith (Eds.), *Nursing management in Canada* (2nd ed., pp. 351–367). Toronto: W.B. Saunders Canada.

Thomas, J. & Waluchow, W. (1998). *Well and good: A case study approach to biomedical ethics* (3rd ed.). Peterborough, ON: Broadview Press.

Webster, G.C. & Baylis, F. (2000). Moral residue. In S.B. Rubin & L. Zoloth (Eds.), *Margin of error: The ethics of mistakes in the practice of medicine.* Hagerstown, MD: University Publishing Group.

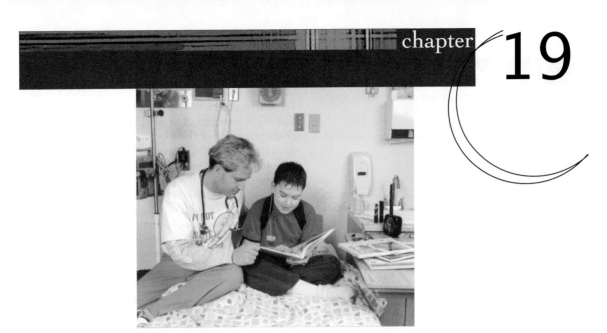

chapter 19

The identification of nursing as a gendered occupation is nothing new. A man who chooses nursing as a profession is inevitably identified as a "male nurse," whereas a woman is rarely referred to as a "female nurse." (Photograph by Larry Arbour. Used with permission from Faculty of Nursing, University of Calgary.)

Issues of Gender and Power: The Significance Attributed to Nurses' Work

Carol McDonald

Critical Questions

As a way of engaging with the ideas in this chapter, consider the following:

1. How have you come to hold the views you hold of gender and gendered roles?

2. How is it that historically some work has been thought of as women's work?

3. How does value get assigned to particular work?

Chapter Objectives

After completing this chapter, you will be able to:

1. Identify ways of thinking about power structures, including ideologies, social discourses, and the discursive process.

2. Understand the conceptualization of gender as socially constructed, the process of naturalizing knowledge, the idea that gender resides both within and beyond the individual, and the ways in which gender knowledge is bound by cultural, temporal, and social realities.

3 Recognize gender as one of a number of intersecting identities, including race, class, age, ethnicity, and sexual orientation, through which we are uniquely constituted as individuals.

4 Articulate the nature of nurses' work, nurses' knowledge, and nurses' public representation as gendered, and discuss the historical social discourses of women's work and nurses' work that have contributed to this understanding.

5 Discuss the barriers that interfere with the resolution of issues that arise from relations of power and gender and the significance attributed to nurses' work.

6 Identify strategies that will serve to interrupt the taken-for-granted notions of gendered work that underlie the devaluing of nurses' work.

This chapter presents opportunities to consider the idea that societally derived concepts about gender are inherent in claims about the value of nurses' work and the importance of nursing knowledge. The chapter challenges readers to look beneath the taken-for-granted assumptions about what is called women's work in general and nurses' work in particular. In reconsidering what we think we know, we come to see the web of social discourses through which work, knowledge, and nursing itself are inscribed with meanings of gender.

Ideas about women and women's work and whether this work requires significant knowledge, responsibility, and skill contribute to the devaluing of nurses' work by society. This chapter examines historical changes in the valuing of work that is ordinarily performed by women. It suggests that the devaluing of nurses' work and knowledge stems from cultural power arrangements. The impact of discourses of care, or ideas about care as central to nursing practice, on the value attributed to nurses' work are examined as well (Box 19.1).

GENDER AND POWER: ARTICULATING THE ISSUE FOR NURSING

How do concepts of gender and power arise in a discussion of the issues currently affecting Canadian nurses in education and in practice? Gender is a concept in our society that is simultaneously taken for granted and poorly understood. In this chapter, *gender* refers to the ways in which a person lives a life that demonstrates or reflects masculinity and femininity. As the chapter explores, gender can be thought of as constructed through social influences outside of a particular individual. And although there is undoubtedly some interrelationship between biologic sex and gender, this chapter addresses gender as distinct from the categories of biologic sex.

As nurses, we seldom think about the preponderance of female practicing nurses. When we do reflect on the gender division in nursing, we may think no further than "the numbers," that is, the distribution of genders in the profession. However, the issues of gender and power, as they relate to nursing, are more complicated than the biologic sex of those who practise nursing. Moreover, gender itself is not an "issue" in nursing. The fact that most practicing nurses are women is not in itself problematic. What is problematic for the profession is that gender is inextricably linked to relations of power. This connection of gender and power underlies and fuels issues related to the devaluing of nurses' work and the subordination of nurses' knowledge.

The discussion of power, and particularly relations of power as they affect nursing, may rouse a certain discomfort within nurse-readers in view of the societally ingrained reluctance to examine our own power (Falk Rafael, 1996). However, because nursing as a profession has been largely composed of women, who are socialized to avoid discussions of power, we must venture into this deliberation.

This chapter explores and raises questions about value and worth, particularly the value and worth attached to the gendered nature of work, of knowledge, of nursing. These concepts of value and worth are the commodities of power. When we talk about the value of nurses' knowledge or the ways in which work that is called women's work is devalued, we are talking about power.

BOX 19.1 Glossary of Terms and Definitions

This list describes the way some terms are used in the content of this chapter. They should not be taken as absolute definitions of the words.

Complicity—our own participation in, for example, supporting or reinforcing societal norms that undermine the value of women's work.

Essentializing—seeing something as representative of all members of a particular group or category. For example, essentializing nurses' work in a woman's domain implies that there is something about nursing that could only be performed by women.

Discourses—social practices, values, and cultural beliefs that prevail in a given culture or subculture at a specific historical moment and shape a collective sense of what is right, proper, worthwhile, or valuable (Thorne, McCormick, & Carty, 1997, p. 2).

Discourses of care—the ways in which ideas about care have been represented in nursing, particularly the values and beliefs that have placed care central to nursing practice.

Discursive process—how we learn to be and to behave in particular ways through the messages received in social discourses.

Gender—the ways in which femininity and masculinity are reflected in the lived life. Gender is distinct from the biologic sex of a person. Culturally, there is value attached to particular genders and the way in which that gender is performed.

Ideologies—not merely ideas, but a powerful and authoritative voice in society that tells us who we are and how we are to behave.

Location of gender—gender is constructed through the interaction of the person with the social realities, values, and beliefs of a culture at a particular time in history. In this sense, gender resides both within and beyond the individual.

Naturalized—when some quality is taken to be innately, or obviously "the way it is," without questioning the beliefs on which that assumption is formed. For example, the symbol of a "woman" (wearing a dress) and a "man" (wearing pants) have become naturalized in our culture to represent the washrooms in public places to be used by women or men. Although there is nothing innately natural about these symbols representing men or women, we have come to interpret them unquestioningly in this way (Fig. 19.1).

Reinscribing—reinforcing or reproducing a concept or belief, at times without the thoughtful intention of doing so.

Social construction—ideas, concepts, and roles that are understood to be formed or built up through the agreed-on ideologies of a society.

Transparency—the ways in which we can see something clearly, or obviously (high transparency), or in which something is obscured from our view. For example, increasing our awareness of material and social realities that contribute to gendering of nurses' work will improve our ability to see, or make transparent to us, the manner in which nursing is undervalued because it is "women's work."

In exploring the significance of gender in relation to nursing practice, nursing knowledge, and nurses themselves, we may begin by acknowledging the complexity of gender per se. Then we need to explore ways of thinking about gender beyond distribution, beyond the numbers of nurses who are female or male (Box 19.2.) These ways of thinking about gender will anchor us in the world of social realities where nursing is practised and where concepts of gender and gender practices are formed.

The first section of this chapter explores the theories that support an understanding of the gendered nature of work, knowledge, and the individual nurse. Grounded in feminist thought, this way

BOX 19.2 Exploring Gender in Nursing

Since the original publication of this text, I have received this inquiry from an undergraduate student. We thought including the question and my response might be a good point of discussion for other students:

Hello Dr. McDonald,

Do you genuinely believe that men should be in the nursing profession? I don't know if it's my imagination but I think you believe that the nursing profession is a feminist movement—"this book is unapologetically feminist, shows respect for our history and is deeply invested in our future" p.xvi. I don't understand.

David (personal communication)

Here is my response:

Hi David—Thanks for your inquiry about the text. In response to your questions:

I don't see the nursing profession either historically or currently as a feminist movement. Feminism is one of the theoretical approaches or lenses through which we examine the issues raised in the text. Feminism in this sense is meant to explore the gendered nature of issues. The notion that nursing has been historically constructed through a feminized approach (i.e., nurses as handmaidens) has not done anyone any favours, least of all the men who enter the profession. I do support the idea of men in nursing and feel particularly supportive of men who, recognizing the gender issues nurses have faced historically, work alongside women to strengthen the discipline and the profession for all people.

I hope this is helpful to you—I would welcome any further comments or questions.

Best, Carol (personal communication)

of conceptualizing gender and its effects in the social world is useful in understanding the significance of nurses' work.

Understanding Gender

As concepts, gender, women's work, and nursing itself derive their meaning in society through social construction. Social construction means that ideas, concepts, and roles are understood to be formed or built up through the agreed-on ideologies of a society. Ideologies, in this sense, are not merely ideas; they are imbued with power. They become the authoritative voice in society through which we come to understand ourselves. Ideologies tell us who we are, what we are to think, and how we are to behave (Althusser, 1971).

The power of ideologies lies in the authority that has us view much of our world as "natural" (obvious). *Nurse*, for example, is not a naturally occurring phenomenon, but the concept of *nurse* may become naturalized through ideologies about what constitutes or makes up the role of nurse. Although we may acknowledge intellectually that there is no natural role or personality attributable to *nurse*, we often, unthinkingly, act as if the opposite is so. The opportunity and the challenge in considering the social construction of nursing, gender, and "women's work" is twofold:

- to disrupt the thinking that supports taken-for-granted notions
- to question the source of ideologies on which the "natural facts" are based.

Thinking in a way that interrupts that which is taken for granted helps us to recognize our own participation and complicity in supporting (reinscribing) ideologies that contribute to the undervaluing of nurses' work and nursing knowledge (Fig. 19.1).

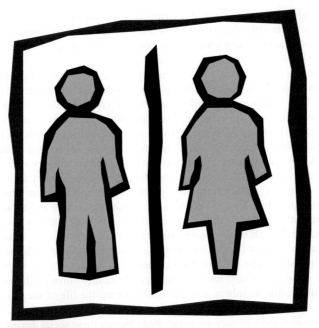

Figure 19.1

The symbols of a "woman" (wearing a dress) and a "man" (wearing pants) have become naturalized in our culture to represent the washrooms in public places to be used by women or men. Although there is nothing innately natural about these symbols representing men or women, we have come to interpret them unquestioningly in this way.

Gender as Social Construction

What does it mean to think of gender as socially constructed? How does this way of understanding gender benefit one's thinking about issues of gender and power in nursing as a profession and in nursing practice?

That people are gendered is taken for granted in everyday life and, although central to our experience of the world, is seldom thought about beyond the surface level. The lack of clarity between concepts of gender and biologic sex supports the tendency to keep our understandings of gender superficial. From the moment of birth, the biologic sex of the newborn is announced in a public way. This proclamation, biologically driven, determines much of the future of the child's life. Or does it?

In *Revisioning Gender*, Nakano Glenn notes that "feminist scholars adopted the term *gender* precisely to free our thinking from the constrictions of naturalness and biological inevitability attached to the concept of sex" (2000, p. 4). In this sense, gender moves us to a broader understanding of what it is to live one's life in ways that reflect masculinity and femininity. Butler (1990), a prominent feminist thinker, discusses gender not as the expression of an internal identity but rather as a performance in which the person acts a script that is written in and through social discourses. In this context, discourses are "social practices, values and cultural beliefs that prevail in a given culture or subculture at a specific historical moment and shape a collective sense of what is right, proper, worthwhile or valuable" (Thorne, McCormick, & Carty, 1997, p. 2).

Through these social discourses, we are inscripted with the knowledge of what it is to live a particularly gendered life. Although Butler maintains "that there is nothing about a binary gendered system that is given" (1990, p. 282), the scripts that are currently provided and normalized through social discourses offer little alternative to the categories of male and female. A concept of gender that surpasses biologic determinism provides the possibility, at least, of recognizing and valuing the masculine and the feminine that reside within each of us.

Crucial to this understanding is what may be called the *location of gender*. Although the biologic anatomy of an individual resides with that person, gender as a social construction is located in a more complex way, both within and beyond the individual. The construction of gender, meaning the ways in which gender identities are acted out and the value attached to gender, originates outside of the individual person, in society. Notions of gender are constructed through the ideologies of the culture; they become known to us through social discourse. Gender knowledge is situated in particular temporal and social realities that are largely taken for granted by members of the culture. This taken-for-grantedness reflects our participation in the ideologies of the society in which we reside. In other words, we are complicit in reinforcing the ideas that define and structure what are accepted as normal, gender-appropriate behaviors and beliefs in our immediate culture and time.

The commonly unexamined evidence of the ways in which gender knowledge is bound by cultural, temporal, and social realities surrounds us. When a child is born, how others respond to "It's a girl!" or "It's a boy!" is heavily influenced by the gender knowledge of the particular culture in a particular time in history. The proclamation communicates not only the sex of the child but also the meaning and value that is held for this young gendered life. Through the powerful ideologies of the culture, parents, family members, and strangers take up the life of the child as gendered, in effect, teaching the child to be in the world in gender-appropriate ways. As adults, we come to perform our gender roles, in large part, as they are prescribed through these social discourses.

Gender as Part of Identity

In recognizing how dominant social discourses influence who we are to be, the production of identity becomes a discursive process (Scott, 1992). The term *discursive process* refers to how we learn to be, in particular ways, through the messages we receive in social discourses. Our concept of ourselves as gendered is one way in which we become subjects with particular identities. As we move on to consider some of the implications of what it means to be gendered subjects, we need to bear in mind that gender is but one component of our identity that is formed through discursive processes.

The gendered self is one of a number of the selves or identities through which we are uniquely formed as people. The gendered self intersects with other identities, such as race, class, age, ethnicity, and sexual orientation, in the constitution of each individual. The experience of living one's life as a Black, young, middle-class, heterosexual, male nursing student may be quite different from the experience of living as a white, middle-aged, poor, lesbian, single-mother nursing student. The difference of experience, although influenced by gender and what it means to be gendered in particular ways, is also constructed through material realities, such as economics and availability of social resources, as well as through the influence of dominant social discourses.

The idea of the intersecting identities of nurses is addressed in Reverby's (1987) historical critique of American nursing. In her exploration of some of the historical unrest in the discipline, Reverby suggests that class differences among individual nurses and between groups of nurses with diverse training contributed to an internal hierarchy within nursing. Although the oppression of women was a reality for these nurses, they were also bound by their own participation in classist assumptions and ideologies. In this case, the "commonalities of the gendered experience could not become the basis for unity as long as hierarchical filial relations, not equal sisterhood, underlay nurses' lives" (Reverby, 1987, p. 201). Reverby describes a situation in which the class identities of these nurses held more influence than their shared gender identity.

In essence, ideologies that become imbued with power carry societal authority to tell us who we are. Allen, writing of the postmodern critique in nursing, calls us to notice and to question "the ways in which discourses function as regimes of power, where knowledge and power interact to normalize or legitimate specific interests" (1992, p. xiv). The power attributed to particular social positions and particular identities, including gender, is neither random nor benign. Collins, a black feminist scholar, reminds us that "race, gender, social class, ethnicity, age and sexuality are not descriptive categories applied to individuals. Instead these elements of social structure emerge as fundamental devices that foster inequity in resulting groups" (1997, p. 376). In other words, the meanings that are attached to these identities and social positions shape what is possible: the ways in which we live our lives and the ways that others see us. And while it is important to remember that not all of these differences matter in the same way, we are challenged to keep in our awareness the difference that the meanings attributed to gender makes.

THE EFFECTS OF GENDER IN NURSES' LIVES

Once we think of people as gendered through a discursive process influenced by the social and material realities of a culture at a particular time, we can see that the gendering process extends beyond individuals—to institutions, organizations, and bodies of knowledge. Although it may be obvious that gender does not explicitly reside in these locations, it is also true that gender attributes are assigned to, or play themselves out in, various institutions. In this way, particular work becomes gendered in our minds. The implications of gendered institutions and gendered knowledge are profound. Gender in our society is not value neutral; thus, the gendered nature of knowledge, work, and institutions impacts the value given to that knowledge or work in our society.

The Gendered Nature of Work

"The gendered division of labor in the home and in the work place is part of a negotiated order that is accomplished within the social context of a prevailing set of normative conceptions or ideologies, about what activities are appropriate for men and women" (Angus, 1994, p. 24).

In exploring the working lives of Canadian women, Angus notes that the "labor force is characterized by marked horizontal (occupational) and vertical (hierarchical) gender divisions" (1994, p. 32). What this means is that women in preponderate numbers enter a limited subdivision of the workforce: a subdivision understood to be gender-typed as "women's work." Among these occupations is nursing, which composes part of about 80% of women workers who are "employed in labor-intensive occupations . . . concentrated in the public sector . . . where cost containment has produced additional burdens and frustration" (Angus, 1994, pp. 32, 38).

Angus' (1994) work also comments on the vertical division of labor by gender in certain occupations. This division refers to the socially created reality that occupations dominated by men are better rewarded than those dominated by women. According to Angus (1994), this phenomenon is attributable to the dominant discourses in our society that support the valuing of technical skill over interpersonal skill. It is also evident that, within many occupational groups, women are less likely to be promoted to administrative positions or to be financially rewarded as generously as their male counterparts.

Although this argument within the nursing profession is open to debate, the challenges that women often negotiate as the primary caregivers in their personal or familial situations along with the demands of professional nursing practice are rigorous. The requirements of personal responsibilities may be experienced as incompatible with the additional demands of administrative work or participation in professional or union organizations, thus limiting the participation of nurses—in particular, women nurses—from positions of power and politics (Angus, 1994). This is not to suggest that men in nursing may rise to particular positions by virtue of being men, but it does open questions about the social landscape on which the realities of the demands of labor reside. Other questions may be raised as well. How do these social arrangements contribute to what some have called an "over-representation (of men) in top positions compared with their minority status in the profession" (Davies, 1995, p. 9)?

A feminist critique would suggest that we resist the temptation to assign responsibility for the work-life choices that women are forced to make to the individual nurse. Instead, we might examine the social conditions of nurses' lives, such as primary caregiving responsibilities and a lack of childcare resources, and the incompatibility of these social realities with the career demands of nursing.

Nursing practice has long been equated with "female virtues"—the virtues of care, nurturance, and altruism. In an exploration of classism, genderism, and racism in nursing, Turkoski notes that, historically, nursing has been "described in purely genderised terms as: 'women's mission, ministry, humanitarian service,' a 'service of womanly duty and conscience,' and 'the noblest and most womanly of professions'" and reminds us that these descriptions "reinforced the assumption that nursing is essentially related to one's biological makeup" (1992, p. 162). "Gentleness and quietness were required of Nightingale's nurses, and many nurses in today's work force that 'trained' in the 1960s and earlier can attest to the importance attached to those virtues" (Falk Rafael, 1996, p. 9). Some of those nurses, who are still in practice, were expected to demonstrate as their "professional" behavior unquestioning deference to physicians, for example, standing when physicians entered the room, vacating chairs and opening doors for them, as well as obediently, even unthinkingly, carrying out physicians' orders. Abbott and Wallace argue that although "nurses no longer see themselves as handmaidens to doctors, they have remained trapped in their status as subordinate to doctors" (1990, p. 22). In support of this argument, Abbott and Wallace remind us of nurses being accountable for administering medication that they are not authorized to prescribe.

In an article discussing the tensions between power and caring in the nursing profession, Falk Rafael itemizes the characteristics traditionally associated with femininity and masculinity as follows (1996, p. 5):

Femininity	Masculinity
Submissiveness	Strength
Helplessness	Aggression
Dependency	Mastery
Tenderness	Independence
Nurturance	Logic
Altruism	Being unemotional
	Competitiveness
	Ambition

Falk Rafael (1996) notes that these traditional notions of femininity and masculinity have been constructed in a way that associates the masculine with power and the feminine with care. She reminds us that knowledge is developed and propagated in particular ways to maintain power. The "scientification" of knowledge over the past several hundred years demonstrates the systematic devaluing of the feminine. The "denigration of women and that which is feminine has been entrenched in all of civilisation's major institutions" (Falk Rafael, 1996, p. 6). In this conceptualization, *care* is constructed as a female virtue and one that holds little esteem in Western society. How do we reconcile this devaluing of care with the centrality of it to the nursing profession?

Fisher, in exploring gender and power in nursing, locates a discourse of care as having "played a central role in the constitution of nursing as a gendered profession" (1993, p. 117). The association of nursing with care is complicated by the social belief in care as an innately female quality. When viewed as natural or essential—meaning innately residing in all women—the idea of care may contribute to undermining the value of nurses' work. When care is undervalued, as a feminine virtue, the devaluation extends beyond the individual nurse, be that nurse a woman or a man, to the work itself.

How is it that the value of care has been so compromised by society? A feminist historical analysis connects the value attached to work ordinarily performed by women in the public sphere to the changing value attached to work performed by women in the private sphere (Bunting, 1992). In preindustrial times, before the advent of large-scale productivity and commercialization, the work ordinarily performed by women was associated with the maintenance and care of home and family and was more closely aligned, in worth, to the work ordinarily performed by men. The refocusing of modern society on a production- and wage-oriented economy resulted in a devaluation of the care work ordinarily performed by women in the private sphere. Women were placed in the "position of performing services and producing products for the family that have no recognised market value" (Bunting, 1992, p. 58). Along with Bunting, we might wonder about the "connections between the devaluing of women's care in the home and the difficulty of gaining recognition for *nurses'* contributions of care" (1992, p. 60). Bunting (1992) finds a relationship between the invisibility and taken-for-grantedness of caregiving in the private sphere, based on the absence of financial remuneration, and the low status of nursing as a profession. Are there, then, in the social discourses of care, blurred boundaries between work that is "recognised, valued, and paid for . . . [and] work [that] is treated as a labor of love or duty" (Bunting, 1992, p. 61)?

Condon suggests we consider the feminist understanding of Fisher and Tronto that appreciates caring as a "positive dimension of our lives that has been socially devalued by a patriarchal and capitalistic order" (Condon, 1992, p. 73). In this way, the concept of care continues to be valued, and the effort is directed toward interrupting the social discourses that contribute to the devaluing of care. In contrast to duty and calling, which she calls "old masculine metaphors," Condon maintains that care provides an "infinitely more authentic metaphor grounded in the experience of women and capable of being practiced by anyone who chooses it as a social, as well as a professional, ethic" (1992, p. 81).

The Gendered Nature of Knowledge

"Ideas about women, about women's work and how it does or does not require significant knowledge, responsibility, and skill are embedded in nursing and become part of nursing's taken-for-granted reality" (Ceci & McIntyre, 2001, p. 121).

In considering the gendered nature of knowledge, and particularly the impact of gendered knowledge on nursing practice, we may ask, what counts as knowledge? Who decides what counts as knowledge? How might we understand the significance of knowledge gendered in particular ways? McIntyre suggests that "nursing knowledge is inextricable from the assumptions and values underlying its generation. Explicating the assumptions underlying different approaches to knowledge generation in nursing . . . helps nurses avoid unquestioning conformity to existing knowledge" (1999, p. 46).

Through time, nurses have been influenced by the discourses around several bodies of knowledge. Before the industrialization of nursing, women healers and caregivers were privileged to gynocentric (feminine-centered) knowledge, for example, midwifery and herbal pharmacology, as well as the knowledge necessary for the care of home and family (Ginzberg, 1999). These areas of knowledge have lost value in the foreground of Western science and scientific knowledge, which was produced with an androcentric (masculine-centered) focus. Critiques of science in the 20th century suggest that "knowledge produced by the sciences is part of the social and political tradition within which it is produced" (Welch, 1999, p. 423). Such critiques support the notion that particular "women's activities haven't been called 'science' for *political* reasons, even when those activities have been model examples of inquiry leading to knowledge of the natural world" (Ginzberg, 1999, p. 441).

In her work *Gender and Science*, Fox Keller, a scientist and feminist, explores the "historically pervasive association between masculine and objective, more specifically between masculine and scientific" (1999, p. 427). She addresses this notion as having reached near-mythical status as "it has simultaneously the air of being 'self-evident' and 'nonsensical'—the former by virtue of existing in the realm of common knowledge and the later by virtue of . . . conflicting with our image of science as emotionally and sexually neutral" (Fox Keller, 1999, p. 427). She cautions, however, of the potential for unexamined myths to subversively affect our thinking. How, for example, might the masculinity associated with the knowledge we call science influence what counts as nursing knowledge?

The kinds of knowledge that are valued and prioritized in nursing education are clearly reflective of the gendered nature of the profession. The association of early nursing education with "womanly virtues," as discussed earlier, continues to be relevant in what Rafferty calls the "intellectual and social subordination of nurses" (1996, p. 1) and in the "deep anti-intellectual prejudice attached to woman's work in general" (1996, p. 1). The concept of the mandate of nurses' education toward producing graduates of a particular moral character remains covertly present in social discourses and reinforces the location of nursing within the "natural" domain of womanhood.

In discussions of Project 2000, regarding nursing education in Britain, Davies found among healthcare professionals the "distinct echoes . . . of the historical equation of nursing with the female sex, of the view that a good nurse is born, not made, that a good woman is a good nurse" (1995, p. 114). Davies (1995) reports, in her gender analysis of the profession, on the belief held by nurses and other healthcare professionals that the work of nursing is a practical skill that does not require advanced education in the sciences or in theory but is best developed through an apprenticeship model of learning. Mackay also argues that there is a "tension between a vocational and a professional view of the nurse" (1998, p. 62) in Britain. She notes that although this may not be directly acknowledged by nurses, the "concept of vocation is embedded in many of the accepted practices and attitudes within nursing, such as being of service to others and putting others first" (Mackay, 1998, p. 63).

Is this discussion relevant to Canadian nurses and to the education of nursing students in Canada? Although some may argue that the Canadian Nurses Association has advocated the baccalaureate entry to practice since 1993, the view of nursing as a vocation may be held by numbers of nurses in practice. In discussing the situation in Canada, Armstrong (1993) presents student nurses as apprentices and points out the financial inequities between these students and apprentices in male-dominated occupations. Despite the endorsement of baccalaureate entry to practice and the increasing academic preparation of nurses, the gender issues of nurses remain.

These conflicted ideals regarding the meaning and methods of nurse education raise resounding questions. Whose purpose is being served through the deintellectualization of nurses' education? How does the apprenticeship model serve the economic and labor needs of hospitals and the healthcare system? What is the meaning for nurses of an education that prepares them to develop "character" and practical skills while undervaluing the development of intellectual pursuit in independent thinking, analysis, and problem solving, to say nothing of the theoretical knowledge underlying the practice of manual or technical skills? How does the intellectual devaluing of nurses' knowledge, reinscribed by particular healthcare professionals, contribute to the marginality of the nurse's position in the healthcare system?

The Gendered Nature of the Nurse

"Nursing has always been a much conflicted metaphor in our culture, reflecting all the ambivalences we give to the meaning of womanhood" (Reverby, 1987, p. 207).

At any given point in time, there may be multiple discourses participating in the construction of the nurse as subject. Put another way, social discourses present an image of what it is to be and to practise as a nurse. "Just as the cosmetic and fashion industries created the 'ideal woman,' so nursing texts, be they in popular press, television, or textbook form, create images of the ideal nurse" (Cheek & Rudge, 1994, p. 589). These idealized images of nurse are by no means unified. Part of the complexity of attaining the ideal is that it comprises mixed and conflicting messages and changes over time.

Regardless of the variables that form this ideal—including race, ethnicity, age, and sexuality—"both the nurse and the work of nursing are firmly associated in the public mind with the female sex" (Davies, 1995, p. 2). The naturalness of a woman performing as a nurse is reflected in the fact that "a man in the same job will be described not just as a nurse but as 'male nurse'" (Davies, 1995, p. 2). As suggested by Davies in the introduction to her text *Gender and the Professional Predicament in Nursing*, "a closer acquaintance with nursing, however, shatters any cozy image of women doing work that is somehow *natural* to them and hence being entirely comfortable in and satisfied with the role they have chosen" (1995, p. 2; emphasis added).

A current American television portrayal of an emergency room nurse as an autonomous, independent, respected, and compassionate professional conveys a particular appeal to nurses entering the profession. The actual social and material realities of this nurse's professional world may, in fact, be as much of a fabrication as the professionally submissive representation of the fictional Dr. Welby's nurse several decades ago. Both of these media portrayals of the nurse reflect an idealized image of "woman" formed through the prominent social discourses of the day. Although these images differ vastly from one another, they both present an idealized image of nurse-woman.

Is it possible that the public propagation of these ideals serves to undermine a more accurate representation of the nurse's lived experience, both in the eyes of the public and in the eyes of nurses themselves? Kalisch and Kalisch (1987) would concur that through the 19th and 20th centuries, media representations of the nurse have contributed to a narrow and undervalued image of nursing, drawing strongly on a received view of the nature of woman. We are challenged by nursing scholars to "raise questions about those discourses and ways of thinking, in the world or in us, which diminish nursing" (Ceci & McIntyre, 2001, p. 121). Among the discourses that require our ongoing interrogation are those that present a gender-idealized image of the nurse.

BARRIERS TO AND STRATEGIES FOR ISSUE RESOLUTION

Several barriers to resolving the issue of gender-related devaluing of nursing practice and the nursing profession need to be identified before strategies for change can be devised.

Identifying Barriers: Furthering Our Understandings

"The dilemma of nursing is too tied into the broader problems of gender and class in our society to be solved solely by the political efforts of one occupational group" (Reverby, 1987, p. 207). The barriers to the resolution of issues of gender and power in nursing are embedded in societal ideology. As nurses, we require both the knowledge and the willingness to critique and to challenge these social discourses. In particular, we can consider the following barriers that impair movement toward understanding the issues:

1. The gendered nature of work in general, and nurses' work in particular, is concealed—or implicitly present—in nursing practice. Although the effects of gendering on nursing practice are part of our experience, there is a lack of discussion that identifies these experiences as the problematic effects of gender and power.

2. The effects of power and gender in nurses' work and nursing knowledge are taken for granted in nurses' practice and education. The lack of transparency regarding the gendered nature of nurses' work (see barrier 1) contributes to our inability to question the embedded assumptions regarding gender and nurses' work.

3. Historically, nurses have lacked a critical feminist analysis that provides a framework to critique and question the taken-for-granted social discourses of gender, nurses' work, and the valuing of care in society.

4. Although the gendered divisions of labor have long been ingrained in society, only recently has the gendered nature of work been called into question in academic discourses that are accessible to nursing.

5. Understandings of the gendered nature of nurses' work are impaired by the larger lack of clarity and articulation of the nature of nurses' work in general. The inaccurate and limited public representations of the nurse and nurses' work contribute to the limited understanding and devaluing of nurses' work and nursing knowledge.

6. Individual efforts to disrupt the taken-for-granted ideas of gender require one to challenge social discourses and dominant views. This necessary strategy produces a barrier for the individual by placing her or him in a tension with commonly held societal views.

Devising Strategies: Voice and Action

1. Several of the barriers to resolving issues of gender and power, and their impact on the significance attributed to nurses' work, could be broken down by providing knowledge regarding the gendered nature of nurses' work both historically and as it is currently embedded in nursing practice. The knowledge necessary for a thorough understanding of gender and power issues is complex and requires familiarity with a structure that can be used to critique and challenge the taken-for-granted assumptions embedded in these issues. Knowledge of the gendered nature of nurses' work may be supported by feminist analysis, which focuses on the idea of power embedded in ideologies and the formation of gendered subjects through social discourses. This knowledge and the means to illuminate and question assumed truths belong in nursing curricula early in undergraduate nursing education. Much of the complexity of this knowledge lies in our lack of familiarity with concepts of gendering and social construction. As nurses become fluent in knowledge and language, the transparency regarding the gendered nature of nurses' work will be improved.

2. As identified in the aforementioned barriers, there is a tension generated between the origin of social discourses of gender and the value of particular types of work in society, and the disruption of these discourses must begin at an individual level. Important strategies to interrupt discourses that undermine the significance attributed to nurses' work begin with increasing our own awareness of these taken-for-granted discourses in our daily lives. Influencing these discourses in ways that call into question the way things have always been or the way things have always been done requires confidence and courage for the individual nurse.

3. The action required to change or disrupt large social ideologies can begin with wondering about the following:

   - what it is we think we "know"
   - the effects of taken-for-granted "truths" on the valuing of nurses' knowledge and practice
   - the ways in which we reinscribe social discourses of gender in our own practice.

4. As members of society, nurses and women have been socialized to suppress difference. To challenge effectively what is taken for granted about the role of gender and its powerful influence on nurses' work, we must be willing to notice difference and to acknowledge the way that differences, such as gender, class, race, ethnicity, and sexual orientation, matter in the ways our identities are lived and viewed by the world.

5. Social discourses of gender are more than ideas. They are intimately connected to the social and material realities of our lives. Exerting influence that will change or disrupt discourses of gender necessitates action that will improve, in particular, the material realities of women's lives. This means, for example, advocating for changes in the workplace that support the lives of women as they negotiate family and work responsibilities and demands. Adequate resources for childcare and family responsibilities are gendered workplace issues. Attending to these needs influences the value and respect attributed to women's multiple roles, including the significance attributed to nurses' paid work.

SUMMARY

This chapter explores multiple issues associated with the gendered nature of nurses' work, of nursing knowledge, and of the public representation of the nurse. Central to the issue are the social discourses about gender that are inherent in the value attributed to nurses' work and the importance attached to nurses' knowledge.

One question examined is this: Is the value accorded to nurses' work representative of the societal devaluing of work that is ordinarily performed by women? The exploration extends our understanding of gender and power in nursing beyond the idea of the distribution of gender in the profession. The significance of nurses' work and the value accorded this work are steeped in societal structures and ideologies that surpass the particular gender of the nurse who is performing the work.

The gendered nature of nurses' work and education has been with us since the inception of nursing. The gendered division of labor has historically placed nursing in the realm of women's work, a division that was supported through the early educational program for nurses that focused on "womanly virtues" and "moral character." The legacy of this account of nursing has been the conceptualization of care as both an innately feminine virtue residing in all women and a discourse central to nursing practice. The significance of nurses' work parallels the devaluing of care in a society that has increasingly valued science and a production-focused economy.

Given the early image of nursing as a natural extension of feminine virtues, we may be tempted to assign responsibility for "gendering" to the pioneering women of nursing practice and education. This chapter argues that the gendering of work occurs not with particular individuals but through society's discourses, which are embedded with ideologies.

The current and perhaps more difficult challenge is to recognize the less overt but no less present discourses of gender that structure current nursing practices. These discourses of gender—the nature of the work called "women's work" and the value that is afforded to caregiving in our society—underlie the significance of nurses' work.

In locating the discourses of gender in society, we need not look beyond ourselves. Our complicity is evident as we participate in the reinstatement of gendered discourses birthed in the societal ideologies from which we cannot extricate ourselves. The challenge, then, is to look for opportunities to recognize and to disrupt the taken-for-granted notions that define and constrain the possibilities for gendered people who are practising and being nurses.

REFLECTIONS on the Chapter...

❶ How do you understand gender as socially constructed? What are the implications of your understanding for nurses, for nurses' work, and for nursing as a profession?

❷ What does a feminist analysis of gender add to our understanding of the value and conditions of nurses' work?

❸ What are the benefits and limitations of placing gender in a central place in our analysis of nurses' work? How does gender intersect with other realities and conditions of nurses' lives?

❹ From your own nursing experience, provide an example of your participation in a taken-for-granted, socially sanctioned norm regarding gender. In retrospect, how might you have acted to interrupt this particular social discourse around gender?

References

Abbott, P. & Wallace, C. (Eds.). (1990). *The sociology of the caring professions.* London: Falmer Press.

Allen, D. (1992). Introduction. In J. Thompson, D. Allen, & L. Rodrigues-Fisher (Eds.), *Critique, resistance and action: Working papers in the politics of nursing* (pp. xi–xvi). New York: National League for Nursing Press.

Althusser, L. (1971). Ideology and ideological apparatuses. In B. Brewster (Trans.), L. Althusser (Ed.), *Lenin and philosophy and other essays* (pp. 123–172). London: New Left Books.

Angus, J. (1994). Women's paid/unpaid work and health: Exploring the social context of everyday life. *Canadian Journal of Nursing Research, 26*(4), 23–42.

Armstrong, P. (1993). Women's health care work: Nursing in context. In P. Armstrong, J. Choiniere, & E. Day (Eds.), *Vital signs: Nursing in transition.* Toronto: Garamond Press.

Bunting, S. (1992). Eve's legacy: An analysis of family caregiving from a feminist perspective. In J. Thompson, D. Allen, & L. Rodrigues-Fisher (Eds.), *Critique, resistance and action: Working papers in the politics of nursing* (pp. 53–68). New York: National League for Nursing Press.

Butler, J. (1990). Performative acts and gender constitution: An essay in phenomenology and feminist theory. In S. Case (Ed.), *Performing feminisms: Feminist critical theory and theatre* (pp. 270–282). Baltimore, MD: Johns Hopkins University Press.

Ceci, C. & McIntyre, M. (2001). A "quiet" crisis in health care: Developing our capacity to hear. *Nursing Philosophy, 2*(2), 121–127.

Cheek, J. & Rudge, T. (1994). The panopticon revisited? An exploration of the social and political dimensions of contemporary health care and nursing practice. *International Journal of Nursing Studies, 31*(6), 583–591.

Collins, P.H. (1997). Comment on Hekman's "Truth and method: Feminist standpoint theory revisited": Where's the power? *Signs: Journal of Women in Culture and Society, 22*(2), 375–381.

Condon, E. (1992). Nursing and the caring metaphor: Gender and political influences on an ethics of care. In J. Thompson, D. Allen, & L. Rodrigues-Fisher (Eds.), *Critique, resistance and action: Working papers in the politics of nursing* (pp. 69–84). New York: National League for Nursing Press.

Davies, C. (1995). *Gender and the professional predicament in nursing.* Philadelphia: Open University Press.

Falk Rafael, A. (1996). Power and caring: A dialectic in nursing. *Advances in Nursing Science, 19*(1), 3–17.

Ferree, M.M., Lorber, J., & Hess, B. (Eds.). (2000). *Revisioning gender.* New York: AltaMira Press.

Fisher, S. (1993). Gender, power, resistance: Is care the remedy? In S. Fisher & K. Davis (Eds.), *Negotiating at the margins: The gendered discourses of power and resistance* (pp. 87–121). New Brunswick, NJ: Rutgers University Press.

Fox Keller, E. (1999). Gender and science. In E.C. Polifroni & M. Welch (Eds.), *Perspectives on philosophy of science in nursing: An historical and contemporary anthology* (pp. 427–439). Philadelphia: Lippincott Williams & Wilkins.

Ginzberg, R. (1999). Uncovering gynocentric science. In E.C. Polifroni & M. Welch (Eds.), *Perspectives on philosophy of science in nursing: An historical and contemporary anthology* (pp. 440–450). Philadelphia: Lippincott Williams & Wilkins.

Kalisch, P. & Kalisch, B. (1987). *The changing image of the nurse.* Menlo Park, CA: Addison-Wesley.

Mackay, L. (1998). In P. Abbott & L. Meerabeau (Eds.), *The sociology of the caring professions* (2nd ed.). London: University College of London Press.

McIntyre, M. (1999). The focus of the discipline of nursing: A critique and extension. In E.C. Polifroni & M. Welch (Eds.), *Perspectives on philosophy of science in nursing: An historical and contemporary anthology* (pp. 46–54). Philadelphia: Lippincott Williams & Wilkins.

Nakano Glenn E. (2000). The social construction and institutionalization of gender and race: An integrative framework. In M.M. Ferree, J. Lorber, & B. Hess (Eds.), *Revisioning gender* (pp. 3–43). New York: AltaMira Press.

Rafferty, R. (1996). *The politics of nursing knowledge.* London: Routledge.

Reverby, S. (1987). *Ordered to care: The dilemma of American nursing, 1850–1945.* Cambridge, UK: Cambridge University Press.

Scott, J. (1992). Experience. In J. Butler & J. Scott (Eds.), *Feminists theorize the political* (pp. 22–40). London: Routledge.

Thorne, S., McCormick, J., & Carty, E. (1997). Deconstructing the gender neutrality of chronic illness and disability. *Health Care for Women International, 18*(1), 1–16.

Turkoski, B. (1992). A critical analysis of professionalism in nursing. In J. Thompson, D. Allen, & L. Rodrigues-Fisher (Eds.), *Critique, resistance and action: Working papers in the politics of nursing* (pp. 149–166). New York: National League for Nursing Press.

Welch, M. (1999). Science and gender. In E.C. Polifroni & M. Welch (Eds.), *Perspectives on philosophy of science in nursing: An historical and contemporary anthology* (pp. 423–426). Philadelphia: Lippincott Williams & Wilkins.

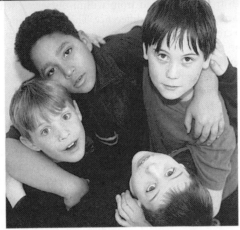

chapter 20

In what ways do differences matter and to whom? Although these boys appear to be friends of the same age, they may come from different cultures, economic levels, and belief systems. (Photography by Larry Arbour. Used with permission from the Faculty of Nursing, University of Calgary.)

When Difference Matters: The Politics of Privilege and Marginality

Christine Ceci

Critical Questions

As a way of engaging with the ideas in this chapter, consider the following:

1. Consider the assumptions that you hold about people who are different from you in relation to age, race, gender, education, and sexual orientation.

2. Take a moment to consider how you might have come to hold such assumptions.

3. As you begin to read this chapter, consider how these assumptions position you in your nursing practice.

Chapter Objectives

After completing this chapter, you will be able to:

1. Discuss multiple interpretations of difference.

2. Discuss social, political, and historical influences on our understanding of difference.

3. Explore the concept of difference as a relationship.

4. Critique the concept of difference as deviance.

5. Identify assumptions underlying ideas of normality.

This is a chapter about difference or, more specifically, about the challenges and resistances we encounter, both from others and from within ourselves, when we try to move beyond the superficial in our efforts to understand difference. The obvious approach calls on us to define differences, to list them, to create categories, to suppose that the significance or meaning of any particular difference is clear or uncontested. The obvious approach often assumes that the meanings of various "basic differences," reflected in categories, such as sex, race, or class, are already known to us—that trusting the evidence of our senses, we can read off the surface the difference of another. This thinking is the kind we want to let go of in this chapter—the thinking that says to us that difference is simply a characteristic, a trait, or a description easily assigned to another whose difference is obvious to us.

This is not to say, however, that activities of defining or categorizing are not sometimes useful but rather to suggest there are effects—some acceptable, some not—from the ways we draw boundaries that create differences. Although we may need to begin by organizing our observations, these definitions, categories, labels, and lists are inadequate in and of themselves for understanding difference. In fact, in this chapter, the tendency these activities have of locating difference outside ourselves and the processes of our own understanding is conceptualized as a problem. Further, this tendency poses a particular problem for nurses because of the opportunities we have to influence the kinds of experiences that people will have in healthcare systems. As nurses, we encounter people in their most vulnerable moments and so have opportunity to cause harm by unthinking adherence to the false and damaging beliefs and assumptions often contained in categories and labels. A willingness to question our own thinking, then, seems an obviously necessary task for nurses.

A PHILOSOPHICAL APPROACH TO UNDERSTANDING DIFFERENCE

The need to raise questions about the implications of the meanings of difference is supported by exploration of the various ways difference has been constructed in historical and contemporary situations. By reflecting on the examples explored in this chapter, we can ask who has defined difference in various situations and for what purposes have particular boundaries between groups been inscribed? On what basis are claims to difference made? How have the meanings of particular differences been contested? In what ways do differences matter and to whom? The historical examples allow us the distance to reflect on how particular ideas of difference have played themselves out and also, when considered alongside contemporary situations, enable us to trace similarities and extend our analyses from one context to another. For the same reason (i.e., so we may observe the similarity in processes of differentiation), a variety of what are commonly viewed as differences are explored. In each case, however, the difference discussed (e.g., race or sex) is not understood as a thing in itself but rather as an outcome of social processes of differentiation. In these terms, difference is understood not as a thing in itself but as a social relationship, and the meaning of any particular difference will depend on this relationship and context. What we want to keep in mind, then, is how difference operates in different areas of life.

Admittedly, this is a more philosophical approach to difference than some readers may be expecting, but if we wish to understand the complexity of ideas of difference, we must be willing to raise questions of meaning, a project that requires from us a certain amount of thoughtfulness. As used here, *thoughtfulness* refers to a conscious and critical engagement with our current understandings of difference, an engagement that encourages us to question what we think we already know. This, then, is the purpose of this chapter: to "problematize" difference. We will proceed by exploring the discourses and ways of thinking that define difference and consider the social contexts and conditions through which differences come to matter.

Historical and Contemporary Considerations

Accounting for difference among people, in situation and status, in privilege and power, has long been a preoccupation of Western societies. From at least as early as Plato's argument for the naturalness of unequal social status for men, women, and slaves, the purpose of these narratives has been, with few exceptions, to explain and justify the prevailing social order. Throughout Western history, dominant belief systems suggested that people were positioned in particular ways in society because of inborn differences in capacities and worth. These differences were often understood as determined by what were considered unalterable laws of nature. The differences in situation between men and women, rich and poor, and races and cultures were all informed by ways of thinking that assumed the properness and inevitability of existing social roles and hierarchies. These ways of thinking, which interpreted selected anatomic, biologic, and phenotypic differences as signs of inherent worth, were typically generated by people who occupied positions of privilege in the same social order they sought to justify. For example, even as late as 1919, the American psychologist H.H. Goddard could publicly argue that "the people who are doing the drudgery are, as a rule, in their proper places" (cited in Gould, 1996, p. 191).

The Significance of Marginalized Perspectives

Understanding and explaining difference, and arguing the grounds on which differences are seen to lie, continue to be major concerns in Western societies—but with one significant change. Many of those theorizing difference today have a stake in transforming rather than justifying existing social arrangements. For some, challenging what are considered inadequate interpretations of difference is related to awareness of the growing complexity of our societies, to increasing racial and ethnic diversity, and to the persistence of social inequities. In some respects, the presence of oppositional social movements (i.e., groups organized around a shared commitment to eradicate social, political, and economic inequities) has placed the need to rethink difference on the public agenda. Oppositional social movements question the validity of social norms and challenge ideas and practices viewed as contributing to the oppression, exclusion, and exploitation of marginalized groups. Marginalized groups—those that have been excluded from the social mainstream, including groups representing the interests of women, people of color, people living with poverty, gays and lesbians, and people with disabilities—pose alternative explanations for their experiences and positions in the social world. In doing so, they challenge the seeming naturalness of existing social roles and arrangements.

The challenges these movements offer are practical and material, having to do with access to resources and opportunities. They are also philosophical, having to do with how we perceive and interpret our worlds. Part of the challenge of oppositional social movements is the challenge they present to our commonsense understandings of society. For example, a challenge people living with poverty may pose to members of dominant groups is whether, in doing the "drudgery," they are, in fact, in their proper places or whether larger social and economic processes limit their opportunities. To understand this situation adequately, we need to ask who is doing what jobs in society. Are some groups disproportionately responsible for the dull, menial, and fatiguing work? How do we explain this? Similarly, some women have argued that it is not a law of nature that they be primarily responsible for the care of children and have instead raised questions about how the caring work of society is allocated and rewarded.

When given voice, members of marginalized groups point out the inaccurate and limited nature of many dominant social narratives—those common, familiar stories we draw on almost unthinkingly to understand our world. For example, there are dominant social narratives that explain the presence of poverty in our society. Chief among these are those that suggest that poor people are responsible for their poverty by virtue of their own inadequacies—this is the "flawed character" view of poverty (Banyard & Graham-Bermann, 1995). This explanation of poverty is partial and inadequate because it locates the "problem" of poverty inside the person and obscures the social, political, and economic arrangements that create and sustain poverty.

Marginalized groups also question the ability of those in positions of privilege to know or understand the experiences of less powerful groups. By contesting the adequacy of dominant perspectives and, hence, their reasonableness as the justification for existing social relations and by offering alternative perspectives, marginalized groups challenge the authority of those in positions of privilege to speak for all of society. Developing more inclusive interpretations of society and more just practices involves taking these concerns of marginalized people seriously. It also involves recognizing that the experiences of many members of society are ignored or distorted by dominant social narratives. Although these narratives are commonly held to explain or describe all of reality, they more often depict only the experiences or situation of a particular social group.

The Insufficiency of Dominant Perspectives: False Universals

History holds many examples of these ostensibly universal discourses revealed instead to refer only to the experience of particular dominant groups. For example, understanding "man" as equivalent to "human" has, in many cases, been demonstrated to be a false universal. The falseness becomes apparent when excluded groups claim the benefits of these discourses or positions for themselves, but, because they are not members of dominant groups, their claims are disallowed or unacknowledged.

In 1929, to cite a well-known example from Canadian history, a particular group of Canadian women demanded to be considered persons under the law. They argued that, in practice, the apparently inclusive and gender-neutral legal concept "person" excluded women. Their argument demonstrated that their femaleness was, in this case, a difference from a male standard that mattered in terms of their rights and privileges in society. Yet, many of those who successfully argued that this gender difference should not matter and who advocated for the legal personhood of Canadian white women did not similarly champion the legal rights of, for example, Aboriginal women. In this case, "gender" for Aboriginal women was inflected by race in a way that mattered for the status of First Nations women, whose right even to vote was not achieved until many decades after that of other Canadian women.

Similarly, in the late 19th century, when American white women organized to gain the right to vote, their failure to include women of color provoked ex-slave Sojourner Truth to ask, "ain't I a woman?" Although she was, of course, biologically female, the dominant social ideology concerning women merged the term *woman* with particular and culturally specific ideals of femininity. "Real" women were gentle, passive, physically frail, in need of male protection, and white. "Real" women did not work the fields, never "plowed and planted, and gathered into barns" (Truth, 1851, cited in Trinh, 1989, p. 100). Truth's words challenged the then-dominant conceptualization of "woman" because an affirmative answer to her challenge would have required a rethinking of what being a woman, in that time and place, meant. Her blackness and her experiences as a black woman were differences that mattered in terms of her rights and privileges in society.

These two examples from "women's" history demonstrate how a supposedly neutral and inclusive category such as "woman" often disregards the experiences of entire groups of women who do not fit the tacit conceptualization on which it is based. These examples also suggest that practices of exclusion have adverse consequences for the status of those excluded.

Nursing and Exclusionary Practices

Organized nursing in Canada, particularly through the early 20th century, was not immune from this kind of exclusionary practice. In their efforts to elevate the status of nursing, the nursing profession and healthcare administrators promoted nursing as a bastion of feminine respectability. They defined nursing according to a particular paradigm of appropriate femininity that drew on racist and classist stereotypes to exclude certain women from education and employment. Canadian historian of nursing Kathryn McPherson (1996, p. 17) writes, "Because nursing relied on an image of feminine respectability to legitimate nurses' presence in the health care system and their knowledge of the body, respectability was constructed in a racial and national context." She also claims, based on the evidence of historical records, that "nurses' respectability and definition of gentility were European in origin. White, native-born Canadian women were expected to bring their superior sense of sexual and social behaviour to the bedside" (McPherson, 1996, p. 17). Although some women of color and immigrant women were able to obtain nursing training, they were expected to provide service only to their "own" communities. "In the eyes of hospital administrators and nursing leaders, Canadian women of non-European heritage could not be relied on to reflect the morality of health at the bedside" (McPherson, 1996, p. 17). In fact, until after World War II (WWII), "administrators remained convinced that the very presence of non-White attendants might exacerbate the health problems of White patients" (McPherson, 1996, p. 17). As McPherson argues, these kinds of beliefs suggest that nursing's exclusivity was "not merely the innocent by-product of objective standards" (McPherson, 1996, p. 17).

As a result, nursing in Canada was "the preserve of white and Canadian-born women" for most of the 20th century (McPherson, 1996, p. 17). Although nursing shortages since WWII have necessitated an opening of occupational boundaries, issues of racism and workplace discrimination persist in nursing. In 1992, for example, a group of African-Canadian nurses successfully argued in front of the Ontario Human Rights Commission that they experienced racial discrimination and harassment in their workplace (McPherson, 1996). This discrimination suggests that, although the face of nursing has changed significantly in recent decades, nursing is also a product of a society in which whiteness is systematically privileged (Dyer, 1997). Differences that matter, then, often arise at the intersections of social categories in the ways that people live the experience of being, for example, simultaneously gendered, raced, and classed. The meanings and implications of these differences and others are considered in this chapter.

THE CHALLENGE OF DIFFERENCE

Part of the challenge that difference offers us is that our knowledge of the world is always limited by our positioning within it. This limitation means that where and how we are located in the social world influences our experiences, our ways of thinking, and the discourses available to us to shape and express our understanding. Discourses consist of beliefs, assumptions, and statements that, although rarely conscious, form our possibilities for knowledge. A discourse of nursing, for example, includes the ways we speak of nursing as well as the ideas, rituals, practices, and social power relations that make nursing a recognizable entity. However, at any point in time, nursing is intersected and influenced by many, sometimes competing, discourses. For example, there are discourses that define nursing as caring, as vocation, or as skilled women's work, and there are others that emphasize the instrumentality or technical nature of nursing work.

To add to this complexity, our positioning in the world is often ambiguous, characterized by multiplicity rather than singularity. For example, a particular woman's understanding of what it means to be a woman is determined not only by her gendered difference from men but also by her differences from other women. The meaning of being a woman will always be inflected by all the other things a particular woman is and does, whether she is poor; whether she is a mother, a refugee, or a lesbian; whether she works as a nurse, an engineer, or a prostitute; or whether she receives social assistance. All of the features of her life texture what being a woman means, just as being a woman changes the meaning of all else that she is and does. What is significant here are the ways in which our circumstances and situations affect the nature of our experiences, what we take as fact, what we consider to be normal or natural, and the ways this changes over time and across society (Ceci, 2000).

The Canadian population is stratified by many relations of difference, and encountering difference is part of everyday life. But not all differences matter in the same way. Rather, it is our interpretations of difference, our attributions of relevance—not specific differences in themselves—that commonly influence whether and how they will matter. That our perspectives are limited and partial is not a problem, particularly not one that we can overcome. Limitedness is simply the character of our situation. However, in light of the limitedness of our perspectives, it seems important to think carefully about the ways in which recognizing and attributing difference as such may have both liberating and discriminating effects. To respond to this concern, we can explore various interpretations of difference and hope to develop new understandings of what difference means in our lives and in our practices. Although difference as an issue is not resolvable, we can explore what it means to name difference. We can consider what it means to practise nursing with respect for difference. Our concern here is with both the meanings attributed to difference and the implications of these meanings in people's lives.

THEORIZING DIFFERENCE

We begin with two related questions. First, what does the term *difference* mean? And, second, what does it mean to theorize difference? A difference, to our common sense at least, is that which distinguishes one thing from another. Although this seems a fairly straightforward definition, it does not tell us whether difference is a feature of the thing itself or if distinguishing difference is a function of our habits of perception. That is, do we assign difference because something is different or because we are accustomed to perceiving it as different? Is it even possible to discriminate between these two activities? This is where theorizing enters the picture. Theories shape our seeing and our possibilities for interpretation. They "provide us with a way of ordering, understanding and capturing aspects of reality" (Cheek & Purkis, 1997, p. 160). Although theories can guide us in picking out features of the world that we then treat as significant, they can also blind us to other, equally important aspects of reality.

Theories organize the way in which a phenomenon, such as difference, will be perceived and represented (Cheek & Purkis, 1997). Described in these terms, theory is not just something located in books or classrooms; rather, all of our seeing and understanding should be thought of as theoretical. Our interactions with the world should be understood as informed beforehand by our beliefs, assumptions, and expectations. Like scientists, researchers, and others who consciously use theory, we too are guided in our lives, in our practices, "by a certain conception of the way things are" (Caputo, 1987, p. 215), by theories. For example, the primacy of race in social classification systems can be understood not simply as a reflection of a reality that contains people who have skin of various shades but as a testament to theories that say this must be important. Or, as Ahmed (1998, p. 27) writes, "bodies are never simply bodies: they are always inscribed within a system of value differentiation," a system that asserts which features of the body, which of its diverse aspects, are worth paying attention to.

The Influence of Theories on Perception: Race as a Category

A good example of how particular theories influence our perceptions of the world is found in theories that suggest that racial differences are important units of analysis. Those who hold these views, consciously or unconsciously, will assume that just knowing a person's race can tell us important things about them. Race becomes a category that is "internalized into ways we think about other people . . . and ourselves" (Allen, 1996, p. 99), and stressing its significance leads us to perceive people initially and, sometimes, chiefly in terms of skin color and phenotype. Race, understood as visible difference, becomes one of the first things we see and interpret as meaningful when we look at a person. But is race, aside from the meanings we attribute to it, an important difference? And how do we know this? And then, how do we incorporate into our analysis the contemporary scientific evidence that demonstrates that race, as a meaningful biologic category, is not real (Alcoff, 1999)?

In societies that continue to categorize, classify, and rank people according to a conception of race that suggests innate, immutable differences among groups, how do we account for the fact that the "overall genetic differences among human races is astonishingly small" (Gould, 1996, p. 353)? How do we account for the fact that there are no such things as "race genes," or genes that are present in certain races but lacking in all others? Does knowing of this "remarkable lack of genetic differentiation among human groups" (Gould, 1996, p. 352) alter our understanding of what we have become accustomed to perceive as intrinsically and biologically distinct groups?

These are important questions because they ask us to reconsider the long-held belief that race constitutes an obvious and important biologic difference among people. However, though race as a category has lost its biologic legitimacy, because of the tenacity and long history of categorizing and ranking people in our society by race, race persists as a significant social, economic, and conceptual category. Though the science of race has changed, the social practices of ascribing qualities based on beliefs about the meaning of race has not.

The Classification of Bodies in History

A useful location from which to begin to rethink race and racial classification systems is history. Here we can see that race has not always been understood as especially relevant, even though in Western societies skin color and phenotype are possibly still considered important signifiers of difference (Weedon, 1999). Rather than disclosing fixed and stable natural categories, the salience of race as a significant social difference has changed over time. And because it has a history, we can see how human beings have made it. Specifically, its history reflects the development of the natural sciences in the 18th and 19th centuries. Racial categories were constructed by biologists and anthropologists as part of a project to order and classify the entire natural world (Alcoff, 1999; Gould, 1996; Weedon, 1999).

In addition, early scientists did not simply describe the realities they observed but rather interpreted difference in light of their pre-existing values, beliefs, and judgments. They ranked perceived differences in body type and appearance according to preconceived notions of character and worth. "The meanings attributed to nineteenth-century racial categories included value judgements about beauty, intellect, morality, emotionality, sexuality and other physical capacities" (Weedon, 1999, p. 153). These judgments, which always assumed the inherent superiority of the white race, came in handy because they "justified colonialism, the slavery of Africans, and the appropriation of African, Asian, and American land and human resources by whites" (Essed, 1996, p. 7). These practices came to be seen as the natural outcome of inborn inequalities between the races.

In addition to interpretations of the meaning of skin color, 18th-, 19th-, and 20th-century scientists theorized links between particular physical features and what were believed to be inborn characteristics, such as intelligence or criminality. High foreheads, low brows, small heads, large jaws, and big arms as well as skin color were all interpreted as direct and uncomplicated reflections of character and capacity. Yet there are literally thousands of ways to measure the human body, and any investigator convinced beforehand by a theory, such as the hierarchic ordering of races, could easily choose the measurements, inadvertently or not, that would subsequently prove his or her theory true (Gould, 1996). These theories of the meanings of racial difference, which can be grouped under the general heading of biologic determinism or sociobiology, take bodies as "their referent and guarantee" and view bodies as the definitive and transparent source of differences among groups (Weedon, 1999, p. 13). Particular features were chosen from a range of possibilities and orders of worth constructed from this starting point.

A CONTINUING PRACTICE

Although one might expect this kind of thinking to have disappeared by now, in some ways, it has simply become more sophisticated. As outmoded and offensive as these views are, publications such as Herrnstein and Murray's (1994) *The Bell Curve: The Reshaping of American Life by Differences in Intelligence* and Rushton's (1995) *Race, Evolution, and Behavior* suggest that, no matter how often these concepts are exposed as vacuous by reputable thinkers, there will be someone—charlatan, fraud, or disingenuous scientist, politician, or social commentator—who is convinced that race and other physical features are important explanations and guarantees of social difference.

The Significance of Theorizing Difference

Recognizing that our understanding is theoretical and, therefore, that our interpretations of difference are informed beforehand by theory is important for at least three reasons.

First, this recognition allows us to appreciate that certain features of the world, particularly those we tend to take for granted as naturally occurring, are, in reality, shaped by our pre-existing theoretical commitments and assumptions—commitments and assumptions we have simply by virtue of being born into a culture. For example, we may assume that race is an important biologically based difference among groups not only because of the "evidence" of our senses but also because our cultural and social experience supports this theory. It is, at some level, obvious to us.

Second, awareness of what we take for granted allows us to attempt to make the beliefs and assumptions that inform our theoretical views explicit rather than implicit. The theoretical perspective informing our assumption about the significance of racial categories is often called *biologic determinism*. This theory supports several propositions, including that of H.H. Goddard, which was mentioned earlier in this chapter: "The people who are doing the drudgery are, as a rule, in their proper places" (cited in Gould, 1996, p. 191). People are believed to be located where they are in the social world essentially for biologic reasons.

Third, consciousness of the specific ways of thinking that influence our understanding allows us to consider the reasons we might choose to hold one theoretical position rather than another. We might ask: What are the views of the people doing the drudgery concerning their proper place? Are their views even available to us? Why might people in positions of privilege hold the views they do? In what ways do social arrangements and the allocation of privileges and resources work to justify a particular social order and the ways of thinking that support it? If race is not an important biologically based category, what kind of category is it? Social? Political? What purpose does it serve?

DIFFERENCE AS DEVIANCE: A CASE OF BIOLOGIC DETERMINISM IN PRACTICE

Different theories—meaning different ways of ordering and interpreting the world—are more than just words. Theories have tangible effects in the world because of the ways in which they shape institutions and practices. The way something is understood, including the kind of problem it is seen to be, has implications for how we think it should be addressed. By focusing in some detail on a particular episode in Canadian history—the pre- and post-WWII preoccupation with the discourses and practices of social hygiene and eugenics—we hope that we can achieve some insight into how this happens. We can then take our understanding of this situation and use it to create new understandings of how issues of difference are theorized in our current contexts.

Part of the usefulness of knowing our own history lies in the ways it can help us to understand how others have attempted to respond to complicated issues, and perhaps even to locate the origins of our own ways of thinking. If we can do this, we can begin to recognize our beliefs as a particular way of thinking, rather than the truth, and reflect on how ideas we may hold have played themselves out in other times and places. Understanding how and why particular ideas may resonate for us or seem so obviously true offers us the opportunity either to take these ideas up more consciously and deliberately or to develop alternative points of view.

Eugenics and Social Hygiene in Canadian History

Eugenic discourses advocating the necessity of intervening in the course of human reproduction flourished openly in many Western countries for the first half of the 20th century fueled by the fears and uncertainties of a rapidly changing world and "consuming concern about the health and welfare of the race" (Dowbiggin, 1997, p. 165). In Canada, the social problems and public health challenges associated with increased immigration and urbanization led many prominent political figures and public health advocates, respected physicians, and psychiatrists to preach a gospel of social hygiene and racial purity rooted in the widespread fear that "traditional Canadian ideals, values and attitudes . . . were disappearing" (Dowbiggin, 1997, p. 134). Erroneously claiming that science could correct the hereditary "deficiencies" believed to cause poverty, crime, and vice, many influential public figures across the country advocated sterilization, segregation, and eugenic immigration restrictions as essential strategies for both public health and social reform (Dowbiggin, 1997). Swept up in the limitless possibilities for advancement that science seemed to offer, and by the expanding authority of medical and scientific discourses to pronounce on all areas of human life, claims that these measures would improve public health were claims that almost no one doubted (Paul, 1998). Faith in science, in its neutrality and objectivity, convinced many proponents that their positions were purely objective, inevitable, and rational responses to the "facts" of scientific knowledge. Such certainty did more than merely mask the cultural values latent in eugenic discourses; it made dissent seem both irrational and irresponsible.

As a pseudoscientific theorizing of difference, eugenic thinking was and is an argument for the biologic innateness of particular defining traits, most notably a belief in the hereditary determination of intelligence and character. Thriving particularly during the economically troubled 1930s, eugenic discourses explained social problems in terms of individual inadequacies, inadequacies defined in terms of, and relying for meaning on, pre-existing social structural relations of class, gender, and race (Valverde, 1991). The physically and mentally subnormal, the different, the deviant, the feebleminded, the unfit, and the defective were categories encompassing those with actual physical and mental illness as well as children who merely performed poorly on standardized tests, unmarried mothers, labor activists, Aboriginal people, immigrants of color, and other non-whites. These groups were assigned the blame for many social problems and were viewed as posing a threat to the smooth functioning of society through their supposedly inborn propensity for violence, crime, and aberrant sexual behavior. So widespread was this way of thinking that even labor unrest was understood by some not as the product of problematic social arrangements but as the result of defective brains (Dowbiggin, 1997).

During these years, it was clear to many influential Canadians that if a particular class of human life was to be preserved and enhanced, then preventive measures to control and contain those who threatened the existing social order, both through their dangerous behaviors and the economic burden their care represented, must be undertaken. This, a social argument, attained greater legitimacy and authority when it was rendered in scientific terms—terms that transformed complex social problems into mere matters of health and disease inviting medical intervention.

Although eugenic thinking could be found everywhere in Canada, only 2 of 10 Canadian provinces enacted sterilization acts—Alberta in 1928 and British Columbia in 1933. Other provinces debated these issues but chose not to create legislation, which is not to say that involuntary sterilization procedures were not performed across Canada without benefit of a law (McLaren, 1990). Eugenic policies, often framed in the language of social hygiene or cleanliness, were directed toward creating stronger, healthier societies through weeding out those deemed unfit in the dominant discourses of the day (Pernick, 1997). Across Canada, there was a general consensus, among dominant groups at least, that controlling the reproduction of some groups, segregating those deemed defective, and restricting immigration on eugenic grounds were warranted public health measures.

It is clear that the problems that eugenic policies were meant to address were very much problems of difference. As Canadian society was becoming more and more obviously heterogeneous, the fear that Canadian values and ideals were being lost was prevalent among more established groups. Eugenic policies were articulated from this center (i.e., by members of dominant groups) and had their greatest effects on society's weakest and most marginalized members. Differences that mattered were clearly framed by categories of class, race, and gender.

For example, in the case of eugenic sterilizations, the supposedly scientific and rational decisions made by eugenic boards clearly revealed the decided influence of social criteria of normality and value

(Dowbiggin, 1997; McLaren, 1990; Paul, 1998; Pernick, 1997). Those sterilized tended to be female, young and inexperienced, poor, rural, a member of a racial or ethnic minority group, and unmarried. In other words, those referred for sterilization procedures were rarely members of the dominant group; rather, as Pernick (1997, p. 1770) observed, "race, class, ethnic, religious and sexual prejudices determined who was defined as unfit."

Difference as Deviance: Assumptions of Normality

As noted previously, eugenic discourses explained social problems in terms of individual inadequacies, inadequacies that were thought to be reflected in and confirmed one's proper position in society. These arguments typically focused on individual deviance from a supposed norm and gained legitimacy when they were communicated in scientific and medical terms that diagnosed those outside the dominant social order as diseased. Thus, complex social problems were transformed into matters of health and illness.

Although it is common to treat concepts of health and illness as matters of fact (Caplan, Engelhardt, & McCartney, 1981), ideas of both health and illness are only meaningful in relation to some prior conception about what is normal (Susser, 1981). And *normal* is not a neutral term with clear and self-evident meaning; rather, ideas of normality are constructed within particular sociohistorical contexts and always contain an evaluative element concerning what is understood to be usual, acceptable, and valued. Features defined as normal achieve a normative status, providing a framework and basis for making comparative value judgments.

Concepts of normality require value judgments to be made, and their use implies the presence of a regulative structure that produces both the "normal" and the "not normal." Because ideas of normality are most often produced and employed by those in positions of social dominance, the experience and values of dominant groups tend to represent that which is then thought to be normal for everyone. For example, many school-aged children were labeled feebleminded or subnormal in the early decades of the 20th century after failing to pass standardized intelligence tests. These tests contained what we now recognize as "arbitrary norms of intellectual achievement" (McLaren, 1990, p. 38). Rather than providing objective, scientific measures of intelligence as it was then believed, these tests reflected the experiences and values of the dominant group who produced them. Children who were not members of this group were less likely to perform well because the questions asked of them were outside their experience. In some instances, then, what is conceived of as deviance from normality might be more usefully and accurately understood as a distant or marginal relation to a powerful center. This marginalization was certainly the experience of many Canadians labeled different or deviant during the years when eugenic policies and practices were prevalent.

Eugenic Practices and Public Health: Nursing Roles

In considering the role of nursing in the implementation of eugenic practices and policies, it is important to recognize that there were links between eugenic discourses and public health goals, beliefs, and values—what has been called "the convergence between genes and germs" (Pernick, 1997, p. 1769). With very little tolerance for difference, the supposedly defective, unfit, and subnormal were constructed in dominant discourses as deviant and diseased. And because public health nurses were concerned with protecting the health of society in general from any number of sources of disease, their goals were apparently congruent with those of the eugenicists whose interpretations of health and illness dominated public discussions.

Segregation, institutionalization, and restrictive immigration were all conceptualized as necessary social and mental hygiene measures intended to stop the spread of an unseen contagion, and to sterilize meant, in eugenics as in bacteriology, "to eliminate agents that cause disease" (Pernick, 1997, p. 1769). In some ways, nurses' actions in implementing these policies and practices, actions that included assessing children in homes and schools, identifying candidates for sterilization, making referrals to eugenics boards, providing operating-room assistance, and assisting in the "Canadianizing" of new immigrants (Mansell & Hibberd, 1998), were simply extensions of the nursing role to care for the health and welfare of the population, at least as that task was then defined.

NURSING PRACTICE AND DOMINANT THINKING

This last point, however, is where difficulties for nurses may arise. Nursing and nurses are constituted within the dominant society and within the possibilities and constraints of particular sociohistorical contexts. The conduct of nurses, in this time and place, should be understood in relation to the lesser status of women in society, the subordination of nurses in the healthcare hierarchy, and the rewards nurses received for compliance as well as the absence of an alternative discourse or way of thinking about difference. Nurses consented to what was dominant in medical and societal thinking and to a particular understanding of difference influenced by the tenets of biologic determinism, a theory that we now clearly understand as informed by false beliefs and assumptions and as having caused significant harm to vulnerable people. This consent was not particular to nurses but rather a reflection of prevailing attitudes and beliefs or, as Mansell and Hibberd (1998, p. 9) have written, "nurses handled, managed, and controlled individuals in order to maintain a society that adhered to the wishes of the dominant group, of which they were part."

Significance for Contemporary Nursing

The purpose here, however, is not to suggest that nurses were right or wrong in terms of their participation but rather to consider the implications for ourselves, as nurses, of the possibility that we also may become the means through which social and moral harms are perpetrated. Nurses must consider these issues simply because they are often in the position of implementing policies not necessarily of their own making and of supporting and sustaining particular social and political arrangements of healthcare. It is a dilemma for nursing that, although much of our work, particularly in the area of public health, involves the care of socially, economically, and politically marginalized or disadvantaged people, the dominant voices in defining health and healthcare policies rarely come from these groups. In their roles as "conduits into the lives and social spaces of groups otherwise beyond the reach of social agents of authority" (Rafferty, Robinson, & Elkan, 1997, p. 3), nurses may have a special responsibility to be attuned to the differences of marginalized perspectives.

DIFFERENCE AS RELATIONSHIP

The meanings given to difference, whether that difference is named in terms of gender, race, class, intellectual ability, or sexual orientation, assume immediate significance for people because these meanings are used to circumscribe and explain experience and to influence both the lived meanings and material realities of their lives. The meanings given to femaleness, for example, have been important to women "because they were used to determine and limit the social and economic spheres to which women had access" (Weedon, 1999, p. 10). Consider these words of the late 19th-century founder of social psychology, Gustave Le Bon: "All psychologists who have studied the intelligence of women, as well as poets and novelists, recognise that they represent the most inferior form of human evolution and that they are closer to children and savages than an adult, civilized man" (Le Bon, 1879, cited in Gould, 1996, p. 137). Le Bon goes on to describe women, with rare exception, as being typically and naturally illogical, irrational, childish, capricious, and unreliable. Given that this is, in Le Bon's view, the nature or essence of woman's being, education for women, as well as any role for women outside the home, was seen not only as a wasteful indulgence but also as against nature and, therefore, dangerously aberrant.

As ludicrous as this now sounds, the importance for women lies not only in the aspersions cast on their characters and capacities, although these are not insignificant, but also in the ways in which these types of views have limited and constrained women's access to resources and opportunities for so many years. Women, in all their various social locations, have learned "who [they] are and how to think and behave through discursive practices" (Weedon, 1999, p. 104). As these social and political practices of thinking and theorizing have become entrenched through institutions, such as psychology (or medicine, religion, philosophy, and law), the difference of being a woman has come to matter in ways that have had and still have real material consequences for women. The meanings attributed to sex differences have justified the social, political, and economic inequality of women. These kinds of practice have had similar consequences in the lives of others who are marginalized and diminished on the grounds of their difference from a dominant group.

The difference of women, which is clearly meant to be understood as the difference between men and women, and most probably the difference between men and women of a particular race and class, is articulated by Le Bon as naturally occurring inferiority and lack. This difference is clearly not a neutral one (e.g., one that would mean, simply, "not the same"). Rather, difference is organized in terms of a relationship in which one side is understood as being or setting the standard the other fails to achieve, a process still quite common in Western thinking.

Dualism and Difference

Western societies have tended to arrange many important features of the world into oppositional and exclusive dualities, necessary hierarchies whose meaning both reflects and sustains clear and pervasive differences in social power and status. Male versus female, white versus black, rich versus poor, and straight versus gay are examples of dualisms that organize difference in crude, yet highly effective, structures in which one side of the duality is clearly meant to be understood as superior to the other. The other in each case is named and defined in relation to the dominant group, whose power in some respects resides in the very capacity to create the kind of relationship that establishes "us here and them over there" (Trinh, 1990, p. 371) and to name and to define those not themselves as "other." In the case of Le Bon, the claim is made that "us here men" are plainly the natural social betters of "them there women"—a crude but unquestionably effective process of differentiation and social categorization. This process of boundary drawing creates a difference that is a difference between the included and excluded and the accepted and rejected—and it is never neutral.

LIMITATIONS OF DUALIST THINKING

In dualistic thinking, difference is organized into simplistic, oppositional, and exclusive categories. This organization occurs despite the limited explanatory power such frameworks for understanding hold. As well as reducing our understanding of men and women, for example, to terms of difference and suggesting that women and men should only be understood in opposition to one another, dualistic thinking tends to erase differences among women and suggests that women should be understood only in terms of sameness—both clearly inadequate proposals. Strictly dualistic conceptualizations of difference limit our understanding of the multiple and shifting ways we are positioned in relation to others. A white middle-class or affluent woman may find herself and her opportunities limited in relation to the men in her life but she may exercise power in her relation to other, less advantageously positioned men and women. Sometimes, the difference of gender may be in the foreground; at other times, race, class, and sexual orientation may be the differences that matter—sometimes singly, sometimes all at once.

Difference as a Relation Between Margin and Center

It is important to recognize that when we are perceiving difference, a relationship of some sort is being inferred, although the fact of relationship is often assumed rather than plainly stipulated. That is to say, there is a norm or a standard to which we refer, consciously or unconsciously, implicitly or explicitly, when we identify someone or something as different. The identification and production of differences, then, are bound up with assumptions concerning the socially, culturally, and politically relevant features of persons, which, in Western societies, have generally corresponded to the ways in which we are categorized according to gender, race, sexual orientation, and class. These differences mark people as different in relation to a dominant and presumably unmarked group, a group that in Western societies has tended to be composed of white, propertied, able-bodied, heterosexual males.

In this way, our identification of difference can be understood as the recognition of a particular relation between margin and center and between dominant and subordinate groups, with the differences that matter most arising in the context of relations of power. Relations of power are intrinsic to all social relations, but of particular interest are those that establish access to such things as resources, opportunities, and knowledge: "Power takes many forms, affecting access to material resources as well as questions of language, culture and the right to define who one is" (Weedon, 1999, p. 5).

Thus, besides trying to understand the processes through which difference is produced, understanding who defines whom as different is also always significant. These relations of difference attain their significance for us when they result in structures of inequality or patterns of disadvantage: "Differences between individuals and groups—between sexes, classes, races, ethnic groups, religions and nations—become important political issues when they involve relations of power" (Weedon, 1999, p. 5).

Processes of Differentiation

Difference is produced through social processes of categorization. Some feature of a person is selected as significant and defined against a backdrop of dominant assumptions, beliefs, and values and in relation to that which is believed to be usual or traditional, normal, or natural. These activities of selection and interpretation, however, cannot be thought of as politically neutral: "Both the construction of commonality among subjects and the assertion of difference between subjects are rhetorical and political acts, gestures of affiliation and disaffiliation that emphasizes [sic] some properties and obscures others" (Felski, 1997, p. 17). For example, designating income level as a person's most significant characteristic brings to the fore a single aspect of a person's identity, while rendering invisible much else that the person is and does. Income level stands in for a more particularized explanation of life and circumstances and allows people living with poverty, for example, to appear as an undifferentiated mass. Conceptualizing difference as a relation rather than a thing in itself, and instead of a feature of people that exists independently of our theorizing about it, encourages us to inquire into the social relations through which differences that matter are produced.

For nurses, coming to understand the ways in which marginalized populations are related to the dominant social center means theorizing how apparently neutral differences are the result of structures of inequality or patterns of disadvantage affecting particular groups in particular ways. The prevalence of poverty among women provides a good example because women's poverty is both disproportionate and relatively intransigent. At all ages, and across most categories, women's incomes are lower than men's, and, although women have made gains in recent years in many areas of life, these income disparities remain relatively unchanged. In 2003 in Canada, for example, 1.9 million women, or 12% of the total female population, were living in low-income situations (Statistics Canada, 2006). Although improved access to education, increased participation in the labor force, smaller family sizes, and changes in the structure of family living have improved the lives of many women, women in all age categories and family types are still much more likely to be poor than are men.

Single mothers and elderly women continue to be those with the greatest likelihood of living in poverty, and there is an especially high incidence of poverty among women of color, immigrant women, First Nations women, and women with disabilities. Each of these groups, in addition to being female, departs in some way from a dominant societal norm circumscribed by a white, middle-class, male, heterosexual, youth-oriented, able-bodied perspective. Not only is the other defined and named in relation to this dominant group but also relations of power and privilege are structured or shaped by this relationship.

For both women as a group and women with particular differences, distance from this center can be seen as having the power to shape both social relations and individual experience. Poverty, given this situation, could be theorized as being neither inherent nor accidental but rather as centrally about power, and society's economic organization could be one way in which relations of power are enacted in many women's lives, determining their success in obtaining both material and social resources. This type of thinking would stand in opposition to views that suggest women are disproportionately poor because they are flawed in some way. We can see through this example that how a problem is defined will influence how we think it should be addressed. In this case, improving the character of those who are poor versus addressing older women's poverty by working to change economic arrangements, i.e. recognizing the value of unpaid labour and instituting better pensions for homemakers.

Differences and Relations of Power

The social relations that work to construct the lived meanings as well as the material realities of differences such as gender, race, sexual orientation, and class need to be understood as relations of power. In fact, to raise the question of difference in the context of social relationships requires that we recognize that our interpretations of difference are always and in every case the "effects of many types of power relations" (Weedon, 1999, p. vii).

Attending to power means understanding that activities of labeling, defining, and categorizing are power moves and often result in some members of society being subjected by the power of others: "Those who claim a dominant position can presume the right to determine which aspects of identities are core, and by which aspect others will be known" (Kaplan, 1997, p. 34). The power exercised by dominant groups to name the differences that matter includes the capacity to determine the kind of difference something is understood to be. That is, is a particular named difference cultural, political, natural, or biologic? Is it normal or pathologic? Acceptable or perverse? Power is what makes differences matter—the power to impose definitions, to determine meanings, and to shape reality.

For example, in a context in which heterosexuality is assumed dominant and is believed to be "normal," sexuality for gay men and lesbian women, whether they wish it to or not, may become their significant defining feature, the feature by which they will be known. To say of someone that "she is a lesbian" has a different meaning and effect than to say "she is heterosexual" because, in our society at least, heterosexuality is assumed; it is not to be different at all. In naming a woman "lesbian," which must be understood as different than naming oneself, a particular difference is called into being, a difference that matters in part because of its relation to a dominant center and to ideas of normality. In addition, a different kind of knowledge of the person is assumed, a knowledge that seems to be saying that the most important thing about this woman is her sexuality, and it is important not because of the meanings it holds for her but because it differs from a supposed norm. For those who are marginalized in relation to a dominant center, the consequences of being categorized in this way can be quite serious and range from having reduced access to resources and opportunities to the failure to have one's understanding or interpretation of one's own experience matter. A peculiar silencing occurs when what becomes most important about a person is how they are defined by others and by their perceived relation to the dominant group, to a supposed norm or center.

THE DISTINCT REALITIES OF OTHERS

It has become a cliché to suggest that, as a society, we must learn to live with difference. This can mean anything from halfheartedly agreeing to merely tolerating difference, to the desire to embrace and celebrate diversity among people. Where we locate ourselves in this situation will depend, to some extent at least, on how we have chosen to interpret difference.

In the case of racial differences, for example, we have seen that, although many continue to believe that the meaning of race is located in biology, actual genetic differences between races are insignificant—the meaning of racial difference is not self-evident in the sense of being directly attributable to nature. Yet, although race is a constructed rather than a natural category and whether we are privileged or marginalized because of it, it remains a compelling force in all of our lives, shaping our understandings of ourselves, our relationships with others, and our possibilities and constraints.

Race in our social worlds is important because we attribute particular meanings to it. We should probably be willing to ask ourselves what it is, exactly, that we think race means. As we notice a person's skin color or his or her appearance, what do we think we already know about that person? Is reading off the surface in this way anything more than a reflection, not of the person but of ourselves, of our own and our society's beliefs, assumptions, and biases?

Similarly, the meanings of gender, sexuality, and economic status, to name only a few of the differences that constitute our social worlds, can also be understood in this way, as constructed within social relationships and as deserving of the same kind of questioning. These are categories that, like race, have the effect of seeming natural but that, to be realized, virtually always require value judgments backed up by the authorizing practices of various institutionalized discourses, such as those of medicine or law or religion. And these are only some of the most obvious differences, those that are enforced and reinforced by relations of power.

As nurses, in our privileged and intimate relationships with others, we must not only resist racist, sexist, classist, and heterosexist definitions of people, we must also be willing to reconcile the innumerable significant and insignificant ways we may differ from one another. Naming difference is not simply a descriptive act but one that creates a relationship that is commonly, although not always, a relation between margin and center and dominant and subordinate groups. In part because of the power we hold to influence events and experiences, we must take the distinct realities of others seriously. Nursing and nurses are embedded in a larger social world, and, because of this positioning, we are not free of the constraints and prejudices that shape all of society. Yet "consequences are enacted by nurses, not as individuals, but because they are part of a larger system" (Liaschenko, 1998, p. 76). We have, perhaps, a greater responsibility than others for a critical consciousness of the beliefs, values, and assumptions that shape our thinking and inform our actions.

But what does this mean, this challenge that nurses practise with respect for the distinct realities of others? In the first place, it means that nurses must understand that many competing discourses exist that make truth claims about people, that these truth claims do not exist equally, and that some versions of the world and some voices are privileged over others (Weedon, 1999). If, as Sherwin (1992, p. 222) has suggested, people's health needs "vary inversely with their power and privilege in society," then nurses need to recognize that quite commonly the people who are the focus of their attentions are also the ones whose voices are silent or silenced in determining the practices and processes of healthcare. Respect for difference, for the distinct realities of others, requires, at the very least, a willingness to reevaluate what will count for us as important sources of knowledge and meaning. We must develop a capacity to hear the voices of the least powerful.

Second, nurses need to understand that they themselves are socially, culturally, economically, and politically situated. We are "located at particular positions, each of which enables and constrains the possibilities of experience" (Grossberg, 1996, p. 99). Our "situatedness" means we are not necessarily going to be able to understand the experience of others, and this knowledge of our limitations is simply the unavoidable character of our situations. But knowing of the partiality and limitedness of our own perspective can compel us to seek other views, to acknowledge that our own understanding is rarely adequate or sufficient (Strickland, 1994). Practising with respect for the distinct realities of others means recognizing that the singular significant characteristic of nursing practice is that someone else is there, someone who must be allowed to speak to us, to really tell us something.

Difference for nurses can mean diversity, a recognition of plurality and multiple points of view. This meaning is important, but there is another facet of difference that may be even more meaningful for nursing, a meaning of difference that has its roots in the essential alterity of others—the inescapable otherness of others. This otherness is what Caputo (1993) calls the "difference that makes a difference" (p. 56), wherein "everything turns on a respect for difference, for the other one" (p. 60). This is difference that is singular, focused on a person, a particular other who is before me, here and now. The ethic of a nursing relationship is such that the presence of this particular other is fundamental, rather than incidental, to how we will proceed, an ethic that is compromised whenever we assume we already know the meaning of another person's life.

SUMMARY

In this chapter, difference has not been presented as an issue to be resolved but rather as a feature of the world that we must consciously consider. Difference is conceptualized as a relationship, the meaning of which is determined in part by how we choose to interpret our worlds. Familiar frames of reference, such as definitions or categories, have been presented as inadequate for truly understanding difference. These have been critiqued for the ways they mask complex and changing social relationships and conceal social processes of differentiation.

What has been raised for consideration in this chapter is how particular differences are constructed and how the meanings attributed to them come to matter in economic, social, and political domains. We are asked to think about how various categories of difference become invested with particular meanings rather than take the meanings of what are named as important differences to be self-evident.

Online

Add to your knowledge of this issue:	
Canadian Nurses Association	www.cna-nurses.ca
National Anti-Racism Council of Canada	www.narcc.ca
Positive Space campaigns on most university and college campuses	i.e. www.positivespace.utoronto.ca; www.positivespce.ubc.ca; www.mtroyal.ab.ca\positivespace
Class Action—Classism Issues	www.classism.org
Canadian Centre on Disability Studies	www.disabilitystudies.ca
National Anti-Poverty Organization	www.napo-onap.ca

REFLECTIONS on the Chapter...

1. From your practice experience, identify differences that seem to matter. Who has named and identified these differences as significant? In what ways do they matter and to whom?

2. Explore how difference is a concern or feature of your practice. What difference does it make to conceptualize difference as a relationship rather than a characteristic or trait?

3. Because difference is not an issue to be resolved, how would you proceed in your practice, given that the world is full of difference? Identify the assumptions and beliefs that influence your understanding and interpretation of difference.

References

Ahmed, S. (1998). *Differences that matter: Feminist theory and postmodernism.* Cambridge: University Press.

Alcoff, L. (1999). The phenomenology of racial embodiment. *Radical Philosophy, 95,* 15–26.

Allen, D. (1996). Knowledge, politics, culture, and gender: A discourse perspective. *Canadian Journal of Nursing Research, 28*(1), 95–102.

Banyard, V. & Graham-Bermann, S. (1995). Building an empowerment policy paradigm: Self-reported strengths of homeless mothers. *American Journal of Orthopsychiatry, 65*(4), 479–491.

Caplan, A., Engelhardt Jr., H., & McCartney, J. (Eds.). (1981). *Concepts of health and disease: Interdisciplinary perspectives.* Reading, MA: Addison-Wesley.

Caputo, J. (1987). *Radical hermeneutics: Repetition, deconstruction, and the hermeneutic project.* Bloomington: Indiana University Press.

_____. (1993). *Against ethics: Contributions to a poetics of obligation with constant reference to deconstruction.* Bloomington: Indiana University Press.

Ceci, C. (2000). Not innocent: Relationships between knowers and knowledge. *Canadian Journal of Nursing Research, 32*(2), 57–73.

Cheek, J. & Purkis, M. (1997). "Capturing" nursing? Theories concealed in writings about nursing practice. *Social Science in Health, 3*(3), 157–163.

Dowbiggin, I. (1997). *Keeping America sane: Psychiatry and eugenics in the United States and Canada, 1880–1940.* Ithaca, NY: Cornell University Press.

Dyer, R. (1997). *White.* London: Routledge.

Essed, P. (1996). *Diversity: Gender, color, and culture.* (R. Gircour, Trans.). Amherst: University of Massachusetts Press.

Felski, R. (1997). The doxa of difference. *Signs, 23*(1), 1–21.

Gould, S. (1996). *The mismeasure of man* (Rev. ed.). New York: W. W. Norton.

Grossberg, L. (1996). Identity and cultural studies: Is that all there is? In S. Hall & P. Du Gay (Eds.), *Questions of cultural identity* (pp. 87–107). London: Sage.

Herrnstein, R. & Murray, C. (1994). *The bell curve: The reshaping of American life by differences in intelligence.* New York: Free Press.

Kaplan, A. (1997). How can a group of white, heterosexual, privileged women claim to speak of "women's" experience? In J. Jordon (Ed.), *Women's growth in diversity: More writings from the Stone Centre* (pp. 32–37). New York: Guilford Press.

Liaschenko, J. (1998). Moral evaluation and concepts of health and health promotion. *Advanced Practice Nursing Quarterly, 4*(2), 71–77.

Mansell, D. & Hibberd, J. (1998). "We picked the wrong one to sterilize": The role of nursing in the eugenics movement in Alberta, 1920–1940. *International History of Nursing Journal, 3*(4), 4–11.

McLaren, A. (1990). *Our own master race: Eugenics in Canada, 1885–1945.* Don Mills, ON: Oxford University Press.

McPherson, K. (1996). *Bedside matters: The transformation of Canadian nursing, 1900–1990.* Toronto: Oxford University Press.

Paul, D. (1998). *The politics of heredity: Essays on eugenics, biomedicine, and the nature–nurture debate.* Albany: University of New York Press.

Pernick, M. (1997). Eugenics and public health in American history. *American Journal of Public Health, 87*(11), 1767–1772.

Rafferty, A., Robinson, J., & Elkan, R. (Eds.). (1997). *Nursing history and the politics of welfare.* London: Routledge.

Rushton, P. (1995). *Race, evolution, and behavior.* New Brunswick, NJ: Transaction.

Sherwin, S. (1992). *No longer patient: Feminist ethics and health care.* Philadelphia, PA: Temple University Press.

Statistics Canada. (2006). *Women in Canada: A gender-based statistical report* (5th ed.). Ottawa: Author.

Strickland, S. (1994). Feminism, postmodernism and difference. In K. Lennon & M. Whitford (Eds.), *Knowing the difference: Feminist perspectives in epistemology* (pp. 265–274). New York: Routledge.

Susser, M. (1981). Ethical components in the definition of health. In A. Caplan, T. Engelhardt, & J. McCartney (Eds.), *Concepts of health and disease: Interdisciplinary perspectives* (pp. 93–106). Reading, MA: Addison-Wesley.

Trinh Minh-ha, T. (1989). *Woman, native, other: Writing postcoloniality and feminism.* Bloomington: Indiana University Press.

_____. (1990). Not you/like you: Post-colonial women and the interlocking questions of identity and difference. In G. Anzaldua (Ed.), *Making face, making soul: Creative and critical perspectives by feminists of color* (pp. 371–375). San Francisco: Aunt Lute Books.

Valverde, M. (1991). *The age of light, soap, and water: Moral reform in English Canada, 1885–1925.* Toronto: McClelland & Stewart.

Weedon, C. (1999). *Feminism, theory and the politics of difference.* Oxford: Blackwell.

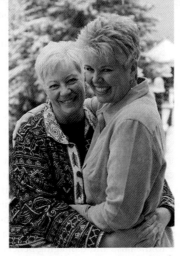

A same-sex couple celebrate their marriage in 2005, having lived together for years previously. (Photographer Bonny Johannson. Used with permission.)

Orientating to Difference: Beyond Heteronormative Sexualities

Carol McDonald

Critical Questions

As a way of engaging with the ideas in this chapter, consider the following:

1. How would you describe your current knowledge of nonheterosexual people?

2. What do you imagine might be the issues for nonheterosexual people in the healthcare system?

3. How do you understand the difference between sexual orientation and gender identity?

Chapter Objectives

After completing this chapter, you will be able to:

1. Identify relevant issues for nonheterosexual people.

2. Understand the idea of the social construction of the categories of sexual orientation.

3. Describe the impact of medical discourses and classification for nonheterosexual people.

4 Understand the complexity of disclosure for gay, lesbian, bisexual, two-spirited, and trans-gendered (GLBTT) people.

5 Identify barriers to reducing assumptions and practices based on **heteronormativity**.

6 Articulate strategies to lessen stigmatization and discrimination.

This chapter presents the opportunity for you to consider the ways we have historically thought about ideas of sexuality in society, how ideas are changing, and the ways in which both historical and newer understandings influence nursing practice. Knowledge of different interpretations of sexualities and genders opens possibilities for us to provide healthcare informed by the realities of people's lived experience. As we delve into the knowledge of sexuality and gender, we are required, I would suggest, to question the assumptions that we hold about these topics. To have this conversation about sexuality, beyond what is commonly seen as the norm of heterosexuality and the binary genders of woman and man, we will necessarily rely on the use of categories. To draw on categories in our conversation is at once useful and problematic. While the use of categories or labels gives us language to talk about differences, we simultaneously run the risk of essentializing, meaning that we would view all people within the category as the same. In the previous chapter that explores difference as a feature of the world of nursing, Ceci reminds us, "As nurses we encounter people in their most vulnerable moments and so have the opportunity to cause harm by unthinking adherence to the false and damaging beliefs and assumptions often contained in categories and labels" (2009, p. 358). And so while categories and labels are used as a way of understanding differences, it is always more important to see the gender and sexual identity of people as individually constituted; in other words, each person's life is formed through a particular set of experiences, and the meanings of those experiences are decided by the individual.

BEYOND HETERONORMATIVE SEXUALITIES: ARTICULATING THE TOPIC FOR NURSING

One place to enter this conversation is to establish a shared understanding of what is meant, for the purposes of this chapter, as heteronormative and nonheteronormative sexualities. In this process I would also hope to disrupt or to challenge the dual notion of sexual orientation as heterosexual and homosexual and the limited binary understandings of genders as woman and man and, instead, consider plural possibilities for the ways in which sexuality and gender are experienced and expressed (Box 21.1.).

Sexuality Beyond the Binary

Sexuality is described by Health Canada as a "central aspect of being human throughout life and encompasses biological sex, gender identities and roles, sexual orientation, eroticism, pleasure, intimacy and reproduction" (Public Health Agency of Canada, 2007). This description helps us to think of sexuality in a holistic way when we consider individuals of any sexual orientation. Consequently, while your sexual orientation may indicate the gender of the person you are sexually attracted to (object of desire), it is also intertwined with many other important aspects of your self and of the ways you relate to others in the world. Experiences of sexuality cannot be thought of as the same for all people who name themselves heterosexual, lesbian, bisexual, or gay. Some people who currently name themselves gay or lesbian may have, or have had, previous relationships with someone of the opposite sex. People who name themselves heterosexual may also engage in sexual behavior with someone of the same sex. There are people who name themselves heterosexual, gay, lesbian, or bisexual who are celibate (McDonald, in press; McDonald, 2006). However, in the face of these multiple expressions and

BOX 21.1 Glossary of Terms

This list describes the way some terms are used in the context of this chapter. They should not be taken as absolute definitions of the words.

Gender identity: One's sense of oneself as feminine or masculine, commonly associated with categories of woman, man, or transgender.

Heteronormativity: The assumption of heterosexual relationships as representative of all sexuality underlies the idea of heteronormativity; the belief that all people are or wish to be in sexual and intimate relationships with a person of the opposite sex or gender.

Heterosexism: Oppressive action that privileges heterosexual people and positions nonheterosexual people in a position of "other."

Homophobia: The irrational fear or hatred of, or aversion to, or discrimination against anyone who is not heterosexual.

Internalized homophobia: When a nonheterosexual person accepts society's stereotypes and negative labels and internalizes them. The person is not always consciously aware of internalized homophobia.

Intersexed people: People who have physical bodies outside the relatively narrow chromosomal, endocrinal, genital, and other physiological ranges associated with male or female. People may be born intersexed or become intersexed as a result of a medical intervention.

Sexual Orientation: The capacity to develop intimate emotional and sexual relationships with people of the same gender (lesbian or gay), the opposite gender (heterosexual), or either gender (bisexual). As these categories are limited, it is sometimes more useful to talk about nonheterosexual as the **sexual orientation**. In addition, some nonheterosexual people have reclaimed the word queer to identify their orientation as an inclusive term for all nonheterosexual people. Sexual orientation is distinct from gender and gender identity.

Transgender: People whose sense of their gender (woman or man) is not congruent with the sexual characteristics of their physical body (female or male). People sometimes choose to transition to another gender while others opt to remain in the "gender-flux."

experiences of sexuality, the overwhelmingly dominant interpretation of sexuality in Canada is of heterosexuality, signifying the sexual and intimate relationships between women and men. The assumption of heterosexual relationships as representative of all sexuality underlies the idea of heteronormativity, the belief that all people are or wish to be in sexual and intimate relationships with a person of the opposite sex or gender. Oppressive action that privileges heterosexual people and positions nonheterosexual people in a position of "other" is understood as **heterosexism** (Gray et al., 1996; Irwin, 2007). An important consideration for this chapter is that experiences of discrimination against GLBTT people continue to exist in contemporary society, both within and beyond the healthcare setting (Chinn, 2008; Irwin, 2007; McDonald, 2006; McDonald, 2008; Morgan & Stevens, 2008; Stevens, 1995; Stevens & Hall, 1988).

Gender Beyond the Binary

As I have discussed in Chapter 19 of this text, gender can be understood as the individual experience of femininity and masculinity and in addition to the expression of that inner experience (McDonald). While there is undoubtedly a relationship between biological sex and gender, we can consider gender as distinct from the biological sex of a person and as constructed through experiences of an individual in the social, physical, and discursive context of their life. The discursive contexts are the discourses we hear, full of assumptions about the "appropriateness" or "correctness" of particular ideas and expressions of gender. These discourses are, of course, reflective of the dominant values and beliefs at a particular time in a culture, and are by no means universal "truths." Beginning very early in our lives we each heard stories that conveyed to us what it meant to be a girl or a boy in our family and cultural setting. Throughout our lifetime we continue to receive messages from the media, popular culture, and many diverse sources, depicting gender identities and gender expression. For the most part, the gender identities that are foregrounded in society are expressions of the binary categories of woman and man.

In reflecting on this dualistic or binary construction of gender, Butler suggests, "there is nothing about a binary gendered system that is given" (1990, p. 282). Rather, we have come to rely on this association of gender with biological sex that supports the dominance of heterosexual reproduction. If, however, we move beyond this biologically driven system, "there is space to recognize the realities of people's lives that do not fit in the polarized and constructed categories. One example of people living beyond the binary understanding of gender is those who would name themselves transgendered" (McDonald, in press). As we begin to move beyond the historical binary system of gender, the use of categories and labels become even less reliable. The label of *transgendered,* for instance, can mean different things to different people who take on the label. One common understanding of transgendered suggests that it represents people whose sense of their gender (woman or man) is not congruent with the sexual characteristics of their physical body (female or male). Drawing on research conversations with transgendered people, Morgan and Stevens (2008) caution us about the complexity of transgendered people's experiences suggesting that we should not simply assume people are "in the wrong body" (2008, p. 585). While some transgendered people are interested in aligning their physical bodies or presentation more closely with their sense of their gender through surgical, endocrine, or cosmetic actions, other people live in the gender flux, avoiding the reinstatement (or compliance to) the historical gender dualism.

A couple of hypothetical examples might help to clarify: Jake was born as a biological female but self-identifies his gender as a man. He is in the process of transitioning to a male through the use of hormone therapy and plans to have a double mastectomy and chest reconstruction surgery. Kim was also born as a biological female but does not associate with the **gender identity** of "woman." Kim identifies with "trans" as gender, avoids aligning with either woman or man as a category, avoids the use of a gendered pronoun, such as "he" or "she," and presents with an androgynous appearance. It is, of course, beyond the scope of this chapter to explore the many possibilities of gender expression. A final thought for this section is a reminder that gender identity and sexual orientation are separate from one another. This reminder encourages us to avoid heterosexist assumptions with people of all genders and appearances; there is every possibility, for example, that a person who transitions from a feminine to a masculine gender is intimately and sexually attracted to men.

 ## ARTICULATING THE TOPIC AS AN ISSUE

The preceding conversation is a useful way of establishing a shared understanding of the topics of sexual orientation and gender. The topic itself, however, is not an issue. The issue to be unpacked (systematically explored) in the chapter is that of heterosexism, in the healthcare setting and beyond, and the deleterious effect of such social conditions to health (Box 21.2.).

The dominance of heteronormativity, in addition to the presence of actions fueled by systemic and individual heterosexism, is becoming increasingly well documented in the nursing literature (Chinn, 2008; Irwin, 2007; McDonald 2006; McDonald, 2008; Morgan & Stevens, 2008; Stevens, 1995; Stevens & Hall, 1988). While we might hope that individual acts of discrimination against nonheterosexual people are decreasing, literature suggests that full acceptance of nonheterosexual people varies considerably according to context and location. I would suggest that the assumptions of heteronormativity are so deeply entrenched in society, including in healthcare settings, that even

BOX 21.2 Sexuality in the Healthcare System

"The health of a nation, physically and emotionally, can only be as good as the health of its most vulnerable and stigmatized citizens. While culture, class and religion are known to affect how illness may appear and be understood, sexual orientation has been less well researched or understood as a mediator of health and illness."

(Source: Forstein, M. (2003). In A. Peterkin & C. Risdon, *Caring for lesbian and gay people: A clinical guide.* Toronto: University of Toronto Press.)

when we intellectually accept the realities of GLBTT people, we continue to practice based on an assumption of heteronormativity. Systemic heteronormativity is reflected in the language and depictions used to convey sexuality, gender, and family life on forms, posters, and pamphlets in healthcare settings, in the textbooks of nursing education, and in the way we structure our conversations with clients, families, and one another.

The second important consideration in framing this topic as an issue is the idea that the social conditions of a person's life influence the experience of health and illness. In particular, Wilkinson and Marmot (2003) remind us that the World Health Organization states, "continuing anxiety, insecurity, low self-esteem, social isolation and lack of control over work and home life have powerful effects on health" (p. 12). We should specifically note that social exclusion resulting from "discrimination and stigmatization" has an injurious effect on health (p. 16). The Gay and Lesbian Medical Association put forth the following view: "Many avoid or delay care or receive inappropriate or inferior care, because of perceived or real homophobia, biphobia, transphobia and discrimination by health care providers and institutions" (retrieved July 20, 2008 from www.glma.com).

Given this knowledge, how might we influence the practice of nurses and other healthcare providers, which is underpinned by unconscious and unquestioned assumptions of heteronormativity and actions depicting heterosexism?

 ## ANALYZING THE ISSUE: WAYS OF UNDERSTANDING

An analysis of the issue surrounding heteronormativity and heterosexism in healthcare begins with a historical analysis, raising questions for consideration in relation to the origin and evolution of the issue. Significantly for this chapter, a historical approach to analysis opens to questioning our taken-for-granted understanding of the issue, rather than simply recounting events as they have been recorded.

An ethical and legal analysis of the issue looks at the influence of Canadian law and the sections within the "Code of Ethics for Registered Nurses" (Canadian Nurses Association, 2008) that directly address gender and sexual orientation. The social and cultural analysis of the issue looks at the influence of language and culture on understandings of nonheterosexual orientations. Political analysis explores the relationship between knowledge and power. In the political analysis of nonheterosexual orientations, questions of disclosure, who to tell and when, are raised and explored. Lastly, the issue will be viewed from a critical feminist perspective through which we question the value attached to particular sexual orientations and question the role of institutional power in our lives.

Understanding the Issue Historically

Have you ever wondered if there were lesbians around when your grandmother was a child? Do you imagine that the early immigrant settlers to Canada were all paired up in heterosexual relationships?

How might people in same-sex relationships have been thought of in the early 1900s, or were they thought about at all?

It is fascinating for me to think of how much has changed for nonheterosexual people in my lifetime; as a young woman in the process of naming myself as gay in the 1970s I would never have imagined that I would one day legally marry a woman. Nor could I have imagined that my grandchildren would grow up in a society in which same-sex marriage would be a reality since before their birth. This reminder of recent history shows the way in which history is not just an account of events, but a view into the way categories and realities are shaped and remembered. Looking back on the accounts of intimate relationships, while holding in our awareness the recent changes for nonheterosexual people, the actual construction of what we currently accept as the categories of sexual orientations and genders come into focus. This look at historical evolution is not intended as a history lesson in dates but rather as an opportunity to think about the discourses and commonly held beliefs of society that influence and shape the way things come to be known or accepted.

Foucault (1990), in his book, *The History of Sexuality,* suggests that the very idea of sexualities came into language in the 19th century, shaped as they were by the efforts of institutionalized religion and the early practice of medicine, with the intention to persuade people to disclose or to confess the details of their intimate activities. As Foucault tells us, "sex was driven out of hiding . . . to lead a discursive existence" (p. 33). The medicalization of sexuality continued through the 19th and 20th century. In a medical practice that created a category of people, names long forgotten to us, such as "auto-monosexualists," were attached to nonheterosexual people. Through the influence of medical classification a category of people was constructed.

This categorical naming of a group of people is different, of course, than another historical reality that intimate practices and relationships have taken place between people of the same gender, likely for centuries. The names and the meanings of categories of sexual orientation have changed over time. The process, however, of the medical categorization and classification of people continued until late in the 20th century.

Nonheterosexual people have suffered from the medicalization of their health, including the pathologization of their relationships, and the oppressive experience of "curative" conversion therapies (Blackwell, 2008; Stevens & Hall, 1991). The medical construction of nonheterosexual people as psychopathological propagated and legitimated stereotypes of GLBTT people that fueled much of the discrimination against them. Under increasing pressure from the gay liberation movement and its supporters with new research findings, in 1973 the American Psychiatric Society removed homosexuality per se from the list of disorders in the *Diagnostic and Statistical Manual of Mental Disorders* (American Medical Association, 2002). What is less known, however, is that a number of related "disorders," including ego-dystonic homosexuality, remained in this influential medical text until as late as 1987.

As you begin your professional nursing practice in 2010 or beyond, the contents of a medical text published in 1987 might seem irrelevant or even obscure to you. Nonetheless, I would ask you to consider that many nurses you will encounter in practice, and an even larger number of citizens, were indoctrinated in the 20th century with the belief that homosexuality was pathological. Given the dominance of medical discourses in western society, it is in some ways remarkable that the ethical, legal, and social fabric of our society has changed as much as it has over the past 3 decades.

Ethical and Legal Understandings

Perhaps the Canadian law concerning the issues for nonheterosexual people that you are most familiar with is the national legalization of same-sex marriage in July 2005. This legislation followed several years of controversial activism and resistance, between and among individuals, political and religious organizations, and the provinces and territories, making Canada the fourth country in the world in which people of the same sex or gender can marry. And while this momentous legislation is changing the legal and social landscape of the country, at least one earlier piece of legislation can be seen as similarly notable. Any guesses what this socially relevant legislation might be? Perhaps you have heard the much quoted 1969 words of Pierre Elliot Trudeau, Justice Minister at the time in the liberal federal government: "There's no place for the state in the bedrooms of the nation." The government had just instituted sweeping changes in Canada's criminal law, which included decriminalizing homosexuality. Prior to that time, homosexuality was a criminal offence in Canada, which could result in long prison terms. Trudeau, speaking for the government stated: "It's bringing the laws of the land up to contemporary society I think. Take this thing on homosexuality. I think the view we take here is that there's no place for the state in the bedrooms of the nation. I think that what's done in private between adults doesn't concern the Criminal Code" (Makarenko, 2007).

While these legal advances have had both immediate and long-term influences on the people of Canada, I want to be clear to not conflate legal discourses with social acceptance. This distinction in part lies with the differences between legalization and socialization. Some people recognize same-sex marriage as an acknowledgment of equal rights for nonheterosexual people (Lannutti, 2005). On the other hand, real acceptance cannot be legally mandated—discrimination and prejudice are still lived realities for many GLBTT people. And further, there are many people who identify as nonheterosexual for whom marriage is not part of their reality, so we have to be careful not to view the legalization of marriage as evidence that the issues complicating the lives of nonheterosexual people have been resolved.

This complexity raises the question of where do we as nurses look for direction to mediate the tensions of the social and legal realities in this changing landscape? In the recent release of the "2008 Code of Ethics for Registered Nurses," section F: Promoting Justice clearly outlines the ethical responsibilities for practicing nurses (Box 21.3). As you might well know, codes of ethics are written to speak broadly to a profession; it is, however, up to each nurse to live this ethic as they work to understand difference.

 ## BOX 21.3 Promoting Justice

Nurses uphold principles of justice by safeguarding human rights, equity, and fairness and by promoting the public good.

Ethical responsibilities:

1. When providing care, nurses do not discriminate on the basis of a person's race, ethnicity, culture, political and spiritual beliefs, social or marital status, **gender, sexual orientation**, age, health status, place of origin, lifestyle, mental or physical ability or socio-economic status or any other attribute. (Emphasis added).
2. Nurses refrain from judging, labeling, demeaning, stigmatizing, and humiliating behaviors toward persons receiving care, other healthcare professionals and each other.
3. Nurses do not engage in any form of lying, punishment, or torture or any form of unusual treatment or action that is inhumane or degrading. They refuse to be complicit in such behaviors. They intervene, and they report such behaviors.
4. Nurses make fair decisions about the allocation of resources under their control based on the needs of persons, groups, or communities to whom they are providing care. They advocate for fair treatment and for fair distribution of resources for those in their care.
5. Nurses support a climate of trust that sponsors openness, encourages questioning the status quo, and supports those who speak out to address concerns in good faith (e.g., whistle-blowing).

Source: Canadian Nurses Association. *Code of ethics for registered nurses (2008 centennial edition)*. Retrieved July 17, 2008 from www.cna-nurses.ca.

Social and Cultural Understandings

As members of society, nurses and other healthcare professionals internalize the dominant discourses of the larger society. That said, nurses are, of course, not a homogenous group, but a very diverse group of people who are themselves influenced by their ethnic and cultural beliefs. It is these assumptions and beliefs that shape our intentional and unintended interactions with nonheterosexual people.

I would suggest that we are not only talking about *other* people belonging to nonheterosexual orientation, we are talking about ourselves—nurses, physicians, and other healthcare professionals who may identify as nonheterosexual. In an article speaking to the stigmatization of gay and lesbian nurses, Chinn (2008) suggests that "we will not realize our full potential as nurses, nor the full potential of our discipline as long as we allow the stigma of lesbian or gay identity to prevail within our own profession" (p. 552).

The language of the healthcare system, as we have touched on earlier, is based on the social norms of heterosexuality. The language is both based on and reinscribes, or reinforces, assumptions about the way things are in the world. These assumptions include the taken-for-granted assumptions of what constitutes a family, who might be a partner, and the gender of parents. Nonheterosexual people talk about the importance of seeing the realities of their own lives and relationships reflected in their environment (McDonald, 2006). It is difficult to know how to respond on a form in which your own reality is not reflected; further, it is difficult to have confidence in a system in which one is excluded by language. This exclusion extends to charts, admission forms, bathroom door signage, and even so-called "innocent" inquiries or conversations (Box 21.4).

Understanding the Political Nature of the Issue

A political analysis explores the relationship between knowledge and power in a situation. We might think of a people's genders or sexual orientations to be their personal knowledge, although increasingly this is knowledge that comes into the public domain. The holder of knowledge that is perceived of as personal and controversial is seen to hold, along with that knowledge, a component of power.

The idea of telling yourself or others of a nonheterosexual orientation has come to be known as "coming out." And, while coming out can be thought of as a one-time event in life, the action of disclosure of sexual orientation or of a transgendered reality is an ongoing, repetitive experience. Every time GLBTT people meet someone new or encounter someone from their distant pasts, a decision is made of whether or not to disclose their current orientations. In everyday conversations with strangers, interviews with potential employers, and encounters with colleagues and healthcare providers, GLBTT people must decide how much to disclose about their lives (McDonald, 2006). These decisions are not really

BOX 21.4 Reducing Heteronormative Bias

Language that reduces heteronormative bias includes questions such as:

Are you in a relationship or partnership?
Who is that with, and how do you define your relationship?
Who do you consider your immediate family?
Over your lifetime have your sexual partners been women, men, or both?
How would you like your partner or family to be involved in your care?

Source: McDonald, C. (In press). Sexuality and sexual practices. In B. Kozier, G. Erb, & A. Berman, et al. (Eds.). *Fundamentals of Canadian nursing: Concepts, process, and practice* (2nd ed.). Toronto: Pearson Education Canada.

about what we might call their "sex lives" at all; they are about sharing what they did on the weekend and with whom, the people who are important in their lives, and who they consider family.

And so how do people make decisions to disclose and how might we support people in these decisions? It's important to know that GLBTT people disclose for many different reasons. Although a considerable focus in the mental health literature associates disclosure with improved self-esteem, emotional health, and improved relationships (Jordan & Deluty, 1998; Morrow, 1996; Radonsky & Borders, 1995; Taylor, 1999), more recent studies suggest that each decision of disclosure must be made in the context of the lived life of the person disclosing (McDonald, 2006, 2008). That is to say that given the continued reality of discrimination and the heterosexual assumptions that influence safety, employment, and housing, the risks of disclosure must always be considered. Some people advocate disclosure as a political action that would disrupt taken-for-granted heteronormativity and, in a sense, reclaim our personal power (Chinn, 2008). "There is a belief that heteronormativity would topple and discrimination against homosexuals would plummet if people discovered that their mother/teacher/sister/friend/neighbor/professor/aunt/roommate/minister was a lesbian" (McDonald, 2006). Nonetheless, I would encourage you to keep in mind that disclosure is never unequivocally the right thing to do, and that the decision for disclosure always rests with the individual. As healthcare providers, we often have privileged access to personal knowledge of individual lives; with this privilege and power comes an obligation to understand the potential consequences of unintended disclosure.

Critical Feminist Understandings

To engage in a feminist critique of the issue, several important ideas come to mind. The first is the conflation that is often made between feminism and sexual orientation (lesbianism), often by people who value neither. To suggest that feminist thought, based on a body of knowledge, and what it means to be lesbian are interchangeable, is to undermine the possibilities for understanding both. Not only are there many feminists who are heterosexual, there are likely proportionally more lesbians who do not subscribe to feminist ideas. Indeed, confusing these two groups raises the question: Whose purpose is being served by this conflation?

A second point of feminist analysis brings to awareness the invisible power that institutional structures and hierarchies hold over nonheterosexual people. For example, accomplished nurse theorist Peggy Chinn relates an incident in which she was "advised by my chairperson that it would be prudent of me not to discuss openly the fact that I am a lesbian" (Chinn, 2008, p. 551). "Even in an academic community where the prevailing ethic is freedom of expression" nonheterosexual people can be silenced and manipulated to conform to heterosexual assumptions (p. 552). A feminist analysis asks, "Is expert power given authority over personal power and the right to be the subject of one's life?" Reflecting on the influence of the historical construction of categories and the power that medical discourses and institutional structures have exerted over nonheterosexual people, I would suggest that the answer is a resounding "yes!" In other words, heterosexism and heteronormativity in the healthcare system and beyond rob people of the right and the opportunity to be the subject of their own lives.

BARRIERS TO RESOLUTION

Given what you have read so far, can you imagine what some of the barriers are to the resolution of discrimination based on heterosexism and heteronormativity? Identifying these potential barriers is an important step in the process toward resolution of the issues.

1. There is a lack of visibility of the everyday life of nonheterosexual people in healthcare and in society generally.

2. Stigmatization reduces the safety for people in vulnerable positions to disclose nonheterosexual orientation.

3. A failure exists to understand all sexual orientations from a holistic view.

4. There is an absence of the knowledge needed about the lives of nonheterosexual people to provide professional care in the curricula of healthcare providers.

5. This lack of knowledge leads to decisions about the provision of care being based on assumptions that derive from heteronormativity and fuel heterosexism.

6. The dominant language of heteronormativity in the healthcare system does not reflect the realities of nonheterosexual people.

7. Outdated assumptions of the pathologization and medicalization of homosexuality remain present in healthcare.

8. The legalization of homosexuality is conflated with social acceptance of nonheterosexual relationships and lives.

9. There is continued reliance on the binary of genders (woman and man) and sexuality (heterosexual and homosexual).

 ## STRATEGIES FOR RESOLUTION

"We cannot 'fix' the larger societal stigma associated with being GLBTT but we can make a commitment to address the internalized oppression of **homophobia** that affects us all. If for no other reason, our societal mandate to care for those who are sick, regardless of who they are, demands that we know, understand, and overcome the barriers of social stigma that affect health and well being" (Chinn, 2008, p. 552).

1. Position statements by professional organizations on gender and sexual diversity have the potential to positively inform and influence their membership. See Box 21.5 for an example.

2. Include knowledge regarding the everyday lives of nonheterosexual people in curriculum, faculty, and staff development in institutions, such as hospitals and universities, where outdated assumptions influence what is informing curriculum development and healthcare practice.

3. People in authority have the obligation to initiate policy reform including changes in the language used in forms and signage.

4. All nurses have the obligation and the opportunity to create social and relational space for the realities of nonheterosexual people.

5. Because of the impact of heterosexism on the health of nonheterosexual people, nurses have the obligation wherever possible, to influence public policy related to the provision of safe and dignified care, access to employment, and housing.

SUMMARY

In this chapter we have explored and analyzed some of the issues facing people of nonheterosexual orientation. In particular, the assumption of heteronormativity and discrimination fueled by heterosexism has been discussed. The key notions in this chapter include the social and historical construction of categories of sexuality and the reality that many healthcare professionals are unwittingly complicit in heterosexism through practices based on inaccurate and outdated assumptions.

Unlike some issues, which require involvement from governments and authorities to make significant change, nurses in everyday practice can influence the issues faced by nonheterosexual people. By

BOX 21.5 Policy Statement on Sexual Diversity and Gender Identity—2002

1. Sexual Diversity in Society

1.1 Homosexuality is defined as the sexual and emotional attraction to members of the same sex, and has existed in most societies for as long as sexual beliefs and practices have been recorded. The proportion of the population that is not exclusively heterosexual has been estimated at between 8 and 11 percent.

1.2 Societal attitudes towards homosexuality have had a decisive impact on the extent to which individuals have been able to express their sexual orientation. In 1973 the American Psychiatric Association removed homosexuality from the *Diagnostic and Statistical Manual of Mental Disorders*. Subsequently, homosexuality was recognized as a form of sexual orientation or expression rather than a mental illness.

1.3 Strong family connections are important to the health and well-being of individuals, and recently there has been greater recognition of the diversity of family structures that exist in our society. These family structures could include nuclear families, single parents, blended families from remarriages, as well as gay and lesbian parents.

2. Discrimination

2.1 The term "heterosexism" has been used to describe the discrimination against gay, lesbian, bisexual, **transgender**, and **intersex** (GLBTI) populations. Heterosexism encompasses the belief that all people are and should be heterosexual and that alternative sexualities pose a threat to society. In this way heterosexism includes homophobia, a fear of alternative sexualities, and transphobia, a fear of alternative gender identities. It may also include a fear of intersex people who do not fit neatly into the binary categories of male and female.

2.2 Discrimination may be overt as in verbal abuse and physical violence or as covert as the silence that surrounds talking about GLBTI issues. This affects all members of society as individuals comply with gender role stereotypes in order to avoid homophobic discrimination. It is a constraint on human behavior that serves to diminish individual potential for development as well as diversity in our community.

2.3 The common experience of discrimination means that the health of GLBTI populations differs from that of the general population. For GLBTI individuals the impact of this discrimination can lead to a poorer general health status, diminished utilization of healthcare facilities, and a decreased quality of health services.

(Source: Australian Medical Association. Retrieved July 18, 2008 from www.AMA.com.au).

questioning our assumptions and being willing to examine our language and practices, nurses can reduce the dominance of heterosexism in the healthcare systems. Nursing students and new graduate nurses are perhaps in the best position to educate and mentor others, to question the historical assumptions that continue to be prevalent in educational and healthcare institutions.

Add to your knowledge of this issue:	
Health Canada, Status of Women	**www.lesbianhealth.ca**
Gay and Lesbian Medical Association (GLMA)	**www.glma.org**
Parents and friends and lesbians and gays (PFLAG)	**www.pflag.org**

Online

REFLECTIONS on the Chapter...

1 How has the information you have read in this chapter affirmed or challenged the assumptions that you held prior to reading it?

2 Given what has been discussed in this chapter, what knowledge do you believe healthcare providers need to provide safe and dignified care to nonheterosexual people?

3 Explore the index in the back of at least three of your nursing textbooks, looking for information on transgender, gay, lesbian, or bisexual people. Does the nonhetero-sexual content in the text disrupt or reinscribe the idea of heteronormativity?

4 What other readings or resources have assisted you in understanding this issue?

5 After reading the chapter "Creating a Welcoming Clinical Environment" in *Guidelines for Care of Lesbian, Gay, Bisexual and Transgender Patients* at www.glma.org, assess your practice environment for its welcome of GLBTT people.

6 Referring to the same guidelines, how would you assess your school as a welcoming environment for GLBTT people?

References

Australian Medical Association. (2002). *Policy statement on sexual diversity and gender identity.* Retrieved July 17, 2008 from www.ama.com.au.

Butler, J. (1990). Performative acts and gender constitution: An essay in phenomenology and feminist theory. In S. Case (Ed.). *Performing feminisms: Feminist critical theory and theatre* (pp. 270–282). Baltimore: John Hopkins University Press.

Canadian Nurses Association. (2008). *Code of ethics for registered nurses* (2008 centennial edition.) Retrieved July 17, 2008 from www.cna-nurses.ca.

Ceci, C. (2009). When difference matters: The politics of privilege and marginality. In M. McIntyre & C. McDonald, (Eds.). *Realities of Canadian nursing: Professional, practice, and power issues.* Philadelphia: Lippincott Williams & Wilkins.

Chinn, P. (2008). Lesbian nurses: What's the big deal? *Issues in Mental Health Nursing, 29*(6), 551–554.

Forstein, M. (2003). In A. Peterkin & C. Risdon, *Caring for lesbian and gay people: A clinical guide.* Toronto: University of Toronto Press.

Foucalt, M. (1990). *The history of sexuality: An introduction.* New York: Vintage.

Gray, P., Kramer, M., & Minick, P., et al. (1996). Heterosexism in nursing. *Journal of Nursing Education, 35*(5), 204–210.

Irwin, L. (2007). Homophobia and heterosexism: Implications for nursing and nursing practice. *Australian Journal of Advanced Nursing, 25*(1), 70–76.

Jordan, K. & Deluty, R. (1998). Coming out for lesbian women: Its relation to anxiety, positive affectivity, self esteem, and social support. *Journal of Homosexuality, 35*(2), 41–63.

Lannutti, B. (2005). For better or for worse: Exploring the meanings of same-sex marriage within the lesbian, gay, bisexual and transgendered community. *Journal of Social and Personal Relationships, 22*(5):5–18.

Makarenko, J. (2007). *Same-sex marriage in Canada.* Retrieved July 19, 2008 from www.Mapleleafweb.com/features/same sex marriage.

McDonald, C. (2006). Lesbian disclosure: Disrupting the taken for granted. *Canadian Journal of Nursing Research, 39*(1), 42–57.

_____. (2008). Unpacking disclosure: Interrupting unquestioned practices. *Issues in Mental Health Nursing, 29*(6), 639–649.

_____. (2009). Issues of gender and power: The significance attributed to nurses work. In M. McIntyre & C. McDonald (Eds.)., *Realities of Canadian nursing: Professional, practice, and power issues.* Philadelphia: Lippincott Williams & Wilkins.

_____. (In press). Sexuality and sexual practices. In B. Kozier, G. Erb, & A. Berman, et al. (Eds.). *Fundamentals of Canadian nursing: Concepts, process, and practice* (2nd ed.). Toronto: Pearson Education Canada.

Morgan, S. & Stevens, P. (2008). Transgender identity development as represented by a group of female to male transgendered adults. *Issues in Mental Health Nursing, 29*(6), 585–599.

Morrow, D. (1996). Coming out for adult lesbians: A group intervention. *Social Work, 41*(6), 647–656.

Public Health Agency of Canada (2007). Retrieved July 17, 2008 from www.phac-aspc.gc/publicat/cgshe-ldnemss/cashe.

Radonsky, V. & Borders, L. (1995). Factors influencing lesbians direct disclosure of their sexual orientation. *Journal of Gay and Lesbian Psychotherapy, 2*(1), 49–63.

Stevens, P. (1995). Structural and interpersonal impact of homosexual assumptions on lesbian health care clients. *Nursing Research, 44*(1), 25–30.

Stevens, P. & Hall, J. (1991). A critical historical analysis of the medical construction of lesbianism. *International Journal of Health Services, 21*(2), 291–307.

Stevens, P. & Hall, J. (1988). Stigma, health beliefs and experiences with health care in lesbian women. *Image: Journal of Nursing Scholarship, 20*(2), 69–73.

Taylor, B. (1999). Coming out as a life transition: Homosexual identity formation and its implications for health care practice. *Journal of Advanced Nursing, 30*(2), 520–525.

Wilkinson, R. & Marmot, M. (Eds). (2003). *Social determinants of health: The solid facts* (2nd ed.). Copenhagen: World Health Organization. Retrieved July 16, 2008 from www.who.dk/ documents/e81384.pdf.

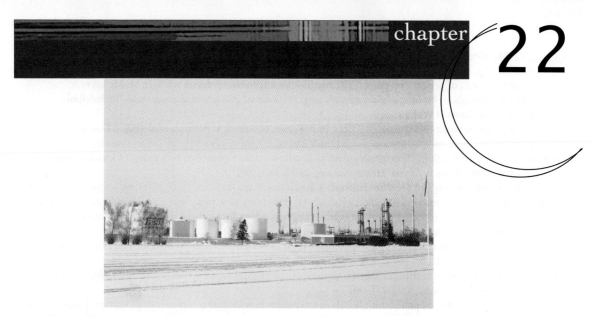

chapter 22

Across Canada, the relationship of the environment to the health of individuals and families is a serious concern. Emissions from gas plants and other environmental pollutants are just a few of the potential hazards to health. Individual nurses and the nursing profession can promote greater societal health through the traditional routes of nursing practice, education, and research.

Environmental Health and Nursing

Carol McDonald
Marjorie McIntyre

The authors of this chapter acknowledge the significant contribution Elizabeth Thomlinson made to an earlier version of this chapter.

Critical Questions

As a way of engaging with the ideas in this chapter, consider the following:

1 What assumptions do you hold about the role of professional nurses in environmental health?

2 What knowledge would you need as a nurse to make a significant contribution to environmental health?

3 How might you account for the scarcity of knowledge in nursing curricula to support this area of nursing practice?

4 Given what you have read in earlier chapters, what contribution would you anticipate that professional organizations would play in creating healthy environments?

After completing this chapter, you will be able to:

1 Identify some common environmental health hazards in your geographic region.

2 Examine the nursing profession's impact in addressing environmental issues.

3 Generate ideas about how individual nurses can affect issues of environmental health.

4 Evaluate how nursing curricula integrate health and the environment.

This we know . . . the earth does not belong to man, man belongs to the earth. All things are connected, like blood which connects one family. Whatever befalls the earth befalls the children of the earth. Man did not weave the web of life; he is merely a strand in it. Whatever he does to the web, he does to himself.

—*Chief Seattle, 1854 Suqwamish and Duwamish*

In a world that is increasingly affected by globalization and global warming, humans are as closely linked to the health of their environments as they were at the dawn of human history. Environmental hazards, the health of the earth, and the health of the earth's inhabitants are inseparable. The interdependence of all species on the earth and the physical environment cannot be overemphasized.

Although this chapter does not focus on the conservation of natural resources, it does underscore how environmental hazards contribute to adverse health outcomes for humans. We hope that readers will examine the regions and communities where they live and work to gain awareness of the connection between their own environments and the health of the people who live there. The need to be aware of how environmental hazards impact human health is important for nurses regardless of their practice settings—community, long-term, acute institutional care, or occupational health. Tragedies, such as the deaths from *Escherichia coli (E. coli)*, bacteria resulting from contaminated water sources in Walkerton, Ontario (Ahluwalia, 2000), raise concerns for other communities about the possibility of similar events in their own neighborhoods.

There is no doubt that human health is affected when the environment or ecosystem is damaged (Canadian Nurses Association [CNA], 2008b, 2005) The term *environmental health,* as used in this chapter, refers to freedom from illness related to exposure to environmental contamination, hazards, and toxins that are detrimental to health. In the discussions that follow, the term *environment* includes the physical, social, political, legal, psychological, and cognitive environments of individuals, families, and communities. As scientific knowledge increases and social and political values change, the definition of, and factors related to, environmental health will also change. And further, "as our knowledge progresses about the etiology of disease, evidence of environmental contributions to disease also grows, particularly the environmental link to a number of chronic diseases" (CNA, 2005, p. 1). The disciplinary concepts of person, environment, health, and nursing, which form the metaparadigm of nursing, underscore the interdependence of the environment and health but a perusal of nursing curricula and textbooks uncovered a lack of focus on issues related to environmental health.

In 2005 the Canadian Nurses Association (CNA) developed a backgrounded paper titled, "The Ecosystem, the Natural Environment, and Health and Nursing: A Summary of the Issues," in which they made central the following issue: "The natural environment has a significant impact on our quality of life, our health and the sustainability of our planet. Increasing population, urbanization and industrialization . . . affect the quality of air we breath, the water we drink and the food we eat" (p. 1). The World Health Organization (WHO) (2007) reminds us "to a large extent, public health depends on safe drinking water, sufficient food, secure shelter, and good social conditions. A changing climate is likely to affect all of these conditions." Recently, as part of the Centennial Celebrations (2008e), the CNA launched a project to support work in environmental health for nursing education, practice, research, and policy development. A group of nurses from across the country, the Environmental Health Reference Group, have guided and developed this impressive project. Their work includes a background paper, educational module, and video presentation on several important focused areas of environmental health. This information can be readily accessed through the CNA Web site. (See Online Resources.)

HISTORICAL LINKS BETWEEN ENVIRONMENT AND HEALTH

The effect that a healthy or, conversely, an unhealthy, environment has on human health is not a recent discovery. Early civilizations were aware of the impact of the environment on health. The Minoans (3000 to 1430 B.C.), Mycenaeans (1430 to 1150 B.C.), and Romans (509 B.C. to 476 A.D.) all built extensive drainage and water systems as well as baths and toilets (McGuire & Eigsti-Gerber, 1999) in response to related environmental health hazards of pestilence and disease. Early Hebrew writings included a code on hygiene, and the ancient Egyptians (3100 B.C. to 600 A.D.) developed safe water and sewer systems. As civilizations rose and fell, this knowledge and the systems that had been developed were often forgotten or destroyed.

Plagues resulting from contamination of water sources and the spread of disease through animal vectors have been documented throughout history. Through the introduction of public health measures, such as providing a clean source of drinking water and disposing safely of sewage and other wastes, great improvements were made in the health of populations; these key elements remain as important as ever (Clark, 1999; McDevitt & Wilbur, 2002).

A major turning point in history, however, was the Industrial Revolution that began in Great Britain in the early 1700s and spread to Europe and North America. Industrialization resulted in a shift from what had been a rural, agricultural economy to one that was urban and factory-based with concomitant problems of pollution from large steel foundries and the burning of fossil fuels. The impact of the Industrial Revolution extended far beyond the production of goods and material to changes in governments, the use of resources in the world, material benefits for some of the world's population, and wars and exploitation of many populations. Modern transportation and communication, the globalization of markets, and the even more rapid destruction of habitats are evident today. Nurses have been integral participants in examining and changing some of the harmful environmental conditions to improve public health.

In *Notes on Nursing*, Florence Nightingale (1860, p. 5) observed that environmental factors had a key impact on health and disease:

> *In watching diseases, both in private homes and in public hospitals, the thing which strikes the experienced observer most forcibly is this, that the symptoms or the sufferings generally considered to be inevitable and incident to the disease are very often not symptoms of the disease at all, but of something quite different—of the want of fresh air, or of cleanliness, or of punctuality and care in the administration of diet, of each or of all of these.*

Further, Nightingale noted that there were "five essential points in securing the health of houses" and, by extrapolation, the health of the population: "pure air, pure water, efficient drainage, cleanliness and light" (1860, p. 14).

Other nurses who actively advocated for safe water, sewage, and sanitation systems, which they incorporated into their health promotion and education practices, included Lillian Wald (1915) and Mary Breckenridge (1952 [Eigsti-Gerber & McGuire, 1999]). Wald was the founder of modern public health nursing, working in New York to improve the health of children in particular. Breckenridge incorporated principles of environmental health in her community health practice in rural Kentucky, which lowered infant mortality rates. Before the establishment of large hospitals and the focus on care in hospitals, most early nursing practice was carried out in the community. Nurses were cognizant of the environmental conditions in which their patients lived and worked. The shift to the majority of nursing practice being concentrated within institutions separated nurses from the environmental effects that had been more readily apparent.

Current environmental debates center on global warming as a result of the burning of fossil fuels (Foley, 2001; Last, Trouton, & Pengally, 1998), destruction of habitat around the world (Malcolm et al., 2002), and the potential for unrestrained population growth to outstrip the ability to produce enough food to feed the world's citizens (Brown et al., 2001). Multiple charters, agreements, summits, and conventions have been held to examine the health of the world's citizens, globalization and global issues related to the environment, access to safe water and food, global warming, the sociopolitical causes and impact of poverty, and the economic disparity that exists among nations within the context of a "sustainable global ecosystem" (Hilfinger Messias, 2001, p. 10). A proliferation of treaties and accords since the 1970s has resulted in more than 240 international agreements (Brown et al., 2001).

Brown and colleagues (2001) noted that the 1987 Montreal Protocol on Substances that Deplete the Ozone Layer led to the gradual phasing out of the use of chlorofluorocarbons that damage the stratosphere. The 1997 Kyoto Protocol to the 1992 United Nations (UN) Framework Convention on Climate Change was much more contentious, when the United States refused to ratify the treaty that required industrialized nations to cut carbon dioxide emissions by 6% to 8% between 2008 and 2012. Going into the more recent July 2008 G8 nations Summit on Climate Change, environmentalists were hopeful that the scientific evidence would influence world leaders to address the increasingly urgent issues around climate change. Although Russia and the United States did agreed to some reduction in emissions by 2050, the conditions surrounding this agreement (the buy-in of China and India, for example) and the timeframe for implementation have drawn significant criticism from environmentalists. A major concern remains regarding the ability to police these agreements and end environmental crime that is fueled by greed and the self-interests of individuals, corporations, and governments.

While recognizing positive global effects linked to health, sanitation, and urban reclamation, Berlinguer (1999) raises concerns regarding pollution, depletion of natural resources, global warming, and the declining quality of life—particularly in urban centers and in developing nations. He notes that people in the lowest socioeconomic classes suffer the greatest damage because they lack the resources and facilities to preserve their health. Put another way, it is the wealthiest countries and the wealthiest citizens of those countries who have benefited the most from industrialization.

In all nations, the poorest residents tend to live in substandard housing in densely populated communities in close proximity to industrial areas where the potential for contamination and hazardous waste leakage is the highest (Chaudhuri, 1998). Within Canadian society, members of First Nations communities are especially at risk for health problems related to unsafe drinking water, lack of adequate sanitation, and substandard housing (Health Canada, 1999b). Environmental contaminants such as polychlorinated biphenyls (PCBs) used in electrical and hydraulic equipment, dioxins from bleaching wood pulp with chlorine, and mercury from old industrial practices and long-range transport have been found in fish and marine mammals throughout the country. The result is a contaminated food supply, particularly for Aboriginal people in the north and those who follow a traditional diet.

ENVIRONMENTAL HEALTH HAZARDS

Around the world, life expectancy has increased and morbidity and mortality have decreased as a result of significant improvement and the availability of safe water and sewage systems and better nutrition and housing. Individuals, communities, and governments need to be conscious that these gains do not overshadow current and developing environmental problems. WHO notes that about 2 million children younger than 5 years of age die annually because of unsafe drinking water and lack of sanitation. Air pollution is responsible for up to 20% of childhood mortality (World Health Organization [WHO], 2001). A WHO task force has been established to promote the identification, assessment, mitigation, and prevention of environmental hazards specifically "to prevent disease and disability in children associated with chemical and physical threats" (WHO, 2001).

Various UN agencies participated in a global environmental assessment by providing data and information on environmental issues within their particular mandates (United Nations Environment Programme, 1999). This assessment was undertaken in response to the need to build a consensus on priorities regarding the environment. According to this report, increased industrialization around the world has contributed to environmental deterioration resulting from air and water pollution, waste dumping, and increasing ill health, especially among the poor. Environmental contaminants include biologic agents, inorganic and organic chemicals, radiation, and particulate matter (Box 22.1).

Contaminants follow pathways from the time they are released into the environment until people, animals, or plants come in contact with them. These exposure pathways consist of five components that need to be examined when tracing sources of contamination (Health Canada, 1998). The components are:

- source of contamination (e.g., emissions, waste water and disposal sites, volcanoes, fires, and household products)
- medium through which the contaminant travels (e.g., water, soil, air, and food products)
- point at which people come into contact with the contaminant
- person, animal, or plant that is the receptor of the contaminant
- route of exposure (e.g., inhalation [gases, vapors, or particulate matter], dermal contact [working in contaminated soil or swimming in contaminated water], or ingestion [contaminated food or water]).

Many symptoms exhibited by people exposed to environmental contaminants can be attributed to other causes, making it difficult to establish an exact cause and effect. Therefore, it is important when assessing exposure to environmental contaminants to take as broad a perspective as possible to include all potential environmental factors.

Water Safety

Water is fundamental to all life on the planet. Uneven distribution of this resource around the globe means that some regions, such as Canada, have an abundance of fresh water, whereas other regions, such as the Middle East and northern Africa, suffer from a shortage. It is estimated that 500 million people in the world live in countries that are short of water and that, by 2025, this number will dramatically rise to 3 billion (Mitchell, 2001). Water use worldwide has risen sixfold between 1900 and 1995, more than double the population increase.

BOX 22.1 Selected Environmental Contaminants

Biologic Agents
Bacteria, such as *Escherichia coli*, protozoa, viruses, fungi, algae, molds, house dust mites, and pollen grains

Chemical Contaminants
Organic substances, such as fluorine, chlorine, bromine, iodine, nitrogen, sulfur, phosphorus, carbon, polychlorinated biphenyls, DDT, dioxins, benzene, malathion, toluene, and dioxane inorganic substances, such as ozone, nitrogen oxides, sulfur dioxide, lead, mercury, cadmium, arsenic, uranium, beryllium, and chromium

Radiation
Microwaves, ultraviolent light, low-frequency electromagnetic fields, and sound

Particulate Matter
Fine dust, smoke from forest fires, burning stubbles and wood burning fires, asbestos, and cigarette smoke

Internationally, the United Nations Children's Fund and WHO (2008) report that tremendous progress has been made in access to improved water supplies worldwide. Told as a "good news story," in relation to the more dismal reality of adequate sanitation facilities, the number of people without an improved drinking water source now numbers below one billion (WHO/United Nation's Children's Fund, 2008, Special focus on drinking water and sanitation, p. 58).

In countries such as Canada, the abundance of water has led to waste and increased pollution of this resource. Although water is the ultimate renewable resource, major problems now exist in that water sources are polluted with chemicals, fertilizers, heavy metals, hydrocarbons, and raw sewage (Robson & Schneider, 2001; UN Environment Programme, 1999; Wanke & Saunders, 1996). Industrial waste, runoff from large-scale farming operations, and the dumping of garbage in uncontrolled waste sites lead to continued pollution.

In nature, water is actually never "pure." As water flows, it gathers tiny pieces of everything it contacts, including minerals, earth, plants, fertilizers, and agricultural runoff. Even in what might seem like pristine locations, water in its natural state will likely require some type of treatment before it is safe to drink. However, you might be surprised to learn that the water you drink is a minor source of most pollutants; the largest percentage of our daily intake of pollutants is from food sources. Nonetheless, water is still the principle source of exposure to some microorganisms (CNA, 2005).

Drinking water in Canada comes either from surface water, such as lakes and rivers, or underground sources such as aquifers. Most Canadians get their drinking water from public water systems. Provincial and territorial governments set requirements for water quality for these public water sources. People living in rural and remote locations may get their drinking water from wells or from surface water sources on their own private property and are individually responsible for the safety of the drinking water (Health Canada, 2008).

Aquifers, underground sources of water, are being drained more quickly than they are being replenished. Global warming has caused the atmosphere to retain more water in the form of vapor, which decreases the volume of water returned in the form of rain. An example of the overuse of subterranean water is the High Plains Aquifer that extends from South Dakota to Texas. The level of water has dropped by more than 40 m as the population uses the water for irrigating land that was once barren. Solutions to this water depletion suggested by United States politicians and entrepreneurs are the bulk sale of water from Canada and the desalination of ocean water for human use. The short-term and long-term effects on the environment of either of these proposals are not known.

The need to provide a safe drinking water supply has been highlighted by outbreaks of E. coli in the water supply at Walkerton, Ontario and Cryptosporidium species found in the water in North Battleford, Saskatchewan. The E. coli outbreak led to multiple gastrointestinal illnesses and, ultimately, to the deaths of nine people (Ahluwalia, 2000). Contamination of the water sources from manure from cattle farms in the area and the inadequate treatment of the water are suspected causes of this outbreak. The impact of these outbreaks has heightened public awareness and increased the need to examine and question water safety in the communities.

Cryptosporidium, although not a new organism, is becoming more prevalent. Animals and humans shed this protozoan parasite in their feces. The consumption of contaminated water or food, ingestion of recreational water, or contact with infected people can lead to infection. There are potentially life-threatening consequences for immunosuppressed people who become infected (Physicians for Social Responsibility, 2001b). Proper filtration, distillation, or reverse osmosis processes must be used to ensure that the organism has been removed from the water supply. Giardia lamblia (G. lamblia) is another parasite endemic to the ecosystem. G. lamblia causes gastrointestinal infections and can also produce life-threatening effects in an immunocompromised person. Contamination of water supplies with various microbial contaminants leads to multiple "boil water" alerts annually in all provinces.

In 2001, a government roundtable found that, although water quality is a serious problem throughout the country, there is particular concern regarding water supply to First Nations communities. A Health Canada report in 1995 signaled that 171 communities (1 in 5) had water systems that could negatively affect the health of the citizens (MacKinnon, 2001). Minimal improvements have occurred during the intervening years. As of 2001, there were no national regulations in Canada regarding water protection and safety, an indication that disasters can and will continue to occur.

Air Pollution

Many regions of the world suffer from air pollution that leads to illness and death. In South America, about 4,000 premature deaths are estimated to occur annually in Sao Paulo and Rio de Janeiro as a result of severe air pollution (UN Environment Programme, 1999). The very young and the very old suffer a greater burden from air pollution than do people in the interim age ranges. The risk from air pollution for children increases because they breathe more rapidly and inhale more pollutants per pound of body weight than do adults. A wide range of negative effects from air pollution include impaired pulmonary function; reduced physical performance; multiple visits to physicians, emergency rooms, and hospitals; and premature death (Health Canada, 1998; CNA, 2008a).

Air pollutants are generated from burning fossil fuels, such as oil, coal, gasoline, and diesel fuel, in vehicles and power generators. Industries, such as pulp and paper mills, oil refineries, and ore smelters, contribute to air pollution (CNA, 2008a). Oil, natural gas, and coal production has resulted in Alberta emitting 30% of the carbon dioxide, 26% of the nitrogen oxide, and 23% of the sulfur oxide emissions generated in Canada (Environment Canada, 2000). Asthma is a respiratory disease that can be triggered by airborne contaminants. Air pollutants, such as ground-level ozone, sulfur dioxide, and particulate matter, are believed to be key factors in increased asthma rates (CNA, 2008a). Pope and colleagues (2002) analyzed the mortality statistics of participants in the Cancer Prevention Study II who resided in United States metropolitan areas where pollution data were available. They demonstrated that fine particulate air contamination is associated with cardiopulmonary and lung cancer mortality (Pope et al., 2002, p. 1137) and is a significant risk factor to population health.

An exponential increase in the incidence of asthma in children in Canada occurred in the 1990s. Rates of hospitalization for boys increased by 27% and for girls by 18% (Health Canada, 1997). This raised annual hospital admissions of children to more than 60,000. According to Last and associates (1998), hospital admissions in Ontario for acute bronchitis, bronchiolitis, and pneumonia in children younger than 1 year of age "can be attributed to the summer pollutants, ozone and sulphates" (p. 21). According to the Canadian Lung Association, airborne contaminants including tobacco smoke and mold can cause or exacerbate asthma and other respiratory conditions; asthma now affects roughly 3 million Canadians (CNA, 2005).

Some authorities suggest that it would cost $6 billion to implement a program to decrease air pollution by developing cleaner vehicles and fuels in Canada (Health Canada, 1998, p. 121). On the other hand, savings to the healthcare system are estimated to be $24 billion as a result of eliminating many of the negative health effects of air pollution. Improving ambient air quality in Canada alone could amount to $8 billion in healthcare savings over the next 20 years (Last et al., 1998). Last and associates (1998) suggest that the reduction of motor vehicle emissions would result in savings to the forest and agricultural sectors of the Canadian economy of between $11 billion and $30 billion.

Although chemically the same, ground-level ozone (found within 11 km of the earth's surface) and the "ozone layer" (found between 11 and 47 km above the earth in the stratosphere) need to be differentiated from each other. The ozone layer acts as a barrier against ultraviolet (UV) radiation (particularly UVB rays) from the sun (Health Canada, 1998). As this layer is damaged or destroyed by chlorofluorocarbons, more radiation penetrates to earth. The result is an increase in skin cancer, particularly melanomas. There is also evidence that UVB exposure increases the risk for cataracts (Institute of Medicine, 1995).

Ground-level ozone, or smog, forms when nitrogen oxides and volatile organic compounds react in the presence of sunlight (Health Canada, 1998). This reaction occurs on hot, still, summer days, and the resultant air pollution can lead to adverse cardiac and respiratory effects. Again, those most affected are elderly and very young people. As the earth's average temperature rises, it is expected that more hot summer days with smog advisories or warnings will occur.

PCBs, dioxins, and other organic compounds can travel long distances through the air before being deposited on the land or in bodies of water. These toxins accumulate in the food chain, where they become a hazard to people who consume fish and wildlife as food, particularly when they are ingested faster than they can be excreted (Health Canada, 1998). There is grave concern that seals and other Arctic animals are contaminated and pose a risk to Inuit communities that rely on these animals as a source of food.

Chemical Pollution

Humans are slowly coming to realize the effects of the huge quantities of man-made chemicals that have been discharged into the environment since the 1940s (Physicians for Social Responsibility, 2005). Excessive use of fertilizers, pesticides, and heavy metals such as arsenic, cadmium, lead, and mercury has polluted the land (UN Environment Programme, 1999). Local sources of contamination, such as sewage and waste disposal, and industrial discharge can be more readily identified. More diffuse contamination occurs through runoff from fields and lawns, motor vehicle emissions, and the long-distance contamination of acid rain (which develops from sulfur dioxide and nitrogen oxides from coal-fired power plants, smelters, and vehicular emissions). Once again, environmental contamination is an issue that disproportionately affects the health of children. Children, relative to their size, eat, drink, and breathe more than do adults. Children are in closer contact with the environment through increased hand-to-mouth activity. Children absorb more chemicals through their skin and intestines than do adults. Certain contaminants can have a major effect as children pass through critical developmental stages. Additionally, children and families living in poverty are likely to have increased exposure and less access to resources (i.e. nutrition and healthcare) to mitigate the negative effects of exposure to environmental contaminants (CNA, 2005).

Many of these chemical pollutants remain in the environment for long periods. They can be ingested and then accumulate in the tissues of humans if their excretion does not occur as quickly as their intake. Dioxins, furans, and PCBs build up in fatty tissue, whereas metals such as lead, mercury, and cadmium are stored in the liver, kidney, and bone. Mercury can be found in many lakes and rivers, where it converts to methyl mercury, a toxic substance that can affect the nervous systems of humans and animals (Health Canada, 2007). An additional concern is long-term arsenic ingestion (through drinking water), which increases the risk for skin, bladder, lung, kidney, and other cancers (Physicians for Social Responsibility, 2001a). The impact on human health of long-term low-level exposure to many chemical pollutants is unknown. Concerns focus on immune system suppression, neurologic and behavioral changes, and the role that chemical toxins play in initiating cancer.

The term *pesticide* refers to a variety of chemicals that control weeds (herbicides), bacteria (disinfectants), fungi (fungicides), insects (insecticides), and rodents (rodenticides). Pesticides are widely used in agriculture and forestry to protect crops and forests. Large amounts of fertilizer and herbicides are used annually in urban and suburban environments in the care of lawns and golf courses. According to a review of the literature completed by the CNA (2008d), a large body of research evidence has identified risks associated with pesticide use, particularly for children. The CNA (2008a, p. 21) document, "The Environment and Health," references the Toronto Health Department (p. 1, 2002) statement that, "These substances [pesticides] are intended to be harmful to living organisms and because they are released into the environment, they pose an exposure and potential health risk to other organisms, including humans."

In Canada, more than 500 active ingredients have been registered for use as pesticides (Health Canada, 1998). There is a growing movement within some municipalities across Canada to ban the use of herbicides because of the risk to human health. As of May 2008, there were 146 towns and cities with active pesticide ordinances, the largest of these being Toronto. A list of these communities can be found at http://www.flora.org/healthyottawa/BylawList.pdf.

Of grave concern are the implications for the health of residents who live in the immediate vicinity of toxic waste sites or who now live in what was once a contaminated industrial site (Carruth, Gilbert, & Lewis, 1997). There are no biologic markers by which the level of exposure can be determined for many of the chemicals that are discharged into the environment. Further, the long-term impact of long-term exposure to some contaminants, such as malathion, is not known. Key concerns related to long-term exposure include the following:

- Those in lower socioeconomic conditions are often the people who live in areas closest to polluted sites.
- As knowledge of chemical pollutants grows, standards may change (i.e., norms or levels that were once considered safe may be now considered a health risk).
- Exposure to toxins may occur and may be undetected over extended periods of time.
- Exposure to contaminants may occur through multiple pathways (e.g., air, water, and soil) and enter the food chain in numerous ways, making detection more difficult.
- Action to curb exposure to contaminants has not kept pace with society's abilities to detect contamination (CNA, 2000).
- Canada is without longitudinal research regarding the effects of individual contaminants as well as the combined effects from multiple sources of contamination (CNA, 2000).

Inside Environments

The Ottawa Charter for Health Promotion (1986) credits adequate shelter as having a major effect on health. According to the report from the federal, provincial, and territorial governments, "Toward a Healthy Future: Second Report on the Health of Canadians," 1 in 5 Canadians who rent accommodations is living in substandard housing (Health Canada, 1999b). The people who most often live in these conditions are single-parent families, particularly ones in which parents are younger than 30 years old; people with mental health problems; and senior citizens living alone. Of grave concern are the inadequate housing and crowded living conditions in which Aboriginal people live. This may be a major contributor to the fact that Aboriginal children suffer from much higher rates of respiratory and other infectious diseases than do non-Aboriginal children (Health Canada, 1999b).

Health Canada estimates that Canadians spend up to 90% of their time indoors in their homes, work sites, and other buildings. In addition to outdoor contaminants, which can also be found indoors, the inside air may contain tobacco smoke, formaldehyde, vapors from household products, carbon dioxide, and biologic agents, such as bacteria, fungi, molds, viruses, and mite byproducts (Health Canada, 1998). The health of the residents may be adversely affected if the concentrations of any of these contaminants rise too high. The growing trend toward weatherizing homes and buildings in the interest of conservation may result in a lack of adequate air exchange because the ventilation systems were not designed for these well-insulated and sealed buildings. Therefore, the potential for contaminant buildup increases.

A principal contaminant in indoor environments is tobacco smoke, including sidestream smoke emitted from cigarettes, pipes, and cigars between puffs and mainstream smoke exhaled by smokers. It is estimated that there are 300 deaths from lung cancer in nonsmokers annually in Canada as a result of environmental tobacco smoke (ETS [Health Canada, 1998, 1999b]). In addition, ETS is considered a significant cause of cardiovascular disease and death in nonsmokers.

Canadian children are at an increased risk for health effects from ETS because they spend more time indoors than do children in many other countries. As mentioned previously, children have smaller airways and breathe more rapidly than do adults, thus inhaling more pollutants per kilogram of body weight. In the United States, authorities estimate that 11% of asthma cases, about 350,000 cases of bronchitis, and 152,000 cases of pneumonia are a consequence of ETS (Health Canada, 1998). More than one third of households with children younger than 15 years of age also have a smoker in the family. Authorities suspect that exposure to ETS during childhood may be associated with increased pulmonary disease and cancer (Health Canada, 1998).

There is a wide variation among provinces in the control and restriction of smoking in public areas. Restrictions against smoking range from being limited to designated smoking areas to a total ban on smoking on public premises. As the public becomes more aware and concerned with the health risks attributed to ETS, smoking bans are increasingly stringent. In 2008 the majority of the provinces and territories have legislated complete bans on smoking in public buildings.

Contaminated Social Environments

If consideration of environmental health risks is confined to the effects of pollution and hazards within the natural environment, a key component of the settings in which individuals and families live will be ignored. Impoverished neighborhoods with substandard housing, abject poverty, homelessness, visible signs of people who are substance abusing and drug dealing, and violence and crime within the community are examples of contaminated social environments. The impact on the physical, psychological, and emotional health of individuals living in such environments can be severe.

If the social environments in which people live are violent, degrading, and impoverished, there is a significant negative impact on the health of the residents. These negative effects are compounded by the toxic waste sites and heavy industry that are often near these communities. Healthcare professionals need to take into account the entire environmental context of the people and communities in which they are working.

BARRIERS AND STRATEGIES

One of the largest barriers to achieving environmental health has been the lack of public knowledge or education about the reality of increasing health risks connected to the environment. The more we know about and understand the links between the environment and human health, the more willing we are as a society to provide the economic support and the political will to make the changes that are needed.

One way to overcome this lack of knowledge in the public domain is for professional organizations to take a position on the issues and to make public their position statements. The CNA position statement titled, "The Environment Is a Determinant of Health," states that "the CNA will work with others in the health and social sectors to influence decisions that impact the environment and thus human health" (CNA, 2000). Of particular concern are the long-term health effects of contaminants on children. In a joint statement, the CNA and the Canadian Medical Association indicate that "a healthy environment is fundamental to life, and attention to the effect of the environment on human health is imperative if we are to attain the goal of health for all" (1996). Through the revised "2008 Code of Ethics for Registered Nurses," the CNA (2008c) has made the position of the profession in Canada even stronger, by obligating nurses in "supporting environmental preservation and restoration and advocating for initiatives that reduce environmentally harmful practices in order to promote health and well-being" (p. 20) (Box 22.2).

In Canada, nurses and other healthcare professionals have the power to influence political decision making directly through lobbying members of parliament and also indirectly through publishing position statements that exert pressure on politicians, governments, and health authorities. In taking this public stance we must first recognize and address the impact that the waste from healthcare facilities has on the environment. Finally, all nurses are in a position to raise awareness of environmental issues that affect the health and well-being of their clients (Box 22.3). Nurses have the capacity to participate and even to lead in the needed efforts to address environmental issues; the change in smoking practices in Canada over the past 20 years is an informative exemplar of overcoming what once seemed to be insurmountable barriers to change.

BOX 22.2 Why Are Environmental Health Issues Important to Nurses?

Nurses in all settings should be well prepared to identify and assess potential environmental health issues related to workplaces, neighborhoods, houses, and schools.

Given that environmental health is a rapidly evolving field, nurses should know where to go to find current and credible scientific information.

Nurses are considered to be trusted sources of information regarding environmental health risks. As such, they are often in a position to translate information from other experts in fields such as toxicology and epidemiology.

Nurses are often in a position to identify environmental health issues because they may recognize patterns of symptoms in people who live or work in the same areas. Nurses should be prepared to investigate and act when they see such patterns.

Source: Canadian Nurses Association. (2005). *The ecosystem, the natural environment, and health and nursing: A summary of the issues* (p. 5).

BOX 22.3 What Can Nurses Do about Environmental Health Issues?

Primary Prevention

- Counsel women of childbearing age about reducing their exposure to environmental hazards.
- Support the development of exposure standards for toxins and other contaminants.
- Advocate for safe air and water.
- Teach avoidance of ultraviolet exposure and use of sunscreen.
- Support programs for waste reduction and recycling as well as energy conservation in your community and workplace.

Secondary Prevention

- Assess homes, schools, worksites, and communities for environmental hazards.
- Screen children under 5 years of age for blood lead levels.

Tertiary Prevention

- Support cleanup of toxic waste sites and removal of other hazards.
- Refer homeowners to approved programs that eliminate contaminants, such as lead and asbestos.

Source: Canadian Nurses Association. (2005). *The ecosystem, the natural environment, and health and nursing: A summary of the issues* (p. 6).

SUMMARY

Water safety, air purity or pollution, chemical spills and spread, the growing contamination of inside environments, and violent surroundings are serious environmental concerns across Canada, as is the relationship of the environment to the health of individuals, families, and populations whether in the home, community, or workplace. The information in this chapter represents a snippet of the volumes of literature available on the topic. Box 22.4. provides some strategies that nurses can use in reducing waste.

BOX 22.4 Nursing Strategies for Reducing Waste

- Introducing recycling programs for hospital waste, 45% of which may be paper
- Supporting the purchase of re-usable linens in hospital and clinic settings
- Lobbying and supporting suppliers willing to reduce packaging
- Ensuring that only material needing incineration goes to the medical incinerator by educating staff and making waste receptacles available and accessible
- Working with other members of hospital staff to purchase healthcare products that do not contain toxic substances such as mercury, so they do not end up in the waste stream

Modified from Canadian Nurses Association. (2008). The role of nurses in greening the health system (p. 6).

Add to your knowledge of this issue:	
Canadian Nurses Association	www.cna-nurses.ca/cna
Canadian Association of Physicians for the Environment	www.cape.ca
Environment Canada	www.ec.gc.ca
Canadian Cancer Society	www.cancer.ca
International Council of Nurses	www.icn.ch
International Development Research Centre	www.idrc.ca/ecohealth/indicators
Canadian Health Networks Web sites for Environmental Health, Workplace Health	www.canadian-health-network.ca
Pollution Probe	www.pollutionprobe.org
Physicians for Social Responsibility	www.psr.org
Canada Health Portal	www.chp-pcs.gc.ca
World Health Organization	www.who.int/peh
Worldwatch Institute	worldwatch.org

Online

REFLECTIONS on the Chapter...

1. Cite specific examples from courses in your nursing program that link health and environmental conditions.

2. Name three health issues related to environmental factors that have been in the news recently in your local region and in your province or territory. Were nurses evident in the discussions?

3. What evidence is there that global climate change will affect the health of individuals and communities across the globe?

4 What legislation has your provincial and territorial government or the federal government passed in the last year regarding pollution and contamination in the environment?

5 What types of medical waste might have an impact on the environment? What is the potential for contamination or pollution to occur from medical waste? Where and how might this contamination or pollution happen?

References

Ahluwalia, R. (2000, May). *Ontario's rural heartland in shock* [Television broadcast]. CBC TV News. Toronto.

Berlinguer, G. (1999). Globalization and global health. *International Journal of Health Services, 29*(3), 579–595.

Brown, L., Flavin, C., & French, H., et al. (2001). *State of the world 2001*. New York: W.W. Norton.

Canadian Nurses Association. (2000). *The environment is a determinant of health: Position statement* [Online]. Retrieved from http://www.cna-nurses.ca.

_____. (2005). *The ecosystem, the natural environment, and health and nursing: A summary of the issues.* Ottawa: Author.

_____. (2008a). *The environment and health: An introduction for nurses.* Ottawa: Author.

_____. (2008b). *The role of nurses in greening the health system.* Ottawa: Author.

_____. (2008c). *The code of ethics for registered nurses* (2008 centennial edition). Ottawa, Author.

_____. (2008d). *Nursing and environmental health.* Retrieved July 29, 2008 from www.cna-aiic.ca/CNA/issues/environment/default_e.aspx.

_____. (2008e). *Nursing and environmental health.* Retrieved July 29, 2008 from www.cna-aiic.ca/CNA/issues/environment.

Canadian Nurses Association/Canadian Medical Association. (1996). *Joint CNA/CMA position statement on environmentally responsible activity in the health sector* (pp. 1–6). Ottawa: Author.

Carruth, A.K., Gilbert, K., & Lewis, B. (1997). Environmental health hazards: The impact on a Southern community. *Public Health Nursing, 14*(5), 259–267.

Chaudhuri, N. (1998). Child health, poverty and the environment: The Canadian context. *Canadian Journal of Public Health, 89*(Suppl. 1), S26–S30.

Clark, M.J. (1999). *Nursing in the community: Dimensions of community health nursing* (3rd ed.). Stamford, CT: Appleton & Lange.

Eigsti-Gerber, D. & McGuire, S.L. (1999). Teaching students about nursing and the environment. Part 1: Nursing role and basic curricula. *Journal of Community Health Nursing, 16*(2), 69–79.

Environment Canada. (2000). *Clean air* [Online]. Retrieved April 14, 2005 from www.ec.gc.ca/air/introduction_c.html.

Foley, D. (2001, May). *Fuelling the climate crisis: The continental energy plan.* Vancouver: David Suzuki Foundation.

Health Canada. (1997). *Health and environment: Partners for life* (Cat. H49-112-1/1997E). Minister of Public Works and Government Services Ottawa Canada.

_____. (1998). *The health and environment handbook for health professionals* (Cat. No. H46-2/98-211-2E). Minister of Public Works and Government Services, Ottawa, Canada.

_____. (1999a). *A second diagnostic on the health of First Nations and Inuit people in Canada* [Online]. Retrieved from http:www.hc-sc.gc.ca/fnihb/cp/publications/second-diagnostic_fni.htm.

_____. (1999b). *Toward a healthy future: Second report on the health of Canadians* (Cat H39-468/1999E). Minister of Public Works and Government Services, Ottawa, Canada.

_____. (2007). *Mercury and health.* Retrieved August 1, 2008 from www.hc-sc.gc.ca/ewh-semt/pubs/contaminants/mercury.

_____. (2008). *Canadian drinking water guidelines.* Retrieved August 1, 2008 from www.hc-sc.gc.ca/ewh-semt/water-eau/drink-potab/guide.

Hilfinger Messias, D.K. (2001). Globalization, nursing, and health for all. *Journal of Nursing Scholarship, 33*(1), 8–11.

Institute of Medicine Committee on Enhancing Environmental Health Content in Nursing Practice. (1995). *Nursing, health, & the environment.* Washington, DC: National Academy Press.

Last, J., Trouton, K., & Pengally, D. (1998). Taking our breath away: The health effects of air pollution and climate change. Retrieved from http://www.davidsuzuki.org.

MacKinnon, M. (2001, July 18). Vital to improve water quality on reserves, group says. *The Globe and Mail,* p. A5.

Malcolm, J., Liu, C., & Miller, L., et al. (2002). *Habitats at risk: Global warming and species loss in globally significant terrestrial ecosystems.* Gland, Switzerland: World Wide Fund for Nature.

McDevitt, J. & Wilbur, J. (2002). Locating sources of data. In N. Ervin (Ed.), *Advanced community health nursing practice* (pp. 109–148). Upper Saddle River, NJ: Prentice Hall.

McGuire, S.L. & Eigsti-Gerber, D. (1999). Teaching students about nursing and the environment. Part 2: Legislation and resources. *Journal of Community Health Nursing, 16*(2), 81–94.

Mitchell, A. (2001, June 4). The world's "single biggest threat." *The Globe and Mail.*

Nightingale, F. (1860). *Notes on nursing: What it is and what it is not.* (Reprinted London: J.B. Lippincott Company. 1992: Philadelphia)

Ottawa Charter for Health Promotion. (1986). *First international conference on health promotion.* Ottawa. Retrieved April 14, 2005 from http://www.ldb.org/inhpe/ottawa.htm.

Physicians for Social Responsibility. (1994). *What you should know about* avoidable *risks of birth defects and other reproductive disorders.* Retrieved April 14, 2005 from http://www. envirohealthaction.org/upload_files/ NEWBirthBro.pdf.

_____. (1997). *Asthma and the role of air pollution: What the primary care physician should know* [Online]. Retrieved from http://www.envirohealthaction.org/upload_files/asthmap01.pdf.

_____. (2001a). *Arsenic: What health care providers should know* [Online]. Retrieved from http://www. envirohealthaction.org/upload_files/arsenicfs.pdf.

_____. (2001b). *Cryptosporidium: What health care providers should know* [Online]. Retrieved from http://www. envirohealthaction.org/upload_ files/cryptofs.pdf.

Pope, C.A., Burnett, R., & Thun, M., et al. (2002). Lung cancer, cardiopulmonary mortality, and long-term exposure to fine particulate air pollution. *Journal of the American Medical Association, 287*(9), 1132–1141.

Robson, M. & Schneider, D. (2001). Environmental health issues in rural communities. *Environmental Health, 63*(10), 16–20.

United Nations Environment Programme. (1999). *Global environment outlook GEO-2000* [Online]. Retrieved from http://www.unep.org/geo2000.

Wanke, M.I. & Saunders, D. (1996). Survey of local environmental health programs in Alberta. *Canadian Journal of Public Health, 87*(5), 345–350.

World Health Organization. (2007). *Climate and health fact sheet.* Retrieved August 1, 2008 from www.who.int/ mediacenter/factsheets/fs266/en/index/html.

World Health Organization/United Nations Children's Fund. (2008) *Report on special focus on drinking water and sanitation.* Retrieved August 1, 2008 from www.who.int/water_sanitation-health/monitoring/jmp2008/en/index.html.

chapter 23

Interpersonal Violence and Abuse: Ending the Silence

Colleen Varcoe

With acknowledgment of Elizabeth Thomlinson who authored an earlier version of this chapter.

Critical Questions

As a way of engaging with the ideas in this chapter, consider the following:

1 What do you think might be the prevalence of violence or abuse in your own community?

2 How do you think most people understand the causes of violence or abuse and who is held responsible based on that understanding?

3 Consider the actions of professionals that might silence the disclosure or reporting of experiences of violence or abuse.

4 Think of some reasons why professionals might be reluctant to address violence or abuse.

Chapter Objectives

After completing this chapter, you should be able to:

1 Understand the complex relationships among the many forms of violence and abuse.

2 Analyze political, legal, and ethical factors related to violence and abuse.

3 Relate the effects of violence and abuse to the health of individuals.

4 Evaluate the impact of violence and abuse on society, including the healthcare system.

5 Examine factors that contribute to the continued silencing of victims of violence and abuse.

6 Differentiate facilitators and barriers to resolution of various issues and generate strategies to address violence and abuse.

This poem is reproduced with permission from Mabel Cook, a member of Mosakahiken Cree Nation, who has spent many years working to prevent abuse and violence within Aboriginal communities. Her primary focus has been the youth of the communities. She has been a magistrate and currently is a community mediator in northern Manitoba.

Waiting to Be Seen and Heard

There are so many of us that cry out in agony
To no-one in particular because nobody cares to hear
People pass us by and never look beyond our exterior
Our bodies grow simply because it's the cycle of life.
When you look at us with contempt and mistrust
We feel that all you see is potential problems
Of young people not knowing how to be responsible
For you think we solve life's problems with violence.
Has it ever occurred to you to ask me how I feel?
We cry in vain in hopes that you will actually see
See the chaotic mess we strive to untangle
Trying to understand why you chose to hurt us.
Why don't you look deep within our very being
To find small defenseless children cowering in fear
Our growth was stunted because of a violent episode
One we did not ask for but received anyway.
You talk about us so negatively because we react in anger
Anger because we cannot tell anyone of our secret
Anyone who can take us on a journey of healing
Anyone who wishes to make us understand this cruelty.
You shattered what faith we had in humanity
For now we have built a wall around us where we cower
Cowering in fear wondering when you will come for us
To shatter our already battered and imprisoned spirit.
You have done much work on compiling information about us
Information that makes for good reading but does very little
We need you to take it to people who want to fight for us
Even the government sends men to war to kill others for freedom.
What about us? We are being killed Spiritually, Emotionally
Physically, Mentally, Sexually, and it is a slow death
We feel every fiber of our soul quivering in pain wanting freedom
Wondering who will see and hear to finally end this abuse.

— Mabel V. Cook

Interpersonal violence is a social problem of epidemic proportions around the world. Since the late 1970s, there has been a growing recognition that interpersonal violence and abuse have a significant impact on the health of individuals specifically and on Canadian society in general, including the healthcare system.

Violence consists of exerting power over another person to control, disempower, or injure the other. As a social act, violence crosses legal, ethical, and healthcare boundaries with serious moral, sociocultural, political, and personal ramifications for society (Hoff, 1994). Violence is perpetrated against people of all ages, in every socioeconomic sector of society, and in all societies around the globe. However, violence is deeply gendered, and is perpetrated along various axes of power. Violence is enmeshed with sexism, racism, ableism, and homophobia. Women, young people, elderly people, people from racialized groups, and people with disabilities are often among the most vulnerable. The long-term negative effects of violence have enormous implications for the victims as well as for all facets of society.

Discussion of violence is an everyday occurrence in the media. Although Canadian culture officially condemns violence, it is often glorified in film, television, books, and music. The long-held myth that the family is a safe haven for all of its members has been dispelled through frequent accounts highlighting the magnitude of the violence and abuse within that setting. In the workplace, there are ever-increasing numbers of stories of violent occurrences leading to injury and even death.

It is not possible in one chapter to present in-depth coverage of this complex topic. Rather, this chapter highlights some forms of violence, the association with the health of individuals, and the role nurses and the nursing profession can and should take to address issues of violence and abuse. There is a vast array of multidisciplinary sources of information, including print, film, and audio, on the topic of violence. This chapter is meant to stimulate a rudimentary recognition of the topic, and readers are encouraged to expand their knowledge and understanding through the numerous other sources that are available. To begin, definitions of the multiple forms of violence and abuse are presented in Box 23.1.

 ## THE MANY FORMS OF INTERPERSONAL VIOLENCE

Interpersonal violence encompasses much more than single physical acts of violence. First, such acts rarely occur without other forms of violation. Second, very harmful abuse can be perpetrated without any physical violence. Third, interpersonal violence and abuse usually occurs as part of a pattern of relating. The word *violence* is derived from the Latin infinitive *violare*, to violate, rape, or injure. Violation of another person may result not only in visible physical harm but also in emotional trauma that may be at least as harmful as physical battering and have more long-lasting effects. Within this chapter, the terms *violence* and *abuse* are used interchangeably, although abuse may not entail physical trauma.

- *Interpersonal violence* includes violence that occurs within relationships as well as that experienced from strangers and acquaintances. All types of violence are encompassed by this term, including violence against children, women, and elders; abuse of spouses or partners; violence within the context of dating; violence witnessed by children; and abuse and neglect of frail and vulnerable persons. Abuse may also be perpetrated by professionals. While violence associated with state violence (for example, war) is not the focus of this chapter, it is important to recognize that such violence is also interpersonal. Health professionals provide care to many people who have experienced such violence (veterans, refugees, immigrants).

- *Violence in relationships* of kinship, intimacy, dependency, or trust can take the form of physical assault, emotional abuse, intimidation, sexual assault, neglect, deprivation, and financial exploitation. Violence in relationships is commonly referred to as intimate partner violence (IPV).

BOX 23.1 Forms of Violence and Abuse

Physical
Slapping, kicking, hitting with a fist, beating, choking, shoving
Using a weapon against another
Forcibly restraining, confining, or kidnapping another

Sexual
Forcing another to perform sexual acts, e.g., fellatio
Forcing another to have sexual intercourse

Psychological
Name calling, humiliating another, verbally degrading another
Harming property or pets
Creating an atmosphere of fear and terror
Using threats and coercion
Witnessing assault or abuse of another (parent, grandparent, sibling, friend, etc.)
Infantilization

Financial
Taking or withholding money
Extorting funds or property
Taking control of all expenditures
Forcing another to stop working and become dependent
Selling the home or possessions of elderly people without their consent

Social
Imposing (forced) isolation from friends and other family
Monitoring all phone calls and connection with others

Physical Neglect
Failing to provide food, clothing, shelter, or medical care
Failing to supervise children or elders appropriately

The multiple definitions of violence and abuse influence how we view violence and where we place emphasis. Terms such as *family violence, domestic abuse, interpersonal violence,* and *violence in relationships* tend to downplay the gender relationships in violence and phrase the behavior in gender-neutral language. Holly Johnson, the primary researcher focused on violence at Statistics Canada notes that "Men's and boys' experiences of violence are different than women's and girls' in important ways. While men are more likely to be injured by strangers in a public or social venue, women are in greater danger of experiencing violence from intimate partners in their own homes. Women are also at greater risk of sexual violence" (Johnson 2006, p. 1). According to the 2004 Canadian General Social Survey (GSS) in the years between 1995 and 2004, males perpetrated 86% of one-time incidents, 94% of repeat (two to four) incidents, and 97% of chronic incidents of spousal violence (Statistics Canada, 2006). In Canada and globally, most perpetrators of violence in families are heterosexual males, and the victims of the most violent crimes are women and children (Bunge & Locke, 2000; Johnson, 2006; Statistics Canada, 2006; World Health Organization, 2002). Terms such as *family violence* locate abuse within the family, and draw attention away from society's influence and effects. Nurses must be aware of how the terminology used affects the perceptions of professionals and society at large. Using language that downplays gender relationships and societal influences emphasizes the responsibility of individuals and victims over the responsibility of society.

HISTORICAL PERSPECTIVES ON VIOLENCE AND ABUSE

The abuse of children and of female partners has deep historical roots. Even today, abuse is condoned within many societies in the world. Throughout history, children have been sacrificed to appease the gods, killed if they suffered handicapping conditions, and beaten and tortured to "rid them of demons" or to educate them (Humphreys & Ramsey, 1993). It was only in 1962 that Dr. Henry Kempe coined the term *battered child syndrome* (Helfer & Kempe, 1968), which was the impetus for educational campaigns and increased efforts in America and Canada to protect children from violence and abuse.

Humphreys and Ramsey (1993) noted that it was the interaction of several factors that focused societal attention and helped raise public concern regarding child abuse. They suggested that the public was affected by the violence in Southeast Asia, namely the Vietnamese conflict, and the rising homicide rates in the United States. Other factors that heightened public awareness of violence were the women's movement and the interest demonstrated by social scientists studying the phenomenon. The combination of these variables led to multiple studies on violence and abuse, with resultant books and articles on the topic. Social agencies were formed, the Society for the Prevention of Child Abuse and Neglect was developed, and laws mandating the prevention of the abuse and neglect of children were updated. In Canada, child abuse and exploitation are prohibited by the Criminal Code (Department of Justice Canada, 2007). Most provinces and territories have legislation that makes the reporting of child abuse by the public, including health professionals, mandatory. "Child Welfare in Canada 2000" (Human Resources and Child Welfare Canada, 2000) outlines the roles and responsibilities of provincial and territorial child welfare authorities in the provision of child protection and preventive and support services. If you are working with children, you should review the specific requirements for the jurisdiction in which you are working.

Equally, the abuse of female partners has deep historical roots. Within Christianity, the Bible provides "the earliest prescription for physical punishment of wives" (Campbell & Fishwick, 1993, p. 73). According to these authors, documentation of wife beating can be found throughout European literature—women accused of adultery could be killed with impunity, and instructions for "correcting" wives by beating were available. While violence against women remains a significant problem around the world, the World Health Organization's (WHO's) "World Report on Violence and Health" (2002, 2005) found that rates varied considerably among different countries, and describes violence against women as both a manifestation and cause of gender inequity, emphasizing the importance of economic inequity. The WHO Summary Report (2005) notes that risk factors for violence against women related to the immediate social context "included the degree of economic inequality between men and women, levels of female mobility and autonomy, attitudes towards gender roles and violence against women, the extent to which extended family, neighbours, and friends intervene in domestic violence incidents, levels of male-male aggression and crime, and some measure of social capital" (p. 4). While forms of violence against women may have culturally specific features, such as "dowry deaths" in India, the use of wood axes to kill women in Canada, or the stoning of women in some countries, it is important to remember that these are manifestations of gender inequality.

The prevalence of elder abuse only began to be recognized in the 1970s with initial efforts to "identify the kind and extent of abuse and neglect of seniors" (MacLean & Williams, 1995, p. xi). The Manitoba Association on Gerontology was the first provincial association to begin addressing this subject by developing guidelines to identify elder abuse and protocols for practice (Interdepartmental Working Group on Elder Abuse and Manitoba Seniors Directorate, 1993). In Canada, Elizabeth

Podnieks, a nurse, provided early leadership in the study of elder abuse (Podnieks, 1985; Podnieks & Baillie, 1995; Podnieks et al., 1990). The national prevalence study that she undertook emphasized the scope of elder abuse in Canada and laid the groundwork for further research and intervention efforts.

Increasingly, violence and abuse are seen from an intersectional persepective that moves beyond a gender-only analsysis to take into account how class, racialization, colonization, heterosexism, homophobia, and other forms of inequity shape the extent and impact of violence and have particular effects for groups such as Aboriginal women, immigrant and refugee women, women of colour, people with disabilities, gay men, and lesbians. Hankivsky and Varcoe (2007) argue that an intersectional perpective:

- shifts from individual to social explanations of violence
- shifts away from assigning blame and responsibility to victims of violence
- turns attention to structural inequalities as causing and perpetuating violence
- focuses on the importance of social policy in reducing and ending violence.

An intersectional perspective on violence is used throughout the remainder of this chapter.

STATISTICS IN THE CANADIAN CONTEXT

Multiple factors contribute to the underreporting of violence and abuse. Widespread ideologies about the causes of violence ("don't some women just ask for it?") and personal responsibility ("why doesn't she just leave?") contribute to misunderstandings and silencing. Shame on the part of the victim and the perpetrator, dependency of the victim on the perpetrator, ignorance of resources, fear of repercussions, and an inability to seek help because of forced restraint all contribute to a code of silence. Judgmental, blameful, incredulous, and other unhelpful or inappropriate responses by potential helpers, including friends, family, and professionals, further such silencing (e.g., Cooper et al., 2004; Lempert, 1997; Tower, 2007). For women living in rural and remote regions of the country, distance and a lack of resources hinder attempts to escape abusive relationships (Biesenthal, Sproule & Plocica, 1997), factors that are compounded for Aboriginal women by racialized discriminatory policies and practices (Varcoe & Dick, 2008). This remoteness helps keep the true number of incidents of violence concealed. These factors compound the difficulties for young people, elderly people, people with disabilities, and immigrants and other women who may not know where to seek help, may not have the physical means to do so, and may fear and encounter judgment and other inappropriate responses.

The study of violence is hampered by the same factors that lead to underreporting and is also hampered by the way violence is measured and such data is collected. To date, the most comprehensive national study of violence against women remains the 1993 Violence Against Women (VAWS) study, conducted by Statistics Canada and analyzed by numerous researchers (e.g., Johnson, 1996; Kaukinen, 2002). The study used a large random sample and made special efforts to ensure safety so that a range of women could respond. Findings from this study indicated that 29% of women had experienced at least one episode of violence and that two thirds of these women reported that it had happened more than once. Since that time, Statistics Canada primarily has relied upon modules within the Canadian GSS to obtain data on violence (Johnson, 2006). This data is collected within a more general survey, and does not employ the same safeguards. Johnson notes that because the VAWS was a dedicated survey it focused exclusively on matters relating to violence against women and employed only female interviewers. The 1999 and 2004 GSSs, on the other hand, are general victimization surveys with a special module of questions based on the VAWS related to spousal violence. The GSS employs both male and female interviewers, although respondents are offered the opportunity to switch to an interviewer of the other sex if they are uncomfortable responding to sensitive questions during the interview. As a result of these methodological differences, comparisons between the two surveys must be made with caution. Seven percent of women who were living in a common-law or marital relationship reported to the 2004 GSS that they had been physically or sexually assaulted by a spousal partner at least once during the previous five years, which is a small but statistically significant drop from 8% in 1999, and a decline from the 12% reported in the 1993 VAWS.

Violence Against Women

Criticisms regarding the use of the terms *spousal abuse, conjugal violence, partner violence,* and *domestic abuse* center on the implication that the abuse that women direct against male partners is equal, in nature and degree, to that committed by men against female partners (Campbell & Fishwick, 1993). There remains a consensus in the statistics on violence and abuse that women continue to suffer the most severe, repetitive, protracted forms of abuse, often resulting in injury and requiring medical attention (Bunge & Locke, 2000; Dobash & Dobash, 1979; Statistics Canada, 2006). There is also concurrence in the research that female-to-male violence results from acts of self-defense (DeKerseredy & Kelly, 1993). This is consistent with the fact that in Canada men reported far greater incidents of hitting, kicking, biting, and having objects thrown at them than did women (Bunge & Locke, 2000; Johnson, 2006). The concerns regarding the impact of terminology in focusing attention away from the reality of who constitutes the majority of abusers must be kept at the forefront while reading the following statistics.

Findings of the 2004 GSS suggest that, within the previous 5 years, 7% of people who were married or in common-law relationships experienced some form of violence from their intimate partners, with the rates for women and men being similar. However, both the report "Family Violence in Canada: A Statistical Profile 2000" and the more recent "Family Violence in Canada: A Statistical Profile 2006," continue to emphasize that the most severe and consistent forms of violence were reported by women. In general, women are more frequently subjected to severe forms of violence from men than men are from women. For example, Statistics Canada (2005) reported that of 78 spouses killed in Canada in 2004, 62 were women killed by male spouses. In 2004, twice as many women than men were beaten by their partners; four times as many were choked; and twice as many female as male victims of spousal assault reported chronic, ongoing assaults (10 or more). In 2000, women made up the vast majority of victims of sexual assault (86%) and other types of sexual offences (78%) (Statistics Canada, 2001). While 23% of women who report being sexually assaulted are assaulted by strangers (Matas, 2001), based on anonymous surveys, it has been estimated that as many as 90% of sexual assaults are never reported.

Violence in Gay and Lesbian Relationships

Until recent decades, there have been relatively few studies of violence in gay and lesbian relationships. Ristock (2001) conducted a multisite qualitative study of violence experienced in lesbian relationships. Service providers (counselors, shelter workers, and social workers) who participated in focus groups noted that basing their efforts on heterosexual dynamics limited their practice. Ristock highlighted that some concerns were raised—chief among them that drawing attention to violence in lesbian relationships will detract from feminist efforts to raise awareness that violence perpetrated by men continues to be a significant social issue.

Although the focus on gender-based violence is challenged by the reporting of same-sex violence, these reports emphasize the need for the further examination of power and control as key factors in violence and abuse. Key questions that may be asked are, "where is power held within a society?" and "what is the relationship between gender and power?" Of importance in this discussion is the relationship to the social context in which this violence occurs. Victims of same-sex violence may fear being stigmatized as gay or lesbian and may expect their complaints to be trivialized (Duffy & Momirov, 2000). In a society that remains largely homophobic, the dynamics of violence within same-sex relationships are even more complex than those of opposite-sex relationships. This complexity will continue to contribute to the silencing of the issues in violent and abusive same-sex relationships.

Abuse and Neglect of Older Canadians

Elder abuse and neglect encompasses IPV that continues into older adulthood and forms of abuse and neglect that arise as persons become more vulnerable with age. As with any form of IPV, IPV in older adults is gendered—that is, older women are at higher risk than men. One of the leading studies on the abuse and neglect of older Canadians found that 4% of respondents reported financial, material, and verbal abuse by family members and other people (Podnieks et al., 1990). Ten years later, 7% of older adults in the GSS reported experiencing emotional abuse in the form of name calling, being put down, being isolated from friends and family, or being taken advantage of financially by a spouse, caregiver, or child (Bunge & Locke, 2000). One must keep in mind that older people may be reluctant or afraid to report abuse by family members for various reasons, among them dependency, feelings of shame, and fear of retaliation.

Elder abuse and neglect includes violence in the home, violence in institutions, and self-neglect (McDonald & Collins, 2000). Older adults who become frail and require medical or other health-related services may experience abuse. In this context, abuse of older adults may involve failing to facilitate their access to medical or health services, failing to provide medical attention due to age, or conducting a procedure or providing treatment without the informed consent of the patient or their recognized substitute. Although age can increase vulnerability, it is important to note that other factors such as economic dependence; disabilities, such as developmental, mental, and physical; and rural isolation also increase vulnerability to violence, intersecting with age and gender. Importantly, as elder care is increasingly shifted to family care providers, nurses must consider how their expectations for family caregiving might contribute to conditions that give rise to abuse.

Little research has been undertaken on the violence and abuse of elderly people living in institutions. Anecdotal and case study reports have been the source of information on abuse within residential care settings. Overt acts of physical abuse included extensive use of restraints as well as hitting, pinching, and shoving (Wiehe, 1998). Limiting freedom and choice, providing inadequate nutrition, and isolating people were among the more covert acts of abuse. In these cases, it was people who had responsibility for the care of the residents—the people who were in power—who commonly were the abusers.

In police-reported statistics of elder abuse, most offenders are strangers and people outside the family. According to statistics from the "Incident-Based Uniform Crime Reporting Survey," older Canadians were 67% more likely to be abused by strangers than by family members (Bunge & Locke, 2000). Although the numbers are relatively small, people who deliberately target elderly people in home invasions and fraud figure prominently in the media.

Violence Against Children and Youth

Child maltreatment is an all-encompassing term that includes the physical, sexual, and emotional abuse and neglect of children. Although child maltreatment is recognized as a significant problem in Canada, no data set consolidates all of the provincial statistics to present a comprehensive national picture. Data on cases of child maltreatment are based on child welfare caseloads, police files on assault and homicide, and hospitalizations for violence-related injuries (Bunge & Locke, 2000). Child welfare is a provincial responsibility, and, although each province has legislation defining child abuse and neglect, a lack of common definitions across jurisdictions precludes the formation of a single national data set.

Understandings of child abuse often focus on the problem as though it occurs in isolation from other forms of abuse and wider social conditions, and often focus on severe forms of physical abuse or more sensational incidents of sexual abuse, rather than on the more common forms of child maltreatment—neglect and emotional abuse. It is important to note that child abuse often overlaps with IPV against women with estimates that children are abused in up to 70% of families in which women are abused (Edleson, 1999; Folsom et al., 2003). It is also important to note that perceptions of what constitutes abuse shift over time and are shaped by changing class and social attitudes. For example, in many Canadian jurisdictions, children who witness violence (usually against their mothers) are considered to be abused, and in such cases fear of child apprehension by the state may be a barrier to women seeking help in relation to abuse. Finally, it is critical to note that there is a high rate of unsubstantiated reports of child abuse.

Estimates of child abuse are difficult to make because they largely rely on *reported* cases. Based on data from child welfare authorities, the "Canadian Incidence Study of Reported Child Abuse and Neglect" estimated that there were 135,573 child maltreatment investigations in Canada in 1998. This was a rate of 21.52 investigations of child maltreatment per 1,000 children. Forty-five percent of these investigations were substantiated; 22% remained suspected; and 33% were found to be unsubstantiated (Public Health Agency of Canada, 2001). The greatest proportion of both reported and substantiated child abuse cases were of neglect. This report suggests that insufficient attention has been paid to neglect in comparison with the attention to risk assessment and urgent intervention for severe physical abuse and in comparison to sexual abuse, possibly in part because it is more sensational (McLean, 2001). Trocmé et al. (2003) argue that because 96% of substantiated cases did not involve severe physical harm, assessment and investigation priorities need to be revised and include consideration of long-term services needs. Importantly, socioeconomic status has been consistently shown to be related to parenting effectiveness (Wekerle et al., 2007), also suggesting that assessment for longer-term, broader social support is required.

Although there are mandatory reporting laws for child abuse, it is accepted that official accounts of child maltreatment underestimate the prevalence because of the failure to report by perpetrators and victims, by community members who observe abuse, and by professionals who fail to recognize the maltreatment (MacMillan et al., 1997). It is thought that as many as 90% of cases are not reported to child welfare authorities (MacMillan et al., 1997). At issue is why, with mandatory reporting laws for child abuse and neglect, underreporting persists. A question for professionals and for society is why and how this silence regarding a significant social and health problem continues.

Children and youth represented 60% of sexual assault victims and 20% of physical assault victims reported in Canada in 1999 (Bunge & Locke, 2000). Acquaintances were the primary abusers (52%), with the remaining perpetrators being family members (24%) and strangers (19%). Girls were victimized more often than boys in 80% of sexual assault cases and 53% of physical assault cases.

Violence in Aboriginal Communities

Violence in Aboriginal communities must be understood in the context of historical and ongoing colonization of Aboriginal people in Canada. Aboriginal people in Canada have been systematically stripped of their lands, ways of living, culture, language, and freedoms, with extensive effects on their health and well-being. These colonizing practices and the system of confining Aboriginal people to reserves and requiring children to attend residential school has had extensive long-term effects (Adelson, 2005; Smith, Varcoe, & Edwards, 2005). Aboriginal people face ongoing discrimination and racialization, including in their experiences of healthcare (Bourassa, McKay-McNabb, & Hampton, 2004; Browne, 2007; Fiske & Browne, 2006). Aboriginal women have been particularly disadvantaged through gender-biased policies and face disproportionate socioeconomic burdens—such as poverty and isolation—that magnify the difficulties they face in dealing with violence (Dion Stout, 1998; MacMillan, MacMillan, & Offord et al., 1996).

High rates of violence experienced by Aboriginal people generally, and women and children particularly, and social responses to their experiences of violence are shaped by these colonizing processes (Brownridge, 2003; Statistics Canada, 2006). According to Statistics Canada, 24% of Aboriginal women experienced spousal abuse in the 5 years preceeding the 2004 GSS, compared with 7% of women in the general population. Aboriginal women in Canada are eight times more likely than non-Aboriginal women to be killed by their partners and experience more severe IPV than the rest of the population (Statistics Canada, 2006). Aboriginal children are much more likely to be investigated for maltreatment, and investigations are more likely to be substantiated, more likely to be kept open for ongoing services, and more likely to result in children being placed in out-of-home care (Blackstock, Trocmé, & Bennett, 2004).

While all victims of violence face possible judgment, disbelief, and discrimination, Aboriginal people in particular can anticipate such responses, responses that operate as barriers to help. In one community survey, 63% of respondents reported they had experienced violence and abuse, whereas 76% were aware that family members had been abused (Thomlinson, Erickson, & Cook, 2000). However, only 37% disclosed that violence to people in authority. Fear of repercussions and a lack of trust that reporting would introduce a change contributed to this lack of reporting.

According to the "Report of the Royal Commission on Aboriginal Peoples," although it is impossible to ascertain the full extent of violence in Aboriginal communities, the topic is distinctive from other communities in that "[violence] has invaded whole communities and cannot be considered a problem of a particular couple or an individual household" (1996, p. 56). The interrelationship of poverty and social and economic marginalization of many Aboriginal communities is believed to contribute to an increase in violence and abuse (Hamby, 2000). Without efforts that will substantially change conditions in the community, attempts to address violence will continue to experience only minor success.

Dating Violence

As they do in other forms of violence, women suffer more severe, pervasive, and systematic victimization in dating relationships (Canadian Public Health Association, 1994) than do men. The "Department of Justice Canada's Fact Sheet" (2007b) on dating violence summarizes the few available studies and concludes that although it is difficult to know the prevalence with any accuracy, violence in dating relationships is common. According to a survey of college and university students, 45% of women had been sexually assaulted while in a dating relationship, 79% had been psychologically abused, and 35% had been physically abused (DeKerseredy & Kelly, 1993). DeKerseredy and Kelly caution that although this survey pointed to high percentages of dating violence, these statistics should be regarded as underestimates for reasons similar to those of other forms of violence and abuse.

Violence in the Workplace

Violence in the workplace, including sexual harassment, is also deeply gendered (Hinch & DeKeseredy, 1994). According to Mireille Kingma, nurse consultant with the International Council of Nurses, "72% of nurses do not feel safe from assault in their workplace," and "97% of nurse respondents in a British survey knew a nurse who had been physically assaulted in the past year and up to 95% reported having been bullied at work" (International Council of Nurses, 1999b). In the United States, Carroll and Morin (1998) reported that one third of nurses working in general areas were affected by workplace violence. In Sweden, Arnetz, Arnetz, and Soderman (1998) found that the incidence of violence toward practical nurses was 31 incidents per 100 person years. Poster (1996) found that 75% of 999 psychiatric nursing staff in Canada, the United States, the United Kingdom, and South Africa reported being assaulted at least once during their careers.

In Canada, the Canadian Public Health Association (1994) concluded that up to 70% of nurses have been abused or threatened on the job, including being hit, kicked, verbally abused, and sexually harassed. A survey of hospital nurses in British Columbia and Alberta found that 46% of those surveyed had experienced one or more types of violence in the last five shifts worked, including emotional abuse 38%, threat of assault 19%, physical assault 18%, verbal sexual harassment 7.6%, and sexual assault 0.6%. (Duncan et al., 2001).

One of the issues that is relevant to the safety of nurses and that ultimately affects the recruitment and retention of nurses in the workplace is the continued lack of reporting and tolerance of abuse against nurses. Of the 5,000 nurses who responded to a survey by the Manitoba Association of Registered Nurses (1989), between one fourth and one third noted that they chose to ignore abusive behavior directed toward them in the workplace. Factors affecting this decision are relevant to the analysis of this issue. More recently, Duncan et al. (2001) found that 70% of those who had experienced violence indicated they had not reported it.

 ## UNDERSTANDING VIOLENCE: THEORETICAL PERSPECTIVES

Since the 1970s, a number of theoretical approaches have been proposed in the attempt to understand factors related to the violence and abuse of people, mainly women and children (Campbell & Fishwick, 1993; Duffy & Momirov, 2000; Gelles, 1980; Hankivsky & Varcoe, 2007). Gelles classified three different types of models: the psychiatric or intraindividual model, the social-psychological model, and the sociologic model. The focus of assessments and interventions varies depending on the type of model to which one subscribes: individuals, individuals in context, or society at large. Beliefs and myths regarding violence and abuse that arise from the underlying theoretical framework will affect how one chooses to interact with individuals who are experiencing abusive situations.

From Inside the Individual

Intraindividual explanations tend to pathologize abusive men as psychopaths and female victims as masochists. Innes and associates (1991) noted that studies focusing on the mental health of men and women in abusive relationships demonstrated a bias against women by blaming the victims. Campbell and Fishwick (1993) contend that vestiges of the masochism myth remain today when authors suggest that a woman provoked a man to batter her. As early as 1979, Walker (1979) stated that by blaming the victims, men are ultimately excused of their abusive behaviors. Innes and associates (1991) further noted that men rarely demonstrate the same violent actions outside the home but confine their abuse to where they will avoid castigation, thus pointing to the importance of the social environment.

Environment and Interaction

The social-psychological model focuses on the interaction of the environment and the individual and the family. In child abuse cases, Helfer and Kempe hypothesized that an interaction occurs between the child, the caretaker, and the circumstance that predisposes toward violence (Helfer & Kempe 1968). Social learning theory (Bandura, 1969) is the basis for the suggestion that growing up in violent homes predisposes children toward violent behavior (Duffy & Momirov, 2000). This model has been used to explain the intergenerational transmission of violence in which the members of each generation of a family continues the violent and abusive behaviors that were perpetrated against them or that they observed against others in the family; however, the evidence for this theory is questionable (Ozturk Ertem, Leventhal, & Dobbs, 2000).

Tolerance of Violence

Sociologic models contend that violence and abuse occur in environments that tolerate, and even foster, violent actions. Garbarino's ecologic model of child abuse stresses the effect of the continued support of force in the care of children and multiple factors that affect the family (Garbarino, 1977;

Garbarino, 1995; Garbarino & Kostelny, 1992; Garbarino & Sherman, 1980). A key component of this model is the incorporation of societal beliefs and values along with other factors that affect the family, such as housing, poverty, social supports, and reactions of others in the family and community.

Feminist Perspective

Feminist analysis emphasizes the role of patriarchal culture in legitimizing male violence against both women and children (Duffy & Momirov, 2000). The power and control that men hold in the corporate world, in government, in religious institutions, and in society as a whole facilitate male use of power and control in the home (Wiehe, 1998). Violence and abuse ensure continued control over women and children. Feminist analysis has contributed to the exploration of violence through examination of how race, culture, disability, social class, age, and sexual orientation affect the experiences that women of all ages have in society. Duffy and Momirov (2000) suggest that inclusion of violence in lesbian relationships in this dialogue has forced feminists to focus more attention on the issues of power and control rather than remaining concentrated on gender-based relationships.

Intersectional Analysis

As outlined at the beginning of this chapter, an intersectional analysis (which is a sociological model) explicitly examines how multiple forms of oppression and privilege operate simultaneously to shape experiences of violence (Crenshaw, 1994; Mosher, 1998; Hankisky & Varcoe, 2007). This perspective overlaps with feminist perspectives, which often treat gender as the most salient aspect of social location. However, while gender is important, we are all shaped by the privileging and marginalizing processes of class, racialization, sexual orientation, ability, and so on. Taking larger societal variables, including historical and cultural perspectives, into account helps explain why certain groups of women (e.g., Aboriginal women, rural women, immigrant women, women of colour, women living with disabilities, and women living in poverty) face more violence and more barriers to social support in relation to violence. Prejudice, economic marginalization, and social powerlessness are key factors in the lives of both the abused and the abusers.

IMPACT ON HEALTH AND THE HEALTHCARE SYSTEM

Violence and abuse present formidable costs to the health of individuals and families and to society. The short- and long-term effects of violence on health are well established. IPV against women is associated with *direct effects* of physical injuries such as bruises and fractures (Muellman, Lenaghan, & Pakieser, 1996); *chronic physical health problems,* such as chronic pain, arthritis, frequent headaches and migraines, visual problems, unexplained dizziness and fainting, sexually transmitted infections, unwanted pregnancies, gynecological symptoms, hypertension, viral infections such as the flu, peptic ulcers, and functional or irritable bowel disease (Campbell & Lewandowski, 1997; Kendall-Tackett, Marshall, & Ness, 2003; Letourneau, Holmes, & Chasedunn-Roark, 1999; Wuest et al., 2007); and *mental health problems,* including clinical depression, acute and chronic symptoms of anxiety, serious sleep disturbances, symptoms consistent with post-traumatic stress syndrome (PTSD), substance use and dependence, and thoughts of suicide (Campbell, 2002; Cascardi, Daniel O'Leary, & Schlee, 1999; Eby, Campbell, & Sullivan et al., 1995; Fischbach & Herbert, 1997; Sleutel, 1998; Wiehe, 1998). These health effects lead to significant suffering for women and incur significant interference with their lives. For example, various sources estimate that abused women suffer losses of up to $7 million annually in wages and productivity (Duffy & Momirov, 2000).

Violence also incurs expenditures for the state, including the Canadian healthcare system, when victims seek medical care. Financial costs to police, child welfare and victim counseling services, the court system, social services, shelters, and foster-home care as well as costs incurred for imprisoning offenders, for second-stage housing, and the incalculable costs in human suffering, contribute to the impact of violence and abuse on individuals and society. Greaves, Hankivsky, and Kingston-Riechers (1995) used the Canadian Violence Against Women study to calculate the proportion of some costs attributable to violence in three forms of violence—sexual assault, violence in intimate partnerships, and incest and child sexual assault—and estimated 4.2 billion dollars spent in four policy areas—health and medicine, criminal justice, social services and education, and labour and employment. In 1996, Kerr and McLean estimated that the health costs in British Columbia were at least $385 million annually. Estimates have been made that more than 100,000 inpatient hospital days can be attributed to violence (Canadian Public Health Association, 1994). With hospital bed costs ranging from $400 to $800 a day, this would result in expenditures between $40 and $80 million annually in Canada as a result of violence.

Child maltreatment can lead to severe, long-term emotional and academic problems. Abused children have difficulty concentrating, have little anger control, may suffer from eating disorders, and are at high risk for dropping out of school (Wiehe, 1998). Koniak-Griffin and Lesser (1996) found that child maltreatment was a significant predictor of self-injurious behavior and attempted suicide. In Canada from 1997 to 1998, childhood admissions for acknowledged cases of assault and other maltreatment such as battering, rape, fighting, strangulation, firearms, and stabbings were 2,359 per 100,000 population (Bunge & Locke, 2000). A total of 38 in every 100,000 children under the age of 1 year were admitted to a hospital as a result of child abuse. Considering that many more cases of abuse are never reported or go unrecognized, these are significant numbers. The cost to the healthcare system and in lost human potential and suffering because of the maltreatment of children and youth is incalculable.

As noted previously, there is a growing awareness that even if they themselves are not abused, children who live in a home where mothers are battered and where violence between parents occurs experience PTSD (Humphreys, 1993). Behavioral responses of these children include truancy, disturbed sleep patterns, decreased school performance, lack of positive peer relations, increased worry for their mothers, and fear. Children who are exposed to violence and abuse learn that violence is the way to settle problems and achieve their own ends (Beauchesne et al., 1997). Pynoos and Nader (1990) examined four main types of symptoms experienced by children who have observed violent and abusive incidents: PTSD, grief reactions, separation anxiety symptoms, and exacerbation or renewal of previous symptoms. They found that exposure to violence may have long-term detrimental effects on a child's cognitive development.

ISSUES FOR NURSES AND THE NURSING PROFESSION

Nursing associations at all levels, provincially, nationally, and internationally, advocate that nurses take an active role in addressing problems of violence by increasing their knowledge of issues associated with violence and abuse (Alberta Association of Registered Nurses et al., 1999; American Nurses Association, 1994; Canadian Nurses Association, 1996). The associations advocate zero tolerance for interpersonal violence and violence in the workplace. What issues, then, should nurses be informed of and what information should they incorporate into their nursing practice?

Language

The use of gender-neutral language in discussing all types of interpersonal violence erroneously creates the impression that violence and abuse are committed equally by men and women in society. A careful examination of the statistics on the types and circumstances surrounding any violence and abuse provides a more comprehensive picture of what actually is occurring. Nurses, as professionals and as members of society, have a role to play in recognizing that the use of a particular language can obscure and slant perceptions of what really is happening in violent and abusive relationships. Further, language that labels (e.g., "battered women") reduces the person to their experience of violence. Hence, it is important to use language that acknowledges the person, not just the problem (e.g., "women who have been battered").

Lack of Understanding

A second issue arises from a lack of understanding about the pervasiveness of violence. Multiple myths about violence and abuse affect how healthcare professionals respond to and treat people involved in violent situations. One myth that continues to pervade society is that it is mainly people living in poverty who act violently toward others. Healthcare providers, then, do not consider that professionals and people from upper socioeconomic brackets could be victims or perpetrators of violence within their families. The effect of holding onto this perception is that poor people may be stereotyped as violent and the effects minimized as being part of the culture, whereas others receive little intervention because "[violence] cannot possibly be happening in that home." A related myth is the idea that people from certain racialized groups are inherently more violent. It is critical for nurses to recognize that it is mistaken to use population statistics, such as higher rates of violence experienced by Aboriginal women, to predict individual behaviours such as anticipating violence when caring for a particular Aboriginal person. For example, in one Canadian study, nurses acting on stereotypes and inappropriate application of population statistics tended to anticipate IPV among poor and racialized people and to anticipate child abuse in Aboriginal families (Varcoe, 2001).

Other Issues

Other issues that require analysis include the following:

- the persistent underreporting of child abuse cases
- the need for prevention and recognition of abuse of elders who live in their own homes or the homes of family members, not in institutions, especially as more families are expected to provide care
- the need for comprehensive approaches to interpersonal violence within healthcare settings
- the ongoing lack of reporting of violence against nurses in the workplace.

 ## BARRIERS TO RESOLUTION

The pervasiveness of abuse and violence through all ages, classes, cultures, and ethnicities and across genders and national and international political boundaries underlies and hampers efforts to address the issues surrounding the topic. This pervasiveness means that victims of violence, as well as the perpetrators, exist in all sectors of society, including the healthcare professions. The strong need to deny abuse, to keep silent, pervades society. This social and political reality counters efforts for change. The silence that has permitted and even encouraged violence and abuse is complex, not easily understood, and universal.

A key factor that reinforces the silencing of abuse is a societal belief in the sanctity of the family: what occurs within the walls of the home is private. A belief that parents and spouses are permitted to control what goes on in the family and to discipline family members is another component. Power differences based on age, gender, ability, ethnicity, class, geography, citizenship, langue, and sexual orientation that underlie society, as noted previously in the chapter, affect relationships at all levels. The perpetrators of abuse may be in positions of power in government, justice, and throughout the rest of society. Secrecy permits them to continue to abuse. Power in relationships such as nurse–patient interactions contributes to the opportunity for abuse to occur; there is sometimes little recognition given to the type and amount of power that health professionals hold over their patients. Indeed, failure to recognize and counter barriers to social support, such as using interpreters for those who cannot adequately communicate in the dominant language, recognizing the dynamics of economic dependence, and countering racial stereotypes, can directly contribute to the continuation of abuse.

Another element may be the helplessness that professionals may feel regarding their inability to understand and to intervene. It is easier not to ask questions about violence than to ask questions that might reveal an abusive relationship and not know how to interact and intervene. Professionals may subvert their assessments by the manner in which they ask questions regarding violence. Those who choose to speak out may be silenced by coworkers and others who wish to have the abuse and violence remain secret. The complex interactions that yield this ongoing silencing suggest that there may be no easy solutions.

 STRATEGIES FOR RESOLUTION

No one profession can successfully work toward ending the silence about abuse and violence in isolation from others. Developing partnerships with victims of violence will require a concerted effort by professionals to gain the confidence and trust that victims must achieve before alliances can be established. Although this is a time-consuming process, effective intervention programs can develop out of these alliances. To aid in developing understanding, interdisciplinary courses in the education setting are a beginning.

Interdisciplinary Education and Intervention

More than a decade after the federal government convened interdisciplinary consultations across the country to address violence and abuse, the persistent lack of interdisciplinary education programs and intervention protocols for health and social service professionals remains a key issue. This issue is particularly relevant to nurses because they are in key positions to advocate for patients, to educate others, to promote healthy relationships, to identify abuse and violence, and to intervene. To act, nurses must be knowledgeable about the topic; they must comprehend the level of education attained by the professionals with whom they work; and they must understand the roles that each has in addressing violence and abuse.

A curriculum guide for nurses was developed by Hoff and Ross (1993) and then followed by an interdisciplinary curriculum guide for healthcare professionals (Hoff, 1994). Although some education on violence and abuse has been incorporated into curricula of healthcare professionals, the need for interdisciplinary courses to aid in developing a comprehensive prevention and intervention program remains.

Victims of violence continue to report that healthcare professionals focus on the injuries that have been sustained, yet ignore any other aspects of the situation (Sleutel, 1998). Additionally, nurses and doctors acknowledged that they defer asking questions that may lead to disclosure of violence and abuse (Campbell & Fishwick, 1993). Moreover, victims have consistently reported that healthcare providers are judgmental, uncaring, and often the least helpful category of professionals to whom they have gone for assistance (American Academy of Nurses Expert Panel on Violence, 1993; Bacchus, Mezey, & Bewley, 2003; Gerbert, Abercrombie, & Caspers et al., 1999; McCloskey & Grigsby, 2005; Tower, 2007).

The Canadian Nurses Association's "Code of Ethics" (2002), the practice standards and expectations for nurses across the country, and the International Council of Nurses (1999a) have set guidelines for zero tolerance of violence and abuse. This unanimity across all levels of nursing highlights the importance given to the problem presented by the diverse types of violence. Other associations and organizations have also recommended the need for the education of healthcare professionals (MacLean & Williams, 1995; MacLeod, 1991; McCullough, 1994). Despite this convergence of opinion and the consensus that everyone has the right to a life free of violence and abuse, the development of interdisciplinary curricula has been slow.

Political Action

The societal and cultural issues underlying the reticence to deal with issues involving violence and abuse are key factors affecting the procrastination in developing joint curricula. The approach of healthcare professionals to focus on the short-term treatment of the signs and symptoms of violence places the onus on the individual to correct the problem and does not demand change within society. Compartmentalization and a focus on the physical effects of violence and abuse also, then, do not require that professionals accept responsibility to address the broader implications of abuse and violence.

Continued joint efforts of the professional associations at the national and provincial levels are needed for developing interdisciplinary curricula on abuse and violence. As with all other issues, there must be individuals within the various organizations who will advocate for these education programs. The efforts to lobby faculties of nursing, medicine, dentistry, physiotherapy, and occupational therapy must be undertaken by those who recognize and believe in the need to address this issue. An example of an organization that could be used in this lobby in western Canada is RESOLVE (Research and Education for Solutions to Violence and Abuse), an interdisciplinary community and academic organization working across Manitoba, Saskatchewan, and Alberta toward ending abuse and violence (http://www.umanitoba.ca/ resolve). Joint research and education organizations exist in other regions of the country (see Online Resources at the end of the chapter for several addresses and links), and the involvement of professionals from multiple disciplines working with community members strengthens the efforts and potentiates success. Importantly, the Nursing Network On Violence Against Women International is an organization that brings together women, nurses, and researchers from around the world. The commitment of time and energy to establish working relationships with members of other disciplines can facilitate efforts to address this issue.

SUMMARY

The enormity and pervasiveness of violence and abuse across society are emphasized and validated by the thousands of books and articles on the topic. The financial and human costs of violence are incalculable but extensive, affecting intimate relationships and all segments of society, particularly the people who are most vulnerable: elderly people, disabled people, Aboriginal people, immigrant people and those from racialized minorities, and children. Violence in the workplace affects nurses and other health professionals.

Nurses are in strategic positions to address issues of violence and abuse because they are among the most trusted professionals, are accessible to the public, and are often the first professionals met by those seeking healthcare.

Nurses, therefore, must become knowledgeable about violence and abuse, develop the skills to assess and intervene in cases of violence and abuse, and work in interdisciplinary teams to provide comprehensive care. To do any less is a disservice to patients and the profession.

Add to your knowledge of this issue:	
British Columbia Institute Against Family Violence	www.bcifv.org
Center for Research on Violence Against Women and Children	http://www.crvawc.ca/
Family and Intimate Partner Violence Prevention Team	www.cdc.gov/ncipc/factsheets/ipvfacts.htm
Family Violence in Canada	www.statcan.ca/english/freepub/ 85-224-XIE/free.htm
Hot Peach Pages	www.hotpeachpages.net
Muriel McQueen Fergusson Centre for Family Violence Research	www.unbf.ca/arts/CFVR
National Clearinghouse on Family Violence	www.hc-sc.gc.ca/hppb/familyviolence
National Council Against Domestic Violence	www.ncadv.org
National Council on Child Abuse and Family Violence	www.nccafv.org
Nursing Network On Violence Against Women International	http://www.nnvawi.org/
Research and Education for Solutions to Violence and Abuse	www.umanitoba.ca/resolve

REFLECTIONS on the Chapter...

1 What images do you have when you hear the terms *family violence, woman abuse,* and *abuse of the elderly*? Who are the main characters in your images and what are they doing?

2 Compile a list of accounts from newspapers, television, and radio from the past week that dealt with violence and abuse. How do these reports counter or reinforce harmful stereotypes? What impact would these incidents have on the health of the population? Were health issues addressed in these accounts?

3 If you have had a patient divulge that she or he had been abused, what steps did you take to assist this person? What steps might you take having read this chapter? What resources could you draw on to guide your actions?

4 What attitudes have you heard expressed that would provide a caring atmosphere for any person (patient or nurse) who divulges abuse? What attitudes would hinder or suppress disclosing this type of information?

5 On which of the many facets of violence and abuse would you choose to focus your attention if you were asked to undertake a project of prevention? Where would you begin your efforts?

6 What resources are available in your work environment that would help you care for and deal with the emotional impact of working with victims of violence?

References

Adelson, N. (2005). The embodiment of inequity: health disparities in Aboriginal Canada. *Canadian Journal Of Public Health. Revue Canadienne De Santè Publique, 96 Suppl 2*, S45-61.

Alberta Association of Registered Nurses, College of Licensed Practical Nurses, & Registered Psychiatric Nurses of Alberta. (1999). *Joint statement on family violence* [Online]. Retrieved from www.nurses.ab.ca/pdf/ Joint_Statement_on_Family_Violence.pdf. Edmonton, AB: Author.

American Academy of Nurses Expert Panel on Violence. (1993). Violence as a nursing priority: Policy implications. *Nursing Outlook, 41*(2), 83–92.

American Nurses Association. (1994). *Workplace violence: Can you close the door on it?* (WP-5). Retrieved April 18, 2001 from http://www.nursingworld.org/dlwa/osh/wp5.htm.

Arnetz, J.E., Arnetz, B.B., & Soderman, E. (1998). Violence toward health care workers: Prevalence and incidence at a large regional hospital in Sweden. *AAOHN, 46*(3), 107–114.

Bacchus, L., Mezey, G., & Bewley, S. (2003). Experiences of seeking help from health professionals in a sample of women who experienced domestic violence. *Health & Social Care in the Community, 11*(1), 10–18.

Badgley, R.F., Allard, H.A., & McCormick, N. (1984). *Sexual offences against children* (Catalogue No. J2-50/1984E). Ottawa: Department of Supply and Services.

Bandura, A. (1969). Social-learning theory of identificatory processes. In D.A. Goslin (Ed.), *Handbook of socialization theory and research* (pp. 213–262). Chicago: Rand McNally.

Beauchesne, M., Kelley, B.R., & Lawrence, P.R., et al. (1997). Violence prevention: A community approach. *Journal of Pediatric Health Care, 11*, 179–188.

Biesenthal, L., Sproule, L.D., & Plocica, Z. (1997). *Violence against women in rural communities in Canada: Research project backgrounder*: Research and Statistics Division, Department of Justice, Canada.

Blackstock, C., Trocmé, N., & Bennett, M. (2004). Child maltreatment investigations among Aboriginal and non-Aboriginal Families in Canada. *Violence Against Women, 10*(8), 901–916.

Bourassa, C., McKay-McNabb, K., & Hampton, M.R. (2004). Racism, sexism, and colonialism: The impact on the health of Aboriginal women in Canada. *Canadian Woman Studies, 24*(1), 23–29.

Browne, A.J. (2007). Clinical encounters between nurses and First Nations women in a Western Canadian hospital. *Social Science & Medicine, 64*(10), 2165–2176.

Brownridge, D. (2003). Male partner violence against Aboriginal women in Canada: An empirical analysis. *Journal of Interpersonal Violence, 18*(1), 65–83.

Bunge, V.P. & Locke, D. (2000). *Family violence in Canada: A statistical profile 2000* [Online]. Retrieved from http://www.statcan.ca (Catalogue 85-224-XIE Canadian Centre for Justice Statistics). Ottawa: Minister of Industry.

Campbell, J.C. (1999). *Safety planning based on lethality assessment for partners of batterers in treatment.* Paper presented at the Partnerships to Enhance Victim Safety Conference: Criminal justice & advocacy responses to domestic violence, Troy, NY [Online]. Retrieved from http://www.opdv.state.ny.us.

_____. (2002). Health consequences of intimate partner violence. *The Lancet, 359*, 1331–1336.

Campbell, J.C. & Fishwick, N. (1993). Abuse of female partners. In J. Campbell & J. Humphreys (Eds.), *Nursing care of survivors of family violence* (pp. 68–106). St. Louis, MO: Mosby.

Campbell, J.C. & Lewandowski, L. (1997). Mental and psychical health effects of intimate partner violence on women and children. *Psychiatric Clinics of North America, 20*(2), 353–374.

Canadian Nurses Association. (1996). *Interpersonal violence* [Online]. Retrieved from http://www.cna-nurses.ca.

_____. (2002). Code of Ethics. Ottawa: Canadian Nurses Association.

Canadian Public Health Association. (1994). *Violence in society: A public health perspective* (Issue Paper). Ottawa: Author.

Carroll, V. & Morin, K.H. (1998). Workplace violence affects one-third of nurses: Survey of nurses in seven SNA's reveals staff nurses most at risk. *American Nurses, 30*(5), 15.

Cascardi, M., Daniel O'Leary, K., & Schlee, K.A. (1999). Co-occurrence and correlates of posttraumatic stress disorder and major depression in physically abused women. *Journal of Family Violence, 14*(3), 227–249.

Cooper, H., Moore, L., Gruskin, S., & Krieger, N. (2004). Characterizing perceived police violence: Implications for public health. *American Journal of Public Health, 94*(7), 1109–1118.

Crenshaw, K.W. (1994). Mapping the margins: Intersectionality, identity politics, and violence against women of color. In M.A. Fineman & R. Mykitiuk (Eds.), *The public nature of private violence* (pp. 93–118). New York: Routledge.

DeKerseredy, W.S. & Kelly, K. (1993). The incidence and prevalence of woman abuse in Canadian university and college dating relationships. *Canadian Journal of Sociology, 18*(2), 137–159.

Department of Justice Canada. (2007a). Child abuse fact sheet. *Journal.* Retrieved from http://www.justice.gc.ca/en/ps/fm/childafs.html.

_____. (2007b). Dating violence: A fact sheet from the Department of Justice Canada. *Journal.* Retrieved from http://www.justice.gc.ca/en/ps/fm/datingfs.html#head2.

Dobash, R.E. & Dobash, R.P. (1979). *Violence against wives.* New York: Free Press.

Dion Stout, M. (1998). *Aboriginal Canada: Women and health—A Canadian perspective.* Retrieved April 29, 1998 from http://www.hc-sc.gc.ca/hl-vs/alt_formats/hpb-dgps/pdf/indigen_e.pdf.

Duffy, A. & Momirov, J. (2000). Family violence: Issues and advances at the end of the twentieth century. In N. Mandell & A. Duffy (Eds.). *Canadian families: Diversity, conflict, and change* (pp. 290–322). Toronto: Harcourt Canada.

Duncan, S., Hyndman, K., & Estabrooks, C., et al. (2001). Nurses' experience of violence in Alberta and British Columbia hospitals. *Canadian Journal of Nursing Research, 32*(4), 57–78.

Eby, K.K., Campbell, J.C., & Sullivan, C.M., et al. (1995). Health effects of experiences of sexual violence for women with abusive partners. *Health Care for Women International, 16*(6), 563–576.

Fischbach, R. & Herbert, B. (1997). Domestic violence and mental health: Correlates and conundrums within and across cultures. *Social Science & Medicine, 45*(8), 1161–1176.

Fiske, J.-A. & Browne, A. (2006). Aboriginal citizen, discredited medical subject: Paradoxical constructions of Aboriginal women's subjectivity in Canadian health care policies. *Policy Sciences, 39*(1), 91–111.

Garbarino, J. (1977). The human ecology of child maltreatment: A conceptual model for research. *Journal of Marriage and the Family, 39,* 721–735.

_____. (1995). Growing up in a socially toxic environment: Life for children and families in the 1990s. In G.B. Melton (Ed.), *The individual, the family, and social good: Personal fulfillment in times of change* (Vol. 42, pp. 1–20). Lincoln: University of Nebraska Press.

Garbarino, J. & Kostelny, K. (1992). Child maltreatment as a community problem. *Child Abuse and Neglect, 16,* 455–464.

Garbarino, J. & Sherman, D. (1980). High-risk neighborhoods and high-risk families: The human ecology of child maltreatment. *Child Development, 51,* 188–198.

García-Moreno, C., Jansen, H.A.F.M., & Ellsberg, M., et al. (2005). *WHO multi-country study on women's health and domestic violence against women: Initial results on prevalence, health outcomes and women's responses* Geneva: World Health Organization.

Gelles, R.J. (1980). Violence in the family: A review of research in the seventies. *Journal of Marriage and the Family, 42,* 873–885.

Gerbert, B., Abercrombie, P., & Caspers, N., et al. (1999). How health care providers help battered women: The survivor's perspective. *Women & Health, 29*(3), 115–135.

Hamby, S.L. (2000). The importance of community in a feminist analysis of domestic violence among American Indians. *American Journal of Community Psychology, 28*(5), 649–669.

Hamilton, A.C. & Sinclair, C.M. (1991). *The justice system and aboriginal people.* Winnipeg: Queen's Printer.

Hankivsky, O. & Varcoe, C. (2007). From global to local and over the rainbow: Violence against women. In M. Morrow, O. Hankivsky, & C. Varcoe (Eds.), *Women's health in Canada: Critical perspectives on theory and policy* (pp. 478–507). Toronto: University of Toronto.

Helfer, R. (1973). The etiology of child abuse. *Pediatrics, 51,* 777–779.

Helfer, R. & Kempe, C.H. (1968). *The battered child.* Chicago: University of Chicago Press.

Hoff, L.A. (1994). *Violence issues: An interdisciplinary curriculum guide for health professionals* (H72-21/129-1995E). Ottawa: Mental Health Division Health Canada.

Hoff, L.A. & Ross, M.M. (1993). *Curriculum guide for nursing: Violence against women and children.* Ottawa: University of Ottawa.

Human Resources and Child Welfare Canada. (2000). Child Welfare in Canada. Retrieved from http://www.hrsdc.gc.ca/en/cs/sp/sdc/socpol/publications/reports/2000-000033/page00.shtml.

Humphreys, J. (1993). Children of battered women. In J. Campbell & J. Humphreys (Eds.), *Nursing care of survivors* of family violence (pp. 107–131). St. Louis, MO: Mosby.

Humphreys, J. & Ramsey, A.M. (1993). Child abuse. In J. Campbell & J. Humphreys (Eds.), *Nursing care of survivors of family violence* (pp. 36–67). St. Louis, MO: Mosby.

Imam, A. (2001, April). *Nigerian women's group condemns whipping* [Online]. Retrieved from http://www.web.net/~matchint/en/apr01/nlapr01_3.htm.

Innes, J.E., Ratner, P.A., & Finlayson, P.F., et al. (1991). *Models and strategies of delivering community health services related to woman abuse.* Edmonton: University of Alberta.

Interdepartmental Working Group on Elder Abuse and Manitoba Seniors Directorate. (1993). *Abuse of the elderly: A guide for the development of protocols.* Winnipeg: Government of Manitoba.

International Council of Nurses. (1999a). *Abuse and violence against nursing personnel* [Online]. Retrieved from http://www.icn.ch/psviolence00.htm.

_____. (1999b, March 8). *Increasing violence in the workplace is a threat to nursing and the delivery of health care* [Online]. Retrieved from http://www.icn.ch/prviolence_99.htm.

Johnson, H. (1996). *Dangerous domains: Violence against women in Canada.* Scarborough, ON: International Thomson Publishing.

_____. (2006). *Measuring violence against women: Statistical trends.* Ottawa: Statistics Canada.

Kaukinen, C. (2002). The help-seeking of women violent crime victims: Findings from the Canadian violence against women survey. *International Journal of Sociology and Social Policy, 22*(7/8), 5–44.

Kendall-Tackett, K., Marshall, R., & Ness, K. (2003). Chronic pain syndromes and violence against women. *Women & Therapy, (26)*, 45–56.

Kerr, R. & McLean, J. (1996). *Paying for violence: Some of the costs of violence against women in BC.* Victoria, BC: Ministry of Women's Equality.

Koniak-Griffin, D. & Lesser, J. (1996). The impact of childhood maltreatment on young mothers' violent behavior toward themselves and others. *Journal of Pediatric Nursing, 11*(5), 300–308.

Langford, D.R. (1996). Predicting unpredictability: A model of women's processes of predicting battering men's violence. *Scholarly Inquiry for Nursing Practice: An International Journal, 10*(4), 371–385.

Lempert, L.B. (1997). The other side of help: Negative effects in the help-seeking processes of abused women. *Qualitative Sociology, 20*(2), 289–309.

Letourneau, E., Holmes, M., & Chasedunn-Roark, H. (1999). Gynecologic health consequences to victims of interpersonal violence. *Women's Health Issues, 9*, 115–120.

MacLean, M.J. & Williams, R.M. (1995). Introduction. In M.J. MacLean (Ed.), *Abuse & neglect of older Canadians: Strategies for change* (pp. ix–xii). Toronto: Canadian Association on Gerontology and Thompson Educational Publishing.

MacLeod, L. (1991). *Freedom from fear: A woman's right, a community concern, a national priority* (C91-099010-7E). Ottawa: Secretary of State Canada; Multiculturalism and Citizenship Canada.

MacMillan, H.L., Fleming, J.E., & Trocmé, N., et al. (1997). Prevalence of child physical and sexual abuse in the community. *Journal of the American Medical Association, 278*(2), 131–135.

MacMillan, H.L., MacMillan, A.B., & Offord, D.R., et al. (1996). Aboriginal health. *Canadian Medical Association Journal, 155*(11), 1569–1578.

Manitoba Association of Registered Nurses. (1989). *Nurse abuse report.* Winnipeg: Author.

Matas, R. (2001, March 24). "He said if I ever told anyone, he will kill me when he gets out." *Globe and Mail,* pp. A9–10.

McCloskey, K. & Grigsby, N. (2005). The ubiquitous clinical problem of adult intimate partner violence: The need for routine assessment. *Professional Psychology: Research and Practice, 36*(3), 264–275.

McDonald, L. & Collins, A. (2000). *Abuse and neglect of older adults: A discussion paper.* Ottawa: Health Canada.

McCullough, I. (1994). *A challenge for health: Making connections within the family violence context* (Discussion papers on health/family violence issues H39-292/1-1994E). Ottawa: Health Canada.

Mosher, J.E. (1998). Caught in tangled webs of care: Women abused in intimate relationships. In C.T. Baines, P.M. Evans, & S.M. Neysmith (Eds.), *Women's caring: Feminist perspectives on social welfare* (2nd ed., pp. 139–159). Toronto, ON: Oxford University Press.

Muellman, R.L., Lenaghan, P.A., & Pakieser, R.A. (1996). Battered women: Injury locations and types. *Annals of Emergency Medicine, 28*(5), 468–492.

Ozturk Ertem, I., Leventhal, J.M., & Dobbs, S. (2000). Intergenerational continuity of child physical abuse: How good is the evidence? *Lancet, 356*(9232), 814.

Podnieks, E. (1985). Elder abuse: It's time we did something about it. *Canadian Nurse, 81*(11), 36–39.

Podnieks, E. & Baillie, E. (1995). Education as the key to the prevention of elder abuse and neglect. In M.J. MacLean (Ed.), *Abuse & neglect of older Canadians: Strategies for change* (pp. 81–93). Toronto: Canadian Association on Gerontology and Thompson Educational Publishing.

Podnieks, E., Pillemer, K., & Nicholson, J.P., et al. (1990). *National survey on abuse of the elderly in Canada.* Toronto: Ryerson Polytechnical Institute.

Pynoos, R.S. & Nader, K. (1990). Children's exposure to violence and traumatic death. *Psychiatric Annals, 20*(6), 334–344.

Report of the Royal Commission on Aboriginal Peoples. (1996). *For seven generations* (Vol. 3). Ottawa: Libraxus.

Ristock, J.L. (2001). Decentering heterosexuality: Responses of feminist counselors to abuse in lesbian relationships. *Women & Therapy, 23*(3), 59–72.

Sleutel, M.R. (1998). Women's experiences of abuse: A review of qualitative research. *Issues in Mental Health Nursing, 19,* 525–539.

Smith, D., Varcoe, C., & Edwards, N. (2005). Turning around the intergenerational impact of residential school on Aboriginal people: Implications for health policy and practice. *Canadian Journal of Nursing Research, 37*(4), 39–60.

Smylie, J. (2001). A guide for health professionals working with aboriginal peoples: Health issues affecting aboriginal peoples. *Journal of the Society of Obstetricians and Gynecologists of Canada, 100,* 54–68.

Statistics Canada. (1997). Graphical overview of crime and the administration of criminal justice in Canada, 1997 (Catalogue No. 85F0018XIE). Ottawa: Minister of Industry.

_____. (2005). Statistics Canada—The Daily. *Homicides.* Retrieved from http://www.statcan.ca/Daily/English/051006/d051006b.htm.

_____. (2006). *Family violence in Canada: A statistical profile 2006.* Ottawa: Canadian Centre for Justice Statistics.

Thomlinson, E.B., Erickson, N., & Cook, M. (2000). Could this be your community? In J. Proulx & S. Perrault (Eds.), *No place for violence: Canadian aboriginal alternatives* (Vol. 1, pp. 22–38). Halifax: Fernwood Publishing and RESOLVE (Research and Education for Solutions to Violence and Abuse).

Tower, M. (2007). Intimate partner violence and the health care response: a postmodern critique. *Health Care for Women International, 28*(5), 438–452.

Varcoe, C. & Dick, S. (2008). Intersecting risks of violence and HIV for rural and Aboriginal women in a neocolonial Canadian context. *Journal of Aboriginal Health, 4,* 42–52.

Walker, L.E. (1979). *The battered woman.* New York: Harper & Row.

Wiehe, V.R. (1998). *Understanding family violence: Treating and preventing partner, child, sibling, and elder abuse.* Thousand Oaks, CA: Sage.

World Health Organization. (2002). *World report on violence and health.* Geneva: World Health Organization.

_____. (2005). *WHO multi-country study on women's health and domestic violence against women: Summary report of initial results on prevalence, health outcomes and women's responses.* Geneva: World Health Organization.

Wuest, J., Merritt-Gray, M., & Lent, B., et al. (2007). Patterns of medication use among women survivors of intimate partner violence. *Canadian Journal of Public Health, 98*(6), 460–464.

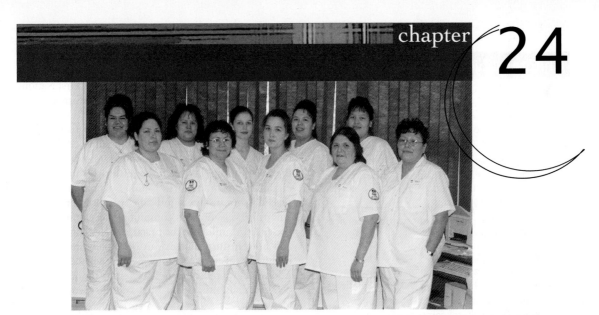

Nursing students from the University of Manitoba Baccalaureate Nursing Program, Norway House, are dedicated to advancing healthcare among the First Nations. Front row (l-r): Cheryl McKay, Georgina Henry, Tena Flett, Harriet Hart, and Barb Queskekapow; back row (l-r): Tracy Fosseneuve, Allison Saunders, Kim Cooper, Glenda Muskego, and Stacy Dixon. (Photograph by Lorraine Robertson. Used with permission from the University of Manitoba.)

Challenges for the New Millennium: Nursing in First Nations

Fjola Hart Wasekeesikaw

Critical Questions

As a way of engaging with the ideas in this chapter, consider the following:

1. Begin to think about the assumptions that you hold about nursing in First Nations communities.

2. How have you come to hold these assumptions?

3. What might be the influence of these assumptions and beliefs on the provision of healthcare to First Nations people?

Chapter Objectives

After completing this chapter, you will be able to:

1. Describe the relationship between the colonization of First Nations people and health-related issues.

2. Analyze the significance of concepts of population health in addressing issues of inequity.

3. Examine some different views of health held by the First Peoples in Canada, the First Nations.

4 Interpret the significance of cultural resurgence, community development, and the expressed need to widen the scope of health and transfer of healthcare services to First Nations communities.

5 Evaluate the role of nurses and nursing in the delivery of healthcare services to First Nations communities in Canada.

6 Examine the following issues confronting nurses in the provision of healthcare services to First Nations people:

- population demographics and the relationship to the healthcare needs
- transfer of healthcare services in relation to nursing issues
- need for cultural competence
- educational needs for nurses working in First Nations communities.

This chapter introduces the reader to issues related to health, healthcare, and nursing for First Nations people in Canada and presents basic information to facilitate greater understanding of First Nations people. Key to understanding is recognition of the great diversity among First Nations communities and the views of health held by First Nations members. Also discussed are the relationship between the historical attempts for enfranchisement of First Nations people and health-related issues and the significance of cultural resurgence among First Nations in community development. How these factors influence the practice of nursing in Canada and how, in turn, nurses can potentially influence the healthcare of First Nations people will be explored. Additionally, current issues related to the nursing and delivery of healthcare to First Nations people will be identified.

DIVERSITY OF THE FIRST PEOPLES

The 560 First Nations in Canada constitute a diverse population of descendants of the First Peoples of North America. Many of these nations are further grouped into tribal councils, which provide unity and greater political power as well as combined resources among nations. Each First Nation has its own reserve land base, traditional territories, culture, and language.

First Nations are part of a larger group of Aboriginal people. As defined in the Canadian Constitution Act, the term *Aboriginal* refers to First Nations, Inuit, and Metis. All Aboriginal people originate from 11 different language families (Smylie, 2000, p. 1072): Algonkian, Athapaskan, Haidan, Iroquoian, Kutenaian, Salishan, Siouan, Tlingit, Tsimshaian, Wakashan, and Inuit.

According to the Indian Act, an act of the Canadian Parliament, First Nations members are legally defined as "Indians." The Indian Act, first passed in 1876, was designed to administer programs to Indians for the purpose of assimilating them into Canadian society; the act also determined who was legally defined as an Indian. There have been many revisions to the Indian Act since its inception, but the purpose remains the same. Each person who is deemed to be legally Indian has a registration number to reflect her or his population number within her or his band or First Nations community.

Some First Nations members are also referred to as having "treaty" status. This term applies to those First Nations that signed treaties with the British or Canadian governments. Between 1817 and 1929, the First Nations conducted negotiations with the British government or with Canada in the right of the Crown, resulting in the signing of more than 20 international treaties. Through this treaty process, the Treaty Nations agreed to cede certain lands for use and settlement in return for specific guarantees. These guarantees are the treaty rights of First Nations. The treaties reserved lands and resources for continued use and existence as First Nations. The treaties also guaranteed specific social and economic rights to ensure continued strong First Nations governments. For example, the Natural Resources Transfer Agreements of 1930 guarantee that First Nations people residing in Manitoba, Saskatchewan, and Alberta have the right to hunt, trap, and fish—except for commercial purposes (Indian and Northern Affairs Canada, www.ainc-inac.gc.ca/index_e.html). Ultimately, the First Nations leadership guaranteed the right to be born and live as a First Nations person.

The term *Indian* originates from early explorers to North America who thought they had discovered India. First Nations members assert that the roots of this term are inappropriate and serve to reflect a history of colonialism. To reflect more appropriately that they are descendants of the First Peoples on this continent, the First Nations have determined that they would be identified accordingly.

EUROPEAN RELATIONSHIP WITH FIRST NATIONS

What is the significance of the impact of colonization on the lives and ways of living of First Nations families and communities in Canada? *Colonialism* (a result of colonization) is considered to be control by one power over a dependent area or people. It also refers to policy based on such control. Before contact with European colonizers, the First Peoples had their own systems of government, trade, and healthcare. After confederation, Canada began to displace the First Nations from their traditional territories to make room for the ever-increasing influx of European settlers. Government policies were developed to protect, civilize, and assimilate the First Peoples into Canadian society. The final outcome of these measures was cultural genocide. The process undertaken to achieve this end would greatly affect the mental, physical, and spiritual health of First Nations. The inherent oppressive and suppressive nature of these policies has had, and continues to have, far-reaching negative effects on First Nation governance and cultural identity.

Because of its extensiveness and the length of time during which colonization took place, this chapter presents no more than a brief overview. The risk in attempting to discuss the historical highlights is the potential to oversimplify the European relationship with the First Nations and the long-lasting negative effects on the population. With this in mind, the history will briefly cover the following key phases:

- cooperation, nation to nation
- colonization and its effects on the health of First Nations members and their communities
- First Nations' cultural resurgence.

Cooperation Among Nations

Colonization did not begin at the point of original contact between the Europeans and First Nations. Unlike the history between the First Peoples and European settlers in the United States, in which wars established the dominance of European culture, the initial relationship between the First Peoples and, first the French, and then the British in Canada was one of mutual tolerance and respect. The social, cultural, and political differences between these societies were maintained. This tolerance reflected how First Nations related to each other. The newcomers came to a continent that was already inhabited by diverse nations of indigenous people who formed alliances and good relations with one another to access and distribute their tribal resources (Dickason, 1994, p. 76).

The First Peoples had their own economic, health, political, and social systems that were developed within their communities according to their traditions and the need imposed by their environments. When the first Europeans came into contact with the First Nations, each thought of the other as distinct and autonomous. Each nation continued to govern its internal affairs. Nations cooperated in areas of mutual interest and were connected in various trading relationships and other forms of nation-to-nation alliances.

The Royal Proclamation of 1763 demonstrates that the partnership between First Nations and the British Crown was one of cooperation and protection. In exchange for cooperation in the partnership that characterized the relationship between them at that time, the king of England extended royal protection to the First Peoples' lands and political autonomy. When Canada was formed in 1867, a legislative basis for dealing with the Indian people as nations had already been established.

Colonization and the Effect on First Nations

The written word reflects an author's attitudes and beliefs, and so it was that the plans of action or policies to carry out the government laws reflected the attitudes of the people who wrote these policies. The Indian Act was the legislative vehicle for implementing policies to civilize, protect, and assimilate the Indian people (Tobias, 1991). No single event marked the beginning of these colonial practices. Rather, they began with the attitudes of the time and laid the foundation for a series of actions that deemed the Indian people as inferior beings. Government laws still reflect these attitudes today; in doing so, these laws perpetuate a colonialistic attitude.

A series of actions led to the proclaiming of the Indian Act. This was one act of many that laid the foundation for the civilization program that was developed in 1828 and gave rise to the reserve system that became a social laboratory designed to enable Indian communities to adopt European values (Tobias, 1991). This program established Indians in isolated, fixed locations where they could be educated, converted to Christianity, and transformed into farmers. The goal was to eradicate the First Peoples' values through education, religion, new economic and political systems, and a new concept of property. Not only was the distinct cultural group to disappear but so, too, was the laboratory where these changes were brought about. It was assumed that each Indian person who became enfranchised would also take his share of the land from the reserve.

The Assembly of the United Canadas of the Gradual Civilization Act of 1857 provided the criteria for determining whether an Indian person qualified to become enfranchised. A special board of examiners determined each applicant's merit based on whether the person was educated, free from debt, and of good moral character. If so, the person was awarded 20 hectares of land within the colony and "the accompanying rights" as a citizen of the Dominion (Milloy, 1991, p. 147). One of the accompanying rights was the opportunity to vote in the country's elections. It was assumed that Indian people would sever ties with their communities and embrace colonial living and values.

The British North America Act of 1867, establishing the Canadian nation, also contained the forerunner of the Indian Act and placed First Nations, and lands reserved for them, under the legislative authority of the Canadian federal government. The Indian Act was amended almost every year to address unanticipated problems in carrying out the government policies. The need for policy revision also reflected resistance by First Nations people to change their values and cultural ways (Milloy, 1991). The amendments persisted on a course to erode the land base of First Nations, wipe out traditional political governance, and smother traditional ways of expression and living. Some effects of the amended Indian Act include the following:

- *The erosion of the protected status of reserve lands.* In 1894, the government leased reserve land held by physically disabled Indian people, widows, orphans, and others who could not cultivate it (Royal Commission on Aboriginal Peoples, 1996a). These tracts of land were neither surrendered nor was approval required by the First Nations communities for the government simply to take over the land and lease it to European settlers. Later, in 1918, the leasing of reserve lands that had not been surrendered was broadened to include any uncultivated lands if the purpose of the lease was cultivation or grazing. Only Indian people who were able to cultivate their land were allowed to keep tracts of reserve land. This practice was in violation of treaty obligations connecting Canada to the Royal Proclamation of 1763, wherein Indian title to land and the need to obtain proper surrender of Indian lands were identified.

- *The undermining of traditional political processes used by First Nations communities.* The federal government determined how First Nations community leadership was to be elected and interfered with the decision-making processes of the communities' affairs. The superintendent of Indian Affairs determined the time, place, and manner in which the elections took place (Milloy, 1991). In addition, the governor could remove a chief or councilor from office if he thought the leader was dishonest, intemperate, or immoral. The interpretation of these terms and how they were applied to each case was left to the governor's advisors and departmental agents. The extent to which community members participated in the elections was limited to all males over the age of

21 years who could vote for their officials. The chief and council were forced to function within a foreign-designed and foreign-controlled system.

Federal authority also set a bureaucratic system of controlling the communities' affairs. The nature of the concerns in which the chief and council could make decisions was preset; in addition, each decision was subject to confirmation by the governor (Cassidy & Bish, 1989). The chief and council functioned within a narrow, federally controlled context, for example, making bylaws for a variety of purposes. Some of these bylaws include the control of band membership; provision of public health; regulation of commerce, traffic, construction, and buildings; assurance of the observance of law and order; prevention of disorderly conduct and nuisances; construction and maintenance of water supplies, roads, bridges, and other public works; regulation of animal populations; and removal of trespassers from reserve land. By interfering with the governing processes of First Nations communities, the federal government undercut the authority of the First Nations communities' leadership.

- *The suppression of the traditions and values of First Nations.* In a concerted effort to extinguish any traditional beliefs and practices in the First Nations community, laws were enacted to ban all traditional ceremonies and to control Indian movement from one reserve to another (Milloy, 1991). It was thought that intertribal gatherings, celebrations, and ceremonies were the primary obstacles to Indian people becoming Christians. In 1884, the potlatch and the Tamanawas dance were prohibited, with a jail term of 2 months to 6 months for any Indian who was convicted of engaging in or assisting with these dances. In later years, further amendments banned the practice of other traditional dances such as the Blackfoot Sun Dance. In part, the system was an attempt to control discussion between political and spiritual leaders living on various reserves. In 1885, Indian people were prohibited from travelling off their reserves without written authorization of the Indian agent on the reserve. These laws were designed to suppress historical, social, and political organization of First Nations societies and governments.

Government laws and policies have systematically assaulted First Nations in their spiritual practices and in their social organization, governance, and economic activities. For many First Nations, the residential school system in which the state and church attempted to capture and socialize First Nations children was the sharpest cut of all (Royal Commission of Aboriginal Peoples, 1996b). The residential school experience left in its wake dislocation and a strong sense of loss for individual students and their families, with rippling, cumulative, intergenerational effects on First Nations communities. Dislocation from one's community effected many losses, including culture, language, spirituality, identity, pride, self-respect, and ability to parent. This dislocation left many communities trapped between what remained of traditional ways of doing things and the fear of importing too much more of mainstream Canadian cultural values into reserve life. The residential school system insult to the spirit of the First Nations people has had, and continues to have, destructive effects on families and communities. It is important to recognize, however, that colonization processes have not been successful in eliminating First Nations. Rather, they have propelled First Nations to embark on reviving traditions and proclaiming their identities.

Attitudes and policies reflecting the colonial system continue today because the present healthcare and government systems exist on a foundation of protection, civilization, and assimilation (Smylie, 2000). This fact has repercussions for the relationships between the First Nations people and their healthcare providers.

CULTURAL RESURGENCE OF FIRST NATIONS AND COMMUNITY DEVELOPMENT

The First Nations cultural resurgence and community development share similar roots and are closely intertwined. In the 1960s, First Nations people demanded the right to set their own cultural course.

They spoke out about indigenous perspectives on development. Their voices were significant in creating a pathway on which community development could be used to bring about economic and social changes in First Nations communities.

Until 1951, when the Indian Act was revised, laws banned First Nations members from attempting to organize themselves. With the revisions to the Indian Act, First Nations members began the enormous task of developing political organizations to strengthen and improve the situations of First Nations people (McFarlane, 2000). Members began travelling from community to community, discussing issues and potential actions to change the conditions within the communities. Over the ensuing decade, tension between First Nations and the government of Canada developed. The early 1960s was a time when government control was so deeply entrenched that policy controlled almost every aspect of First Nations people's lives, interests, and concerns. For example, the Indian Act affected the family unit in that it provided for arbitrary enfranchisement of an Indian woman who married a person who was not registered as an Indian. Within a family unit, women's status as band members could cease depending on whom the female siblings married. Concomitant with this example, the Wildlife Act prohibits any Indian person from giving meat to a non-Indian. The non-Indian person in this case could be a sister who is enfranchised.

First Nations people set out to challenge policies reflecting a belief that Canadian institutions alone could prescribe solutions to the problems faced by First Nations people. They had different ideas about dealing with their own issues. Provincial organizations were developed to deal with concerns facing the status of Indian people. Nationally, the first status Indian organization, the National Indian Brotherhood, was started in December 1968. (*Note:* The term *status Indian* is applied to an Indian person who is registered under the Indian Act.) The National Indian Brotherhood gave a single voice to all status Indian people in Canada (McFarlane, 2000). Of particular significance was the First Nations response to the White Paper, a Canadian government policy statement in 1969 that aimed to abolish all First Nations rights, including rights to reserve lands. The First Nations response shifted the nature of the relationship the First Nations would have with the government of Canada; the response would be key in moving away from a relationship whereby Indian people were the wards of the state. First Nations governing their own affairs would provide a basis for developing community-specific health and healing systems.

MIYUPIMAATISSIIUM: BEING ALIVE WELL

Miyupimaatissiium, or "being alive well," is seen as an interdependent relationship people have with the natural world and with keeping one's spirit strong (Adelson, 1991; Hamilton & Sinclair, 1991; Malloch, 1989). Culture, language, and traditions used to express concepts similar to that of *being alive well* vary from one First Nations community to another. For example, to the members of a First Nations Eastern Ininiwuk—or "human beings"—community, also known as the Cree people, in the province of Quebec, Ininiwuk food is essential to miyupimaatissiium. Game and fish are requirements for miyupimaatissiium and symbolize essential aspects of Ininiwuk life.

To the people in this community, "eating well" means that one has been eating bush food, or food from the land, and from this, it can be assumed that there has been a good hunting season. In turn, a good hunting season signifies that one has the physical strength required to work in the bush. Miyupimaatissiium is evidence of an experienced hunter and of a woman who has the skills and ability required for preparing the meat and hides. The spiritual aspect of eating well is at the moment when the animal chooses to give itself to the hunter. The relationship between an Ininiwuk hunter and the animals hunted for food is based on mutual respect. A cyclical affinity between the Ininiwuk (human being), hunting, the land, and food incorporates all aspects of life and so too, being alive well. Miyupimaatissiium is a holistic concept encompassing people in relation to their environment and all that is within the universe. The Royal Commission of Aboriginal Peoples (1996c) identified that holism is an integral part of Aboriginal health and healing systems.

Health Status of First Nations People in Canada

The First Peoples enjoyed good health in the Americas; then, as result of European contact, the decimation and extinction of many First Peoples followed. The effects of infectious diseases, such as smallpox, were devastating to the health and cultures of the First Peoples. They suffered many losses, ranging from decreased community sizes to a strong sense of personal and collective loss. The epidemics resulted in declining fertility rates because infected women were unable to conceive or carry their pregnancies to term and also in decreased chances of conceiving as a result of population loss and subsequent lack of partners. Loss of relatives and large numbers of community members resulted in loneliness, grief, and depression. Loss of leaders, warriors, and hunters, and the reduced size of communities, made it difficult to protect territorial boundaries (Ray, 1974). This resulted in migratory shifts in the tribal territories and the modification of economic roles from trappers to middleman traders. Canadian historian Olive Dickason presented to the members of the Royal Commission of Aboriginal Peoples reasons for the impressive state of good health of the First Peoples and then related the impact of infectious diseases on their health and well-being:

> Some analysts argue that disease agents themselves were rare in pre-contact America until the tall ships began to arrive with their invisible cargo of bacteria and viruses. What is more likely is that Aboriginal people had adapted well to their environment; they had developed effective resistance to the micro-organisms living along side them and had knowledge of herbs and other therapies for treating injury and disease . . . some . . . died prematurely. But more stayed well. Or recovered from illness, and thus lived to raise their children and continue the clans and the nations. Aboriginal populations fluctuated largely in relation to food supply.
>
> Hundreds of thousands . . . died as a result of their encounters with the Europeans . . . infectious diseases were the greatest killer. Influenza, measles, polio, diphtheria, smallpox, and other diseases were transported from the slums of Europe to the unprotected villages of the Americas. . . . Aboriginal people were well aware of the link between the newcomers and the epidemics that raced though their camps and villages. During the eighteenth and nineteenth centuries, their leaders sought agreements or treaties with representatives of the British Crown aimed at ensuring their survival in the face of spreading disease and impoverishment. In the expectation of fair compensation for the use of their lands and resources and in mounting fear of the social and health effects of Euro-Canadian settlement, many Aboriginal nations, clans and families agreed to relocate to camps, farms, villages or reserves distant from sites of colonial settlement. Many did so in the belief that the Crown would guarantee their wellbeing for all time. Given the gulf that separated Aboriginal and non-Aboriginal cultures, it is not surprising that the meaning of those oral and written agreements has been a matter of conflicting interpretation ever since (Royal Commission of Aboriginal Peoples, 1996c, p. 112).

Use of a Population Health Approach to Address Inequity

Population health includes a study of the determinants of health and disease, health status, and the degree to which healthcare affects the health of the community (Shah, 1998). An examination of the determinants of health helps to identify and then address inequities within the healthcare system (Evans, Barer, & Marmor, 1994). Many First Nations have identified the significance of clean drinking water; safe, uncontaminated food; reliable sanitation; comfortable housing and workplaces; and adequate employment as essential to the health of the population (Royal Commission on Aboriginal Peoples, 1996c). The health of a community is largely determined by the food available, the nature of the environment, and the behavior of its residents.

Human poverty is any fundamental need that is not adequately satisfied. Some First Nations communities have come to know many faces of poverty related to low socioeconomic status. Poverty is also related to marginalization and the imposition of alien values on local and regional culture (Aboriginal Nurses Association of Canada [ANAC], 2001c). Health involves more than physical integrity of the body; it includes social and political concerns and the relationship of individuals to the environment in which they live. Community development is an avenue for facilitating active participation of each member in a community. Resources—both personal and social in nature—to improve the health and social conditions of people may be hidden. One of these resources is First Nations' determination in obtaining community control and adequate resources to design health, social, and political systems that are of their choosing and reflective of their communities' cultures.

The Royal Commission on Aboriginal Peoples articulated in *Gathering Strength* (1996c) that Aboriginal people want to access health and healing services and to achieve health status equal to that of the general Canadian population.

Access to Healthcare: A Fiduciary Responsibility

The federal government has a fiduciary responsibility to ensure the delivery of healthcare to the members of First Nations communities (Venne, 1997). However, the government of Canada has not acknowledged this responsibility. The relationship between the government of Canada and its fiduciary responsibility to deliver health services to First Nations is based on the medicine chest clause of Treaty Six (1876). Treaty Six specifically mentions medical care in two clauses: The first refers to measures to be taken by the Indian agent when Indian people in their charge were subjected to pestilence or famine; the second clause refers to the medicine chest that was kept at the house of the Indian agents.

> *Clause 1—That in the event hereafter of the Indians comprised within this treaty being overtaken by any pestilence or by a general famine, the Queen on being satisfied and certified thereof by her Indian Agent or Agents will grant to the Indians assistance of such character and to such extent as her chief Superintendent of Indian Affairs shall deem necessary and sufficient to relieve the Indians from the calamity that shall have befallen them.*
>
> *Clause 2—That a medicine chest shall be kept at the house of each Indian Agent for the use and benefit of the Indians at the discretion of such Agent.*

Treaty Six process reflected the cultures of its participants—the representatives of the Crown and the leadership of the First Nations people. However, the significance of these cultural contexts, such as the oral tradition, is not reflected in the final agreement.

 # HEALTHCARE IN NORTHERN AND ISOLATED COMMUNITIES

From the end of the 19th century, semitrained government agents, members of the Royal Canadian Mounted Police, and missionaries provided healthcare services. Graham-Cumming wrote in 1967 that the first Department of Indian Affairs, established in 1880, was not originally concerned with First Nations health problems (as cited in Waldram et al., 2006). Then, after decades of ignoring the health of First Nations people, the government of Canada began to develop a system of primary care clinics, a public health program, and regional hospitals. This was done primarily to stave off the threat of tuberculosis epidemics spreading to the general Canadian population. Indigenous healing ways were absent from this healthcare system. Medical personnel devalued the practice of indigenous medicine by determining it to be nothing more than witchcraft and sorcery. As a result of this and government policy, the people who practised traditional medicine feared persecution and went underground with their skills and knowledge.

Nurses and doctors, employees of the federal government of Canada, were integral to delivering healthcare to First Nations. Nurses have served as entry to this Western model of healthcare in First Nations and Inuit communities since the beginning of the 20th century (Young, 1984). In response to the healthcare needs of the First Peoples, the Department of National Health and Welfare established the nursing station model as the center for providing medical services in northern communities (Waldram et al., 2006). In 1922, a mobile nurse-visitor program was implemented to provide both medical and nursing care services in communities. The first nursing station was opened in 1930 on the Fisher River reserve in Manitoba. By 1935, the Medical Branch of the Department of Indian Affairs employed 11 field nurses who joined a team of medical officers and Indian agents with medical training to provide services to First Nations and Inuit communities. Nurses in these stations provided all primary care with only radio contact with physicians, and patients were evacuated to southern urban hospitals for more comprehensive treatment. By the mid-1950s and into the 1960s, a total of 37 nursing stations in northern Canada had become integral to accessing healthcare in First Nations, Inuit, and Metis communities.

Nurses in northern First Nations settings have provided care and continue to practise within the sphere of advanced practice (Lemphers, 1998; Stewart et al., 2005). In addition, many function collaboratively within a community-based health and social team comprising community health representatives and social service workers.

Widening the Scope of Health: A First Nations Perspective

According to *Gathering Strength,* the Report of the Royal Commission of Aboriginal Peoples (1996c), First Nations protested when the government attempted to reduce noninsured health benefits, such as prescription drugs and eyeglasses, dental work, and transportation costs for medical services. They argued that treaty rights were being violated because changes were being made without negotiation with First Nations. In 1979, the federal government had acknowledged the following:

1. community development as a key strategy for improving First Nations health
2. the continuing responsibility of the federal government for the health and well-being of First Nations people and Inuits
3. the essential elements of the Canadian healthcare system, including the federal and provincial jurisdictions.

Justice Thomas Berger (1980), in his Report of the Advisory Commission on Indian and Inuit Health Consultation, proposed mechanisms that included First Nations consultation in the development of community-controlled health and healing systems. His report was described as "radical" by the Royal Commission on Aboriginal Peoples (1996c). Despite the proposed changes, First Nations were cautious of the proposed federal government initiatives on transfer. They expressed their unease at the federally initiated Community Health Demonstration Program, which began in 1981. Why should First Nations have to prove to the federal government that they could manage their own community affairs? The community health projects were implemented to provide information about costs for First Nations control of health services (Health Canada, 1999b). When the demonstration projects were completed in 1987, First Nations communities participated in the federal initiatives for transfer process to administer the control of federally sponsored healthcare programs. The transfer of healthcare services to First Nations communities continued to be fraught with controversy. Culhane Speck (1989) identified gaps in the transfer process. First, the Canadian government refused to accept legal responsibility for Indian health. The evidence for this was the exclusion of noninsured health benefits. Second, in contrast to the understanding that control by First Nations would develop community-based and culturally designed health programs and services, the government's interpretation was that administrative control would be transferred to the First Nations only for certain existing health programs. The education component that would be required to develop culturally appropriate systems would not be funded. Specifically, there would be no upgrading and clinical training for nurses and other community program personnel. This lack of resources would have far-reaching ramifications for nursing services in First Nations communities.

Transfer of Healthcare Services to First Nations

As of March, 2002, 284 First Nations communities—out of 599 communities eligible for transfer—have taken on the administrative responsibility for healthcare services—either individually or collectively—through multicommunity agencies or tribal associations (Health Canada, 2002). In addition, 41 First Nations communities are involved in the pretransfer process. Communities that have completed the transfer process are employers for nurses and other healthcare personnel in their communities.

Every community is unique in the manner in which it establishes its own health and healing system. The extent and manner in which traditional views about health are used in developing the system or in influencing existing healthcare services will lie with each community. The Royal Commission on Aboriginal Peoples (1996c) proposed that new Aboriginal health and healing systems embody the following four essential characteristics:

1. pursuit of equity in access to health and healing services and in health status outcomes
2. holism in approaches to problems and their treatment and prevention
3. Aboriginal authority over health systems and, where feasible, community control over services
4. diversity in the design of systems and services to accommodate differences in culture and community realities.

The key to restoring well-being among Aboriginal people originates from within Aboriginal cultures (Royal Commission on Aboriginal Peoples, 1996c). There will likely be as many variations of healthcare delivery systems as there are First Nations communities in Canada. Self-determination in the development of community healthcare systems is essential.

 ## CLIMATE FOR CHANGE: NURSING IN FIRST NATIONS COMMUNITIES

Nurses have played a vital role in the delivery of health services in First Nations communities over the past century. Nursing is at a critical crossroads in addressing the healthcare needs of people living in First Nations communities. Improving the overall health status of First Nations people is the impetus for creating more effective ways of delivering nursing care services that reflect the health and healing systems determined by each community or tribal council. Aboriginal nursing services are an integral part of a First Nations community's health and healing system. A community's processes for economic development and participation in transfer of healthcare services can serve as vehicles for making these changes. This would require nurses to learn how the First Nations community or tribal council in which they work views health and healing, whether community development is being used, what is being planned, and what changes have been made. Having this information will provide nurses with context and an understanding of the healthcare priorities selected by the community. These are important elements of a population health approach and the use of community development principles in providing nursing care in First Nations communities.

First Nations communities face many challenges, and some of these are barriers to the delivery of effective healthcare services (O'Neil et al., 1999, p. 147). Some of the barriers include the following:

1. *Scarce resources.* Beginning in 1995, the federal government capped increases in spending directed to First Nations and Inuit health services.
2. *No real autonomy for First Nations communities who have assumed administrative responsibility for health services.* Along with limited resources, a lack of planning for the increasing need for trained personnel to fill positions in a community's health and healing system, and a lack of resources to train personnel, communities have inadequate resources to develop new models of health programming. Unless nurses collaborate with community members and communities at large to overcome this major barrier, health programs to address the need will not be realized.
3. *Emphasis on curative services.* The Canadian health system's focus on curative services and the poor health of many First Nations communities mean that the limited health resources are focused on treatment services.
4. *Emphasis on physical health.* The Canadian health system ignores holistic health and culturally based health programming.
5. *Lack of attention to health promotion and disease prevention.* With the emphasis on curative programming, there are few resources for innovative health promotion and prevention.
6. *Lack of health service integration.* There is no single, concerted approach to improve health through addressing the determinants of health, including economic development, employment, housing, and education. This void exists mainly because of the lack of integrated health services between the federal, provincial, and community jurisdictions.
7. *Diminished traditional role of women.* Reflective of western models of governance that have replaced the traditional hereditary system, the role of indigenous women as central in sustaining the health of communities has been weakened.
8. *The legacy of enforced dependency.* Communities have had to rely on Canadian government-directed approaches to health services; thus, members have not had opportunities to develop integrated, effective First Nations health strategies.

Many First Nations face obstacles in delivering healthcare services to their community members. Subsequently, each of these barriers produces challenges for nurses and nursing. Current issues in the provision of nursing care to First Nations in Canada include the following:

- significance of population demographics in relation to the healthcare needs of First Nations
- effect of transfer of healthcare services and community development as a climate for change in providing nursing care to First Nations, including issues faced by nurses
- the need to develop cultural competence in providing meaningful nursing care to First Nations through education, research, and practice
- barriers to accessing services in the healthcare system
- scarcity of First Nations people in the health professions.

Population Demographics

First Nations people are demographically distinctive from the Canadian population. Compared to the Canadian population, significant growth of the registered Indian population (First Nations) is projected well into the future (Indian and Northern Affairs Canada, 2007). Under the medium growth scenario, the total population in Canada entitled to Indian registration is expected to increase by 40% during the period from 2004 to 2029. In addition, the First Nation population will remain extremely youthful in comparision to the Canadian population. During this period, the registered Indian population 15 years of age will decrease from 32% to 24% and the registered Indian population 45 years of age will increase from 21% to 32%. In contrast, about 49% of the Canadian population will be age 45 years or more in the year 2029.

In addition, during this same period, the registered Indian population living on-reserve is projected to rise by about 62%, whereas the registered Indian population living off-reserve is projected to increase by about 12%. Fertility and mortality are some factors affecting current and projected First Nations population growth. The contrast between First Nations and the general population within the scope of current and projected population growth provides a basis for developing an understanding about the healthcare needs of First Nations people.

Regional variations exist in projected population growth among First Nations communities. The overall expected population growth is most prominent in the prairie provinces, whereas declining off-reserve First Nations population are projected in British Columbia and the provinces east of Manitoba. In addition to regional variation, knowledge about the migration patterns of young First Nations women to and from reserves can affect the nature of healthcare services provided both on and off the reserves. Demographic profiling serves as a valuable frame of reference within which to determine appropriate healthcare programming now and in the future.

Fertility and mortality affect the age and sex configuration among First Nations people. Although higher than in the general population, First Nations fertility has been declining since the 1960s. This decline is attributed to the use of contraceptives. Consequently, the size of Aboriginal families is decreasing numerically, and native women are having children later and spacing them farther apart (Romaniuc, cited in Norris, 2000, p. 175; Indian and Northern Affairs Canada, 2007).

Mortality rates for First Nations have declined since the turn of the 20th century. However, the life expectancy of First Nations members continues to be shorter than that of the general population (Canadian Population Health Initiative, 2004). In 2039, the life expectancy in the general Canadian population was 76 years for men and 82 years for women, with cancer being the leading cause of potential years of life lost (PYLL) in 1999. However, in 2000, the life expectancy in First Nations communities was 69 years for men and 77 years for women, with injuries as the leading cause of PYLL. PYLL between ages 0 and 74 years is an indicator used to illustrate the effects of premature death on the population.

The increase of First Nations people's life expectancy is due to the decrease in infant mortality and the influx of Bill C-31 registrants, who tended to be relatively young. In the early 1900s, about 25% of First Nations infants died within 1 year of their births (Norris, 2000). The infant mortality rate continues to be higher among First Nations than among the Canadian population. Infant mortality rate includes all births under 500 grams, and deaths are per 1,000 live births. The infant mortality rate for the registered Indian population was 7.2 in 2001 compared to 5.2 for the total Canadian population (Indian and Northern Affairs Canada, 2005). Infant, child, and teenage health programs are essential to prevent chronic diseases, such as type II diabetes and heart disease, from developing during the middle years in First Nations adults.

Bill C-31 is the prelegislation name of the 1985 Act to Amend the Indian Act. This amended act eliminated certain discriminatory provisions of the Indian Act, including the section that resulted in Indian women losing their Indian status when they married non-Indian men. Bill C-31 enabled people affected by the discriminatory provisions of the old Indian Act to apply to have their status restored. Since 1985, about 105,000 people have successfully regained their Indian status (Department of Indian Affairs and Northern Development, 1997). Bill C-31 contributes to the population growth of First Nations. However, the net effect of migration (in-migrants minus out-migrants) is far less significant.

Most First Nations members who migrate do so between cities and reserves (Norris, 2000; Indian and Northern Affairs Canada, 2007). Migration of registered Indian people is a dynamic process that constitutes bidirectional movement between reserves and large urban centres, rather than simply as migration into cities. Specifically, of those who migrated between 1991 and 1996, about 60% moved from reserves to urban areas and about 70% moved from the cities to the reserves. More First Nations people are moving to the reserves, and, as a result, reserves are serving more people. However, this gain is relatively small in relation to the reserve population. Norris (2000) surmises after the examination of the Department of Indian Affairs and Northern Development's 1996 Indian Register and adjusted census data that about 60% of registered First Nations people live on reserves. The initial percentage was adjusted for undercoverage and incomplete enumeration of reserves. The extent to which First Nations people migrate to and from reserves affects the health needs of First Nations, both on and off reserves.

Young First Nations women are similar to the general population and other Aboriginal groups in that they tend to be the most mobile in a population (Norris, 2000, p. 184). In 1996, First Nations women, especially those between the ages of 15 and 24 years, migrated from reserves to urban areas significantly more so than did men of the same age range. Women who attend postsecondary education influence this pattern. According to an analysis of 1996 Census data, it appears that women, younger families, and lone-parent families are over-represented in the migrant population, especially among those moving to the urbans centres. Consequently, this migration is contributing to larger concentrations of lone-parent families among the Aboriginal population in several major Canadian cities.

Nursing Issues Related to Transfer of Healthcare Services

Many nurses who are employed by First Nations communities that are administering their own healthcare services state the professional administrative structure and standards could no longer be guaranteed in their practice (ANAC, 1995, 2001a, 2001b). When the administration of healthcare services is transferred from Health Canada to a First Nations community, nursing service delivery also becomes the responsibility of that community. However, many communities were inadequately prepared through the transfer process to organize an effective system of nursing services (ANAC, 2000). Subsequently, nursing service structure and processes for supporting nurses at the community level were developed on an individual community or tribal council basis (ANAC, 2001b). The ANAC held nursing roundtables across Canada from 1986 to 1995 in which band-employed nurses clearly identified key issues surrounding health transfer, the delivery of nursing services, and the health of First Nations people in communities. Over the years, as communities completed the transfer process, these concerns became reality to the nurses.

In "Issues Verification: Current Nursing Workplace Issues and Best Practices in Aboriginal Communities: A Literature Review and Analysis," ANAC (2002a) compiled the main workplace issues in the contemporary context by examining literature, surveys, reports, and other information ranging from the time of band nurse workshops to the present. One conclusion, in particular, was clear: Issues that were articulated more than 10 years ago at the ANAC Band Nurse Workshops continue to be pertinent. Indeed, they have now been identified as requiring strategic planning and research in the area of best practices. Issues related to transfer are identified in the following reports of the ANAC:

- "Developing Best Practice Environments. Best Practice Model Development in Aboriginal Communities. Final Report." 2002b.
- "Supervision of Nurses in First Nation Communities: What Are the Gaps? A Literature Review and Analysis. Final Report." January 2002c.
- "Community Orientation for Newly Employed Nurses. Components of a First Nations Community Orientation Template. Final Report." March 2002d.

Since the Indian Health Transfer policy was initiated in 1986, more than 40% of communities that were eligible have signed agreements for the health transfer initiatives. Although Health Canada has the structure and organization for delivering nursing services, First Nations communities had neither the experience and expertise to develop them nor the financial resources to implement them.

Some key components for nursing services are nursing management and supervision, orientation, ongoing education, professional development, and a system of performance appraisal and evaluation. Substantive liability coverage and standards to practise nursing in the advanced role are also required to be available to nursing personnel. Standards of practice are established and regulated by professional nursing organizations. Only a few provincial professional nursing organizations have developed guidelines for use by employers and nurses to address advanced nursing practice.

A lack of understanding regarding the infrastructure required for nursing services may have been partly due to a shift in understanding about jurisdiction, self-government, and the role of the Medical Services Branch (MSB) of Health Canada. It was apparent that the nursing services department that was in place before transfer initiatives did not meet the nursing service needs of a transferred community. Communities gained through trial and error; others may have had the resources to redesign nursing services for their communities. Many communities engaged in the transfer process in isolation and so struggled to create effective community-based nursing services.

In the "Survey of Nurses in Isolated First Nations Communities: Recruitment and Retention Issues" (ANAC, 2000), several leaders from First Nations, who were considering transfer or were in pretransfer stages, and First Nations authorities, who had taken over management of nursing services, provided their suggestions and recommendations to address conditions successfully. One of these was to create mechanisms for First Nations authorities to exchange information and facilitate mutual learning and collaboration as they go through the transfer process. For example, the development of best practice models is one way of sharing solutions between communities and nurses. ANAC has identified a number of key issues directly related to the transfer of healthcare to First Nations communities:

1. Nurses, their employers, and professional nursing associations lack understanding about liability coverage as it pertains to scope of practice. Nursing legislation differs from province to province on the degree of protection provided to nurses who are functioning in advanced nursing practice. What are the implications of this legislation for nurses and employers?

2. Nurses are uncertain about how to support the community in which they are employed in the design of new program initiatives. Many transferred communities choose to take on this type of initiative by reallocating community funds. However, many First Nations communities consider the incorporation of cultural and traditional knowledge into these new health and healing systems as being desirable but unattainable. This unattainability is largely because of the cost of such initiatives and lack of personnel who have the skills to help the community create these kinds of systems.

3. Nurses who are newly employed in a First Nations community are unclear about the manner in which they can become involved with the community, which can be a challenge for the nurse because community members may view nurses as being part of the Western healthcare system. Or they may see that nurses "parachute" into a community to work only for a short time, and then they are gone. The legacy of colonization and illness prevail in some communities, and in others, only remnants are evident.

4. Nurses are not clear about the jurisdictions within which First Nations authorities are operating when considering the delivery of various community programs. In some cases, the jurisdiction rests with the First Nations government, whereas in other cases it may be the federal government. How does a nurse determine where the accountability for a program lies?

5. In some First Nations communities, the nurse reports to a non-nursing supervisor, such as the director of health. The nurse, supervisor, and community leadership may not be aware of the ramifications of this practice. There is potential that the supervisor may lack understanding about the role and function of nurses and may overrule nursing decisions, potentially eroding quality care.

6. Nurses may not be aware that nurse managers are key to creating effective community-based nursing services. Their role is pivotal in working with community leadership, health service directors, community members, and nursing staff to create mechanisms for effective quality nursing care.

Other issues that have been identified include the following:

1. Some band-employed nurses do not believe they have the respect of the community in which they are employed. This lack of respect is evident when there is interference with the nurses' decisions.

2. The retention of nurses in First Nations communities depends on the quality of the practice environment. What are the key elements that need to be in place to ensure this quality is retained in the community workplace?

3. The employers of nurses may not be aware of the need for professional performance appraisal and evaluation.

Cultural Competence and Effective Healthcare Programming

For many nurses, working with First Nations presents an opportunity to provide nursing care in a culture different from one's own. This opportunity, in turn, creates other opportunities to positively affect nurse–patient relationships. Community development principles can affect the development of relationships with a community's leadership and its members (Shuster et al., 2001). Nurses who see themselves as partners with a community recognize that the strengths of the community will form a basis for organizing and improving the health of that community. The development of this kind of relationship could be profound for nurses as well as empowering and liberating for community members. This opportunity for deeper understanding and patience will help to convey an attitude that will foster the kind of relationship that First Nations patients would find helpful as they manage their healthcare needs.

Cultural competence includes an understanding of the perspectives and behaviors patients have about health and illness, family healthcare decisions, treatment expectations, and compliance with healthcare treatment plans (Lester, 1998). Cultural competence moves away from viewing how patients can fit into the nurses' world and way of doing things to examining how nurses may understand and fit into the patient's world (St. Clair & McKenry, 1999). Nursing research reinforces these elements of culturally competent approaches in the prevention and treatment of chronic disease among Aboriginal people. For example, programming and services must take into account the historical, social, and cultural factors surrounding chronic disease (Gregory et al., 1999). Having this understanding influences how one will approach each patient within a community.

Nurse–patient relationships are affected by the perceptions that community members have about nurses and the nursing profession. First Nations people consider nurses and other healthcare providers to be a part of a healthcare system rooted in colonization. Indeed, elements of colonization continue today and affect nurse–patient relationships, in turn positively or negatively affecting access to healthcare services by First Nations members.

Access to Services

First Nations people experience a sense of isolation and marginalization when using general Canadian healthcare services (Dion Stout, Kipling, & Stout, 2001; Saunders, 1999). These experiences prompt many First Nations people to use healthcare services unwillingly or to avoid using them at all. A sense of isolation begins with having to leave one's home and community and, in many cases, travel great distances to access health services for specialized treatment. These distances tend to be geographic, but there are other kinds of distances, too: A key issue identified in the literature on Aboriginal health is that Aboriginal people face racism, prejudice, and insensitivity from the healthcare professionals from whom they are seeking services (ANAC, 2000; Royal Commission on Aboriginal Peoples, 1996c).

One method to ensure that comprehensive care is available to First Nations people is to assess their experiences with mainstream healthcare services. After the barriers and supports for patients have been identified, health policies and practices can be instituted to provide equitable services to all patients. The effectiveness of nurse–patient communication can impose or remove barriers for persons seeking care. Dion Stout and colleagues (2001) compiled findings from the National Workshop on Aboriginal Women's Health Research held in Ottawa, in March 2001, and from results of research affiliated with the Centres of Excellence of Women's Health and Women's Health Bureau of Canada. Some of the most important findings include the following:

1. In an exploration of barriers and supports encountered by pregnant and parenting women entering addiction programs in Vancouver and Prince George, British Columbia, Poole and Isaac (2001) made a series of recommendations to redress the stigma, shame, and prejudice experienced by substance-abusing mothers and pregnant women. A number of supports were identified, ranging from those provided by families to those provided by healthcare professionals.

2. An assessment of the positive and negative aspects of Aboriginal women's experiences with mainstream healthcare services was completed in the Carrier First Nation reserve community (Browne, Fiske, & Thomas, 2000). Health professionals were respectful of this community's cultural heritage and shared knowledge and decision making with patients about their healthcare. However, health professionals also learned that they dismissed or trivialized the women's concerns, judged in stereotypical negative ways, or demonstrated no regard for the patients' personal circumstances. The adoption of health policies and practices that incorporated the concept of cultural safety was among the recommendations made to address these concerns. Evaluation of other health service programs identified the following items as areas to address:

- the importance of asking the Aboriginal clientele themselves about their needs and priorities in accessing healthcare services
- the need to provide support in tandem with services
- the need for culturally appropriate services
- the use of patient health outcomes as indicators for effective services
- the need to be familiar with the socioeconomic issues relevant to patients
- the development of awareness of the daily living contexts of patients
- a knowledge of the history of community social supports.

3. An assessment of the degree to which the service needs of Aboriginal women were met by the Vancouver Native Health Society located in downtown Eastside of Vancouver, British Columbia, was carried out by Benoit and Carroll (2001). Interviews with service providers and a series of focus groups with Aboriginal women helped researchers to identify a number of access barriers, including the following:

- a lack of sufficient security and anonymity while accessing clinic services
- the use of western approaches to counseling and the exclusion of more traditional Aboriginal forms of healing
- a general lack of female healthcare providers on staff.

Guidelines and policy statements originating with health professional organizations can provide insight and significant information about developing culturally appropriate relationships with Aboriginal people. Statements (Smylie, 2001) that have been developed in collaboration with Aboriginal people and endorsed by the national Aboriginal organizations add credibility to the content of the documents. Ethically, nurses are bound to respect culturally diverse clients (Canadian Nurses Association, 2002).

According to the College of Nurses of Ontario, patient-centered care requires that nurses recognize the patient's culture, the nurse's culture, and how both impact the nurse–patient relationship. Consequently, culturally sensitive care is the recognition of the similarities and differences between the patient's culture and that of the nurse. Nurses enhance their ability to provide patient-centered care by reflecting on how their own values and beliefs impact the relationship (College of Nurses of Ontario, 1999).

SUMMARY

Nursing in First Nations communities presents many challenges. At the forefront is the need to understand indigenous history, starting from the time when only First Peoples inhabited North America. The relationship of First Nations with the Crown of England and, later, the government of Canada beginning with the treaties and then the Indian Act, the goal of colonization to obliterate First Nations peoples' cultures and assimilate them into mainstream society, and First Nations' cultural resurgence and determination to obtain self-government are important parts of this history.

Both community development and transfer of healthcare services are integral to the development of culturally specific community health and healing systems. Population health is a way of identifying determinants of health to address inequities in healthcare. Nurses are also challenged to understand the relationship between population demographics and the development of relevant health programs. Nursing issues related to the transfer of healthcare services to First Nations communities will require critical analysis and collaborative efforts to effect optimal resolutions.

Add to your knowledge of this issue:	Online
Aboriginal Nurses Association of Canada	www.anac.on.ca
Assembly of First Nations	www.afn.ca
Educational Links—Pathfinders—Native Studies	http://www2.kpr.edu.on.ca/lvc/ lib/native.htm#Weblinks
Census 2006: Aboriginal Peoples in Canada in 2006	www12.statcan.ca/English/census06/ release/aboriginal/cfm
Indian and Northern Affairs Canada	www.ainc-inac.gc.ca/pr/pub/ywtk/ index_e.html
National Aboriginal Health Organization	www.naho.ca
Population Health Approach	www.phac-aspc.gc.ca/ph-sp/index.thml
Report of the Royal Commission on Aboriginal Peoples	ainc-inac.gc.ca/ch/rcap/index_e.html

REFLECTIONS on the Chapter...

1 How have teachings regarding First Nations healthcare been included in your nursing program? Where are you able to obtain further information?

2 Using the determinants of health, examine the impact on the health of First Nations members and their communities.

3 Name four healthcare needs in First Nations communities. What are some strategies for dealing with them?

4 Using First Nations demographic data, determine two health issues that could become priorities by the year 2020.

5 Identify four approaches that will enhance nurse–patient communication with a First Nations person.

References

Aboriginal Nurses Association of Canada (ANAC). (1995). *Band nurse workshops, Halifax, Montreal, Saskatoon, Vancouver: Summary report, March 1995.* Ottawa: Author.

_____. (2000). *Survey of nurses in isolated First Nations communities: Recruitment and retention issues. Final report, September 8, 2000.* Ottawa: Author.

_____. (2001a). *The Aboriginal Nurses Association of Canada Submission to the Canadian Advisory Committee, November 19, 2001.* Ottawa: Author.

_____. (2001b). *Recruitment and retention workshop. Final Report, May 2001.* Ottawa: Author.

_____. (2001c). *Submission to the commission on the future of health care in Canada. Commissioner: Roy J. Romanow, Q. C.* (November 1, 2001). Ottawa: Author.

_____. (2002a). *Issues verification: Current nursing workplace issues and best practices in aboriginal communities: A literature review and analysis.* Ottawa: Author.

_____. (2002b). *Developing best practice environments* [Online]. Retrieved from http://www.anac.on.ca/ publications.html.

_____. (2002c). *Supervision of nurses in First Nations communities: What are the gaps?* [Online]. Retrieved from http://www.anac.on.ca/publications.html.

_____. (2002d). *Community orientation for newly employed nurses* [Online]. Retrieved from http://www.anac.on.ca/ publications.html.

Adelson, N. (1991). "Being alive well": The praxis of Cree health. *Arctic Medical Research, 50* (Suppl.), 230–232.

Benoit, C. & Carroll, D. (2001). *Marginalized voices from the downtown eastside: Aboriginal women speak about their health experiences.* Toronto: National Network on Environments and Health.

Berger, T.R. (1980). *Report of the Advisory Commission on Indian and Inuit Health Consultation.* Indian and Northern Affairs. Ottawa: Government of Canada.

Browne, A., Fiske, J., & Thomas, G. (2000). *First Nations women's encounters with mainstream health care services and systems.* Vancouver: British Columbia Centre of Excellence for Women's Health.

Canadian Nurses Association. (2002). *Code of ethics for registered nurses.* Ottawa: Author.

Canadian Population Health Initiative. (2004). Improving the health of Canadians. Ottawa: Canadian Institute for Health Information.

Cassidy, F. & Bish, R. (1989). *Indian government: Its meaning and practice.* Oolichan Books: Institute for Research on Public Policy: Lantzville.

College of Nurses of Ontario. (1999). *A guide to nurses for providing culturally sensitive care for registered nurses and registered practical nurses in Ontario.* Toronto: Author.

Department of Indian Affairs and Northern Development. (1997). Definitions [Online]. Retrieved from http://www. ainc-inac.gc.ca/pr/pub/cana/def_e.html.

Dickason, O.P. (1994). *Canada's First Nations: A history of founding peoples from earliest times.* Toronto: McClelland & Stewart.

Dion Stout, M., Kipling, G.D., & Stout, R. (2001). *Aboriginal women's health research, synthesis project.* Final report. Centres of Excellence for Women's Health Program, Women's Health Bureau, Health Canada. Ottawa: Government of Canada.

Evans, R.G., Barer, M.L., & Marmor, R. (Eds.). (1994). *Why are some people healthy and others not? The determinants of health of populations.* New York: Aldine de Gruyter.

Frideres, J.S. & Gadacz, R. (2005). *Aboriginal peoples in Canada.* Toronto: Pearson Prentice Hall.

Gregory, D., Whalley, W., & Olson, J., et al. (1999). Exploring the experience of type 2 diabetes in urban aboriginal people. *Canadian Journal of Nursing Research, 31*(1), 101–115.

Hamilton, A.C. & Sinclair, C.M. (1991). *Report of the aboriginal justice inquiry of Manitoba: Vol. 1. The justice system and aboriginal people.* Winnipeg: Queen's Printer.

Health Canada. (1999a). *A second diagnostic on the health of First Nations and Inuit People in Canada* [Online]. Indian and Northern Affairs Canada. Available from www.ainc-inac.gc.ca/pr/pub/ywtk/index_e.html.

_____. (1999b). *Ten years of health transfer. First Nation and Inuit control. April 1989–March 1999.* Ottawa: Minister of Public Works and Government Services Canada.

_____. (2002). *First Nations and Inuit control.* Annual Report 2001–2002. Retrieved April 24, 2005 from http://www.hc-sc.gc.ca/fnib/bpm/hfa/fnic_annual_report_2001_2002.htm.

Indian and Northern Affairs Canada. Retrieved April 24, 2005, from http://www.ainc-inac.gc.ca/index_e.html.

Indian and Northern Affairs Canada. (2007). *Registered Indian demography. Population, household, and family projections, 2004–2029.* Retrieved July 16, 2008 from http://www.ainc-inac.gc.ca/pr/ra/abd-eng-pdf.

Lemphers, C. (1998). Perspective. Northern nursing: A type of advanced nursing practice. *AARN Newsletter, 54*(1), 11, 23.

Lester, N. (1998). *Cultural competence: A nursing dialogue.* Part one of a two-part article based on a roundtable discussion. *American Journal of Nursing, 98*(8), 26–34.

Malloch, L. (1989). Indian medicine, Indian health. Study between red and white medicine. *Canadian Woman Studies, 10*(2 & 3), 105–112.

McFarlane, P. (2000). Aboriginal leadership. In D. Long & O.P. Dickason (Eds.), *Visions of the heart, Canadian aboriginal issues* (2nd ed.). Toronto: Harcourt Canada.

Milloy, J.S. (1991). The early Indian Acts. In J.R. Miller (Ed.), *Sweet promises: A reader on Indian–White relations in Canada* (pp. 145–154). Toronto: University of Toronto Press.

Norris, M.J. (2000). Aboriginal peoples in Canada: Demographic and linguistic perspectives. In D. Long & O.P. Dickason (Eds.), *Visions of the heart, Canadian aboriginal issues* (2nd ed., pp. 167–236). Toronto: Harcourt Canada.

O'Neil, J., Lemchuk-Favel, L., & Allard, Y., et al. (1999). Community healing and aboriginal self-government. In J.H. Hylton (Ed.), *Aboriginal self-government in Canada* (pp. 130–156). Saskatoon, Saskatchewan: Purich.

Poole, N. & Issac, B. (2001). *Apprehensions: Barriers to treatment for substance-using mothers.* Vancouver: British Columbia Centre of Excellence for Women's Health.

Ray, A.J. (1974). *Indians in the fur trade: Their role as trappers, hunters, and middlemen in the lands southwest of Hudson Bay 1660–1870.* Toronto: University of Toronto Press.

Royal Commission on Aboriginal Peoples. (1996a). *Report on the Royal Commission on Aboriginal Peoples. Vol. 1, Chap. 9.1: Protection of the reserve land base* [Online]. Ottawa: Government of Canada. Retrieved April 23, 2005 from http://www.ainc-inac.gc.ca/ch/rcap/index_e.html.

_____. (1996b). *Report on the Royal Commission on Aboriginal Peoples. Vol. 2: Restructuring the relationship* [Online]. Ottawa: Government of Canada. Available from http://www.ainc-inac.gc.ca/ch/rcap/index_e.html.

_____. (1996c). *Report on the Royal Commission on Aboriginal Peoples. Vol. 3: Gathering strength.* Ottawa: Government of Canada. Available from http://www.ainc-inac.gc.ca/ch/rcap/index_e.html.

Saunders, W. (1999). Cultural sensitivity, a matter of respect. *Canadian Nurse, 95*(9), 43–44.

Shah, C. (1998). *Public health and preventive medicine* (4th ed.). Toronto: University of Toronto.

Shuster, S., Ross, S., & Bhagat, R., et al. (2001). Using community development approaches. *Canadian Nurse, 97*(6), 18–22.

Smylie, J. (2000). Society of Obstetricians and Gynaecologists policy statement. A guide for health professional working with Aboriginal peoples: The sociocultural context of Aboriginal peoples in Canada. *Journal for Society of Obstetricians and Gynaecologists, 100,* 1070–1081.

_____. (2001). Society of Obstetricians and Gynaecologists policy statement. A guide for health professionals working with Aboriginal peoples: Cross cultural understanding. *Journal for Society of Obstetricians and Gynaecologists, 100,* 157–167.

St. Clair, A. & McKenry, L. (1999). Preparing culturally competent practitioners. *Journal of Nursing Education, 38*(5), 228–234.

Stewart, N., D'Arcy, C., & Pitblado, R., et al. (2005). *Report of the national survey of nursing practice in rural and remote Canada.* Retrieved July 10, 2008 from http://www.nuralnursing. unbc.ca/reports/study/SurveyReportEnglish.pdf.

Tobias, J.L. (1991). Protection, civilization, assimilation: An outline history of Canada's Indian policy. In J.R. Miller (Ed.), *Sweet promises: A reader on Indian-White relations in Canada* (pp. 127–144). Toronto: University of Toronto Press.

Venne, S. (1997). Understanding Treaty 6: An indigenous perspective. In M. Asch (Ed.), *Aboriginal and treaty rights in Canada. Essays on law, equality, and respect for difference* (pp. 172–207). Vancouver: UBC Press.

Waldram, J., Herring, D.A., & Young, T.K. (2006). *Aboriginal health in Canada: Historical, cultural, and epidemiological perspectives.* Toronto: University of Toronto Press.

Young, K. (1984). Indian health services in Canada: A sociohistorical perspective. *Social Science and Medicine 18*(3), 257–264.

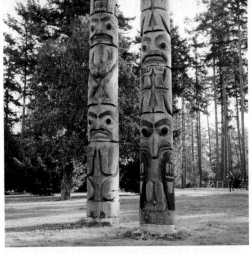

Totems on the University of Victoria campus. (Used with permission, University of Victoria.)

Opening Conversations: Dilemmas and Possibilities of Spirituality and Spiritual Care

Anne Bruce

Critical Questions

As a way of engaging with the ideas in this chapter, consider the following:

1. What are the different ways we speak of our spiritual natures and our philosophies of life? What makes your life worth living?

2. If faced with a life-limiting illness, what do you think you might identify as most important in your life?

3. In the ordinariness of your days, what do you yearn for? Do you see yearning as linked to health?

Chapter Objectives

After completing this chapter, you will be able to:

1. Understand the relevance of spirituality for nursing practice.

2. Reflect on your own assumptions about the meaning of spirituality and the effects of these assumptions in your practice of spiritual care.

3. Articulate barriers to providing spiritual care.

4. Generate possibilities for meeting the mandate of providing spiritual care to patients and families.

INTRODUCTION TO THE TOPIC: OPENING THE CONVERSATION ABOUT SPIRITUALITY

Spiritual is that part of human beings that is responsive to beauty, searches after truth, appreciates kindness and compassion, accepts the obligations to care for fellow beings, motivates our efforts, energizes our lives, and opens the gates to laughter and tears. Spirit has little to do with religion, or as much, as he or she who has it, wishes.

Bevis & Waston, 1989

Spirituality is difficult to contain within language. Some authors see spirituality as a personal journey of discovering meaning and purpose in life (Hermann, 2006). Others feel spirituality as a force like the wind that cannot be seen but is always felt (Cavendish et al., 2004). And yet others hear spirituality in the whispers of forest groves or in music and in the silences before words. I acknowledge a view that no single understanding of spirituality can adequately embrace all human experience (Box 25.1) and yet also recognize that the practice of nurses includes accompanying people during birth, old age, sickness, and death. As nurses, we engage with people during times of extreme vulnerability—when opportunities for spiritual awareness present themselves, and we are called to cultivate our capacities and willingness to engage openly with people at a spiritual level; this I see as integral to nursing practice.

This chapter introduces spirituality and spiritual care in nursing as both a topic of interest and a conundrum with multiple dimensions, dilemmas, and possibilities. As an issue, spirituality is of widespread concern to the general public and poses challenges for nursing practice as we grapple with nurses' roles and capacities in providing spiritual care. However, unlike nursing problems that can commonly be resolved with adequate analysis and consultation, spirituality as a nursing issue is not seen as something to be solved but rather as a multifaceted topic that requires personal awareness, critical analyses, and the powers of curiosity and "unknowing" to open possibilities for understanding and engaging spiritual connectedness.

My intention in writing this chapter is to open a conversation about what I identify as some of the relevant questions that emerge with the topic of spirituality and spiritual care in nursing practice. The purpose is not to convince you, the reader, of anything at all about spirituality but rather to open spaces for you to wonder about and to explore the meaning that the topic of spirituality holds in your nursing practice. My belief is that we bring ourselves to each encounter with clients. Although this may seem an obvious and taken-for-granted idea, the notion that we accompany ourselves to practice holds within it important assumptions that are central to the writing and reading of this chapter.

BOX 25.1 How Other People May Refer to Spirituality

Philosophy of life	Connection
	Love
Search for meaning	Peace
	Contentment
Inner resources	Personal strength
Personal beliefs	Religious beliefs/practices
Faith	Opening to the universe
Relationship with a higher power/god/goddess/nature	

SITUATING THE TOPIC: PERSONAL AND PROFESSIONAL ASSUMPTIONS

Each of us comes to the conversation about spirituality with a history and a particular "situatedness" in the world. Our history is constructed of past experiences, beliefs, and values that have brought us to our current understandings of spirituality. From this position, I hold assumptions about the place and purpose of spirituality in my own life and in the lives of others (Box 25.2). These assumptions are present in my nursing practice. Although some people may believe that we can extricate ourselves as nurses from ourselves as people, it is not always clear that we can or would even want to do this. And so, our assumptions about spirituality and spiritual care are with us in our conversations and in the practice of spirituality and nursing. At this juncture, it may be useful to contemplate the assumptions that are present for you as you engage with this chapter, assumptions derived from your personal and professional histories and your current "situatedness" in the world.

SITUATING THE TOPIC: UNDERSTANDING SPIRITUAL PRACTICES HISTORICALLY

As well as the individual assumptions that accompany us to this conversation, our understandings of spirituality and, in particular, our understandings of the dilemmas that arise when considering spirituality in nursing practice are influenced by the ways in which spirituality and nursing have intermingled historically. You might wonder what this history has to do with your current nursing practice. I would suggest that our history is, in a sense, inescapable and that, although historical practice may not be clearly visible, it remains present and influences the ways in which nursing is understood by nurses and others.

The history of nursing in the Western world has a close alliance with spirituality and spiritual practices. Long before the era of Florence Nightingale, credited with the founding of modern Western nursing, individuals who were organized around religious or spiritual ideals practised care of the sick. According to Nelson (1995), a nurse scholar and historian, nursing's inception can be traced backward through the 19th-century Sisters of Mercy and Sisters of Charity and the 17th-century origins of the Daughters of Charity to the early Christian doctrine of St. Benedict, who elevated the care of the sick as service imbued with spiritual value. Nightingale is said to have studied with the Daughters of Charity in Paris, France, and to have "learned from them, how to become, and how to form a nurse" (Nelson, 1995, p. 37). Nightingale's so-called secular schools of nursing ascribed to ideals originating with Christian ideology. The influence of particular spiritual ideals is readily recognizable in our Canadian nursing history, in which the earliest organized nursing practice arrived in the form of Augustine nuns from France in August 1639, centuries before a Nightingale-model nursing school was established in Canada in June 1874. "For the Augustine nuns, caring and healing work was central to their Christian beliefs" (Carr, 2003, p. 472). The "training regimen" of Nightingale's schools and of

BOX 25.2 Personal Assumptions

The lens through which I view the world is multihued. In part, my world view is shaped by my connection with the natural world and, in part, by my interest and practice in Buddhist interpretations of life and suffering.

nursing schools well into the 20th century sought to build capacity in nursing students for service and duty, building on a thinly veiled Christian morality.

Nelson (1995) asserts that Christian doctrine remains embedded in particular nursing discourse, now reinscribed as ideologies of humanism. "Humanism in nursing has resurrected the religious discourse and the spiritual dimension of nursing . . . Salvation has been redrafted to self-actualization" (Nelson, 1995, p. 37). Entire nursing curricula embrace humanism's ideals as foundational to nursing practice: valuing individual uniqueness, empowerment, freedom, and the caring relationship. Perhaps the most visible reinterpretation of spirituality in nursing from the 20th century onward is the widely held and seldom-critiqued ideal of nursing practice as a "holistic" endeavor.

This cursory look at the history of the alliance of nursing and spirituality is important for a number of reasons, not the least of which is the recognition of the position from which this history has been written. Much of what we take to be an unbiased account of our past can also be understood as an interpretation of historical proceedings, recorded through the lens of people who are situated within particular social, cultural, political, and spiritual realities. Our nursing history has been written and interpreted from a position of Eurocentrism, in this case meaning that history has been interpreted through a Western world perspective that privileges Judeo-Christian ideology. Embedded in this position is the notion that kindness, compassion, charity, faith, hope, and service are primarily Christian attributes. And yet would we actually believe this when faced with the unspoken but implicit assumptions that kindness and compassion originated with Christianity or that these attributes are not esteemed in spiritual, philosophical, or social knowledge systems quite unrelated to Judeo-Christian ideology? How might nursing's history be understood differently through the lens of other positions in the world, positions that have been less privileged in the recorded history of the Western world?

SIGNIFICANCE OF THE TOPIC FOR NURSING: EMBRACING THE TENSIONS

Several considerations underlie the relevance of spiritual practice for nurses, including our position of access to patients' lives during times of spiritual crisis or suffering, the subscription of nursing discourse to "holistic care," and a growing mandate to categorize and account for spiritual care.

As was highlighted in the introduction to this chapter, nurses often have opportunities to be with people during birth, old age, sickness, and death, and, as nurses, we have privileged access to people during times of extreme vulnerability—when opportunities for spiritual awareness present themselves. These opportunities do not necessarily announce themselves as spiritual crises or awakenings, prompting us to plan for or execute "spiritual care," but they unfold in the ordinariness of days and evenings and nights, when we as nurses are already present and engaged with patients as they live out their lives. It is with the knowledge that these occurrences are surely and repeatedly lived by patients and families and nurses that we are invited to cultivate our capacities and willingness to engage openly with people at a spiritual level.

A "holistic" approach to nursing practice is a central tenet in many nursing school curricula and is embedded in the philosophies of practice of countless individual nurses. One interpretation of the beliefs underlying holistic practice is "the mind, body and spirit are interdependent; the human spirit is the core of the person; a person's attitude and beliefs toward life are major etiological factors in health and disease" (Freeman, 2004, p. 165). In spite of the predominant understanding of holistic practice as inclusive of spiritual practices, many nurses do not feel adequately prepared to provide spiritual care to patients—and spiritual aspects of care are poorly represented in Canadian nursing school curricula (McLeod & Wright, 2008; Olson et al., 2003).

Last, the relevance of spiritual practice in nursing is underscored when we recognize the provision of spiritual care as mandated both ethically and through overt and pragmatic means. The

Canadian Nurses Association (CNA) "Code of Ethics" asserts that nurses "take into account the biological, psychological, social, cultural and spiritual needs of persons in health care" (Canadian Nurses Association, 2002, p. 13). The impetus to attend to spiritual care grows as practicing nurses face increasing pressure to categorize and document all nursing practice, including practice that is spiritual in nature. For example, the Joint Commission on Accreditation of Healthcare Organizations in the United States now requires that every patient receive spiritual assessment on admission along with appropriate care for those who request it (Taylor, 2003). See Box 25.3.

ARTICULATING THE TOPIC AS AN ISSUE: PRACTICE DILEMMAS

This chapter also invites you into a conversation on the topic of spirituality and nursing practice. I have selected one particular dilemma around which to focus the analysis and conversation. The issue, reflected in the nursing literature on spirituality, is the *gap between positive attitudes toward spiritual care among nurses and the lack of spiritual care that is actually being provided by nurses*. It seems that, although assessing and attending to the spiritual needs of patients and families is valued by nurses, many of us do not feel comfortable doing so.

Analyzing the Issue: Multiple Understandings

There are multiple ways of understanding the tension that arises between the ideal and the reality of spiritual care in nursing practice. Pesut and Thorne (2007) explore one way by analyzing the issue based on understanding spirituality as a personal and private concept that is being brought into the public domain of nursing care. They view spirituality as primarily a personal concept that must now be engaged publicly, and this tension evokes unique dilemmas and ethical risks for nurses. Olsen and coworkers (2003) present another way of analyzing the issue, which will frame the analysis in this chapter. The issue will be analysed by exploring different ways of understanding what contributes to

BOX 25.3 How People May Identify Spiritual Practice

Yoga		Conversation
Meditation		Reminiscing
Prayer		Being in nature
Practising kindness		Chanting
Listening		Singing
Ceremonies	Rituals	Traditional dance
Silence	Solitude	Sacred space
Making offerings		Sharing meals
Reading sacred text		Sacred art
Celebrations		Listening to/making music
Being close to important others		Mantra repetition

the existing discrepancy between the valuing of spirituality in nursing discourse and the inadequacy of nurses' preparation and ability to address spiritual care in practice. I will engage with three understandings, or positions, that inform this issue. Embedded in each of these positions are barriers to, as well as strategies that will promote, resolution. In the following sections I will analyze the following understandings:

1. The nonscientific nature of spirituality does not easily fit within a science-based approach to nursing care (Price, Stevens, & LaBarre, 1995).

2. There is ambiguity about what is included in spiritual care in nursing (Price, Stevens, & LaBarre, 1995).

3. Nurses do not believe they have the knowledge necessary to adequately approach spiritual care (Chadwick & Piles, cited in Olson et al., 2003).

Engaging in a critical conversation about spirituality and spiritual care requires questioning the assumptions embedded within each of these ways of understanding the issue. I situate this discussion in a constructivist view; that is, knowledge is not perceived as unbiased or detached but as always generated, formed, and constructed within particular social, cultural, political, and material realities. This means that knowledge is never neutral but is always developed and situated within a particular view of the world. One approach to making the "situatedness" of knowledge visible is to identify the taken-for-granted assumptions on which the knowledge is shaped or constructed. My intention, then, is not to resolve the challenges of how to provide spiritual care but to analyze and critique the issue with the view of opening spaces for you to develop your own interpretations.

Ways of Understanding: Scientific and Nonscientific

The non-scientific nature of spirituality does not easily fit within a science-based approach to nursing.

Price, Stevens, & LaBarre, 1995

HISTORICAL INFLUENCES OF SCIENCE: PRIVILEGING A DISPIRITED BODY

Although a spiritual heritage has been claimed in nursing, Wojnar and Malinski (2003) suggest that this spiritual legacy has been challenged by the separation of body from spirit in science. Interestingly, this was not always the case, as, when around the 8th century, the body and spirit were established as connected yet separate in the Christian tradition (Burkhardt & Nagai-Jacobson, 2002). Later, in the 17th century, philosopher René Descartes proposed that the body and spirit are mutually exclusive. This belief became accepted in Western thought and paved the way for biologic and medical knowledge to become the dominant scientific view that persists today in many parts of the world. The body became the exclusive domain of science, whereas the spirit and soul were relegated to philosophers, theologians, and priests. The modern era is marked by an unprecedented growth of scientific knowledge and power of the natural sciences. Indeed, natural sciences have been regarded as the zenith of human achievement (Couvalis, 1997).

This view of the world also reinforced oppositional thinking, a view where binaries or opposites are set up, known as *dualism*. In dualism, emphasis is given to separateness rather than to interconnectedness of phenomena. For example, dualistic thinking sees opposite positions of this versus that: science versus nonscience, body versus spirit, and good versus bad, for example. Although oppositional thinking is useful in distinguishing differences and categories, it is often inadequate when addressing complex human experiences. The complexity of human suffering or spirituality, for example, cannot be contained in simple categories. Instead, the messy, ambiguous nature of living and dying, of feeling health within illness, also needs to be acknowledged and valued. However, ambiguity, uncertainty, and unknowing have not often been valued in nursing.

In the name of science, oppositional thinking has become almost uncritically accepted. Scientism, as distinguished from science, is a matter of putting too high a value on science as a branch of learning in comparison with other ways of knowing (Dzurec & Abraham, 1993). With scientism, the belief is that science is the most beneficial form of learning and, as such, it is good for all domains, including spirituality and philosophy, to be placed on a scientific footing. Consequently, we see that scholars claim to have made history, politics, ethics, or aesthetics into a science and assume that these claims of scientific status are desirable (Sorell, 1991). In nursing, Kikuchi and Simmons (1994) provide examples in which nurse researchers attempt to answer philosophical questions such as, "what is the nature of health?" and "what is the purpose of caring?" using exclusively scientific means, thereby demonstrating nursing's vulnerability to scientism. In recent years, however, many of the long-held tenets of science and ways of obtaining knowledge have been questioned. Previously held assumptions about reality and the nature of truth have been challenged both within traditional scientific communities and by feminists, critical theorists, and postmodern thinkers. Even so, science and, perhaps, scientism remain the dominant view within healthcare professions. The dominance of scientific knowledge has led to almost unquestioned acceptance of technology and secularism in social, political, and educational institutions.

Until recently, spirituality as a human phenomenon that is separate from the body and material world has been neglected by scientific inquiry. Increasingly, however, spirituality is receiving scientific attention as the body–mind–spirit split is challenged and shown to be too limited in understanding human health and well-being. Consequently, spirituality is being conceptualized in ways that promote distinctions and measurements that are congruent with the assumptions of scientific world views. Without minimizing the importance of scientific knowledge, the risk of scientism must also be attended to as we see the call in nursing for standardized language and interventions for spiritual care. Clearly, we must avoid the pitfalls of according science a privileged view at the expense of other ways of knowing spirituality, while at the same time valuing the contributions of scientific knowledge.

In analyzing science, it is not my intention to throw out science or situate spirituality in opposition to science. Nevertheless, different ways of generating knowledge will shape our nursing practice differently. Through critical analysis, we can distinguish what kinds of knowledge and practices are left out, which are ignored or perhaps not legitimized, and where particular beliefs and knowledge become dominant.

NATURAL SCIENCE AND HUMAN SCIENCE: DIFFERING APPROACHES TO KNOWLEDGE

In the academic milieu of the early 1980s, nursing attempted to legitimize its position as a discipline of science by privileging the natural sciences of medicine over what became known as human sciences (Johnson & Webber, 2005). The natural sciences support a view where people are made up of different components continuously interacting with one another and the environment. This concept of person as an assemblage of traits and variables is inconsistent with a human science view. A decade later, the mood had changed; nursing science's position on "the person" (as a bio-psycho-social-spiritual being made up of components) was challenged by nurses valuing a human science perspective. Rather than seeing a person with components, the view from a human science perspective sees the person as a complex, evolving being, interconnected with the universe. The personal meanings of people's realities are considered of central importance in the investigations and practices of human science disciplines.

This is not to suggest that there is a single perspective of nursing theory and practice that draws on the human science view. Numerous nursing theories within human science value spirituality in nursing practice, among them the diverse approaches of Jean Watson, Betty Neumann, Martha Rogers, and Rosemarie Parse. Consider the effect that differences in underlying assumptions have on how spirituality is understood and practiced. For example, to view spirituality as a component of a person would lead to different ways of practising than would seeing each person as spirit and spirituality as integral to our nature.

Ways of Understanding: Clarity and Ambiguity

There is ambiguity about what is included in spiritual care in nursing.

Price, Stevens, & LaBarre, 1995

Embedded in this position is an assumption that clarity is required to overcome current ambiguity about what spirituality means in nursing practice. As with the underlying assumption of the first position, a binary of "clarity versus ambiguity" is inferred in the language of this position. That is, it is assumed that clarity concerning spirituality is preferred over the existent situation of multiple and diverse understandings. Is it possible, or even desirable, to construct a single, clear, concise definition of spiritual practice that will adequately encompass all perspectives from ecologic, Aboriginal, religious, and humanistic views as well as from those views that cannot be easily identified? This assumption and its oppositional thinking are challenged as we explore other ways of approaching this dualism. In particular, I will consider differences between and the interdependence of spirituality and religion followed by differences of spiritual experience from conceptual understandings of spirituality.

Religion and Spirituality: Vehicle and Destination

According to Paley (2008), spirituality as a concept separate from particular religions is a relatively recent shift. Nevertheless, it could be said that religion and spirituality are interconnected for some people some of the time, for some people all of time, and for some people none of the time. Given this variability, it seems important to understand them as separate, yet sometimes related, concepts. A great deal of the research before 2000 has examined *religion* and *spirituality* as if they were synonymous (George et al., 2000). Increasingly, however, nurses and others understand the importance of teasing apart the differences between religious traditions and our many interpretations of spirituality. Although religion and spirituality are seen as related concepts, religion is often linked to formal religious institutions whereas spirituality is seen as a broader idea that does not depend on institutional contexts. Religion is like a train journeying through and toward spirituality in which we are cautioned not to mistake the vehicle for the destination (Borysenko, 1999). While for some, spiritual experience is not separate from religious beliefs and practices, this is not the case for many who consider themselves spiritual yet not at all religious.

Spirituality as a Concept and as Lived Experience

Just as religion and spirituality are closely linked, yet also very different, the interdependence of experience and concept can also be made. The nature of spirituality is complex as an experience and as a concept (Wojnar & Malinski, 2003). This distinction between experience and the conceptual representation of experience—how we understand spirituality through language—is rarely distinguished in current discussions of spirituality. Nevertheless, this distinction is important and may assist us in sifting through the many ways of understanding (conceptualizing) spiritual phenomena.

As with experiences of pain, many authors suggest that the experience of spirituality is unique to each person and can only be known by that person. From this perspective, the understanding of a particular person's spirituality is whatever the person says it is. Although our experiences are unique, at the same time there are also common themes and patterns of spiritual understanding that extend across groups of people. Through systematically examining how people describe their experiences, researchers generate categories and theories to better understand this human experience. The caution, however, is to avoid confusing individual experience (of each distinct patient and family) with a generalized understanding generated in concepts about spirituality. In nursing, we require embodied knowledge from the unique experiences of patients and families along with diverse sources of generalized conceptual knowledge, including nursing knowledge and empirical research.

If we accept the assumption that no single expression of spirituality can embrace all human experience, then it cannot reasonably be anticipated that nurses will know how to recognize or interpret the multiple possible expressions of spirituality or spiritual need. However, what nurses can do (and often do very well) is enter into and engage with the unique experiences of patients. From this standpoint, the central questions may not be, "what is spirituality?" but rather "how is spirituality lived between this patient and family and the illness, and how can we engage there with families?" Nurses do not necessarily need to possess broad understandings of religious practices, theology, or cultural studies to provide spiritual care. Instead, nurses can be willing and able to engage patients with spiritual awareness about values, beliefs, and their experiences of illness.

Paterson and Zderad (1976) also emphasize the relationality of nursing in their focus on where nursing happens rather than what it is. "Nursing is an experience lived between human beings" (p. 3) "and is concerned with, 'the between' of nurses and their others" (p. 44). Here, "the between" refers to a merging of nurse–patient boundaries into a space of authentic presence while maintaining one's capacity to question.

> *When I reflect on an act of mine (no matter how simple or complex) that I can unhesitatingly label "nursing," I become aware of it as goal-directed (nurturing) being with and doing for another. The intersubjective or interhuman element, "the between," runs through nursing interactions like an underground stream conveying the nutrients of healing and growth. In everyday practice, we are usually so involved with the immediate demands of our "being with and doing with" the patient that we do not focus on the overshadowed plane of "the between." However, occasionally, in beautiful moments, the interhuman currents are so strong that they flood our conscious awareness. Such rare and rewarding moments of mutual presence remind us of the elusive ever-present "between" (Paterson & Zderad, 1976, pp. 21–22).*

This perspective resonates closely with definitions of spirituality and notions of spiritual care. According to Paterson and Zderad, it is important to explore and describe the nature of in-between experiences. This exploration is significant, according to Paterson and Zderad, if we are to better understand how our interactions with others can have both humanizing and dehumanizing effects.

How we conceptualize spirituality within nursing discourse also shapes our clinical practice. The way we talk and write about spirituality shapes knowledge about the phenomenon—through writing and reading, we are making real, so to speak, and establishing what spirituality is (Boxes 25.4 and 25.5). However, generating knowledge is not done in isolation, and we see healthcare institutions also mandating nurses to provide spiritual care. What conceptualization of spirituality do we want to support and foster? How might we proceed in a healthcare system and society that privileges "interventions" that can be measured and documented? An all-encompassing definition would be congruent with a science-based approach to nursing while the ambiguity of diverse and multiple definitions would more closely reflect differences encountered in people's experiences.

Is it possible to hold a space open in our thinking, where spirit and spirituality in nursing practice are understood in multiple ways, as experience and concept, rather than narrowing our thinking to reach a clear and concise definition? I would suggest that in our wish to find simple definitions to these complex experiences, we risk generalizing and relying too heavily on the power of already privileged religious ideologies in our society. Rather than creating space for a range of spiritual practice, the search for "clarity" can lead us to marginalize, ignore, or trivialize spiritual practices that fall outside of the dominant norm. Perhaps then, developing comfort with the inevitable ambiguity of complex human experiences is also important.

Ways of Understanding: Knowing and Unknowing

> *Nurses do not believe they have the knowledge necessary to adequately approach spiritual care.*
>
> Chadwick and Piles, cited in Olson et al., 2003

BOX 25.4   Reflection Poem

Momentarily awake, pale gray-blue eyes washed out by morphine.
  Pin-point pupils, beady eyes peering into space.
You didn't want this, but are at the mercy of night guardians.
  Well meaning, yet inattentive . . . or unable to see?

"Good morning Martin".
. . . . You startle,
eyes flitting, seeking recognition,
hands grasping invisible objects in space.

"Hi, how are you" you whisper through dentureless jaws.
About to respond, but you're gone
drifting rudderless
  eyes rolling upward
    and away.

Are you able to be present
for the journey?
  You moaned and groaned too loudly,
so they took away
the/ir pain
  and hushed you into slumber
where we cannot go or witness,
you journey there alone . . . .

Source: Bruce, A. (2002). *Abiding in liminal spaces: Inscribing mindful living/dying with(in) end-of-life care.* Unpublished doctoral dissertation, University of British Columbia. Used with permission.

BOX 25.5   Reflection on Nursing

I am aware of the dance between definitive and non-definitive language. Although the question remains, how is this relevant for nursing practice, I hope to elude the pitfall of prescriptive discourse as my intention has always been otherwise. Death is not a problem to be remedied. Accompanying those in this journeying is also seeing the interplay of y/our dying and the limits of pre-scribed 'doing'. . . . . and yet . . . .

Source: Bruce, A. (2002). *Abiding in liminal spaces: Inscribing mindful living/dying with(in) end-of-life care.* Unpublished doctoral dissertation, University of British Columbia. Used with permission.

Without minimizing the question of what nurses need to know to provide spiritual care, I would like to question the underlying assumptions embedded in this third position that infer an emphasis on knowing versus not knowing. Attending to knowledge, as this question implies, renders a valuing of "doing" and knowing in opposition to "being" and not knowing. The following discussion of these tensions may provide alternative ways of looking at spirituality.

The quest to know and define phenomena can be seen as part of a larger ideology or belief system. As mentioned, the model for generating nursing knowledge and practice has been embedded within a discourse of science. Although this model is changing, the push toward standardization of spiritual care and measurements of spirituality illustrates both the usefulness and continued dominance of this view. Once again, the issue is not that different ways of knowing are beneficial but rather that we need to be aware of and question the privileging of particular views at the expense of others. One such privileging arises in valuing knowing over unknowing and is explored here for other possible interpretations.

Unknowing as a Way of Knowing

Recognizing different modes of reality (such as spirit as supernatural) is difficult within the limited scope of language and ways of knowing in science (Wilber, 1998; Wolfer, 1993). For example, conventional scientific knowledge focuses on what is said, thereby excluding what is unsaid, or unsayable. By concentrating on what is certain and knowable, we often exclude the ambiguous, unknowable, and paradoxical. Conventional models of scientific knowledge depend on exclusion and function to privilege one voice or perspective over another. Through valuing what we can know of spiritual experience within a fixed idea of what is acceptable, we may ignore that which is "unknowable" or indescribable within spiritual experience. When exploring spirituality in nursing practice, careful attention to language and discourses can guide us to help people to live within the reality of their own spiritual experiences.

The question of what nurses need to know to provide spiritual care has practical implications when we consider that many nurses do not feel comfortable attending to the spiritual needs of their patients (McSherry & Ross, 2002), and nursing students seek guidance for developing spiritual awareness and engaging in spiritual discussions with patients and families (Pesut, 2002). Addressing spirituality from a scientific or a modernist view emphasizes knowing through establishing clear definitions that may lead to assessment tools and concept clarification. This could help to differentiate spirituality from other phenomena, such as a sense of coherence, caring, or connectedness. Although these ways of knowing contribute to nursing knowledge and practice, they also raise many other questions, including, "How are definitions determined?" "Who decides what definitions we will rely on?" "What world view or belief system is embedded within this knowledge?" "What happens when patients and families do not fit into particular views of spirituality?" Even though themes related to spiritual experience may be identified across groups and aggregates, if spirituality, as some authors suggest, is whatever people say it is for them (Malinski, 2002), what pitfalls and potential harms do we face in privileging the views that are dominant or most commonly held?

Alternative ways of knowing may complement and yet put into question modernist approaches to spirituality. Whereas the modernist approach is based in a historical era when there was increased growth in the valuing of freedom, individuality, and scientism, views from a postmodern perspective challenge the nature of modern assumptions. Modernism, although largely located in the 19th and early 20th century, continues to inform some schools of thought, particularly those of the natural sciences; whereas postmodernism critiques of modern thought are increasingly prevalent in nursing scholarship.

Munhall (1993) challenges modernist assumptions about knowledge in exploring unknowing as a way of knowing. Munhall introduces "unknowing" as a state of mind and a way of knowing that brings another dimension to understanding complex human experience. Unknowing is viewed not simply as a gap in knowledge that must be filled but as an ability and way of knowing that is interconnected with conventional knowing. After all, knowing that we do not know opens us to learning and new possibilities. Munhall calls for unknowing to be included as another pattern of knowing (Box 25.6).

BOX 25.6 Unknowing May Be a Way of Knowing

Let us not talk *about* death,
Let us talk . . . with/in
. . . . open-endedness
forming and dissolution.
trans/forming, per/forming,
constantly dissolving
becoming anew
abiding in spaces between thoughts.

Let us talk
nursing
as witnessing
mindful of empty spaces and places
   of self/no self
   of birth, old age, sickness and death.
Mindful of basic impermanence
of living and dying,
abiding in spaces
of ceaseless transitioning . . . . .

Source: Bruce, A. (2002). *Abiding in liminal spaces: Inscribing mindful living/dying with(in) end-of-life care.* Unpublished doctoral dissertation, University of British Columbia. Used with permission.

Cultivating Abilities to Engage With Spiritual Openness: A Way of Being

I support the view of nurse scholars who suggest that spiritual care is multifaceted and wide-ranging, much of which does not demand or require specialized knowledge (Chung, Wong, & Chan, 2007; Wright, 2002). If we are practising nursing in an interdisciplinary setting, what aspects of care are within the purview of nursing and what areas can best be referred to other healthcare and spiritual care practitioners, such as Aboriginal healers, pastors, shamans, and priests? And what aspects of spiritual care can be attended to within direct nursing care?

Recent research reports that patients and families appreciate and see spiritual care from nurses more as a way of being rather than as specific interventions (Sellers, 2001). The most frequently identified descriptors of spiritual care included being treated with kindness and respect ("it's the little things"), talking and listening, praying, connecting (e.g., being genuine and showing interest), providing quality temporal care (e.g., keeping the room tidy and not letting the patient suffer), and mobilizing religious and spiritual resources (e.g., providing referrals to clergy and providing spiritual music or readings [Taylor, 2003, pp. 587–588]).

Some patients have reported that they do not want nurses to be spiritual care providers based on the perception that nurses are not qualified and an assumption that differing beliefs between patients and nurses would be a barrier to spiritual care (Taylor, 2003). Other participants in the same study saw nurses as appropriate spiritual care providers because nurses were perceived as those who are there during vulnerable experiences and recognize experiences that would prompt a desire for spiritual care. Patients without family or particular spiritual or religious support were seen to particularly benefit from nurses with spiritual awareness. Taylor identifies several prerequisites to the provision of spiritual care from the perspective of patients in her research (Box 25.7). Most significantly, patients stated that "nurses need to establish some respect and relationship with patients prior to providing spiritual care" (Taylor, 2003, p. 589). This finding supports an understanding that spiritual practice may be most effectively delivered through a "way of being" with patients rather than through the influences of scientific or modernist knowledge.

BOX 25.7 Prerequisites to Spiritual Care

Prerequisites to Spiritual Care

<u>Personal</u>: Having a spiritual awareness; establishing trusting relationships

<u>Relational</u>: Possessing a caring attitude; developing rapport first; conveying warmth and interest; assessing patient receptivity

<u>Professional</u>: Meeting patients' expectations for what nurses might do; having appropriate training if needed

Source: Taylor, J.E. (2003). Nurses caring for the spirit: Patients with cancer and family caregiver expectations. *Oncology Nursing Forum, 30*(4), 585–590.

 ## IDENTIFYING BARRIERS: FURTHERING OUR UNDERSTANDING

The following are some barriers to nurses providing spiritual care:

1. Our lack of knowledge of our nursing history and the influence of this history on our current understandings of spiritual care in nursing practice

2. An unexamined Eurocentric perspective of spirituality that privileges Judeo-Christian ideologies

3. The dilemma of defining *spirituality* and *spiritual care* (Definitions and clarity, regarding both concepts and interventions, lend themselves to accounting for evidence-based practice and meeting mandated requirements for care. However, this kind of clarity is located within a particular world view and understanding of knowledge that may not move us any closer to the actual provision of meaningful spiritual care for patients and families.)

4. The idea that there is, or should be, a single understanding of spirituality and of approaches to spiritual care in the face of the lived realities of multiple understandings and meanings of spirituality.

 ## GENERATING STRATEGIES: FUTURE POSSIBILITIES

The following are some possibilities for nurses to remain open and provide spiritual care.

1. Make clear our personal and professional assumptions about spirituality and recognize the influence that these hold on our practice.

2. Always search for the taken-for-granted assumptions on which knowledge is shaped or constructed.

3. Pay careful attention to language and discourse because it is important in helping others live within their own spiritual realities.

4. Develop curricula and opportunities for nurses in practice to expand their comfort with the inevitable ambiguity of complex human experiences.

 ## SUMMARY

Through this chapter's conversations, poems, and reflections on the literature, I have intended to open the possibilities for multiple understandings of spiritual practice for nurses. One might assume from the language used in the literature regarding spiritual care (*kindness, gentleness, caring*)

that good nursing care is spiritual in nature. However, as you consider this evocative idea, we are left with the notion that it is something more—that spiritual practice involves accompanying patients and families on their journeys of suffering and hope and joy in ways that allow them to be present to the journeys themselves.

Add to your knowledge of this issue:		Online
American Holistic Nurses Association	www.ahna.org	
Canadian Holistic Nurses Association	www.chna.ca	
Canadian Wellness Directory of Alternative Medicine Professionals	www.canadianwellness.com/alternative/alternative_associations.asp	
Care Nurse	care-nurse.com	
International Association for Human Caring	www.humancaring.org	

REFLECTIONS on the Chapter...

1 Does everyone have spiritual experience? What words do you use to refer to your spiritual life and practices?

2 In your practice, what have you observed about the spiritual nature of people and how does that fit with nurses' practice?

3 Identify the assumptions and beliefs you hold about spirituality and the provision of spiritual care to patients and their families.

4 How do your assumptions align or differ from those held by the author of this chapter and the literature she included?

5 Is there a mandate for nurses to provide spiritual care in your province? If so, how does this compare with the CNA "Code of Ethics" mandate?

References

Borysenko, J. (1999). *A woman's journey to God: Finding the feminine path.* New York: Riverhead Books.

Bruce, A. (2002). *Abiding in liminal spaces: Inscribing mindful living/dying with(in) end-of-life care.* Unpublished doctoral dissertation, University of British Columbia.

Burkhardt, M. & Nagai-Jacobson, M.G. (2002). *Spirituality: Living our connectedness.* Albany: Delmar Thomson Learning.

Canadian Nurses Association. (2002). *Code of ethics for registered nurses.* Retrieved April 01, 2008, from www.cna-nurses.ca/cna/documents/pdf/publications/codeofethics2002_e.pdf.

Carr, T. (2003). The spirit of nursing: Ghost of our past or force for our future? In M. McIntyre & E. Thomlinson (Eds.), *Realities of Canadian nursing: Professional, practice, and power issues.* Philadelphia: Lippincott Williams & Wilkins.

Cavendish, R., Luise, B.K., & Russo, D., et al. (2004). Spiritual perspectives on nurses in the United States relevant for education and practice. *Western Journal of Nursing Research, 26*(2), 196–212.

Chung, L.Y., Wong, F.K., & Chan, M.F. (2007). Relationship of nurses' spirituality to their understanding and practice of spiritual care. *Journal of Advanced Nursing, 58*(2), 158–170.

Couvalis, G. (1997). *The philosophy of science.* Thousand Oaks: Sage.

Dzurec, L.C. & Abraham, I.L. (1993). The nature of inquiry: Linking quantitative and qualitative research. *Advances in Nursing Science, 16*(1), 73–79.

Freeman, J. (2004). Holistic healing modalities. In B. Kozier, G. Erb, A. Berman, et al. (Eds.), *Fundamentals of nursing: The nature of nursing practice in Canada.* Toronto: Prentice Hall.

George, L., Larson, D., Koenig, H., et al. (2000). Spirituality and health: What we know, what we need to know. *Journal of Social and Clinical Psychology, 19*(1), 102–116.

Hermann, C.P. (2006). Development and testing of the spiritual needs inventory for patients near the end of life. *Oncology Nursing Forum, 33,* 737–744.

Johnson, B.M. & Webber, P.B. (2005). *An introduction to theory and reasoning in nursing.* Philadelphia: Lippincott Williams & Wilkins.

Kikuchi, J. & Simmons, H. (1994). *Developing a philosophy of nursing.* Newbury Park: Sage.

Malinski, V. (2002). Developing a nursing perspective on spirituality and healing. *Nursing Science Quarterly, 15*(4), 281–287.

McLeod, D.L. & Wright, L.M. (2008). Living the as-yet unanswered: Spiritual care practices in family systems nursing. *Journal of Family Nursing, 14*(1), 118–141.

McSherry, W. & Ross, L. (2002). Dilemmas of spiritual assessment: Considerations for nursing practice. *Journal of Advanced Nursing, 38*(5), 479–488.

Milligan, S. (2004). Perceptions of spiritual care among nurses undertaking post registration education. *International Journal of Palliative Nursing, 10*(4), 162–171.

Munhall, P. (1993). "Unknowing": Toward another pattern of knowing in nursing. *Nursing Outlook, May/June,* 125–128.

Nelson, S. (1995). Humanism in nursing: The emergence of the light. *Nursing Inquiry, 2*(1), 36–43.

Olson, J., Paul, P., & Douglass, L., et al. (2003). Addressing the spiritual dimension in Canadian undergraduate nursing education. *Canadian Journal of Nursing Research, 35*(3), 94–107.

Paley, J. (2008). Spirituality and nursing: A reductionist approach. *Nursing Philosophy, 9,* 3–18.

Paterson, J. & Zderad, L. (1976). *Humanistic nursing.* New York: National League for Nursing.

Pesut, B. (2002). The development of nursing students' spirituality and spiritual care-giving. *Nurse Education Today, 22,* 128–135.

Pesut, B. & Thorne, S. (2007). From private to public: Negotiating professional and personal identities in spiritual care. *Journal of Advanced Nursing, 58*(4), 396–403.

Price, J.L., Stevens, H.O., & LaBarre, M.C. (1995). Spiritual caregiving in nursing practice. *Journal of Psychosocial Nursing, 33*(12), 5–9.

Sellers, S.C. (2001). The spiritual care meanings of adults residing in the midwest. *Nursing Science Quarterly, 14,* 239–248.

Sorell, T. (1991). *Scientism: Philosophy and the infatuation with science.* London: Routledge.

Taylor, J.E. (2003). Nurses caring for the spirit: Patients with cancer and family caregiver expectations. *Oncology Nursing Forum, 30*(4), 585–590.

Wilber, K. (1998). *The marriage of sense and soul.* New York: Random House.

Wojnar, D. & Malinski, V. (2003). Developing a nursing perspective on spirituality and healing: Questions and answers following a letter to the editor. *Nursing Science Quarterly, 16*(4), 297–300.

Wolfer, J. (1993). Aspects of "reality" and ways of knowing in nursing: In search of an integrating paradigm. *Image: Journal of Nursing Scholarship, 25*(2), 141–146.

Wright, M.C. (2002). The essence of spiritual care: A phenomenological enquiry. *Palliative Medicine, 16,* 125–132.

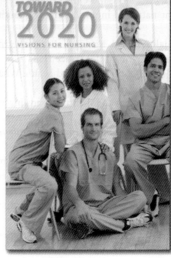

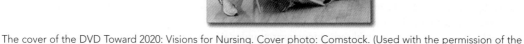

The cover of the DVD Toward 2020: Visions for Nursing. Cover photo: Comstock. (Used with the permission of the Canadian Nurses Association and NurseONE.)

Looking Back, Moving Forward: Taking Nursing toward 2020

Michael J. Villeneuve

With thanks to Carol McDonald, Marjorie McIntyre, and Elizabeth Thomlinson who authored earlier versions of this chapter.

Critical Questions

As a way of engaging with the ideas in this chapter, consider the following:

1. What occurs to you when you think about future or emerging issues for the profession of nursing and the health system at large? What is the point of conducting "futures" exercises?

2. Thinking about your own life, how have recollections of your history influenced your actions or understandings of the future?

Chapter Objectives

After completing this chapter, you will be able to:

1. Describe the way in which any account of history can be understood as a partial interpretation of historical realities.

2. Discuss current and emerging trends that will have an impact on the future of nursing and healthcare.

3. Identify five key issues on the horizon for the discipline of nursing.

History, despite its wrenching pain, cannot be unlived
But if faced with courage, need not be lived again.

Dr. Maya Angelou, 1993

One of Canada's great thinkers, Sister Elizabeth Davis (Board Chair, Canadian Health Services Research Foundation), shares the simple example of the Newfoundland dory when she talks of ways to think about the future of the healthcare system. As she notes so poetically, to row a dory and move it forward, one actually sits backwards, with eyes upon the shore. But importantly, keeping a close watch on the safe and distant harbour is about vigilance and perspective—not about stopping the forward movement.

And go forward we must. What a perfect metaphor to shape our thinking as we conclude this book by talking about the future of human health, the healthcare system, and nursing's role in both. How do we do that strategically? Day and Schoemaker (2005) advise organizations to conduct "periphery scanning," by asking the right questions to learn from the past, examine the present, and envision new futures. They talk about the need to listen to *mavericks*, clients, and those seemingly "out there" on the boundaries—in other words, to have the hard conversations, not just the comfortable ones, and imagine the unimaginable. Canadian futurist and researcher Marc Zwelling says we need to "look long" (look at historical data and trends and extrapolate them forward), "look wide" (at what is going on all around us), and "look deep," (drilling down into the details of any given problem or issue).

So looking and planning forward must happen in the context of understanding—critically, not just casually—our past and the trends that brought us to this point. Those trends, and responses to them, have been well laid out in earlier chapters of this book and in many other resources, so they won't be restated here. But it is important to have that frame in mind as we set forward on what looks to be a precipitous and uncertain road forward.

It is just over 50 years since the First Canadian Conference on Nursing (1956) was convened for nurse leaders to discuss the future of nursing in Canada. Canadian Nurses Association (CNA) leaders and the federal chief nursing consultant at the time, Dorothy Percy, expressed concerns then over shortages of nurses and nurse leaders. Sound familiar? In fact, talk of shortages and a lack of leadership in nursing are two of the most consistent themes expressed in Canadian nursing literature over the past 5 decades.

Now nearly a decade into a new century, the supply–demand mismatch expressed as "nursing shortages" still sits at the core of all our dialogues about the nursing workforce—whirling around the problems of workload, absenteeism, overtime, job satisfaction, and, most urgently, of wait times and access for Canadians. Left unchecked, it seems set to colour all our conversations over the coming decade too; if CNA's predictions are even close to correct (Ryten, 1997; Ryten, 2002), then we are heading toward a shortage of nurses in the 30% range.

Despite an unprecedented, decade-long intensity of effort to study, explain, and strategize around the issue of supply and demand, the profession has been held back by a relative failure to redress the basic issues that seem to drive up dissatisfaction, absenteeism, turnover, and intent to leave the job or profession. And nurses are not alone; there is a worrying picture of shortages, burnout, and dissatisfaction in medicine and in some other health professions within and beyond Canada.

We cannot sustain a healthcare system on that foundation, and on what ethical grounds would we even try? Canadians and their providers can do better and deserve better—and that imperative must underpin all our thinking as we put the pieces in place to build a new and effective 21st century healthcare system.

 ## STUDYING THE FUTURE

The past is a guidepost, not a hitching post.

Thomas Holdcroft

The public healthcare system we enjoy today—still the envy of most countries around the world, it bears remembering—evolved largely from the values, needs, and realities of the mid-20th century. It did an especially good job of meeting demands for access to doctors, hospitals, acute care, and advanced diagnostics and treatment. But Canada in 2008 is a vastly different place than it was 50 years ago. Tinkering with and retooling that system can only go so far to meet the needs of a modern, diverse, technology-driven society based in instant communication, consumer leadership, and high expectations that the vast bulk of health and illness services will be delivered outside of institutions. It was just not set up for those realities.

Canadians will still need care in 2020; all indications are that demands for it are growing. But as today's trends grow forward, it is likely to be a very different kind of care, demanding different kinds of nurses and doctors doing different things. Why would we imagine that future will be any different for us than we are different from 1960? The pace of change is escalating, with futurists like Kurzweil predicting that the 21st century will actually see some 20,000 years of progress. Shorter spans of time are seeing greater and greater change; we've all witnessed that pattern evolving for the past 20 years. As Kurzweil has argued, power and performance of technology basically double every year, at the same time as size and cost drop by half (2001). The sense that the world is speeding up is not just a perception, it really is happening around us.

Futures Frameworks

What the healthcare system should look like in 2020, and how we transform it to be viable, responsive, and sustainable, will be driven by a) what we *want* it to look like and b) the influence of trends shaping the society around it. To organize futures thinking and scenario development, Henchey described a framework based in four imagined futures as follows (Roy, 2000; Ward-Murray, 2000):

- A *possible future* is one that might happen, but for which the probability is very low. This is the kind of future that is difficult to imagine ever happening—even in one's wildest dreams. Such a future would have a real focus on health promotion and disease prevention and the funding support necessary to achieve change. In such a future, community members and politicians fully collaborate with educators and practitioners toward a common goal of health for all.

- A *plausible* future is one that could happen. It might be one in which society and nursing evolve to include governments that work to protect the environment and thereby alter the healthcare needs of the world's residents. Development of a comprehensive home-care system across Canada that permits citizens who wish to remain in their homes during periods of ill health and infirmity is a plausible future.

- A *probable future* is one that is based on current trends and one that is likely to happen. If changes to modify or reverse current situations do not happen, today's realities are likely to be our future realities. Unless there are significant changes in the nutritional and exercise habits of Canadians, for example, the increasing numbers of Canadians now developing diabetes will continue—and so will the concomitant effects on the healthcare system (Zinman, 1998). Some futurists argue that the probable future is always a continuation of the present with no major change of course.

- A *preferable future* is one that is desirable, one that addresses the hopes and wishes of the profession and society. A preferable future is one in which nurses are autonomous, accountable decision makers with both the authority and resources needed to provide competent ethical care to patients and their families. Rogers (1997) suggests that an effective strategy to plan for the future is to develop future scenarios and work back from what has been envisioned. By stepping into the future, we are unencumbered by current and past "experiences, knowledge and the dominant values and beliefs in the socio-cultural environment" (p. 32). Considering the possibilities for what each of these futures could hold provides a vision for the profession and a direction for future goals. By working through the scenarios one has envisioned, each with different consequences, one can make decisions and choices regarding the actions needed to bring about the preferred scenario. Nurses are well positioned to participate in co-creating a vision for health and healthcare for Canadians and members of the global community.

Too often in nursing we have resigned ourselves—or sometimes felt forced—to accept the *probable* future for nursing when we knew it was the wrong course. In 2004, CNA chose to tackle that problem head-on by setting out on a journey to understand global, national, health system, and nursing trends; build scenarios; and shape a national conversation about the *preferred* future for nursing and the health system. The first step in that journey, publication of *Toward 2020: Visions for Nursing* (Villeneuve & MacDonald, 2006) followed 2 years of intense study, dialogue, and reflection. It responded to the need for the nursing profession to take control of its future proactively. It put on the table questions such as what health issues will be prevalent, how will they be resolved, how many nurses will be needed, what their categories and roles should be, and how they might be educated. Other organizations within and beyond healthcare have taken on similar exercises since the turn of the century as they collectively grapple with aging workforces; worker shortages; growing demand; and rapidly shifting, complex business environments.

Trends that Matter

> *The future doesn't just happen: People create it through their action—or inaction—today.*
>
> *World Futures Society, 2006*

Without going into great detail, examples of the leading trends that have shaped Canadian society, the economy, healthcare, and nursing in 2008 bear a quick revisit:

- global HIV/AIDS pandemic and the spread of communicable diseases
- improved health and longevity in most nations
- domination of global politics and public policy by the post-World War II "baby boomer" generation and its values, and especially by the United States
- global economic, business, and cultural influence gradually beginning to shift back from west to east—away from the United States toward the European Union and certainly toward China and India
- slow natural population growth, aging populations, and worker shortages in western and Organisation for Economic Co-operation and Development nations like Canada; booming growth, young populations, and worker surpluses in the southern and eastern hemispheres; and accompanying global migration leading to unprecedented ethnocultural diversity in Canada
- a robust Canadian economy for the past decade after a generation of building up debts and deficits; the North American Free Trade Agreement (1994); and globalization of economies and trade
- global and regional wars and terrorism
- the technology era starting in 1950s, including advances in health sciences
- establishment of the public medicare system and Canada Health Act
- pollution, climate change, and the environment
- the global push for advanced education and greater access to it and increased need for specialty training and specialized workers.

Nursing in 2008 continues to be especially impacted by policy decisions of the 1990s to reduce the size of the nursing workforce—most dramatically by removing about 40% of the seats in schools of nursing and enticing thousands of nurses to retire early during that decade. And the strategy worked: as iconic Canadian economist Robert Evans has said, "sometimes policy is possible" (2005). Canada graduated some two thirds less nurses in 1999 than in 1972, while the country grew by some 10 million citizens during that time. The scene was well set for the service shortages and related problems now playing out across Canada.

Building Nursing and Health System Scenarios: Assumptions about 2020

When it comes to the future, there are three kinds of people: those who let it happen, those who make it happen, and those who wonder what happened . . .

John M. Richardson, Jr.

Putting structures in place to build nursing's preferred future means making some assumptions about the ways past and current trends will play out in the future. Imagine that you could be transported by more than a decade, suddenly finding yourself in the Canada of 2020. Based on CNA's "Toward 2020" study, the following scenarios are offered as assumptions about the world you'd see around you.

SOCIETAL

- Globalization is the norm.

- The world's population was growing by a quarter of a million people every day back in 2008 and has now reached about 8.2 billion. It is predicted to rise to nearly 10 billion by 2050 before levelling off. Nearly all that growth is happening in the southern hemisphere: 96% of world population increase now occurs in the developing regions of Africa, Asia, and Latin America, and that will only rise over the course of the next quarter century (United States Census Bureau, 1999).

- Canada's growth (including the tax base to fund healthcare) depends entirely on immigration; for over a decade the only natural growth has been among First Nations, Métis, and Inuit Peoples, and they are younger on average than Canadians—the latter continuing to age as a result of the large cohort of baby boomers now in their retirement years.

- The year 2008 marked a milestone for humanity—according to the United Nations, it was the first time in history that more than 50% of all human beings lived in cities and large urban areas. The trend has continued, leaving smaller towns aging and short of workers and services globally. Global travel and migration are normal everyday events, although the decaying environment is forcing many people to consider less travel—especially less flying.

- Technology, in all its forms, has dramatically changed how we communicate with each other, deal with illness, and maintain health. Computers are now ubiquitous in public places and are voice activated, eliminating old worries about literacy and keyboard skills!

- Demographic tables have turned and the population of Canada looks dramatically different than it did in 2008. The cultural and ethnic makeup of communities is significantly more diverse. The Aboriginal community has grown sharply in some urban centres and in western Canada. For the first time in Canadian history, the visible minority populations of Toronto, Montreal, and Vancouver consist of European-origin Caucasians.

- The preoccupation with global security and emergency preparedness dubbed the "fear society" back in 2005 has continued in light of ongoing terrorist activity globally.

DISEASE AND CARE DELIVERY CHALLENGES

The healthcare system in 2020 is being confronted with a variety of global health issues, including:

- more virulent infectious diseases that spread more quickly
- more mental health problems, especially related to stress, anxiety, and fear
- the patient safety agenda—an increased focus on complications caused by care interventions and what is needed to reduce and control them

- the health and social needs of migrating populations, including treatment of communicable diseases uncommon in Canada and mental health issues like torture
- the reality that Canadians travel more and farther, and they expect to carry their own complete, computerized health records with them!

THE HEALTHCARE SYSTEM

- Canadian health spending grew slowly to 13.9% of GDP in 2018, then levelled off.
- Exponentially rising costs for pharmaceuticals and other treatments were constrained by 2015 before they completely broke the system. Forums for dialogue about ethical implications of emerging treatments, including who gets what treatment, for how long and at what cost, were established with nurse leadership by 2010.
- The interest of Canadians in health and wellness keeps growing and is reflected in the present focus on healthcare versus illness treatment. Primary healthcare models have been much more fully implemented than imagined in 2008. Canadians want more information and choices in their lives, and this is no different for health. There is a range of personalized choices for patients, a shift towards independence and various provider options, including complementary health practitioners.
- Health is defined very broadly to take into account incomes, poverty, literacy, the environment, and other broad determinants of health.
- Nurses, other providers, patients, and families are being confronted by much more complex ethical issues related to beginning-of-life and end-of-life technologies, treatment options and costs, and the implications of human cloning and artificial intelligence.
- Canadians are actively involved in their healthcare. Self-care is really becoming the norm for all except the oldest Canadians. Health professionals are viewed more as advisors and resources than as the source of "health."
- Health records are all electronic, transferable, and accessible by Canadians.
- Communities, families, and volunteers are formally recognized and supported as critical partners in health promotion and maintenance.

Responding to all these changes, the healthcare system as it was created it in the mid-20th century has really changed. For example:

- Healthcare is much more focused on the places where people live, work, and play—homes, communities, schools, retail settings, and work settings—than on treatment settings. It is less focused on providers and more focused on people, communities, and wellness.
- Healthcare does not first mean hospitals, surgeons, and high-technology diagnostics now; that type of healthcare is becoming the exception that fewer and fewer Canadians experience. The system does a better job than it used to in balancing hospitals, wait times, and diagnostic technologies with strategies and mechanisms that emphasize and improve health.
- To support care in the community, budgets finally have shifted emphasis away from hospitals, physicians, and drugs and toward wellness strategies based in communities, families, and individuals. The push in community settings and homes is on health, illness, and injury prevention, lifestyle modification, literacy, ameliorating the impacts of poverty, and so on.
- Much more illness care and much more complex care, including acute, long-term and palliative care, is now provided in homes, hospices, and other community settings. Hospitals truly are settings only for short-stay and outpatient services, critical and emergency care, and transplant care. There are more long-term care and transitional-care beds in the system than in 2008, including alternative living options for seniors and better supports to keep people in their homes. Hospitals are actually smaller overall, more regional and tertiary in nature, and are essentially short-stay intensive care environments.

- The bulk of surgical and other procedures—much less invasive than in the past—are performed on an outpatient basis with follow-up nursing care taking place in homes. Human donor transplants and artificial replacements are replacing many therapies; cloned organs have been successfully grown and transplanted in animal experiments.

- Improved audio, video, and robotic technologies have enabled tele-health options, reducing the need for surgical and other invasive procedures and the need to travel for such procedures. These technologies have really increased access to health and illness care options for isolated Canadians.

- Clinical, monitoring, and automated diagnostic technologies have finally begun to reduce demands for nurses in hospitals, allowing nurses to follow computer-generated treatment algorithms and focus on care issues beyond technology.

- Technology drove the integration of Canada's 13 "mini health systems" into a more streamlined pan-Canadian system by about 2017. It really forced development of standardized ways to document care, for example, in electronic health records, and standardized ways of recording the costs of care. Other traditions, including regulatory and related professional bodies in each province and territory, have also been greatly streamlined.

- The wait times that used to be in every headline in 2008 have been resolved, but quality, safety, and accountability are still paramount.

HEALTH AND HUMAN RESOURCES

Changing health, disease, and care delivery patterns are reflected in different health and human resources patterns in 2020. For example:

- Care in 2020 is delivered using fewer professionals in models that are more effective for the system, more satisfying to patients, and more rewarding to the workforce.

- Patient and community needs determine the mix of healthcare providers most appropriate for the population.

- Multiple gateways into the healthcare system and points of access to care through a range of providers, including, but not limited to, physicians, are the norm. Nurse practitioners and registered nurses (RNs) with added skills provide the bulk of primary care and health services that used to be provided by general practice physicians; all physicians are now specialists including those in family practice.

- More human and nonhuman (robotic) care partners have been added to the system to deliver nonprofessional aspects of care, allowing nurses, physicians, and others to focus on what they are best prepared to do for patients.

- Shortages are still a problem, particularly in rural, remote, northern, and Aboriginal settings. Interest in working in such settings has not really changed much since 2008 despite lucrative recruitment incentives. Accessing health using audio and video technologies and travelling to access in-person care are the norm now.

- In institutional and community settings, health and illness care are normally delivered by fully integrated, multiprofessional teams who co-care for patients. Accountability is team based; professional care is led by the provider most appropriate for the patient and his or her health issues, and this provider may change over time.

- Complementary and alternative healthcare providers (e.g., acupuncturists, massage therapists, and homeopaths) are integrated members of healthcare teams.

- Assistive and supportive healthcare workers (e.g., personal support workers) are an important part of the healthcare system and more integrated into teams in long-term care, home care, and rehabilitation settings.

Possibilities for Re-Visioning the Future

You may know the right thing. But do you have the discipline to do the right thing? And equally important, to stop doing the wrong things?

Collins, 2005

In a 2005 report, the Conference Board of Canada stated that "Canadians are capable of confronting thorny challenges, discarding long-held views, and getting down to the job of finding solutions." Can we say the same in nursing? The truth is we must. Given the scenarios and assumptions about the future outlined here, what might be the place of nursing, and how do we get there from here?

And looking beyond the details of roles and numbers, what is the potential for social justice in nursing? What would it mean to understand nursing practice as leadership and political activism? (Is it realistic and reasonable to locate the responsibility for leadership and political action with the individual nurse?) How can we understand and address the tension between the expectations placed on nurses and the realities of discordant views and an absence of support from the institutions in which we are educated and practice? What *should* nurses do—and what are we *willing* do to—about the shameful outcome disparities still confronting the publics we serve at home and globally?

Some analysts (e.g., Porter-O'Grady, 1998) have suggested that nurses collectively are reluctant to face issues head on and that we undermine the actions of others inside and outside the profession. An alternative viewpoint suggests that nurses as a group are neither passive nor inactive but that we have been socialized in particular ideologies of what it means to be a nurse and, given our makeup, what it means to be a woman. Conservative ideologies have undermined the initiative of some women to act in direct, challenging, and powerful ways. The challenge is to disrupt discourses that promote and sustain powerlessness and to support one another in raising the profile and the esteem of the nursing profession.

Historically, we also have been fairly well indoctrinated in nursing to follow the rules of our educational, employment, and regulatory hierarchies and particularly to avoid risk—first, of course, because we want to protect those we serve. But the "risk" threat has also been wielded effectively to keep nurses quiet and stymie both innovation and creativity. During her interview as part of CNA's 2020 study, Sister Elizabeth Davis said, "hierarchies are structurally defined to prevent new thinking," adding that they "may be useful in a stable environment but are useless in an unstable one" (cited in Villeneuve & MacDonald, 2006). As Villeneuve and MacDonald wondered in their report, *are* there any stable environments any more?

Former *Disney Studios* icon Michael Eisner put it this way: "When you're trying to create things that are new, you have to be prepared to be on the edge of risk." We've often lived on that edge clinically in the interest of our patients; we have not done that (or sustained it) as well in our collective willingness to take action and "draw a line in the sand" around certain political positions.

Important in all this has been our inability to articulate fully the benefit that nurses bring to the health and healthcare of citizens, and at what cost. The study by Tourangeau and colleagues (2002), for example, finding that having more RNs led to lower mortality (after 30 days) among hospitalized acute-care patients, needs to be interpreted and emphasized to Canadians and their governments. Our challenge is to find ways to make nursing practice and the roles of RNs compelling enough to engage decision makers and the public at large.

In addition, nurses face the attitudes of governments and employers toward a profession that is still female dominated. In this book (Chapter 19), McDonald claims, "Ideas about women and women's work and whether this work requires significant knowledge, responsibility, and skill contribute to the devaluing of nurses' work by society" (p. 344). She reminds us that to "challenge effectively what is taken for granted about the role of gender and its powerful influence on nurses' work, we must be willing to notice difference and to acknowledge the way that differences, such as gender, class, race, ethnicity, and sexual orientation, matter in the ways our identities are lived and viewed by the world" (p. 354).

Given the trends around us, the enablers and barriers in our environments, and in consideration of futures scenarios like the ones proposed here, there are numerous areas in which it is important that nurses and their associations act today if we are going to have a hand in shaping our own future. In Chapter 15, McIntyre and McDonald note that "downsizing and restructuring have undermined existing leadership structures and the vision the CNA documents provide for nursing. Significantly, positions such as the chief nursing officer are being eroded. In some instances, they have disappeared altogether" (p. 280). We need all our remaining nurse leaders to speak clear messages and act in bold, visionary ways to define a new future for nursing and insist on moving the agenda forward. In Chapter 7 we talked about future priorities for the CNA and some of the program areas being undertaken by the International Council of Nurses as part of its 21st century vision. Key messages that must be part of discussions within nursing and between nursing and the larger world of public policy include the following:

- If we stay on track with the same demand, supply patterns, and delivery models, the shortages of nursing services seen in 2008 and projected forward are not resolvable. Something has to give, and given the global population demographics and work patterns we are seeing, it is naive to imagine that "more nurses" is a feasible solution on anything but a very distant and hopeful horizon.

- In a nation with no natural population growth outside of its indigenous peoples, and otherwise relying entirely on immigration for its very future, nurse leaders must be prepared to discuss managed, ethical migration as a strategy to populate the nursing workforce (and indeed other health provider workforces) of the future. "More seats" in Canadian schools of nursing is a necessary but insufficient response in a global, 21st century world. Given young and booming populations of people seeking careers and better lives in nations that are already 30 times the size of our own, set against our education infrastructure and the age of our nursing teachers, innovative models—including the possibility of offshore Canadian schools of nursing that educate nurses in a purposeful, reciprocal education and practice arrangement beneficial to both nations—must be on the table.

- Canada's population health demands must drive the models of care and who will deliver them—not vice versa. Canadian nurses must be prepared to suggest what those models of care delivery should look like and, in turn, what should be the mix and roles of the teams who will provide them.

- A generation of research describing every nuance of a healthy workplace should be translated into vibrant, exciting, and rewarding practice settings for the country's health professionals wherever they work.

- RNs, and not just advanced practice nurses, must be prepared to provide primary care services by the mid-2020s, meaning being prepared for independent assessment, diagnosis, treatment (including prescriptive authority and admitting privileges for patients requiring in-patient nursing care), and follow-up of patients in communities, care teams in clinics, and emergency rooms. The demand exists now, and to meet it, nurses must decide on their place in the new health and illness system and be prepared to take on those roles. RNs in 2020 should primarily be prescribing medications, not delivering them.

- Vastly different responsibilities and accountabilities for Canada's RNs in the 2020s means putting the pieces in place now for a) a new vision of who is recruited into the RN workforce, b) the new competencies and curriculum they will require, and c) a modern and flexible system of regulation.

- As physicians and RNs tailor their roles to new demands and a new system, licensed practical nurses, and those providing the range of ancillary nursing services, also will need to take on new responsibilities and accountabilities; in turn, their recruitment, curriculum, and regulation will need to adapt.

- The leadership and decision-making structures of Canadian nursing at all levels and in all domains of practice must mirror the Canadian population and Canadian communities.

Mechanisms to dismantle the gender and racial segregation of nursing must be generated and implemented now to shape a different-looking nursing workforce made up of different people and ideas by 2020.

- Every possible strategic effort should be made to attract and retain a new generation of nurses and nurse leaders. Strategies must include:
  - establishing programs of reverse, or at least mutual, mentoring (new graduates mentoring nurse leaders)
  - modernizing the fleet of *tools to do the job* in homes, communities, schools, and in-patient settings
  - implementing existing and emerging technological solutions to streamline or replace human functions when they allow nurses and other providers to focus on their patients, residents, clients, and communities.
- Nurses must create the structures to dismantle old silos and imagine areas where nursing can have a common and strengthened future—and then speak courageous and common messages to ourselves, other health professionals, governments, and the Canadian public.
- Nursing must position itself as a solutions-focused, added-value, and informed partner at every policy table in this country, not as a problem to be solved.

SUMMARY

These issues on the horizon, and those beyond our view, will shape the future of nursing as a professional and a practice discipline. The ways in which we articulate, understand, and respond to these issues are open to the individual and collective interpretations of both the history and the future directions of the discipline. Our history, as it is known, has the capacity to help us understand who we are. And our history—still emerging and becoming known—has great potential to inform our directions. A willingness to engage deeply with the salient issues of the discipline includes a critical interrogation of our historical and current realities—professional, practice, and power issues. It is, however, through courage, risk taking, and political action in education, healthcare, and government arenas—and through the recognition of nursing practice as entwined with social justice and our long history of advocacy—that we have the opportunity to make a difference.

Emerging from the chaos of the last decade, the future holds the promise of excitement, innovation, new roles, vigour, and new thinking across the world of nursing—*if* we choose that and act now to make it happen. The opportunity to build a new health system with strong nursing leadership is as real, as exciting, and as desperately needed as it was for our nursing ancestors exactly a century ago. Importantly, Canadians are urging us on. As Villeneuve and MacDonald concluded in closing the "Toward 2020" report (2006), "The public puts far more trust and faith in nurses than nurses sometimes put in themselves. The public is waiting, and looking to nurses to act forcefully. The messages are clear; the ball is now in nursing's court."

Add to your knowledge of this issue:		
Canadian Nurses Association	http://www.cna-aiic.ca	
World Future Society	http://www.wfs.org	

REFLECTIONS on the Chapter...

1 Distinguish among the concepts of *possible, probable,* and *preferred* futures.

2 What are three global socioeconomic trends that have had an impact on shaping Canada's healthcare system in 2008—and what impact they have exerted?

3 Imagine a scenario in which, by 2015, there will be 25% fewer RNs and 20% fewer physicians than required in the city or region where *you* live. If you could lead the team making the decisions, what kinds of delivery models might you put in place to provide access to care for the public? What steps would you need to start putting in place today so that your new delivery model can be implemented by 2015? What are the kinds of enablers, barriers, and issues you are likely to encounter?

4 Review the summary of the six scenarios suggested in CNA's futures document, "Toward 2020," and then read any one of the six in detail in the report. Talk with your colleagues about the scenario. If the scenario seems feasible or maybe even preferable to you, what are its strengths? If you think the scenario "missed the mark," what were its flaws or weaknesses? If it seems improbable to you, then what scenario would you suggest in its place given the trends analysis that led to its development?

Acknowledgement

Sections of this chapter are based on the Canadian Nurses Association's futures document and were used with permission of the authors and publisher. Source: Villeneuve, M. & MacDonald, J. (2006). *Toward 2020: Visions for Nursing.* Ottawa: Canadian Nurses Association.

References

Collins, J. (2005). *Good to great: Why some companies make the leap . . . and others don't.* New York: Harpercollins (CD edition).

Conference Board of Canada. (2005). *The world and Canada: Trends reshaping our future.* Ottawa: Author.

Davis, E. (2005, March). *Dory, rainbow and inukshuk: The journey to a strong health system in Canada.* Paper presented at the Canadian Health Services Research Foundation 7th Annual Workshop—Leveraging Knowledge: Tools & Strategies for Action. Montreal.

Day, G. & Schoemaker, P. (2005). Scanning the periphery. *Harvard Business Review Online.* Retrieved November 14, 2005 from http:/harvardbusinessonline.hbsp.harvard.edu.

Evans, R. (2005). *Keynote address.* Paper presented at the Canadian Association for Health Services and Policy Research Annual Meeting. Montreal.

Kurzweil, R. (2001). *The law of accelerating returns.* Retrieved April, 2008 from http://www.kurzweilai.net.

Porter-O' Grady, T. (1998). A glimpse over the horizon: Choosing our future. *Orthopaedic Nursing, 17*(2), S53–S61.

Rogers, M. (1997). *Canadian nursing in the year 2020: Five futures scenarios.* Ottawa: Canadian Nurses Association.

Roy, C. (2000). The visible and invisible fields that shape the future of the nursing care system. *Nursing Administration Quarterly, 25*(1), 119–131.

Ryten, E. (1997). *A statistical picture of the past, present and future of registered nurses in Canada.* Ottawa: Canadian Nurses Association.

_____. (2002). *Planning for the future: Nursing human resource projections.* Ottawa: Canadian Nurses Association.

Tourangeau, A., Giovannetti, P., & Tu, J., et al. (2002). Nursing related determinants of 30-day mortality for hospitalized patients. *Canadian Journal of Nursing Research, 33*(4), 71–88.

United States Census Bureau. (1999). *World population profile.* Retrieved 2005 from http://www.census.gov.

Villeneuve, M. & MacDonald, J. (2006). *Toward 2020: Visions for nursing.* Ottawa: Canadian Nurses Association. Retrieved 2008 from http://www.cna-aiic.ca.

Ward-Murray, E.M. (2000). Creating nursing's future: Issues, opportunities, and challenges. *Nursing and Health Care Perspectives, 21*(6), 305–306.

Zinman, B. (1998). *Diabetes: The magnitude of the problem.* Proceedings from the National Forum on Diabetes (pp. 5–16). Ottawa: Canadian Diabetes Association.

Zwelling, M. (2005). *Futures thinking and planning.* Paper presented at the Merrickville Stakeholder Consultation for the Toward 2020 Study, Merrickville, Ontario.

Index

Note: Page numbers followed by f, t, and b indicate figures, tables and boxed text, respectively.

A

Aboriginal communities. *see also* First Nations
definition in Canadian Constitution Act, 436
First Nations, Inuit, Metis, 436
healthcare, 22, 24
languages, 436
violence in, 422–423
Aboriginal Nurses Association of Canada, telehealth, 243
Academy of Canadian Executive Nurses, 105
Accessibility, in Canadian health care, 42–45
Action group, formed to address health care issues, 4b
Acute Care Nurse Practitioners (ACNPs), 170
Advanced nursing practice (ANP), 177. *see also* Nurse Practitioner (NP)
Advanced Practice Nurses, in rural and remote communities, 17–34
Alberta
College and Association of Registered Nurses of Alberta (CARNA), 157–158, 161
nurse practitioner regulation, 153t
Alberta Heritage Foundation for Medical Research (AHFMR), 263
Alberta Nursing Research Foundation (ANRF), 263
Allen, Moyra, 261
American Holistic Nurses Association (AHNA), 229–230
American Nurses Association (ANA), classification for nursing care, 140–141
American Society of Superintendents of Training Schools for Nursing of the United States and Canada, 1893, 149
Annual Conference of the Matron's Council of Great Britain and Ireland, 1899, 135
Assembly of the United Canadas of the Gradual Civilization Act of 1857, 438
Associated Alumnae of the United States and Canada, 1896, 149
Association of Registered Nurses of Newfoundland and Labrador, 151
Audioconference delivery, in nursing education, 249
Australian College of Holistic Nurses, Inc., 230–231

B

Bachelor of Science in nursing (BScN) bridging program, 189b
Balance billing, 42
Band-Aid campaign, 108
Barriers to resolution, nursing issues, 10
Basic Principles of Nursing Care (Henderson), core publication of ICN, 137
Begin, Monique, 42
The Bell Curve: The Reshaping of American Life by Difference in Intelligence (Herrnstein and Murray), 375
Benton, David, 142
Best practice, 268
Better Patient Care Through Nursing Research (Abdellah & Levine), 261
Bioethics, 339
Biologic agents, 404b
Bottorff, Joan, 207
British Columbia
healthcare programs, 35
nurse practitioner regulation, 153–154t
British Columbia - Alberta Trade, Investment, and Labour Mobility Agreement (TILMA), 157
British Columbia Nurses' Union (BCNU), 328
British Columbia Royal Commission on Health Care and Costs, 1991, 161
British North America (BNA) Act of 1867, 40, 47–48, 438
Browne, Gina, 97–98
Building the Future: An Integrated Strategy for Nursing Human Resources in Canada (Nursing Sector Study Corporation, 2004), 80
Burlington Randomized Trial of the NP, 169

C

Callan, Mona, 169
Canada Health Act (CHA), 35–47, 124
nurse-influenced amendments, 74b
Canada Health Infoway, 245
Canada Health Transfer, 44
Canada-Russia Initiative in Nursing (2004-2008), CNA, 131
Canada-South Africa Nurses HIV/AIDS Initiative (2003-2008), CNA, 131
Canadian Association of Nurse Researchers, 264
Canadian Association of Schools of Nursing (CASN), 264
position statement on graduate education, 216–218b
Canadian Association of University Schools of Nursing (CAUSN), 80b, 152, 191
doctoral degree programs, 207
Canadian Consortium for Nursing Research, partner of CNA, 121
Canadian Federation of Nurses Unions (CFNU), 105, 316
mission statement, 323b
quality practice environments, 287b
Canadian Gerontological Nurse, 261
Canadian Healthcare Association, member of G-4 collective, 122
Canadian health care system, 34–55
accessibility, 42–45
care for the chronically ill, 38
communicable disease and patient safety, 38–39
comprehensiveness, 36–39
framework for health promotion, 41
government studies and agreements, 42
health human resources planning, 124–126
importance of understanding, 35
National health grants, 36–37
nurses influencing change, 50–51
primary healthcare, 37–38
public administration, 45–47
universality and portability, 39–42
violence and abuse effects, 425–426
what lies ahead, 49–50
worth saving despite flaws, 47–48
Canadian Health Leadership Network, partner of CNA, 121
Canadian Health Services Research Foundation (CHSRF), 46–47, 96, 264
Canadian Holistic Nursing Association (CHNA), 229
Canadian Institute for Health Information (CIHI)
data on variation in services, 42
employment trends of the registered nurse workforce, 332b
on nursing shortages, 95–96
on rural nursing, 21

Canadian Institutes of Health Research (CIHR), 262, 264, 268
structure, 275–276
Canadian International Development Agency, CNA in, 131
Canadian Journal of Cardiovascular Nursing, 261
Canadian Journal of Nursing Leadership, 261
Canadian Labour and Business Centre, 101
Canadian Medical Association, member of G-4 collective, 122
Canadian National Association of Trained Nurses (1908), 122
Canadian Nurse, CNA publication, 132
Canadian Nurse Practitioner Examination, 128, 175
Canadian Nurse Practitioner Initiative (CNPI), 122, 170, 175
Canadian Nurses Association (CNA), 117–146
  advocate of primary healthcare, 37–38
  age of registered nurses in Canada, 294t, 308f
  Code of Ethics for Registered Nurses (2008), 6, 8, 61, 129, 343,
    391, 393, 428
  communication, publications, and administration, 132
  employment predictions, 285t
  environmental health, 401
  Forum on Nurse Practitioner Assessment, 2004, 175
  governance structure, 120–121
  influences on move to unionization, 323b, 1322–323
  information management and technology, 240
  International Policy and Development (IPD), 130–132
  leadership awards, 65t
  levels of education, 290t
  member of G-4 collective, 122
  National Nursing Research Agenda, 126–128
  Ninth Decade, 78b
  Ontario and Quebec nurses, 118–119
  partnerships, 121–122
  power and influence, 120–121–123
  presidents and executive directors since 1980, 121b
  priorities and issues, 133
  provincial and territorial members, 119t
  public policy, 123–126
  quality practice environments, 287b
  on regulatory frameworks, 149
  regulatory policy, 128–130
  sources of empowerment, 71–72
  specialties current recognized, 24b
  student members, 119
  Toward 2020: Visions for Nursing, 132
  vision, mission and goals, 120
  where do Canadian nurses work?, 291t
Canadian Nurses Foundation (CNF), 262
  doctoral degree programs, 207
Canadian Nurses Protective Society (CNPS), 342
Canadian Nursing Advisory Committee, 122
  report, 2002, 80, 125
Canadian Nursing Students' Association (CNSA), 80b, 119
  Leadership Boot Camp, 63
Canadian Patient Safety Institute (CPSI), 39
Canadian Pharmacists Association, member of G-4 collective, 122
Canadian Red Cross Society, remote nursing, 22
Canadian Registered Nurse Examination (CRNE), 128, 158–159
Canadian Registered Nurse Exam Prep Guide, CNA, 128
Canadian Society of Superintendents of Training Schools for
    Nurses, 1907, 149
Caring for Lesbians and Gay people: A Clinical Guide (Peterkin and
    Risdon), 391
Centre for Collaborative Health Professional Education
    (Newfoundland and Labrador), 186
Centres for Excellence for Women's Health (CEWH), 106
Certification

definition, 177
  specialty programs of CNA, 129, 130t
Chemical contaminants, 404b
Child maltreatment, 421–422
Chronic illness, care for, 38
Clients, 177
Clinical Nurse Specialists (CNS)
  definition, 177
  in rural and remote communities, 17–34
Code of Ethics (CNA), 6, 8, 129, 343
  gender and sexual orientation, 391, 393
  nursing leadership, 61
  violence and abuse, 428
College and Association of Registered Nurses of Alberta (CARNA),
    157–158, 161
  MLA Mentorship Program, 106
College of Nurses of Ontario (CNO), 118, 151–152
College of Physicians and Surgeons, nursing regulation and, 150
College of Registered Nurses of British Columbia (CRNBC), 151
Colonialism, effects on First Nations communities, 437
Colonization, European relations with First Nations, 437–439
Commission on the Future of Healthcare in Canada, 2002, 43
*Commitment and Care: The Benefits of Healthy Workplaces for
    Nurses, Their Patients and the System* (Baumann et al), 289
Communicable disease
  in Canadian health care, 38–39
  resurgence of, 39
Community, as a workplace, 291–292
Competencies, definition, 177
Complicity, definition, 357b
Comprehensiveness, in Canadian health care, 36–39
Computerized patient-care records
  holistic nursing and, 233
  nursing and technology, 245–246
Computer literacy, in nursing schools, 247–248
Confidence, in nursing leadership, 59
Conjugal violence, 420
Continuing education, rural nurses, 26–28, 27t
Controlled acts, 160
Correspondence courses, in nursing education, 249
Council of University Programs in Nursing, Ontario, 151
Cryptosporidium, 405
Culturally safe care, First Nation communities, 24

D

Decision making, application of biomedical technology,
    246–247
Difference, 369–386
  challenge of, 373–374
  classification of bodies in history, 375
  as deviance, 376–379
  dualism and, 380
  historical and contemporary considerations, 371
  marginalized perspectives, 371–372
  philosophical understanding, 370–373
  process of differentiation, 381–382
  race as a category, 374–376
  realities of others, 382–384
  relation between margin and center, 380–381
  as relationship, 379–382
  relations of power and, 382
  significance for contemporary nursing, 379
  theorizing, 374–376

Difference dominant perspective, 372
Discourses
    of care, 357b
    definition, 357b
Discursive process, definition, 357b
Distance learning, in nursing schools, 248
Dock, Lavinia L., 135
Doctoral degree programs, 265–268
    CASN position statement, 216217b
    challenges for nurses, 214–215
    evolution of, 207–208
    issues and controversies, 210–213
    lack of employer support for, 290
    strategies for advancement of, 215–218
Domestic abuse, 420
Domestic violence, 417
Dominant groups, false universals, 372
Dualism, 460
    difference and, 380
Ducharme, Francine, 207
    first Ph.D. in nursing, 265

E

Economic analysis
    nurse practitioner issues, 171
    nurses' work, 295–296
    nursing issues, 9–10
    nursing leadership, 61
    nursing shortage, 309–310
    rural nursing, 23–24
Education
    achievements in policy development, 72–73
    adopting technology in, 250–252
    advocating for change, 191–192
    allocation of technology in, 247–250
    authority for approval of programs, 151–152
    basic, 177
    connecting the global and the local, 190–191
    diversity and difference in the 19th Century, 195–196
    entry-to-practice struggle, CNA, 129
    future issues, 198–199
    future of technology in, 252–254
    graduate, 203–222
    for NPs, 173–174
    ICT in, 241
    levels among Canadian nurses, 290t
    mentorship and orientation programs for new graduates, 292
    nurse involvement in policy development, 80
    nurses' work as taught vs. work as practiced, 288
    provincial and territorial colleges, 147–165
    research influence on, 272–273
    specialization and the Canadian welfare state, 197–198
    standards, element of nursing, 6
    undergraduate, 183–202
    uniformed and unified, 1880-1950, 196–197
    violence and abuse, 428–429
Educational Program for Nurses in Primary Care, 169–170
    e-Health, nursing and, 241
    Electronic health records (EHR). see Computerized patient-care records
    Environmental hazards, 403–409, 404b
    air pollution, 406–407
    chemical pollution, 407–408
        contaminated social environments, 409
        inside environments, 408–409
        water safety, 404–406
    Environmental health, 400–413
    barriers and strategies, 409
    historical perspective, 402–403
    importance to nurses, 410b
    what nurses can do, 410b
Environmental tobacco smoke (ETS), 408–409
Epp, Jack, 41
Essentializing, definition, 357b
Ethel Johns Award, 63, 65t
    recipients, 65t
Ethical analysis
    application of biomedical technology, 246
    identifying and articulating issues, 340–342
    nurse practitioner issues, 173
    nurses' work, 295
    nursing issues, 8–9
    nursing leadership, 61
    recognizing issues, 339
    rural nursing, 25–26
    sexuality, 392–393
Ethical issues, 337–352
    barriers to resolving, 349–351
    book reviews, 344b
    identifying and articulating, 340–342
    incorporating into practice, 345
    recognizing, 339
    strategies for resolution, 351–352
Ethics informs law, 341–342
Ethiopian Nurses and Needle Stick Injury Research Project (2006-2008), CNA, 131
Ethnicity
    active education, 190–191
    nursing education 1950-2000, 197–198
Eugenics
    differences and, 376–378
    public health and, 378–379
Eugenic sterilization, 377–378
Evans, Robert, 93
Evidence-based policy, 95–96
Evidence-based practice, holistic nursing and, 232–233
Exclusionary practices, in nursing, 372–373
Expert generalists, rural nurses as, 19–20
Expert practice, 177
Extra billing, 42

F

Family practice nurses (FPNs), 168
Family violence, 417
Federal Commission on the Future of Health Care in Canada, 2001, 81
Femininity, 362
Feminist analysis
    multicultural nursing, 190–191
    nurse practitioner issues, 172
    nurses' work, 295
    nursing issues, 9
    nursing shortage, 311
    rural nursing, 24–25
    sexuality, 395
    violence and abuse, 425
Fenwick, Mrs. Bedford, 135

Financial violence, definition, 417b
First Nations, 435–454. *see also* Aboriginal communities
    colonization and, 437–439
    culturally safe care, 24
    cultural resurgence and community development, 439–440
    demographics, 445–447
        fertility, 446
        life expectancy, 446
        migration, 446–447
        mortality, 446
    diversity, 436–437
    European relationship with, 437–439
    health care
        access to, 442, 449–451
        cultural competence, 449
        northern and isolated communities, 442–444
        nursing, 444–451
        population approach, 441–442
        transfer of services, 444, 447–449
        widening the scope, 443–444
    health status, 441
    Miyupimaatissiium, 440–442
    Office of Nursing Services, 74
    reserve lands, 438
    rural nursing care, 24
    telehealth practices, 243
    traditional political process used by, 438–439
    traditions and values, 439
Fonds de Researche Scientifique du Québec, 263
Future
    disease and care delivery challenges, 474–475
    health and human resources, 476
    healthcare system, 472–473, 475–476
    nursing and health system scenarios, 474–476
    nursing challenges and strategies, 85–87
    nursing education issues, 198–199
    nursing issue priorities, 133–134
    revisioning possibilities, 477–479
    societal scenarios, 474
    trends in Canadian society, economy, healthcare, and nursing, 473
Future of Health Care in Canada (Romanow), 186

G

Gathering Strength, Report of the Royal Commission of Aboriginal Peoples, 1996, 443
Gay, lesbian, bisexual, two-spirited, and transgendered (GLBTT), 387–399
    violence, 420–421
Gay and Lesbian Medical Association, 391
G-4 collective, CNA in, 122
Gender, 355–368
    barriers and strategies, 365–366
    definition, 357b
    effects in nurses' lives, 361–365
    exploring, 358b
    feminist analysis of nursing issues, 9
    feminist analysis of rural nursing, 24–25
    glossary of terms and definitions, 357b
    nature of knowledge, 363–364
    nature of work, 361–363
    as part of identity, 360–361
    power and, 356–361
    as social construction, 359–360

    understanding, 358, 359f
Gender and Science (Keller), 363
Gender and the Professional Predicament in Nursing (Davies), 364
Gender identity, definition, 389
Giardia lamblia, 405
Graduate education, 177, 203–222. *see also* Doctoral degree programs; Education; Masters degree programs
    challenges for nurses, 214–215
    history, 204–208
    issues and controversies, 210–213
    practice realities and, 208–210
    strategies for advancement of, 215–218
Gunn, Jean I., 73

H

Health Action Lobby (HEAL), partner of CNA, 121
Health as Expanding Consciousness (Newman), 226
Health Canada, 262, 264
Health Care in Canada Survey, CNA role in, 121–122
Health care issues
    analyzing an issue, 8–10
    articulating an issue, 7b
    articulation and resolution, 4–5
    contribution of nursing research, 273–274
    northern and isolated communities, 442–444
    sexuality, 391b
    significance for nurses, 5
    situating the topic, 7
    transformations in, 320–321
    violence and abuse effects, 425–426
Healthcare Renewal Accord, 2003, 44, 82, 125
Health Council of Canada, 41
Health policy, 69, 92
Health Policy and Politics: A Nurse's Guide (Milstead), 92, 108–109
Health Professions Act, British Columbia, 152
Health-seeking behaviors, technology and, 244
Healthy Nurses, Health Workplaces agenda, 100
Heteronormativity, 388
    bias, 394b
    gender beyond the binary, 389–390
    sexuality beyond the binary, 388–389
Heterosexism, definition, 389
Historical analysis
    nurses' work, 293
    nursing issues, 8
    nursing shortage, 305–307
    rural nursing, 21–23
    undergraduate nursing education, 195–198
    unionization, 317–318
Holistic Nurses Association of New South Wales, 230–231
Holistic nursing, 223–237
    definition, 224
    international organizations, 231t
    issues and challenges today, 232–234
    modern perspectives, 229–232
    popular culture and interest, 228–229
    20th Century developments, 224–229
    as a way of life, 233–234
    writings, 227
Holistic Nursing: Handbook for Practice (Keegan, Dossey, and Guzzetta), 227
Home care nurse
    isolation of, 291–292

in rural setting, 18
Homophobia, definition, 389
Hospital Insurance and Diagnostic Services Act, 35
Human Becoming (Parse), 226

I

Ideologies, definition, 357b
Indian Act, 1876, 436–440
    1985 Act to Amend, 446
Indian Health Transfer Policy, 1986, 447–449
Information and communication technology (ICT), nursing and, 240
Informed consent, 340–342
    ethics informs law, 341–342
    legal responsibility of nurses, 342
    right to be informed, 340–341
Institutes of Medicine in the United States, report on infection, 39
Institutional policies, 69
Interdisciplinarity, research, 276
Interdisciplinary education, addressing violence and abuse, 428–429
Interdisciplinary team-work, 187
Internalized homophobia, 389
International Classification for Nursing Practice (ICNP), ICN, 141
International Council of Nurses (ICN), 135–146
    advancing nursing practice, 140–141
    early goals, 135–136
    global nursing shortage, 139–140
    goals of regulation, 148
    position statements, 137–138
    regulating nursing, 138–139
    standardizing and credentialing, 139
    in the 21st Century, 141–142
    war years and Great Depression, 136–137
Internationally Educated Nurses (IENs), 189–190, 189b
    Assessment Centre, 159
International Nursing Review, ICN, 136
International Policy and Development (IPD), CNA, 130–132
Interpersonal violence, definition, 416
Interprofessional Education for Geriatric Care (IEGC), 186
Intersexed people, definition, 389
Inuit communities
    Office of Nursing Services, 74
    rural nursing care, 24
    telehealth practices, 243

J

Jacques Chaoulli et al v. Attorney General of Quebec, 44
Jeanne-Mance Award, 63
    recipients, 65t
Jeans, Mary Ellen, 264
Journal of Nursing Scholarship (Image), 262
Jurisdictional Collaborative Project for Entry-level
        Competencies, 158

K

Kamstra, Krista, 63
Kellogg Foundation, master's degree programs, 206
Kirby, Michael, Senator, 43
Knowledge, in nursing leadership, 59

L

Labrador, nurse practitioner regulation, 155t
Lalonde Report, 41
LeaRN CRNE Readiness Test, CNA, 128
Learning distribution systems, in nursing schools, 248–249
Lefebre, Sister Denise, SQM, Ph.D., 207
Legal analysis
    nurse practitioner issues, 173
    nursing issues, 8–9
    rural nursing, 25–26
    sexuality, 392–393
Legal issues
    barriers to resolving, 349–351
    book reviews, 344b
    incorporating into practice, 345
    nurses responsibilities in informed consent, 342
    strategies for resolution, 351–352
    understanding requirements, 343–345
Legislation
    achievements in policy development, 73–74, 74b
    CNA role in, 129–130
    licensing laws, 148
    practice, scope of, 160–161
    umbrella, 161–162
Letters
    to the editor, on nursing issues, 12
    to officials, on nursing issues, 12
Levine, Myra, 225
Licensed practical nurses (LPNs), where they fit in, 186
Licensing laws, 148
Lobbying strategies, 11–14, 11b
    additional resources and political action, 14
    direct and indirect, 11b
    example, 12b
    letters to officials, 12
    letters to the editor, 13
    news releases, 13
    resolutions, 13–14
Location of gender, definition, 357b
Lomas, Jonathan, 96

M

MacKenzie, Mary Ard, 73
Manitoba, nurse practitioner regulation, 154t
Manitoba Law Reform Commission, 1994, 161
Manitoba Nurses Union (MNU), 325
Manitoba's Health Links, telephone technology, 243
Manson, Ethel Gordon, 135
Marginalized groups, 371–372
Marxist model, policy development, 76
Masculinity, 362
Master's degree programs
    CASN position statement, 216b
    challenges for nurses, 214–215
    evolution of, 204–207, 205t
    issues and controversies, 210–213
    lack of employer support for, 290
    practice realities and, 208–210
    strategies for advancement of, 215–218
McGill University, doctoral program, 265
McIntosh, J. W., 41
McMaster University, preparation of NPs, 169–170

Medical errors, 45
Medical Research Council (MRC) of Canada, 262–263
   joint MRC/NHRDP Research Scholar awards, 267
Medicare program, 46–48
Memorial University, School of Medicine and Faculty of Nursing,
   NP program, 168
Meta-analysis, 270
Métis communities, telehealth practices, 243
Michael Smith Foundation for Health Research in British
   Columbia, 263
Midwifery, reintroduction of, 23
Milieu of care, element of nursing, 6
Minister of Health and Long-Term Care (MOHLTC), 108
Miyupimaatissiium, 440–442
Moad, Margaret, 73
Mobility, nurses wishing to move, 157–158
Modeling and Role-Modeling (Erickson et al), 226
Moral integrity, 345–349
   dilemmas, 348
   reflection and, 346–347
Mount Royal College (MRC), Calgary, competence-assessment
   process, 159
Multidisciplinary Collaborative Primary Maternity Care Project
   (MCP), 23
Multidisciplinary cultures, in nursing education, 185–187
Mussallem, Helen K., 63
Mutual Recognition Agreement (MRA), 129, 157, 158b

N

NANDA-International. *see* North American Nursing Diagnosis
   Association (NANDA)
National Forum on Healthcare (1997), 42
National health grants, 36–37
National Nursing Competency Project, 1997, 158
National Nursing Research Agenda, 126–128
National Occupational/Sector Study of Nursing, 122
National Research and Development Program (NHRDP) of Health
   Canada, 262
   joint MRC/NHRDP Research Scholar awards, 267
National Health Scientist Award, 267
National Sector/Occupational Sector Study of Nursing, 2006, 125
National Survey of the Work and Health of Nurses, 2005
   (NSWHN), 101
Naturalized, definition, 357b
Natural Sciences and Engineering Research Council, 263
New Brunswick, nurse practitioner regulation, 155t
Newfoundland, nurse practitioner regulation, 155t
Newfoundland and Labrador Nurses Union, 322–323
Newfoundland Graduate Nurses' Association, 1931, 150
The New Leadership Challenge: Creating the Future for Nursing
   (Grossman and Valiga), 57
News releases, on nursing issues, 12
Normality, difference and, 378
North American Free Trade Agreement (NAFTA), 44
North American Nursing Diagnosis Association (NANDA), 226
Northwest Territories/Nunavut, nurse practitioner regulation, 155t
Northwest Territories Registered Nurses Association, 1975, 150
Notes on Nursing (Nightingale), 402
Nova Scotia Act, 1922, 150
Nurse availability, element of nursing, 6
Nurse Healers Professional Associates, 228
Nurse practitioners (NP)
   acute care, 170
   barriers to resolution, 173–174
   Canadian Nurse Practitioner Initiative (CNPI), 170
   critical feminist understandings, 172
   definition, 177
   economics, 171
   ethical and legal issues, 173
   graduate education, 173–174
   historical analysis of issues, 168–170
   politics of, 170–171
   recurring issues, 166–179
   regulation of, 152, 153–156t
   role in primary healthcare, 37
   social and cultural issues, 171–172
   strategies for improvement, 175
Nurse researchers
   preparation of, 265–268
   shortage, 274–275
Nurses Association of New Brunswick, 119
Nurses Registration Act, 1918, 73
Nurses' work, 283–302. *see also* Workplace issues
   barriers to resolving issues, 296–297
   critical feminist analysis, 295
   economic analysis, 295–296
   employment predictions in 2011, 285t
   ethical analysis, 295
   framing and analyzing nature and conditions of, 292–293
   gendered nature of, 361–363
   historical understanding, 293
   increasing demands, 286–288
   lack of control, 289
   lack of support for, 289–290, 349–350
   nature of, 284
   nurses responsibilities in informed consent, 342
   political analysis, 294–295
   significance of issues, 285–286, 285t
   social and cultural analysis, 293–294
   strategies for resolving issues, 297–299, 298b
   where do Canadian nurses work?, 291t
   work as taught *vs.* work as practiced, 288
Nursing: The Philosophy and Science of Caring (Watson), 226
Nursing: The Science of Unitary Man (Rogers), 226
Nursing Care Partnership Fund, 264
Nursing education. *see* Education
Nursing Enhancement Fund (NEF), 108
Nursing informatics, 241–242
   applications, 242–246
   in curricula, 253
Nursing issues
   analyzing the issue, 8–10
   articulation and resolution, 4–5
   articulation for the profession, 5–6
   barriers to resolution, 10
   constructing bodies, 188–190
   devising strategies for resolution, 10–11
   environmental health, 410b
   eugenic practices and public health, 378–379
   exclusionary practices, 372–373
   First Nations communities, 444–451
   framing the topic, 7
   future priorities, 133–134
   gendered nature of, 364–365
   leader articulation of, 59
   lobbying strategies, 11–14, 11b
   role in Canada's health care system, 50–51
   self-care practices for nurses, 233–234, 234b

technology, 187–188, 188b
violence and abuse, 426–427
workplace problems for students, 192–194
Nursing knowledge and work, status of, 311–312
Nursing language and classification systems, 226
Nursing leadership, 56–67
    attributes, 58–59
    barriers to excellence, 62
    celebrating our leaders, 63–65, 64–65t
    CNA and, 134
    economic analysis, 61
    ethical analysis, 61
    history of, 60
    lack of support for nurses' work, 289–290, 349–350
    management differences, 57–58, 58t
    participation in, 57
    policy developments, 73–74
    political analysis, 61–62, 294–295
    social analysis, 60–61
    strategies for improvement, 62–65
NursingOne, 50
Nursing policy, 68–90. see also Policy
CNA and, 126
Nursing Policy Summer Institute, 2004, 71
Nursing practice. see also Nurses' work
    biomedical technology and, 246–247
    care delivery by telephone, 243
    dominant thinking and, 379
    electronic mail and the internet, 244
    environmental health, 410b
    future of technology in, 252–254
    gender in relation to, 355–368
    health-seeking behaviors, 244
    holistic, 223–237
    impact of foreign-trained nurses, 189–190, 189b
    influence of research on, 268–272
    online support groups, 244–245
    as political action, 6–7
    quality practice environments, 287b
    realities for graduate-prepared nurses, 208–210
    scope, 178
    spirituality and, 459–467
    telepractice, 242–243
Nursing regulation. see also Regulation
    approval of education programs, 151–152
    authority of regulatory bodies, 150–152
    challenges to authority, 162–163
    changing approaches, 160–162
    competencies or credentials for registration, 158–159
    globalization, 152, 157
    guiding principles, 157
    history, 149–160
    mandatory registration, 150
    nurse practitioners, 152
    public participation in, 162
Nursing research, 259–280
    contribution to Canadian healthcare, 273–274
    evolution of, 260–268
    funding, 262–265, 269f
    future, 276–277
    influence on education, 272–273
    influence on practice, 268–272
    issues facing, 274–276
    model, 260
    publishing, 261–262

utilization, 276
Nursing Research, 261
Nursing Research Fund, 79b
Nursing shortage, 303–315
    actions needed to ameliorate, 94–95
    age of registered nurses in Canada, 294t, 308f
    analyzing as a political issue, 5
    barriers to resolution of, 312–313
    critical feminist analysis, 311
    economic analysis, 309–310
    historical analysis, 305–307
    how created, 306–307
    ICN strategies, 139–140
    nature of, 304
    policy development and, 93–95
    political analysis, 310–311
    recruiting international nurses, 189–190, 189b
    researchers, 274–275
    social and cultural analysis, 307–309, 308f
    status of nursing knowledge, 311
    status of nursing work, 312
    strategies for resolution, 313–314
    what counts as shortage, 305–306
    workplace problems, 192–194
Nursing Strategy for Canada, 2000, 125
Nursing telepractice, 242–243
Nursing theory, holistically oriented, 226, 227t
Nursing workforce, aging of, 293–294, 294t, 308f

O

Office of Nursing Policy (ONP), 74, 99
Online support groups, 244–245
Ontario
    CNA federation in, 118
    Council of University Programs in Nursing, 151
    nurse practitioner regulation, 155t
Ontario Health Professions Regulatory Advisory Committee
        (HPRAC), 162
Ontario Maternity Care Expert Panel, 23
Ontario Nurses Association (ONA), 326
Ontario Nursing Act, 2004, 161
Order of Canada, 63
    recipients, 64t
Ordre des infirmiéres et infirmiers du Québec, 108–109, 119, 152
Organizational policies, 69
Organization for Economic Cooperation and Development
        (OECD), 45
    nursing shortages, 93–94
    Ottawa Charter for Health Promotion, 408
    Oulton, Judith, 141–142
    Our Health, Our Future: Creating Quality Workplaces for
        Canadian Nurses (Canadian Nursing Advisory Committee,
        2002), 80
    Outpost nursing, 18, 22

P

Particulate matter, 404b
Partner violence, 420
Patient safety, communicable disease and, 38–39
Personal protective equipment, planning for a pandemic, 328b
Pesticides, 407

Physical neglect, definition
Physical violence, definition, 417b
Pluralistic model, policy development, 76
Policy
    adoption and implementation, 83–84
    advocating for nursing education, 191–192
    avoiding critical situations, 93–95
    communication, 83–84
    future challenges and strategies, 85–87
    impact on nursing, 84–85
    regulatory, CNA, 128–130
    research and, 92–113
    revision of, 84
    vs. politics, 70–71, 70t
Policy agenda, 81–82
Policy cycle, 99–104, 99f
Policy development
    CNA, 120
    conceptualizing the process, 81–84
    discovering reasons for, 82
    evaluating the outcome, 84
    historical perspective, 72–75
    historical significance of, 75
    history and background, 72–81
    instruments for, 82–83
    Marxist model, 76
    nurse involvement, 76–81
        community, 80–81
        educational institutions, 80
        government, 77–78
        professional organizations and unions, 78–79
        workplace, 77
    pluralistic model, 76
    power and, 71–72
    professionalism and, 72
    public choice model, 76
    relevance of a nursing perspective, 84–85
    research and, 92–113
    theoretical perspective, 75–76
    understanding the complexity, 76
Policy networks, 105
Political action, 3–16
    CNA and, 123
    nursing practice as, 6–7
    violence and abuse, 429
Political acumen, 104–106
Political analysis
    advocating for nursing education, 191–192
    nurse practitioner issues, 170–171
    nurses' work, 294–295
    nursing issues, 9
    nursing leadership, 61–62
    nursing shortage, 310–311
    rural nursing, 23
    sexuality, 394–395
Politics, *vs.* policy, 70–71, 70t
Portability, in Canadian health care, 39–42
Power, policy and, 71–72
Practical Nurses Canada, 105
Practice statements, 160–161
Primary healthcare, 37–38
    definition, 124b
Prince Edward Island, nurse practitioner regulation, 156t
Prince Edward Island Nurses Union, 322–323
Principal Nursing Officer, Canadian federal government, 137

Privatization, 43
Professionalism
    integrity, 348–349
    policy and, 72
    practice environments, CNA, 126
Professional organizations
    CASN and CNSA, 80b
    CNA, 117–146
    holistic nursing, 228
    national and international, 117–146
    policy development, 78–79
    provincial and territorial, 147–165
Protected title, 178
Provisional Society of the Canadian Nurses Association of Trained
        Nurses, 1908, 149
Psychological violence, definition, 417b
Public administration, in Canadian health care, 45–47
Public choice model, policy development, 76
Public Health Agency of Canada (PHAC), 39
Public health nurse (PHN), in rural setting, 18, 21–23
Public Health Nurses Act of 1919, 22
Public health services, resurgence of communicable disease and, 39
Public Hospitals Act, 108
Public policy, 69, 92. *see also* Policy; Policy development
    CNA and, 123–126

Q

Qualitative Nursing Research, 262
Quality of care, element of nursing, 6
Quality Worklife—Quality Healthcare Collaborative, partner of
        CNA, 121
Quebec
    Charter of Human Rights and Freedoms, 44
    CNA and other organizations, 119
    history in national programs, 40–41
    nurse practitioner regulation, 156t
    Quebec Nurses' Act, 1946, 150

R

Race, Evolution, and Behavior (Rushton), 375
Racial differences. *see also* Difference
    theories on perception of difference, 374–376
Radiation, 404b
Randomized clinical trial (RCT), holistic nursing and, 232–233
Recruitment strategies, rural nurses, 26–28, 27t
Registered Midwives (RMs), 23
Registered Nurses Act, Nova Scotia, 1910, 149–150
Registered Nurses Association of Ontario (RNAO), 118–119, 151
Registration
    across borders, 159–160
    Canadian vs U. S. model, 159–160
    competencies or credentials, 158–159
    endorsement, 157, 158b
    mobility, 157
Regulation. *see also* Nursing regulation
    definition, 148
    evolution of, 148–149
Regulatory policy, CNA and, 128–130, 134
Reimann, Christiane, 136
Reinscribing, definition, 357b
Relational autonomy, 350

Research. *see also* Nursing research
Burlington Randomized Trial of the NP, 169
National Nursing Research Agenda, 126–128
policy development and, 92–113
realities of, 259–280
Research in Nursing and Health, 262
Research-policy links, 96–97
Resolutions
on nursing issues, 13–14
on rural nursing, 26–28
what to ask, 14b
RESOLVE (Research and Education for Solutions to Violence
and Abuse), 429
Restricted actions, 160
Retention strategies, rural nurses, 26–28, 27t
Rhetoric, defined, 105
Rock, Alan, 74
Rodger, Ginette Lemire, 62–63
Romanow, Roy, 42–43
Royal Commission of Aboriginal Peoples, 1996, 440
Royal Proclamation of 1763, 437
Royal Sanitary Conference, Vancouver (1914), 41
Rural nursing, 17–34
constraints and possibilities, 26–28, 27t
framing the issue, 18–19
as a specialty, 24–25
understanding the issues, 19–26
workplace isolation, 290–291
Russell, E. Kathleen, 73

S

Saskatchewan, nurse practitioner regulation, 156t
Saskatchewan Registered Nurses Association (SRNA), 108, 322
Screening program, tuberculosis, political action results, 4b
Self-care activities, for nurses, 233–234, 234b
*Service Employees International Union v. Saskatchewan Registered
Nurse Association* (SRNA), 79
Sexuality, 387–399
as an issue, 390–391
barriers to resolution of discrimination, 395–396
ethical and legal understandings, 392–393
ethical responsibilities of nurses, 393b
feminist understandings, 395
in the healthcare system, 391b
historical, 391–392
political nature, 394–395
social and cultural understandings, 394
strategies for resolution of discrimination, 396
ways of understanding, 391–395
Sexual orientation, definition, 389
Sexual violence, definition, 417b
Shaman, Judith, 63
Simulated learning, in nursing schools, 248
Sinclair report, 338–339, 341
Snively, Mary Agnes, 122, 135
Social and cultural analysis
nurse practitioner issues, 171–172
nurses' work, 293–294
nursing issues, 9
nursing leadership, 60–61
nursing shortage, 293–294
rural nursing, 24
sexuality, 394

Social construction, definition, 357b
Social hygiene, differences and, 376–378
Social Sciences and Humanities Research Council of Canada
(SSHRC), 263
Social Union Agreement, 42
Social violence, definition, 417b
Specialization
achievements in policy development, 73
education, 1950-2000, 197–198
Specialties recognized by CNA, 24b
Spiritual care, 455–469
barriers to understanding, 467
multiple understandings, 459–460
openness, 466–467
prerequisites for, 467b
strategies for providing, 467
Spirituality, 455–469
concept and experience, 462–465
historical perspectives, 457–458
identification of types, 459b
knowing and unknowing, 463–466
opening the conversation, 456
personal/professional assumptions, 457, 457b
reflection on nursing, 464b
reflection poem, 464b
relevance for nursing, 458–459, 459b
religion and, 462
science and, 460–461
understanding of, 456b, 462
Spousal abuse, 420
Stallknecht, Kristen, 142
Standard, definition, 178
Statistics Canada Labour Survey, 100
Strategies for resolution, nursing issues, 10–11
Strengthening Nurses, Nursing Networks and Association Program
(2007-2012), CNA, 131
Styles, Gretta, 142
Superbugs, patient safety and, 38–39
Surgical waiting lists, 44
Systematic reviews, 270
System-Linked Research Unit on Health and Social Service
Utilization, 97–98

T

Taking Action! Political Action and Information Kit for RNs (2006), 71
Taskforce on Health Care Workforce Regulation, 1995, 148
Taylor, Malcolm, 35
Technology, 238–258
biomedical, nursing practice and, 246–247
nursing education and, 247–254
Telehealth, 242–243
Testing, CNA role, 128
Theory-based practice, 268
Thoughtfulness, in understanding difference, 370
Toffler, Alvin, 60
Toxic waste sites, 408
Transgender, definition, 389
Transparency, definition, 357b
Tuberculosis, screening in homeless population, 4b

U

Umbrella legislation, 161–162
Undergraduate nursing education, 183–202. *see also* Education

historical issues, 195–198
issues in, 185–187
Unionization/collective bargaining, 316–336
CFNU contract comparison, 330t
CNA influences on, 322–323
historical influences, 317–318
issues surrounding, 324–326
moving ahead, 330–331
nurses' thinking about, 324
organizing professional nurses, 319–320
today and tomorrow, 331–333
workplaces, 326–328, 327t
Unions, 316–336
emergence in practices, 320
policy development, 78–79
transformations in, 321–322
workplace issues, 194b
United Nurses of Alberta (UNA), 325–326, 326b
Universality, in Canadian health care, 39–42
University of Alberta, doctoral program, 207, 265

V

Victoria Order of Nursing (VON), 1897, 21, 318
Videoconference delivery, in nursing education, 249
Violence
domestic, 417
family, 417
interpersonal, 416
in relationships, 416–417
Violence and abuse, 414–434
Aboriginal communities, 421–422
barriers to resolution, 427–428
against children and youth, 421–422
dating, 423
elder abuse and neglect, 421
environmental interactions, 424
feminist perspective, 425
forms of, 417b
gay and lesbian relationships, 420–421
historical perspective, 418–419
impact on the healthcare system, 425–426
intersectional analysis, 425
intraindividual model, 424
nursing issues, 426–427
statistics in the Canadian context, 419–424
strategies for resolution, 428–429

theoretical perspective, 424
tolerance of, 424–425
against women, 420
workplace, 423–424
Visibility, in nursing leadership, 59

W

Waste reduction, nursing strategies, 411b
Web-based and blended delivery, in nursing education, 249
Western and Northern Health Human Resource Forum, 159
Western Journal of Nursing Research, 262
Winnipeg nurses, 338–339, 341
Workplace issues, 283–302. *see also* Nursing practice, Nurses' work
barriers to resolving, 296–297
community as a workplace, 291–292
creating a safer moral climate, 298b
disruption, 292
employment trends, 2006, 332b
framing and analyzing of, 292–293
increasing demands, 286–288
isolation, 290–292
lack of support for higher education, 290
mentorship and orientation programs for new graduates, 292
nature of, 284–285
nursing involvement in policy development, 77
personal protective equipment, 328b
problems for students, 192–194
quality practice environments, 287b
strategies for resolving issues, 297–299, 298b
unionization/collective bargaining, 326–328
unions, 194b
World Health Organization (WHO)
definition of primary healthcare, 124b
environmental hazards, 403, 405
ICN and, 137
nursing shortage, 140
PHAC and, 39
primary healthcare approach, 73
violence and health, 418
World War Nursing Sisters, England, 188f

Y

Yukon, nurse practitioner regulation, 156t
Yukon Registered Nurses Association, 119